Dance A While

Handbook for Folk, Square, Contra, and Social Dance

Eighth Edition

Dance A While

Handbook for Folk, Square, Contra, and Social Dance

Jane A. Harris
FORMERLY OF WASHINGTON STATE UNIVERSITY

Anne M. Pittman
FORMERLY OF ARIZONA STATE UNIVERSITY

Marlys S. Waller
FORMERLY OF THE UNIVERSITY OF WASHINGTON

Cathy L. Dark
OREGON STATE UNIVERSITY

ALLYN AND BACON   BOSTON   LONDON   TORONTO   SYDNEY   TOKYO   SINGAPORE

Editor-in-Chief: Paul A. Smith
Publisher: Joseph E. Burns
Series Editorial Assistant: Tanja Eise
Marketing Manager: Rick Muhr
Composition and Prepress Buyer: Linda Cox
Manufacturing Buyer: Megan Cochran
Cover Administrator: Linda Knowles
Editorial-Production Administrator: Mary Beth Finch
Editorial-Production Service: Shepherd, Inc.
Electronic Composition: Shepherd, Inc.

Library of Congress Cataloging in Publication Data
Dance a while : handbook for folk, square, contra, and social dance / Jane Harris . . . [et
al.].--8th ed.
      p. cm.
   Rev. ed. of: Dance a while / Jane A. Harris, Anne M. Pittman, Marlys S. Waller. 7th ed. c 1994.
   Includes bibliographical references and index.
   ISBN 0-205-27936-8
   1. Dancing.   I. Harris, Jane A. II. Harris, Jane A. Dance a while.

GV1751 .H322 2000
793.3--dc21
                                                                  99-049853

Printed in the United States of America

10 9 8 7 6 5 4 3 2 VHP 04 03 02 01 00

Dedication

The Eighth Edition of *Dance A While*
is dedicated to those who continue to share
their wealth of experience and passion for
International Folk Dance.

Contents

Foreword   xvii

Preface   xviii

Acknowledgments   xx

1

History   1

The Beginning   1

Forms   2

Music   2

Cultural Significance   3

   Religion   3

   Education   3

   Health   3

   Fertility   4

Africa   4

   The Continent   4

   European Influence   4

   Slave Trade   4

   Traditional Dance   4

   Art and Dance   5

   Improvisation   5

   Dance Instruments and Objects   5

   Spiritual World   5

   Environmental Influences   5

   Beo and Gnenon Dances   6

   The Future   6

Pacific Rim Perspective   6

   India   6

   China   9

   Korea   13

   Japan   13

   Bali   15

   Maori   17

   Philippines   17

   Hawaii   19

American Perspective   20

2

Effective Group Instruction   23

Why Dance   23

Purpose of Dance   24

Facilities   24

   Floor   24

   Acoustics   24

Equipment   25

   Sound Systems   25

   Camcorder/VCR   26

Music   26

   Recordings   26

   Teaching with Recordings   27

   Live Music   27

   Teaching with Live Music   28

Planning Instruction   28

   Total Dance Program   28

      Program Curriculum   28

      Extracurricular Opportunities   29

   Dance Unit   29

   Goals   29

   Daily Planning Instruction 29

      Daily Lesson   29

   Objectives/Students Outcome 29

   Assessing Group Variables   30

   Content Selection   30

   Lesson Plan   30

Orientation to the Dance Class   31

   Setting the Stage   31

      Etiquette   32

      Social Aids 32

      Fun with Cutting In   32

      Uneven Numbers: Creating a "Ghost Partner"   32

      Teaching Students with Special Needs   33

   First Class Meeting   33

Class Procedure   34

   Strategies for Selecting Material
     and Presentation   34

   General Teaching Points   34

   Teaching a Specific Dance   35

   Evaluation   37

   Practical Test   37

   Written Test   37

      Grading the Class   38

   Enrichment Activities   38

      Class Project   38

      Bulletin Boards   38

      Culminating Activities   38

      Community Resources   39

      Teacher Resources   39

Organizing Special Activities   39

   Family Dances   39

   One-Night Stand   39

   The Special Party   40

   The Theme Party   40

   People with Physical Disabilities   41

   Senior Dances   41

3

Dance Fundamentals   43

Rhythm and Meter   43

Analysis of a Basic Rhythm   46

Fundamental Locomotor
  Movements   47

   Walk   47

   Run   47

   Leap   47

   Jump   48

   Hop   48

   Sissone   48

   Assemblé   48

   Gallop   49

   Slide   49

   Skip   50

   Exercises for Fundamental Locomotor
     Movements   50

Basic Dance Steps   50

   Shuffle, Dance Walk, or Glide   50

   Two-Step or Triple-Step   50

   Polka   51

   Schottische   51

   Waltz   51

   Mazurka   52

Basic Dance Turns   52

   Schottische Turn Clockwise   52

   Two-Step Turn Clockwise   53

   Polka Turn Clockwise   53

   Waltz Turn   54

Suggestions for Teaching Basic
  Dance Steps   55

   Analysis of Rhythm of Basic Step   55

   Method of Presentation   55

   Interdependent Factors Influencing
     Procedure   56

Procedure for Teaching Basic Dance
  Steps and Turns   56

   Schottische and Clockwise Turn   56

   Progressive Two-Step   57

   Two-Step Turn Clockwise   57

   Polka   57

   Polka Turn Clockwise   58

   Running Waltz   58

   Box Waltz and Turn   58

   Waltz Turn Clockwise   58

   Pivot Turn   59

   Spin or Twirl   59

Dance Positions   60

Dance Formations   63

Music in Relation to Dance   64

   Listen to the Beat   64

   How to Recognize Music for Dance   65

   Rhythm Training and Appreciation   65

Dance Style   66

   The Beautiful Dancer   66

   Ear and Ankle Alignment   66

   Good Posture—Key to Body Balance
     and Control   66

   Achieving Appropriate Style   66

   Teaching Style   67

4

American Dance Sampler 69

Dances from the European Courts to the American Ballrooms 70

The Unique Contributions of African Americans 70

The Spanish-Mexican Influence 71

Dances of the People 71
Square Dances 71
Play Party Games 71
Round and Novelty Dances 72
Contra Dances 72
Appalachian Clog Dances 72
Cajun Dance 72

Music 72

Dress 73

A Social Occasion 73

Revival of Folk Traditions 73

The Melting Pot versus Ethnic Identity 74

Conclusion 74

Teaching Suggestions 74
Various Approaches 74

Dances 75
Grand March 75
Virginia Reel 77
Grand Square Quadrille 78
Paul Jones Your Lady 80
Ninepin Reel 81
Portland Fancy 83
Big Circle Square Dance 84
Clogging 88
History 88
Costumes and Shoes 90
Music 90
Style 90
Basic Clogging Steps 91
Teaching Clogging 95

Example of Step Combinations 95
Alabama Gal 96
Nobody's Business 97
Schottische 98
Ping-Pong Schottische 100
Texas Schottische Variations 101
Texas Schottische for Three 103
Salty Dog Rag 104
Boston Two-Step 105
Heel and Toe Polka 106
Cotton-Eyed Joe 107
Blue Pacific Waltz 109
Garden Waltz 111
Varsouvienne 112
Oh Johnny 113
Amos Moses 114
Popcorn 115
Twelfth Street Rag 116
Plain and Novelty Mixers 117
Jiffy Mixer 119
Patty-Cake Polka 120
Mexican Mixer 121
Tennessee Wig Walk 122
Red River Valley 123
Levi Jackson Rag 124

5

Square Dance 125

History 125
Antecedents 125
New England 126
The South 126
Texas Square Dance 127
Early Leaders 128
Post-World War II 128
Standardization of Basic Movements 129
Contemporary Notes 130

Square Your Sets 130
Calling 131
Sight Calling 131
Tips for Sight Calling 131

Keys to Good Calling 132
Calling Sequence 132
Use of Prerecorded Calls 132

Styling 132

Teaching Approaches 133

Planning Units and Lessons 133

Mixers for Square Dance 133

Big Circle Mixers 134

Methods of Squaring Up 134

Methods for Changing Partners
or Moving to a New Square 135

Basic Movements 136

Teaching Progression and Analysis
for Basic Movements of Square Dance 136

Level 1A: Beginner Basics 1–8 137

Level 1B: Orientation to the Square 138

Level 2: Beginner Basics 9–20 139

Level 3: Beginner Basics 21–33 142

Level 4: Intermediate Basics 34–44 146

Level 5: Intermediate Basics 45–50 149

Additional Basics 51–59 151

Mainstream Movements 60–78 153

Patter Calls—Notes on the Dance Figures 157

Dances 158

Promenade the Ring 158

Gents Star Right 158

Bend It Tight 158

Texas Star 158

Arkansas Traveler 158

Easy Bend the Line 158

Split the Ring and Around Just One 158

Arkansas Traveler With a Cross Trail Thru 158

The Route 159

Promenade the Outside Ring 159

Split the Ring Variation 1 159

Roll Away Combo 2 159

Ends Turn In 159

Roll Away Combo 1 160

Box the Gnat—Pull By 160

Split the Ring Variation 2 160

Another Trail 160

There's Your Corner 160

Easy Square Thru 160

Pitt's Patter 3 160

Half-Square Thru Combo 160

Just a Breeze 161

Five Hands 161

Half-Square Thru and Then
Three-Quarters 161

Sail Away 161

Star Thru Square Thru Combo 161

Star Thru—California Twirl 161

Gnat and Flea Combo 1 161

New Star Thru 161

Go the Route 162

Mucho Combo 162

Pitt's Patter 2 162

Sides Break to a Line 162

Duck Then Wheel Around 162

Four in the Middle 163

Now Hear This 163

Eight Chain Combo 1 163

A Long Way Over 163

Turn Thru Combo 163

Inside Arch and Outside Under 163

Easy Wave 163

Ocean Wave—Swing Thru Combo 2 164

Ocean Wave—Circulate 164

Ocean Wave—Swing Thru Combo 1 164

Circulate Sue 164

Supplementary Square Dance Patter 164

Openers 164

Endings 164

Breaks 164

Breaks for Fours 165

Breaks for Eights 165

Western Cowboy Square Dance 166

Dances 166

Bird in the Cage—Seven Hands
'Round 166

Catch All Eight 166

Cowboy Loop 167

Forward Up and Back 167

Forward Up Six 167

Milagro Square 168
Sally Good'in 168
Sides Divide 168
Tea Cup Chain 168

Singing Calls 169

Dances 169

Hurry, Hurry, Hurry 169
Alabama Jubilee 170
Hello Dolly 170
Mañana 170
Just Because 171
Gentle On My Mind 172
Marianne 172
Old-Fashioned Girl 172
Don't Let the Good Life Pass You By 173
Happiness Is 173
Chime Bells 173
Goodbye My Lady Love 174
A Fooler a Faker 174
Tie Me Kangaroo Down 174
Houston 175
If They Could See Me Now 175
Smoke on the Water 175

6

Contra Dance 177

History 177

Playford Collection 177
English, Scottish, and Irish Influence 177
Contra Dance to the New World 178
Contra Dance in California before the Gold Rush 178
French-Canadian Influence 178
Yankee Musicians 178
And Yet They Live 178
National Square Dance Revival and Country Dance 179
The First Contra Dance Revival— Ralph Page 179
The Country Dance and Song Society and Other Organizations 179

The Second Contra Dance Revival 180
Contra Dance Research 180
Contra Dancing Moves into the 21st Century 180

Contra Dance Basics 181

Starting the Contra Dance Set 181
Formations in the Contra Dance 181
Music and Timing 182
The Role of the Caller 182
Dance Sources 182
Card File 182
Music Sources 183
Contra Dance Figures 183
Teaching Suggestions 184
Dance Levels 185
Contra Dance Tunes Composed by Ralph Page 185

Dances 187

Aw Shucks! 187
Becket Reel 188
Brimmer & May Reel 189
British Sorrow 190
Broken Sixpence 191
CDS Reel 192
Chili Pepper #4 193
Chorus Jig 194
Contra for Margie 194
Dance Gypsy 195
Dancing Sailors 196
Delphiniums and Daisies 197
Easy Does It 198
Hull's Victory 198
Jed's Reel 199
Lady of the Lake 200
The Nova Scotian 201
The Other Mary Kay 202
Petronella 203
Pierce's Hall Stroll 204
Roadblock Reel 205
Roll in the Hey 206
Rory O'More 207
Salmonchanted Evening 208
Shadrack's Delight 209

Silver Lake Waltz   210
Small Potatoes   211
Symmetrical Force   212
The Tourist   213
Weave the Line   213
With Thanks to the Dean   214

7

International Folk Dance   217

Introduction   **217**

Folk Dance Movement   **218**
  Dance Sources   218
  Camps   219
  Performing Groups   219
  Research and Advanced Studies   219
  Trends   220
  Future   220

**Understanding Folkways Enhances
  Dance**   **220**
  Eastern and Western Culture   220
  Geography and Climate   220
  Religion   221
  Music   221
  Costumes   222
  Holidays, Festivals, and Special Occasions   222

Africa   **223**

Dances   **223**
  Borborbor   223
  Gahu   224
  Pata Pata   226
  Tant' Hessie   227

**Alpine Region—Switzerland, Austria,
  and Germany**   **228**
  Dance Characteristics   228
  Folk Dancing in Switzerland   228

Dances from the Alpine Region   **230**
  D'Hammerschmiedsg'selln *German*   230
  Dr Gsatzlig *Swiss*   231
  Kanonwalzer *German*   233
  Krüz König *German*   234

  Man in the Hay *German*   237
  Sonderburg Dopplequadrille
    German   240
  Spinnradl zu Dritt *Austrian*   241

Balkan Countries   **243**
  Introduction   243
  Greece   243
  Former Yugoslavia   244
  Bulgaria   245

Dances from the Balkan Countries   **246**
  Hasápikos *Greek*   246
  Lesnoto *Macedonian*   247
  Misirlou *Greek-American*   249
  Pljeskavac Kolo *Serbian*   250
  Rumunjsko Kolo *Serbian-American*   251
  Sarajevka Kolo *Bosnian*   252
  Savila Se Bela Loza *Serbian*   253
  Šetnja *Serbian*   255
  Syrtós *Greek*   256
  Tropanka *Bulgarian*   257

British Isles   **258**
  Introduction   258
  England   258
  Ireland   260
  Scotland   261

Dances from the British Isles   **262**
  Bonny Prince Charlie Crossing
    the Frew *Scottish*   262
  The Bridge of Athlone *Irish*   264
  Butterfly Hornpipe *English*
    (Warwickshire)   265
  Dover Pier *English*   266
  The First of April *English*   267
  Flowers of Edinburgh *Scottish Reel*   268
  Gie Gordons *Scottish*   269
  The Northdown Waltz *English*   270
  Oslo Waltz *Scottish - English*   271
  The Ragg *English*   272
  Road to the Isles *Scottish*   273
  Siamsa Beirte *Irish*   274
  Three Meet *English*   275
  The White Cockade *Scottish Reel*   277
  Willow Tree *English*   279

Canada 281
 Discovery and Settlement 281
 Population 281
 Culture 281
 Cape Breton 281

Dances from Canada 282
 La Bastringe 282
 The Saint John River 283

Czech and Slovakia 285
 Dance Characteristics 285

Dances from Czech and Slovakia 286
 Doudlebska Polka *Czech* 286
 Tancuj *Czech* 287

France 288
 Dance Characteristics 288

Dances from France 289
 Branle d'Ossau 289
 La Montagnarde 290
 La Tournijaire 292
 Mon Père Avait un Petit Bois 294
 Rondeau de Garein 296

Hungary 297
 Introduction 297
 Dance Characteristics 298

Dances from Hungary 299
 Hungarian Motifs 299
 Csárdás Palócosan 300
 Kiskanásztánc 301
 Ugrós 302

Israel 304
 Clarification of Ethnic Names
  and Nationalities 304
 Dance Characteristics 304

Dances from Israel 305
 Cherkessiya 305
 Harmonica 306
 Hava Nagila 307
 Hineh Ma Tov 309
 Hora 310
 Ma Na'avu 311
 Mayim 312
 Vé David 313

Italy 314
 Dance Characteristics 314

Dances from Italy 315
 Il Codiglione 315
 Sicilian Tarantella 316

Lithuania 318
 Dance Characteristics 318

Dances from Lithuania 319
 Kalvelis 319
 Klumpakojis 320

Mexico 321
 The Dance in Mexico 321

Dances from Mexico 323
 El Jarabe Tapatío 323
 Jesucita en Chihuahua 325
 La Cucaracha 327
 La Raspa 328
 Las Chiapanecas 329
 Santa Rita 330

Poland 333
 Dances of Poland 333

Dances from Poland 335
 Tramblanka—Polka Mazurka 335
 Walczyk "Ges Woda" 337

Romania 338
 Background 338

Dances from Romania 339
 Alunelu 339
 Hora De Mina 340
 Itele 341
 Sirba Din Cimpoi 342

Russia 343
 Dance Characteristics 343

Dances from Russia 344
 Alexandrovska 344
 Korobushka 345
 Troika 346

Scandinavia 348
 Introduction 348
 Denmark 349
 Norway 349

Finland   350

Sweden   350

Dances from Scandinavia   **351**

Bitte Mand I Knibe
(Little Man in a Fix) *Danish*   351

Den Toppede Høne
(The Crested Hen) *Danish*   352

Familie Sekstur *Danish*   353

Familjevalsen *Swedish*   354

Hambo *Swedish*   355

Norwegian Polka
(Scandinavian Polka)   357

Seksmannsril *Norwegian*   358

Snurrbocken *Swedish*   359

Swedish Varsouvienne *Swedish*   360

Swedish Waltz *Swedish*   361

To Ting *Danish*   362

Totur *Danish*   363

South America   **364**

Dances from South America   **364**

Carnavalito *Bolivia*   364

Ranchera *Uruguay*   365

8

Social Dance   367

Introduction   **367**

Phases of Social Dance   368

Competition   368

Dancesport   369

Vintage Dance   370

Teaching Social Dance   **370**

Formations   370

Walk-Through   370

The Cue   370

Demonstration   370

Unison versus Free Practice   371

Dance Lesson Preparation   371

Sample Lesson Plan   371

Teaching Progression   371

Technology Aids Teaching   371

Style of Social Dance   **371**

Footwork in Social Dance   372

One-Step/Dance Walk   372

Dance Positions   **373**

Closed Position   373

Trends in Vocabulary and Leading   374

Techniques of Leading and Following   374

Following   375

Foxtrot   **377**

Foxtrot Rhythm   377

Foxtrot Style   378

Fundamental Foxtrot Steps   379

Foxtrot Combos   390

Disco Dance   **390**

Disco Swing   **391**

Hustle with Partner   **392**

Combination of Basic Steps   393

Hustle Variation   393

Charleston   **393**

Charleston Rhythm   394

Charleston Style   394

Teaching Suggestions   394

Fundamental Charleston Steps   394

Swing (Jitterbug)   **397**

Swing Rhythm   397

Swing Style   398

West Coast Swing Rhythm   399

Fundamental Swing Steps   399

Triple Time—East Coast Swing   **405**

Swing Combos   407

West Coast Swing   **407**

Lindy Hop   **410**

Cajun Dance   **413**

Cajun Waltz   **415**

Cajun Two-Step   **415**

Cajun One-Step   **416**

Cajun Jitterbug   **416**

Zydeco Two-Step 417

Tango 418
  Tango Rhythm 418
  Tango Style 419
  Fundamental Tango Steps 419
  Tango Combos 426

Waltz 426
  Waltz Rhythm 427
  Waltz Style 427
  Fundamental Waltz Steps 428
  Waltz Combos 433

Country Western 434
  Country Western Style 434
  Dance Hall Etiquette 434

Traditional Country Western Swing 435
  Traditional Country Western Swing
    Rhythm 435
  Cowboy Swing Style 435
  Cowboy Swing Variations 436

Texas Two-Step Swing 440

Ten-Step 440

Traditional Two-Step 442
  Two-Step Rhythm 442
  Two-Step Style 442

Traveling Cha Cha 444

Sweetheart Schottische 445

Line Dance 446
  Teaching Tips for Line Dancing 446
  Line Dance Style 447

California Hustle 447

Cowboy Boogie 448

El Tango Sereno 449

Electric Slide 450

Freeze 451

Four Corners 452

Para Bailar 453

Saturday Night Fever Line Dance 454

Slappin' Leather 455

Watermelon Crawl 456

Western Wind 458

Cha Cha Cha 459
  Cha Cha Cha Rhythm 459
  Cha Cha Cha Style 459
  Fundamental Cha Cha Cha Steps 460
  Cha Cha Cha Combos 466

Mambo 467
  Mambo Rhythm 467
  Mambo Style 467
  Fundamental Mambo Steps 467

Merengue 469
  Merengue Rhythm 469
  Merengue Style 469
  Fundamental Merengue Steps 469
  Merengue Combos 472

Rumba 472
  Rumba Rhythm 472
  Rumba Style 472
  Fundamental Rumba Steps 474
  Rumba Combos 479

Salsa 479
  Salsa Style 479
  Salsa Steps 480

Samba 480
  Samba Rhythm 481
  Samba Style 481
  Fundamental Samba Steps 481
  Samba Combos 484

Appendixes

Appendix A: Periodicals 485

**Appendix B: Organizations
and Resources** 487

**Appendix C: Record, Cassette, Video
Sources: Distributors and Producers** 489

**Appendix D: Instructional Aids:
Records/Cassettes and Videos** 491

Bibliography 495

Glossary 505

Index of Mixer and Nonpartner
Dances 523

Index of Folk Dances 525

Subject Index 526

Music to Accompany *Dance A While* 533

Dance A While CD: Notes
on the Recordings 535

Foreword

Dance A While is a treasure chest of knowledge shared with us by talented authors. Through their love, dedication, and total awareness of the material, they have compiled a book that has become a legend in the dance field.

During my career, *Dance A While* was a resource that never failed me. From historical background of the dance to the final presentation of teaching, the information was clear and concise, a wonderful tool for experienced and inexperienced dancers and teachers.

With my interest in folk dance, the help I received from *Dance A While* can be given much of the credit for the success of the Brigham Young University International Folk Dance program.

Having gone through similar situations of teaching and writing in my career, I stand in awe of these very talented authors. Their contribution to the dance world is invaluable.

In their eighth edition, they have brought a completeness unique to a single volume on dance. Through the book comes a means of communication into the magic of dance history, group instruction, and fundamentals of social and folk dance, both international and American.

I would like to pay tribute to the authors who have kept their enthusiasm and research up to date to bring to each of us an exciting book for our personal use, for educational use, and for every library collection.

Congratulations on *Dance A While*, for it has enabled us to dance far into the future

Mary Bee Jensen
Professor (retired),
Brigham Young University,
Provo, Utah
Founder, Director, Choreographer,
Brigham Young University
International Folk Dancers

Preface

Anne and Marlys welcome Cathy L. Dark as a member of the team producing the eighth edition of *Dance A While*. Cathy is currently an Instructor of Ballroom and Country Western Dance at Oregon State University and advisor to Cool Shoes, the Ballroom Performing Group. She graduated from the University of Oregon majoring in Dance. Her M.S. degree is from the Laban Center for Movement and Dance, Goldsmith's College, University of London, England, with a thesis on *Invirtita Hoteni, The Social and Cultural Context of Romanian Dance*. She was Artistic Director of Silver Spurs International Folk Dance Youth Group, Spokane, Washington, and instructor of jazz dance, Risseik, Japan. She responds generously to community requests and has leadership positions in dance with AAHPERD.

The CD which accompanies the eighth edition is an exciting and very helpful addition to *Dance A While*. The sampling of American and International favorite folk dances presents opportunities for teachers, leaders, and students to practice, teach classes, offer one night dance parties immediately.

The CD was produced by Stew Shacklette, Director of the Kentucky Dance Institute and President of the Kentucky Dance Foundation. The music is from the vast collection of recordings belonging to the late Michael and Mary Ann Herman. The central purpose of the Kentucky Dance Foundation is to preserve folk music, thus it was most appropriate for that institution to be the recipients of this important and significant Herman collection. In line with the mission and purpose of the Kentucky Dance Foundation this collection enables them to keep alive and available treasured folk dance music for both present and future generations.

Dance continues to be a popular recreational activity for all ages. The benefits include exercise, the opportunity for self-expression, and social relationships within groups. Since dance is closely associated with music, rhythmic development adds to the skill and pleasure of dance.

Social Dance is presently the most popular recreational dance form. With the revival of the Jitterbug/Swing, *Dance A While* is current. The Lindy Hop and West and East Coast Swing are the rage! Country Western, Line Dancing, Tango, Latin Dances, Charleston, Cajun, traditional Waltz, and Foxtrot are all included. Chapter 8, Social Dance, is a gem!

The original format of *Dance A While* continues to be a winner. The fundamentals of teaching dance, lesson planning, testing, rhythm analysis, basic steps, dance positions, and formations are the cornerstone. Current information on sound systems is featured.

Dances are selected for basic steps, group formations, degree of difficulty, mixers, and exhibition. The dances come from many foreign countries. The American Dance Sampler in Chapter 4 represents traditional and contemporary dances. The Square Dance chapter covers Modern and Western Cowboy Squares.

Penn Fix has written new teaching instruction for Contra dance. Three original fiddle tunes by Ralph Page are included. The Contra dances featured in Chapter 6 range from traditional "New England Chestnuts" to contemporary dances.

The cultural significance of dance tradition for the Pacific Rim, Chapter 1, and countries represented in Chapter 7, International Folk Dance, is presented. New countries represented in the eighth edition are Africa, Bolivia, Canada, Romania, Poland, and Uruguay. Mihai David, Romanian specialist, Jacek Marek, Polish specialist, and George A. Fogg and Kate Van Winkle Keller, English Country dance specialists, have contributed material for this edition. Dick Crum, Serbian; Andor Czómpo, Hungarian; Nelda G. Drury, Mexican; George A. Fogg, English; Karen Gottier, German, Austrian, and Swiss; Mary McLaren Lindsay, Scottish; and Marilyn Smith, French, have contributed dances and dance background for previous editions.

Extensive resources are in the Appendices, Bibliography, Glossary, and Indices. As new material is added to *Dance A While*, favorite dances are retired. Therefore, previous editions of *Dance A While* continue to serve as excellent resources.

The eighth edition of *Dance A While* is dedicated to the special group that has contributed to Dance A While, those who continue to share their wealth of experience and passion for International Folk Dance.

The original vision of *Dance A While* by Jane, Anne, and Marlys continues. Cathy adds new sparks. The CD offers immediate opportunities to dance. May the spirit and joy that comes from dancing continue to expand. Like the pebble dropped in the pond, the ripples multiply. Dance has enhanced our lives. We pass this wondrous tradition on through *Dance A While*.

Anne M. Pittman
Marlys S. Waller
Cathy L. Dark

Acknowledgments

The eighth edition of *Dance A While* is very special since it is, indeed, the result of almost fifty years of wisdom shared with us by many outstanding teachers, leaders, and dancers, the refreshing experience of our new colleague, Cathy Dark, and the music of the late Michael and Mary Ann Herman, CD produced by Stew Schacklette, Director of the Kentucky Dance Institute. We would like to express our great appreciation to our original coauthor and colleague, Jane A. Harris Ericson, for her extensive work in developing the format and content of *Dance A While*.

We are honored that our colleague, Mary Bee Jensen, retired Professor, Brigham Young University, founder and former Director of the Brigham Young University International Folk Dancers, has written the Foreword.

Beth Lessard, former chair of the Arizona State University Dance Department, has so willingly shared her knowledge and assisted us in updating the Chapter 8, Social Dance. Kathy DuBois of the University of Wisconsin, La Crosse, and Sue Lipscomb have contributed original Country Western Line Dances and our long-time friend, Henry "Buzz" Glass, contributed two original line dances, a Tango, and a Caribbean rhythm dance.

Penn Fix, Spokane, Washington, has critiqued the Contra Dance chapter, along with Brad Foster, Bob Dalsemer, and Luther Black. The new Contra Dance Basics are to Penn's credit. The estate of the late Ralph Page has given *Dance A While* permission to include three original fiddle tunes by Ralph Page. The following composers have contributed one or more original Contra dances to this edition: Kathy Anderson, Don Armstrong, Erna-Lynne Bogue, Fred Breunig, Bob Dalsemer, Roger Diggle, Fred Feild, Penn Fix, Tom Hinds, Gene Hubert, Jim Kitch, Carol Kopp, Dan Pearl, Steve Schnur, Tony Parkes, Tanya Rotenberg, and Steve Zakon. There are also dances by the late Ralph Page and the late Ted Sannella, with permission by their estates.

Thanks to Dr. Barbara Cusimarro, Oregon State University, for helping transform the mystery of curriculum development and lesson plans into a form relevant to dance.

Chapter 7, International Folk Dance, has been enriched by many. Jacek Marek is a renowned Polish dance specialist living in the Boston area. Born in Krakow, the ancient capitol of Polish culture, he was, from an early age, steeped in the songs and dances of his culture. Jacek has had worldwide experience in teaching and performing the stately and lovely dances of his country. We are honored to be the medium through which these dances can be learned, enjoyed, and perpetuated. Mihai David has contributed several Romanian dances. George A. Fogg and Kate Van Winkle Keller have written a splendid piece on English Country Dance. A number of English Country dances are credited to George A. Fogg.

Andor Czómpo, Hurgarian dance specialist, presents a cultural background and warm-up exercises (motifs) along with several Hungarian dances. Nelda G. Drury, Mexican dance specialist and long-time friend, developed historical notes and selected Mexican dances and dances from Bolivia and Uruguay. Karen P. Gottier's knowledge of German, Austrian, and Swiss dances also has enhanced this section. Marilyn (Walthen) Smith has contributed popular French dances and Mary McLaren Lindsay, Scottish dances. Dick Crum has generously given permission to include several Serbian dances that he introduced to the United States.

Dr. Sandra Gallemore contributed a complete unit on Clogging, along with hours of current information from the Internet. Glenn Bannerman continues as a living treasure on the Big Circle Dance.

Several organizations have been most helpful: The Country Dance and Song Society, The Folk Dance Federation of California, The Mountain Folk Festival, Berea College, The Lloyd Shaw Foundation, and The Royal Scottish Country Dance Society.

With every production there are the ground troops that lend immediate assistance with facts, ideas, and opinions. Luther Black, Hal and Jean Blean, Wayne DeYoung, Brad Foster, Glenn Nickerson, Alice Nugent, Judy Robare, and Mary Sarver have served the eighth edition well. Then there are the relatives who are on constant call: Rick Barnett, Cathy's husband, for his helpful comments, editing, and wonderful support; daughter Kristina Waller Golden and Michael Golden for technical musical assistance and insight of dance for children with physical disabilities; and husband Lynn Waller for editing, second opinions, and constant support. Merci!

A very special thanks to Kathleen Murphy, Lopez Island, Washington, for typing away, deciphering the inserts, and meeting the deadlines.

Finally, we would like to acknowledge again those who have had special impact on this edition and more who have been loyal contributors over the many years.

History

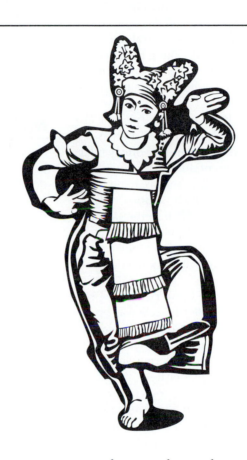

THE BEGINNING

Dance and the dancer have belonged to every age and culture since the beginning of time and thus have reflected the human condition and experience in each succeeding age. In the earliest human experience, dance was a functional means of survival. For primitive societies, dance was a psychological and physiological imperative.

Among primitive peoples everywhere, religion was a highly developed notion of a world of unseen powers. Worship was an expression, in one form or another, of the dependence of humans on powers outside themselves. Fear and a universal dependence on nature for sustenance are the two most conspicuous elements in primitive religion. Humans depended on natural phenomena–on the rain to

grow plants, on the regular succession of seasons, and on the reproduction of animals. Primitive people feared sickness, death, hunger, drought, storms, and the spirits of the dead, both human and animal. The power to communicate with and manipulate the unseen powers that controlled their lives was engendered by the magic of rituals and ceremonies designed to please and appease these forces. It is from these ancient mimetic ceremonies and rituals that the oldest of the arts has emerged–the dance.

Primitive people were one with their environment and, as such, were keen observers of the animal life around them. They reproduced with great fidelity the movements of birds and animals in the art of the period. These dancelike movements were unquestionably models for the mimetic movement used in primitive rituals. The observation of the structured movements of bird and animal groups and individuals gave rise to some of the earliest and oldest dance forms still in use today, namely, Circles, Chains, and Processionals.

FORMS

The *Closed Circle* is perhaps the most ancient of these forms and is believed to have derived from observation and imitation of the sun's rotation. In the early uses of the Closed Circle, dancers entered into the circle equally without regard for differences in gender or social position. Magic was engendered by simple left-and-right movements around a central object that was the focus of the circle. Breaking the circle allowed the evil spirits out and the good spirits in, or vice versa, depending on the culture of the performers.

A second stage, in which the complexity of the circle increases, reflects the effect of cultural change. A dance for alternating genders or for only one gender indicates occupational differentiation. Movement directions, forward and backward and weaving in and out, also increase the complexity of the circle. The elaboration of the Closed Circle into the Double Circle with men on the inner circle, women on the outer circle, either facing center or each other, represents forms used for executing occupational dances and fertility rites.

The *Chain* is derived from the Closed Circle. It first occurred, perhaps, when the Closed Circle was broken. Moving, or traveling the chain from one place to another, allows the magic or good luck engendered by the circle to be distributed over a larger area. Chain dances were generally "gender free"; that is, they could be danced by either gender or by a combination of genders usually placed alternately in line. The Lira vase, modeled and decorated 22 centuries ago by Indo-Europeans, depicts a group of four women linked with three men in a chain who are moving sideways in unison. The *Carole*, a song-dance of the early Middle Ages, was danced in a chain formation. The *Farandole*, a form of Carole, was also danced in a hand-linked line or chain.

The *Processional* consisted of a single or double file of dancers. The latter form was more common and consisted of couples, men in one file and women in the other. The Processional, March, or Promenade was once a complete dance; however, it was more commonly used to begin a program of dancing. The Processional form is said to have originated from two important tribal customs, namely, to clean the community after a hard winter and to ensure its continued fertility. In England, whole communities dance the Processional, moving through the town and in and out of houses, cleaning all before them with a May branch or a green broom. It is from the Processional of couples that first the early Processional Court Dance, then the English Longways set and their continental versions, and finally the Couple Dances developed.

Throughout the ages, forms such as these have functioned to describe something about the society and culture of which they were a part. In the early stages of human development, the forms were as simple as humans imitating animals. As society became more complex, dance forms also became more complex. The effects of cultural changes on dance forms are particularly reflected in gender, occupational, and social-class distinctions. These prehistoric dance forms–the Circle, Chain, and Processional–still exist in present contemporary dance sequences.

MUSIC

Music, the twin sister of dance, has, through the ages, been intimately related to all phases of life–birth, death, love, work, play, war, peace, and religion–and to a myriad of occurrences that arouse human emotions, be they joyous, comedic, or tragic. Because of this intimate relationship with all facets of the human experience, music has had a universal appeal.

Primitive music was spontaneous and improvised, and it was characterized by its nonaesthetic nature and lack of notation. In primitive cultures, music had a magico-functional purpose that served to carry out and perpetuate tribal traditions. The endless singsong of primitive tribal chanters is reflected in early Christian chanting as well as in the droning rhymes of a child jumping rope.

The order in which the elements of music were developed is not known. It is tempting to surmise, however, that primitive humans were not wholly insensitive to the wealth of rhythm in their natural world. The rhythm of seasons, wind, water, and people's own physiological processes were constant cues. There is evidence that primitive people were keenly aware of the two sets of percussion instruments, hands and feet, provided by nature. It is equally tempting to surmise that they vented their feelings of joy and sorrow in bodily motions accompanied by rhythmic noises. These crude rhythmic patterns and raw snatches of melody enacted in pantomime or expressed in grunts and shouts were the antecedents of dance and song.

The origins of instrumental music can be projected on more solid grounds because practically all types of instruments existing today can be traced from primitive and ancient times. Three classes of instruments have evolved: percussion, wind, and string.

Percussion instruments, predominantly the drum, were used to accompany ritual dances and to communicate. In addition to the drum, rattles, seashells, twigs, bond scrapers, and gourds are examples of percussion instruments employed in primitive cultures.

Wind instruments in the form of flutes, trumpets, and reeds date back to the Stone Age. The flute and the trumpet are associated with magico–religious functions. The trumpet is also known to have been used as a signaling instrument in much the same way as it is used today.

In primitive cultures, the *string instruments* were the least developed. The predominant vocal and rhythmic character of primitive music did not require the use of melody or pitch. Primitive cave paintings, dated 30,000 to 15,000 B.C., reveal a human disguised in an animal skin and apparently playing a bow. This gives rise to the possibility that the hunting bow could very well have been the progenitor of string instruments. Whether rhythm preceded melody, vocal music preceded instrumental music, or, in fact, it all happened simultaneously, music was born.

CULTURAL SIGNIFICANCE

Human history attests to the significance of dance as a serious and sacred activity. It was not a mere exuberant display of motor–rhythmic energy separated from the other institutions of a society. It was, indeed, the basis of the survival of the social system in that it contributed significantly to the society's functional and instrumental needs.

■ Religion

Among pre–Christian civilizations, dance was a functional part of religion. In Egypt, dance was an essential part of every religious celebration. Worship was predominantly a ritualized concern for death and rebirth. Egyptian art has left lasting tributes to the importance of dance in wall paintings, reliefs, and literary hieroglyphs. The Egyptians were the first to describe dance movement on paper, and so they are the inventors of the art of choreography.

The Bible, particularly the Old Testament, gives abundant evidence of the importance and place of dance in ancient Hebrew religion. Dance was primarily an act of gratitude for victory or an accompaniment for a hymn of praise. Dances were generally joyous in nature and circular in form. Gratitude, joy, and praise are all found in David's dance in leading the procession of the ark and the canticle of the Israelites after the destruction of the Egyptians led by Miriam and "all the women" (II Sam. VI) and David danced before the Lord with all his might (Exod. 15:20).

■ Education

Dance pervaded the life of ancient Greece, primarily in the form of worship and education. It also penetrated everyday life and achieved perfection as an art form in Greek drama. The Muse of Dance, Terpsichore, was one of the seven Muses. Ancient Greek philosophy defined the soul as the harmony of the body; thus the aim of the Greeks was to develop equally all poses of the mind and the body. Dance, a chief branch of education, was the medium through which total integration of mind, body, and spirit could be achieved.

Dance as it is functionally significant to education has been recognized at various stages throughout human history. The Greeks considered dance a necessary part of education for all people. Plato proposed that all children, boys and girls, be instructed in dance from an early age. He wrote, "To sing well and to dance well is to be well educated" (Lawler 1964; p. 124). The Pyrrhic was the great Greek dance of war. It was accompanied by the flute and danced by armed warriors, who simulated warlike deeds with all the proper maneuvers for attack and defense. Sparta required every child over the age of five to learn the Pyrrhic and to practice it in a public place.

In New England, contrary to popular belief, settlers recommended that the young be taught to dance to learn poise, discipline, and good manners. John Locke, the great commonsense philosopher, wrote of dancing, "Nothing appears to me to give the children so much becoming confidence and behavior . . . as dancing" (Damon 1957; p. 3). Elsewhere in the New World, North American Indian war dances and primitive hunting dances were occasions to teach and practice the skills necessary for war and hunting.

■ Health

The preservation of health and the power to cure ailments through dance rituals are found in every culture. Among primitive people, the *Death Dance* was a united rhythmic effort to remove the ghost, dust the spirits from the house, quiet the emotions, and dispel the fears of those who remained. The 15th century version of the Death Dance was strange in that it happened only in the minds of medical writers and artists. Paintings and woodcuts of the period depict the universality of death, the equality of death, and the vanity of rank and riches. All people, regardless of caste, eventually succumb to the Death Dance. Death also appeared among the living in the form of a skeleton as a warning of impending death.

Captain Cook, of English naval fame, required his crew to dance the *Hornpipe* to ensure immunity from disease. In mid–14th century Italy, the violent, nervous exercise of dancing was believed to relieve the harmful effects or the unreasonable fear of the bite of the tarantula spider.

Devil dances to drive out the ghost of a dead person are thought to be the basis for many funeral dances found throughout history. The Hopi Indians of Arizona use an ancient sand–painting ceremonial for curing purposes. During the four holy days following na ih es, the San Carlos Apache girl's puberty ceremony, the girl's power is believed to be strong enough to cure the sick (Basso 1966; p. 160). So great is the residual power of the dance in this ceremony that it has even been known to cure conditions such as bowed legs (Goodwin 1969; p. 443).

■ Fertility

Dance in the form of fertility rites has been universally used by humans to propagate the species and to secure food. Initiation, courtship, marriage, and birth are themes represented by the dance in these rites. In the initiation rite, youth is danced into adulthood. Fertility of the fields and of humans is abduced by the power generated by encircling a maypole, a tree, or a sword. The three themes symbolized by the dance are (1) passage from one phase to another, as from youth to adulthood or from single to married status; (2) transfer of power (e.g., to carry or decorate with green or to encircle another person); and (3) purification, exemplified by leaping through or running around fire. "Sowing and copulating, germinating and bearing, harvesting and delivering are under one law" (Sachs 1937; p. 67).

Dance and the dancer have belonged to every age and culture since the beginning of time. It is evident that dance and the dancer have played a significant role in the evolution of mankind. In all ages, the human body, as an instrument moving in space and time, has made dance unique among the arts. It is this uniqueness that makes dance older than art and thus explains the antiquity and universality of dance.

AFRICA

■ The Continent

Africa is a vast continent and the home of some of the oldest traces of human existence. As the 21st century approaches, it has captured worldwide attention as a land of newly emerging nation–states.

The Sahara Desert naturally divides the continent into two parts. The north stretches from Morocco to Egypt then up the Nile River to Ethiopia, the cradle of civilization. This area focuses on the Mediterranean Sea and is influenced by Arab culture. To the south, the barriers of the desert, mountains, and tropical forest serve to divide the northern Arab–oriented culture from the greater part of the continent called by the

Arabs "Bilad–as–Sudan," or land of the black people. This area makes up 20 percent of the world's total land area and is the poorest part of the world. It is divided into 40 countries and, except for South Africa, contains two–thirds of the world's least developed nations.

■ European Influence

The desert, mountains, and tropical enviroment served as an impenetrable barrier to interest and knowledge of the area by Europeans until the Portuguese landed at Cape of Good Hope toward the end of the 15th century. Following this opening contact, Africa south of the Sahara was organized into spheres of influence for economic development by Great Britian, France, Spain, Belgium, Portugal, and Germany. Prior to this division the people affected had been organized into ethnic or tribal groups, many with semi–national status. These new boundaries cut across tribes and clans, leading to mutually antagonistic groups within one colonial entity.

■ Slave Trade

National commercial expansion by European countries not only included exploitation of natural resources but more tragically the exploitation of human resources in the form of slaves. The importation of slaves to the New World was not the first incident of enslavement. The Portuguese are said to have begun African slave trading in 1441. Africans were enslaved by Europeans before the time of Columbus's vogage to find the New World. However, the stage was set, and by 1518 slaves were imported to the West Indies. By the end of the 16th century, it is estimated that the number of slaves in the West Indies numbered in the hundred of thousands.

Contrary to some historians, these slaves brought with them a rich mythology, graphic and plastic art, and music with a highly developed rhythmic structure. Dance both secular and recreational came as part of their heritage and was a fundamental element in their aesthetic expression.

■ Traditional Dance

The 21st century finds traditional African dance still an unknown and misunderstood art in the western world. Westerners generally regard it as a spontaneous expression producing gestures and movements lacking any technical mastery or regard for any system. Traditional African dance, on the contrary, has a complete mastery and respect for the precise rules perpetuated and passed down by the society of the Masques de Sagesse, Mask of Wisdon, who have preserved the richness and wisdom of the dance over the centuries.

Masks are not exclusively an African phenomenon. However, nowhere else is their use so widespread and varied. Masks are closely linked to religion, social life, and protection against evil spirits. Secret societies use them to make sure tribal traditions are upheld. Masks are almost exclusively used by males. In many tribes, under threat of punishment, females are not permitted to even set eyes upon them.

Dance is the pervasive and dynamic force in every aspect of African culture and is the living expression of the philosophy and memory of its evolution. Traditional African dance is the result of centuries of perfecting and cannot be danced or understood without the training of the Masques de Sagesse, who are the possessors and protectors of dance knowledge. It is they and they alone who pass this knowledge on to initiates by the centuries–old oral tradition.

■ Art and Dance

The early 20th century saw many conquests of non-European territories, particularly in Africa, which led to a greater exposure and understanding of African culture. In addition, it brought about a revolution in African arts, especially sculpture, and a rediscovery of the powerful force and unity of traditional dance. The general lack of knowledge of these many forms of art was mainly due to the tradition of an oral rather than a written means of communication. Statues and statuettes represented the material knowledge of everyday life and memory existed in the many forms of gestures. These were the manuals for choreographers of traditional dance.

■ Improvisation

Improvisation is the chief characteristic of traditional dance. To achieve the freedom to improvise, traditional dance is taught and learned. Only after the basic movements, gestures, attitudes, and positions are learned is improvisation possible. Gestures learned according to tradition leave the dancer free within the technique to improvise and respond according to his inspiration, which is part of his dialogue with the cosmos. The dancer respects the traditional gestures as "words" of the dance but improvises and creates his own "phrases." The true superiority of African dance lies in the fact that the dance depends on repetition of basic movements and improvisation around these movements.

■ Dance Instruments and Objects

Percussion is the basic rhythm for African dance. The most primitive of all percussion instruments is the stamping and clapping provided by the human body.

Drums are the heartbeat of Africa. They both control and follow movement. They set the tempo and communicate the meaning of rituals and ceremonies. In addition, decorative objects carried or worn by the dancers help mark rhythm or beat time, and each carries its own meaning. These "dance objects" are essential to certain traditional dances, and it is considered a sacrilege to perform certain movements without them. The Bile, made from hair of the tail of a domestic or wild animal, is the oldest. The Gbon, usually a palm branch, is the most common. The Koou, a carved baton featuring scenes of everyday life, serves as a cane or third foot and represents old age. Together the instruments, dance objects, and movements enable African dance to express feelings and convey meanings without resorting to mime and pantomime.

■ Spiritual World

Dance is an intricate part of the daily life in every village. Children are cradled by the rhythm of walking, working, and dancing. Dance is the main avenue of communication and is the expression of life and all its emotions. Every dance tells something and is a link between body, earth, and sky. Its strength is that it draws its resources from the universe and thus recognizes the inseparability of man and the universe. To dance in the African manner is to understand that man is the divine spark indispensable to reaching and conveying the messages of the spiritual world.

The spiritual evolution of man, in African terms, is represented by three concentric circles. The larger or outer circle represents the world, the village, crowds, or body and is the seat of human values. The middle circle represents the intellect or intermediaries, those more detached from the world yet integrated into the world. They search for a more spiritual state. The inner or third circle represents the spiritual world. This is the world of initiates, the Masques. Dance is the common medium of each circle and the privileged form of exchange between the three circles.

As a major component of African culture, dance also depends upon the circle, which is the symbol of both spiritual and temporal life. The spectators represent the outer circle. The dancers represent the second circle and are the necessary intermediaries between the spectators and the spirit of the dance. Thus they are indispensable to reaching and conveying the message of the third circle of the spiritual world.

■ Environmental Influences

Africans live in a variety of environments and, as with other people in other countries, they adapt to their surroundings. That adaptation is reflected in their dance movements. Mountain people live in restricted space; therefore, moves are more prudent and agile. Leaping and climbing are necessary skills. The dance of mountain people is animated and alert, and achieving height is a characteristic. Plains people, peasants who cultivate the land, enjoy extensive space in which to move. Their dance reflects the use of space. The hunters and gatherers of the forest display extensive use of the legs to flex and stretch and to move over and under objects. Their dance tends to be airy, lively yet slow and alert. Coastal people walk in heavy sand and thus place their weight on the flat or complete sole of the foot as they move. Their dance tends to be rigorous and precise, and they walk with deliberation and restraint.

Stilt dancing, although not necessarily environmentally related, is still done in many African countries today. It is an exciting and acrobatic form of dance. Stilts dances are found in neolithic rock paintings in Tassili, which marks it as a very ancient form of dance. Theories abound as to its origin; however, it is generally believed to have begun with forest people who devised stilts to extend their legs, leaving their arms free to gather food from trees. Whatever the origin, dancers perform exciting and perilous exercises in exploring the limits of balance.

■ Beo and Gnenon Dances

Beo and gnenon dances are two gender-oriented categories of dance found throughout Africa. Beo is a highly structured dance for men that has been refined over the centuries and named by whichever ethnic group created it. The traditional movements and basics are accompanied by theoretical instruction in the history of its symbolism and tradition. Because of its strict and traditional heritage, it leaves little or no room for improvisation. The focus of the dance is upon communication with God through harmony of body and spirit.

Gnenon dances are for females. These are far less structured and lend themselves to a high degree of improvisation. They are non-initiating dances of rejoicing and allow the spectators to become freely involved. Dances of this nature performed to modern music and danced in night clubs can be classified as gnenon dances. Unfortunately, these are the kind of dances that Westerners most often see and on which they judge traditional African dance.

■ The Future

For generations Western civilization has been slowly creeping into this vast land and changing both its landscape and its people. As the young have become more accomplished in the manners of the West,

knowledge and respect for the "old ways" of the "knowing ones" have diminished. Since dance is an integral part of the culture as a whole and daily life in particular, it can be a medium for protecting and preserving the cultural heritage of generations past.

PACIFIC RIM PERSPECTIVE

The Pacific Rim is a vast area extending from the southern tip of the western edge of South America north along the western coast of South and North America; west across the Bering Sea to the eastern edge of the former Soviet Union; south along the eastern edges of the three regional groupings referred to as East Asia (China, Japan, North and South Korea), South Asia (India, Pakistan, Afghanistan, Nepal, and Sri Lanka), and Southeast Asia (Myanmar [Burma], Laos, Thailand, Philippines, Indonesia, Malaysia, New Guinea, and hundreds of islands in the South Pacific); to Australia and New Zealand. Historically the area represents the western edge of the 15th and 16th century European expansion and influence and the eastern edge of the Asian expansion and influence. The cultural impact of these two forces is dramatically portrayed in the history of the Philippines, which was dominated by the Spanish; Indonesia, which was greatly influenced by India; and Australia and New Zealand, which are part of the British Commonwealth.

Historically the Western study of the arts, including dance, has been dominated by the arts of European or Western civilization. Until early in the 20th century, little was known of dance as it existed in the eastern part of the European continent, although for centuries it was an important element in the cultures of this portion of the world. In more recent times Western interest, particularly American, has led to increased study and research and extensive exposure to Western audiences by performing groups from many of the East, South, and Southeast Asian countries. This heightened interest in dance as part of the culture of many Asian countries has led to the inclusion in this chapter of brief background sketches of dance in a select group of countries in Asia and the island nations of the South Pacific.

■ India

Dance in India is reputedly the most primitive and at the same time the most sophisticated of the arts. Historical references record that classical dance existed and flourished for centuries before the birth of Christ and, in fact, all India's theater arts were highly developed. The Hindu god Siva is supposed to have created the world by setting its rhythm in motion by dance. Mythology abounds with descriptions of gods and goddesses dancing to produce blessings or to ward off evil.

Classical dance was intrinsically bound to religion. Temple festivals were inseparable from dance and served as the place for the performance. Temple sculpture depicted gods and goddesses dancing and provided a visual legacy of movement for succeeding generations to study. Temple dancers or "devadasis," servants of the deity, helped develop and preserve dance tradition. It has been said that classical dance might never have survived had it not been for these temple dancers and their teachers.

Classical dance in India is in essence dance–drama. The dancer is a storyteller and through dance movements acts out the cast of characters. The elements found in these dance–dramas are song, pantomime, expression, movement, speech, and scenery. The performance may convey ideas, moral values, moods, emotions, and philosophy. The elements vary with the style and historical time of the dance. Aside from their function as entertainment, dance–dramas played an important role in educating the unlettered masses. It was through theatrical spectacles that the ordinary people learned the benefits of virtue, dangers of vices, legends of heroes, and stories of the gods. The theater, often called the bible of the poor, with its color, sound, action, drama, and splendor, gave the people an opportunity to participate in festivals fit for kings and to enter the world of gods and heroes.

Physical training played an important role in all forms of classical dance. Years of arduous training was necessary to acquire the intricate control, skills, and postures required by the dance. Each body part and individual muscle, large and small, was trained to perform separately. Extensive and intensive work was required to control the muscles of the eyeball, eyelids, and eyebrows. In addition, control of the nose, cheek, lips, chin, and neck muscles along with the ability to produce coloration of the face, perspiration, and tears were all to be acquired for dramatic effect. Lastly, the multi–meaning or vocabulary of the hundreds of hand and finger gestures so typical of Indian dance were to be mastered.

The four classical dance styles in India are *Bharata Natya, Kathakali, Kathak,* and *Manipuri.* All four styles are composed of three common elements: pure dance, mime, and a combination of the two. Pure dance is simply dancing to a rhythmical accompaniment without regard for the theme. Pantomime or mime consisted of expressive gestures that communicated the meanings in the story.

All four styles have a common beginning in the system codified by the poet–sage Bharata in the third century B.C. Although each style was conditioned by the environment in which it developed, all share similar techniques, aesthetic principles, and historical and mythological backgrounds. On the other hand, each style differs in language, technique, music, costume, and physical training requirements.

In Bharata Natya the basic geometrical motif is one of three triangles. The movements are angular, measured, and symmetrical. A rectangle forms the basic posture of the Kathakali style. All movements on the floor or in the air are governed by this geometric form. Kathakali movements are violent and expansive. Kathak emphasizes a straight line and preserving gravity. The movements are light, vague, and vacillating. Manipuri dances are based on the figure eight and circular movements in which the body and limbs move in flowing curves.

BHARATA NATYA

The Bharata Natya style of dance is the oldest and most classical in India. Bharata, a combined sage and patron saint of dance, wrote in Sanskrit a treatise on dance and drama in approximately the third century B.C. He codified the knowledge and formulated the theories for the practice and study of dance and drama as revealed to him by the gods. This canonical work is referred to as the Fifth Veda (Holy Book) because of Bharata's sacred relation to art and the Hindu religious concept of dance. The traditions he codified indicated an advanced stage of development in the arts in his time. The Bharata Natya is the most brilliant and classical dance in India and thus is the master form and parent for all dance.

Bharata Natya is the dance style of south India, more specifically, the Tamil Nad region, which encompasses a major portion of southeast India. There it has been preserved and practiced. Originally it contained masculine and feminine roles as taught by the god Siva (male) and goddess Paravata (female). The movements of the dance thus displayed the vigor of the active male and the soft passiveness of the female. Today Bharata Natya is a solo dance that developed independently and is distinct from other dance forms. This solo type is thought to be a direct descendant of the dances of the devadasis.

The basic posture of the Bharata Natya is a triangle, in fact, three triangles. The first is formed by the turned–out feet, as in the first position of ballet, and flexed knees. The line across the knees forms the base with the apex at the heels. The second has the apex at the waist sharing the base line at the knees. The third is formed by the shoulder line sharing the apex at the waist. The knees must remain flexed throughout the dance except during short song sequences whose meanings are danced out by hand gestures and facial expressions. Characteristic movements are terse lines in space and abrupt head and shoulder movements. Outstretched arms and crisp hand movements extend the torso. Leg extensions move from a well–balanced opposite–side base. Leaps are frequent and concise.

Vertical elevations are limited. Bharata Natya is characterized by energy, speed, force, exuberance, clarity, and, above all, physical precision.

KATHAKALI

Kathakali is the dance–drama of Malabar in southwest India. Malabar is a tropical coastline of some three hundred miles lying between coastal hills and the ocean where the Arabian, Indian, and Bengal seas meet. Its excellent harbors attracted the Greeks, Phoenicians, Arabs, and Chinese a millennium before the Christian era; it was the oldest part of India to have contact with the outside world. This mixed ethnic background is reflected in the dance form.

The dance–drama Kathakali is held outdoors and is an all–night performance ending at dawn. It is usually held during periods of the full moon. The performers, all men, also take women's roles. Dancers appear not as human beings, but as gods, demons, and spirits from another world. Their actions create certain moods characteristic of a view of life in the abstract.

Kathakali is the culmination of many different theatrical forms existing over time in south India. The dance style is overwhelmingly dramatic. To achieve this dramatic quality a highly developed, complex, and symbolic system of makeup has evolved. Colors are associated with certain moods and sentiments. In facial makeup, green is the color for virtuous characters. A black moustache drawn on the upper lip indicates an angry mood. The color symbolism is carried out in the colorful costumes and headgear, which represent gods and spirits of the world of myth and legend, not of the real world.

Kathakali technique follows other classical styles in that it uses pure dance, expressive dance, and mime. However, unlike other styles, Kathakali uses both skeletal and large muscle groups of the body. The geometric pattern is a square or rectangle. The basic posture is feet apart, knees turned out. The dancer moves his feet to all corners of the rectangle. The rectangle is used in hand and arm movements as well. Jumps, spirals, and leaps along with some elevation is characteristic. Facial expressions are of major importance. The most exacting part of Kathakali training is learning to control the eyes, eyelids, eyebrows, and lip movements.

The pantomime aspect of the dance sequence is the test of a great Kathakali dancer. This is the creative portion of the dance in which the dancer can embellish a simple line in a poem into a solo improvisation of great dramatic effect. In mime the hand movements are particularly important in setting the dramatic mood. Some 24 hand gestures communicate more than 500 words and word signs.

Kathakali style is energetic, active, violent, athletic, and acrobatic. It is predominantly masculine in feeling. The conditioning of the body requires that dancers begin at an early age and spend up to 10 years in training. Massages and oil baths make the body soft and flexible so that each muscle, joint, and nerve can operate independently when called on. Acrobatics and fencing are used to produce fantastic leg extensions, leaps, jumps, and splits. Eye training is extensive and arduous. The eyes are trained to open to twice their normal size, tremble rapidly, move slowly in tracking an object, and show the whites only. Kathakali training makes the body perform in ways that otherwise seem impossible.

KATHAK

Kathak is the dance style of northern India, a section ruled by the Muslims during the 12th to the 18th centuries. During this period, the otherwise religious and temple–oriented Kathak degenerated into a secular form known as Nautch. The vulgarity of Nautch relegated the dance to brothels and Muslim courts where it was performed to please the overlords, not the gods, and for remuneration rather than spiritual reward. Under Muslim influence and material encouragement large numbers of artists pursued their talents in this environment. Since the revival of classical dance in India, Kathak has resumed its rightful place among other forms.

Kathak is characterized by a wide–eyed stare and a whirl and sudden halt. The dancer's feet are percussion instruments that produce rhythmic pulses to vibrate the ankle bells. The dancer can tap out long, involved meters with or against the drum syncopation. Dancers have been reputed to be able to control all bells but one in a percussion action. Kathak movement is neither violent nor overly dainty, and the mood is soft and sweet. It can be danced, therefore, by male or female. The latter, however, constitute the majority. Aside from these elements, the dance style is much like other classical forms.

MANIPURI

Manipuri dance is at home in the province of Manipur in northeast India along the Myanmar (Burma) border. This small part of India is a beautiful, fertile, self–sufficient valley inhabited by mixed ethnic groups predominantly of the Vaishnavite Hindu persuasion. The area has been isolated both geographically and for political reasons for many years. Until very recently visitors came only by permission from the government.

According to mythology, Manipur was created so the gods would have a place to dance. Therefore, Manipur is a land of amateur dancers! It is a matriarchal society in which men are idle while women take care of the home and business affairs. It is compulsory for women to dance and optional for men.

Manipur is most celebrated for producing polo and *Ras Lila*. Polo is known and played worldwide. *Ras Lila*, a dance of ecstasy in heaven, was created by the god Siva and his wife Parvati. Legend further claims that the imitation Ras Lila for which Manipur was founded was Lai Haraoba.

Lai Haraoba, an imitation Ras Lila, is the oldest dance form in Manipur and therefore the basis for all their dance. It is performed for one month, usually April or May, by each village as a religious obligation. It is at once dance, fertility ritual, religious in context, and village entertainment. In reality it is a small-scale version of the creation of the world.

The dance is accompanied by drums and a small string instrument played with an archery-like bow to which bells are attached to add percussion. Dance training is unnecessary in Manipur. The natural grace of its people and their outdoor life give them enough exercise and training to perform the dance. The people literally dance as soon as they walk!

Religion is the focus of the dance and the body movements are considered the highest dedication of the human body to the gods. The Manipuri consider movements in sports and dance a means of worship. Gods are worshipped in boat racing, polo, hockey, and mountain climbing. The holy book even suggests offering a stick and a ball to the gods in cases of epidemics. To the Manipuri dance is physical culture made more ornamental for the glory of the gods.

Ras Lila is one of India's most outstanding contributions to the arts. Ras Lila is a love dance or love play as conceived by Joy Singh, a Manipur king who saw and heard it in a dream. In contrast to polo, Ras Lila has never been performed outside of Manipur. It is performed after midnight and staged according to season, usually in a mountain area or a remote temple. Ras Lila is in truth a full-scale opera-drama combining dance, choral singing, and religious cantatas. It is a spectacle of color, glittering jewels, flashing mirrors and mica on flamboyant costumes. It is considered a national treasure and is without a doubt a moving and exciting dance-drama with universal appeal.

Classical dance in India has been revived from oblivion and extinction more than once since its codification by Bharata in the third century B.C. Passed along mainly by rote and practice, the details of the dance-drama grew dim or were lost over succeeding generations. In the mid-18th century Vadivela and Ponniah Pillay, brothers of Tanjori, both masters of the dance, music, and Sanskrit, revised and standardized Bharata Natya. Their expertise uniquely suited them to interpret the literature and theatrical background of the dance; thus they were able to crystallize the repertoire and regulate the dance items into a more classical program.

Subjugated by Muslims and the British and later influenced by Christianity, dance in India did well to survive at all. However, with independence came a rebirth of interest in all the arts, including dance. Anna Pavlova's Indian tour in 1929 is credited with stimulating renewed interest in classical dance. Her performance, based on Indian themes and music, along with her inquiries and obvious interest in Indian dance, helped awaken national interest. More importantly, perhaps, was the part she played in enhancing the stature of women artists.

Classical dance in India today is the product of some half a century of activity stimulated partly by American interest and wholly by the dedication of many Indian artists. Interest and support of dance by people of a higher caste, particularly women, coupled with travel and performance abroad have been the major forces moving dance from provincial to national stature. Classical dance is India's most significant and unique gift to the world of dance.

■ *China*

China is a vast country encompassing a civilization dating back more than 4,000 years. Discoveries of late Stone Age sites on the Loess Plateau along the Yellow and Wei Rivers indicate that the Chinese civilization did indeed develop independently of South Asian and Western cultures.

The first Chinese state has been traced by scholars to the Shang dynasty (ca. 1766–1122 B.C.). Priests, scholars, officials, and artisans of the Shang dynasty developed agriculture, formalized religion, set up government and legal systems, produced writing and literature, began the tradition of dynasties, and developed handicrafts and metallurgy. All of these accomplishments clearly distinguished China from other cultural systems of the same period. A common means of communication in the written literature has always been a unifying factor between past and present in Chinese culture.

The dynasty system, which began with the Shang and ended with the Qing (A.D. 1644–1911), is one of China's most interesting and unique cultural developments. The cyclic rise and fall of dynasties over the centuries make it important to understand and cast the study and research of events and the cultural progress of Chinese history against the chronology of this system.

China and India were the two major cultural forces in Asia. As India's influence waned, China, an equally powerful force, began to dominate. China is a gigantic multinational country made up of the Han, the Chinese people, who represent approximately 90 percent of the population, and more than 50 national minorities. It is this mix and the influence they had on one another that created the common cultural tradition of the Chinese people. The bulk of dance before and after liberation has come from the minorities. Unlike the Indians, the Chinese produced little or no dance. China's forte in the arts was the theater, better known as the opera. India cultivated dance and music to the detriment of drama; China developed drama and music to the exclusion of dance.

Despite the domination of the opera there was dance. Thanks to the mountainous bulk of literature the Chinese have produced in written history dating from the most ancient times and to archaeological finds of more recent times, dance has been quite thoroughly researched and studied. Of particular importance have been archaeological digs, cave paintings, and murals. These, combined with accounts in poetry and essays from the Han dynasty (206 B.C.–A.D. 220) and the Tang dynasty (A.D. 618–907), indicate that dance and songs were indeed a part of the life of the primitive people who were the fore-bears of the Chinese people. A Neolithic bowl, one of the oldest finds, depicts a line or circle of dancers holding hands with movement indicated by the angle of the braided hair hanging from their heads. Legends tell of dances developed to serve as fitness exercises and martial dance with weapons to train soldiers. Votive dances related in ancient legends tell of clan or tribal leaders who ordered songs and dances composed to offer as homage to a good harvest, for the pleasure of a god, or to heaven, earth, and the ancestors.

The dynastic system in Chinese history began as a slave society, a period lasting some 1,600 years. As was true in most of the world's emerging human societies, people had no means for understanding natural phenomena and thus resorted to shamans to communicate with the gods. During this period shamans practiced their sorcery by singing and dancing. Rain dances, for agricultural reasons, were especially in demand. Dances of exorcism were also used to drive away the demons of pestilence or devils. Dancers wore masks and performed frenziedly to clear out the evil. These dances enjoyed an unbroken tradition of several thousand years.

Dancing slaves represented the gradual entry of dance into the realm of performing art. Rulers of the time considered dance as entertainment and kept troupes of dancing girls in their courts. Legend tells that groups of slave dancers were killed and buried with their owner so they could continue serving their master after death.

The powerful slave state of the Western Zhou (11th century B.C.) appointed a director of music whose task it was to work out a system of ritual music and dance. He collected songs and dances of various clans under previous dynasties and taught them to the members of the court for ritual ceremonial purposes.

This system included the dances for votive ritual, a martial type of dance, dances costumed with animal tails or plumage relating to hunting, and music and dance of national minorities such as "Music of Border Tribes." Succeeding generations of feudal rulers praised this system of court ritual as "Music of Early Kings" or as "sublime music."

A slave revolt brought an end to the Western Zhou reign and thus ended the cruel regime and along with it organized court dance and music. China entered a period of turmoil and change, and folk song and dance were left to the vicissitudes and vagaries of the general population. During this period, known as the Spring, Autumn, and Warring States period, groups of poor people roamed the countryside offering their services as actors or dancing girls. Many excellent artists were produced during this period. Performers continued to lead harsh lives during the feudal period but despite this these early professional performers preserved and developed dance in ancient China.

China experienced its first multinational unified state during the Han dynasty. Unification led to stability, economic progress, and frequent contacts between nationalities within and outside the borders. Under these circumstances literature, art, and dance flourished. A board of music was established to collect and improve folk song and dance. Variety shows became the vogue for performing and entertaining. These shows included acrobatics, martial arts, comic acts, recitals of music, song, and dance as well as other folk arts. The widespread popularity of the variety shows drew audiences from hundreds of miles around.

Archaeological finds have provided a life-like look at the variety show popular in the Han period. One such group of Han clay figurines on a tray shows the arrangement of musicians, acrobats, and dancing girls. A brick relief shows the *Tray Drum Dance*, an ingenious combination of dance and acrobatics which is a distinctive style in Chinese classical dance. Other artifacts show the *Fish Dance*, *Dragon Dance*, and *Peacock Dance*. The sleeve movements of a dancer's costume, an ancient tradition in Chinese dance, are also found in figurines and in murals. Stone reliefs and other objects depicting dance have been corroborated by contemporary folk dances such as the *Red Silk Dance* and the *Long Silk Dance* created after Liberation.

During the more than 400 years of the Han dynasty artists created many dances. Dancers underwent strict training during this time and were successful in raising dance to a new artistic level. However, the low social status of the dancer was such that only the figurines and stone engravings buried with the feudal nobles remain to tell the story of their work.

The development of cities, institution of the guild system, and increased foreign trade led to a prosperous economy during the northern and southern Song dynasties. The arts flourished and expanded with special venues being set aside in the cities to stage shows for increasingly large, eager audiences. These venues were known as Wazi and Goulan. They were places to display all kinds of skills such as poetic dramas, acrobatics, story telling, comic acts, musical acts, wrestling, and dances.

Although the song and dance pieces given at the Wazi were well received, the most popular were the poetic dramas. Dance performances increasingly included sections depicting stories, and it was in the telling of these stories that the populace found an avenue for expression suited to their needs. This was in essence the beginning of the traditional Chinese opera. Traditional opera continued to grow from the Song dynasty to the Qing dynasty and proved to be the most popular form of art, becoming China's world-renowned art form.

Under the short-lived Sui dynasty the rulers celebrated the end of the latest period of war and set about unifying China once again. They amassed the traditional songs and dances of the Han dynasty, minority nationalities, and materials from abroad into "Seven Books of Music," later increased to "Nine Books of Music." The books were for the populace as well as for court use. They also continued the variety shows of the Han dynasty. The lavish spending and self-indulgence of the Sui dynasty spelled its doom in some thirty short years.

The golden age of the arts followed under the Tang dynasty (A.D. 618). The Tang court set up offices for music and dance and employed noted artists to train professional performers in a systematic manner. These trained professionals were then dispersed all over the country, which helped ancient and traditional dance to attain a new standard of performance and skill.

The "Nine Books of Music" from the Sui dynasty was enlarged to "Ten Books of Music" by incorporating materials from the minority nationalities, the Yan, Qingshang, Xiliang, Indian, Korean, Kucine, Bokhara, Shula, Samarkand, and Qoco. Of the ten books only Yan and Qingshang music were Han music; the other eight were of other nationalities. The "Ten Books" enjoyed great popularity in the Central Plains.

The "Samarkand Music," commonly called *Dervish Dance*, was the dance of the minority from the northwest boundaries of China. The dance featured whirling movements variously described as "gyrating frenzy like flurrying snow." Most of the Dervish Dances were performed by women and were very popular during the Tang period.

Zuobu Arts and *Libre Arts* were two new categories of dance formed in the Tang period. Zuobu Arts were refined movements performed inside by a small number of dancers. Libre Arts were ostentatious displays of dance performed outside by a large number of dancers. Both were based on the artistic tradition of the Central Plains but largely made up of materials of the national minorities and neighboring countries. The "Taiping Music" in the Libre Arts was also known as the *Lion Dance of the Five Directions*. The Lion Dance appears over several centuries in several cultures in the Asian area and has a particularly interesting history as it relates to China. Although not native to China, lions were often brought as gifts to the Han dynasty court from Afghanistan and Persia. They were viewed as symbols of power and strength. The dance, in its many forms, grew out of the imitation of the lion's appearance and actions and was danced to express what the lion symbolized.

Small-scale dances used at less important or ordinary banquets were classified as *Jian Dances* and *Ruan Dances*. The former were robust dances requiring agility; the latter were more sedate and beautiful in their movements. The *Sabre, Mulberry Branch*, and *Dervish* represent the Jian group while the *Green Waist Dance* was the most famous of the Ruan dances.

"Grand Compositions" and "Folk Song and Dance Drama" were two other forms active in the Tang period. The "Grand Compositions" included song, dance, and poetry while the "Folk Song and Dance Drama" combined singing, dancing, and acting to portray set characters and a plot. Most of the latter consisted of one character and a simple plot; therefore, they could not be termed full-fledged song and dance dramas but could be said to be the precursor of China's later world-renowned traditional opera.

Music and dance were the main performing arts during the Tang dynasty. Although based on traditional dance, the choreography was bold and innovative and embraced many national folk dances as well as those introduced from abroad. It is said that whenever the Chinese adapted anything from abroad it was as if they had taken it as a prisoner to do with as they pleased. Tang arts absorbed everything, and given fairly stable political and economic conditions, a golden era in the development of dance in China's feudal society was created.

National minority dances played an important role in the overall mosaic of Chinese folk dance. Their work, life, love, and customs were bound up in their dance, which was largely passed along by oral tradition. Hand-written historical documents carried few records of their dances. The most influential were the Mongol, Tibetan, Uygar, Miao, Korean, Yao, and Dai minorities. The following are some examples of the style and type of minority dance that was popular in central China.

The *Daola* of the Mongols displayed the strong, vigorous, and rapid whirling action characteristic of the northern border neighbor. The *Guozhuang Dance* from Tibet reflected the hunting life of its people by imitating tigers, eagles, and peacocks. The *Xie* or *Xianzi Da*, the graceful sleeve dance, and the *Duixie* or *Tap Dance*, which beat out rhythm with the feet, were well–received dances from Tibet. The *Long Drum Dance* of the Yao was popular through the Song, Yuan, Ming, and Qing dynasties. It is also a present–day favorite of new China. The beautiful *Mynah Dance*, which imitates the movements of the mynah bird, and the *Reed Pipe Dance* of the Miao people are both currently being performed by professional dancers. Other national minority dances known during the feudal periods and which have been drawn upon and used in present–day performances are the Yi people's *Axi Moon Dance*, the Dai *Peacock Dance*, the Li *Money Bell and Double Sword Dance*, the Zhuang *Carrying and Pole Dance*, and the Gaosham *Pestle Dance*.

The Ming and Qing dynasties were the final stages of China's feudal system. Popular thought and action at this time bore the seeds of capitalism and a thriving city life spurred a boon in the arts. Traditional opera, singing, and storytelling flourished while dance performances alone were rare. Popular opposition to feudalism found in the opera a means for communicating resistance to the cruel constraints of everyday life, something that dance alone could not do. Dance merged with opera and thus rarely existed as an independent performing art although a wealth of dance was preserved in the opera. Dance continued in the general populace in the form of small song and dance shows put on by amateur performers of working people during slack seasons. These small touring groups of seven or eight actors developed shows from original song and dance pieces such as *Local Flower Drum*, *Tea Picking Lantern*, and other well-known pieces. The resulting shows were widely popular and provided an outlet for the people to pour out their joys and sorrows and make public note of their resistance to feudal rule.

Although dance performances alone were uncommon in the Ming and Qing dynasties, dances at local festivals were widespread. The traditional Lantern Festival held on the 15th day in the first month of the lunar calendar was a particularly joyous occasion for song and dance. Homes and streets were festooned with lanterns, fireworks were set off, drums and gongs sounded, and the *Lion Dance* and the *Monk with the Big Head Dance* were traditional attractions. Chinese literature in the form of books, poems, accounts, and recollections attest to the continued popularity of dance among the populace at festival times.

In the intervening years after the dynasty system became history and the Republic exited to Taiwan, some efforts were made to collect and arrange folk dance materials but the major effort was left to be done after liberation. Almost immediately the Chinese government seized on folk dance as a means of fostering national spirit and to present the people as happy and cheerful members of the new Chinese society.

In 1951, two years after liberation, a large celebration of song and dance called "Great Unity of the People" was held in Tiananmen Square. It was an opportunity for national minorities to demonstrate their dances as well as a national review of the achievements of professional dancers from the folk art tradition of old China. In 1952 the performance toured all areas of China to demonstrate unity and exuberance for the new society.

Under a policy adopted by the Chinese Communist Party and the central People's Government, national minority art and literature was to be developed. This policy led to extensive research, study, and rearranging of many of the traditional dances throughout China. Specifically, folk dance disciplines were set up in dance schools, dance teachers collected and arranged dance materials and studies of dance in classical Chinese opera were undertaken aided by older performers in the opera. In the mid 1950s Chinese dance leaders created a national dance with a distinct style based on the study of national, traditional, and foreign dance forms. The result was "The Precious Lotus Lamp," the first large–scale dance-drama. A second large–scale dance–drama, "The East Is Red," which was especially supported by Premier Zhou Enlai, required some 3000 dancers. This epic covered the various stages of the Chinese revolution.

Suddenly the Gang of Four headed by Jiang Qing came to power and brought to a virtual halt all the work in dance and other arts. During the 10 years of their influence artists, dancers, singers, and musicians were cruelly treated; they were executed, imprisoned, or sent to the country to do manual labor. In 1976 this foursome was ousted and national art was liberated for the second time. Since the mid '70s, the national art movement has regained its momentum and is once again teaching, practicing, researching, and staging mammoth and spectacular performances for audiences in China and abroad.

China is presently awash in dance. Dances are created in villages, cities, communes, schools, factories, and professional dance schools. It is seen in parks, courtyards, plazas, indoors, and outdoors. A festival held in Beijing in 1972 was reported to have had more than 2000 amateur groups performing. Performers, even eight- and eleven–year–olds, are polished, technically adroit, and project theater–quality proficiency.

Dance in China is an expression by and of the people. It is about them and exists for them. The frames of reference are contemporary situations, historical events, revolutionary themes showing workers, peasants, and soldiers as heroes and heroines, and stories of the crimes of the old society. Movement styles come from minority nationality forms, work techniques of the field and factory, old dances of the Tang and other dynasties, and even a touch of Wu Shu, a traditional style of physical culture. Regardless of the style or content, the dance is always presented in a joyous, happy, and exuberant mode.

Content and style is best reflected in dance titles such as *The Spinners and Weavers Dance, Dance of the Steel Workers, Think of the Consumer When Growing Vegetables, On the Way to Battle,* and *The Bayonet Fight.* Titles of dances for children reflect history, vocational preparation, and acquiring attitudes: *The Long March, The Nurses, Friendship Dance,* and *Washing Clothes.*

The new China is clearly allowing for the fullest expression of people's ideas and feelings through dance. Just as the ancient "Book of Odes" suggests, "If words do not suffice, then sigh; if sighing fails, then sing; if singing is not enough, then let your arms and legs dance it."*

■ Korea

Korean history dates back to 2333 B.C. It is a peninsula strategically located with Manchuria and the former Soviet Union to the north, Yellow Sea to the west, and Sea of Japan to the east. The Chinese and Japanese have invaded and conquered Korea at various times and influenced its culture. The Japanese gave Korea the name "Choson," translated as "The Land of the Morning Calm," a name used by the Koreans. The Western name, Korea, came from the Koryu dynasty (A.D. 935 to 1392). Korea remained under Japanese dominance until after World War II. Then Korea was given to Russia and the United States in trusteeship and consequently divided into two countries at the 38th parallel.

TRADITIONAL KOREAN DANCE

Korea's traditional dance can be divided into three major groups: the religious ritual dances, the stately court dances, and the lively folk dances.

The ritual dances include those of Chinese Confucian origin, Buddhist dances, and Shamanist ritual called *Mudang Dance,* which predated the others, with its roots in Korean animism.

The court dances are graceful, slow, and elegant movements, performed by women, ladies of the court. The costumes reflect the period of each dance and typically influence the dance movement. For instance, long sleeves cover the dancer's hands and the arm movement becomes very elaborate.

Originally a court dance, the Sword Dance has been adapted by the common people and now is considered a folk dance. Some of the Buddhist dances are also considered folk dances. The *Farmers' Dance* and *Changgo* (drum) *Dance* are of purely folk origin. Farmers' musical bands would go out to the fields, with dance and song, to lend support to the workers transplanting and weeding. In earlier days, this was a fertility ritual at Festival time.

Mask dances and folk dramas are enjoying a revival. The mask dances are satires on the nobility of the Yi dynasty or monks who have broken their vows.

MUSICAL INSTRUMENTS

Korea has a large number of musical instruments, mostly introduced from China, along with some invented by Koreans. They were used in the classical music of the royal courts.

The instruments are classified by the Chinese system according to the materials from which they are made: metal (bells, gongs, cymbals), stone (stone slabs), silk (harp, lute, two–stringed fiddle), bamboo (flute, pipe), leather (drums), and wood (clappers, clarinet–like reed pipe). The changgo (two–headed drum shaped like a hourglass) and tae geum (six–hole large flute) are quite popular among the Korean people today.

■ Japan

The three professional classic dance forms in Japan are *Bugaku, Noh,* and *Kabuki.* All three are performed by men, confirming Japanese society as indeed a man's world. Each represents an aspect of three different historical socioeconomic groups found in the cultural life of Japan. Bugaku was developed from dances brought from Asia for the imperial courts during the Heian period (794–1185). Noh was developed under the patronage of samurai rulers and aristocracy during the Muromachi period (1338–1573). Kabuki was a popular form among merchants and townspeople of Osaka and Edo (Tokyo) during the Todugawa period (1600–1867).

Folk dances in general occur as part of the three major religious festivals, Kaura, Ta Asobi, and Obaon. Kagura is the music (god music) and dance of Shinto, the indigenous pantheistic religion of Japan. It includes a wide variety of activities such as dances and ceremonies of the imperial shrines, dances of the Miko or shrine maidens, and numerous regional dance–dramas, martial arts, and animal dances. Ta Asobi or "rice paddy play" refers to a variety of agricultural rites dealing with the cultivation of rice from mid–winter to the fall harvest festivals. Bon dances are performed throughout Japan, generally on the grounds of Buddhist temples. Bon festivals are celebrations of the return of the souls of dead ancestors,

---

*Wand Kefen, *The History of Chinese Dance.* Beijing: Foreign Language Press, 1985, p. 1.

who visit the earth once each year in mid–August. Noh performances are also given as a part of some festivals.

BUGAKU

Bugaku dance style emphasizes pure dance forms over the dramatic elements. Although dramatic elements exist in some dances, they become mostly topical and little or nothing of the story is communicated. Bugaku emphasizes symmetry of the basic movement patterns in solo dances and the frequent use of paired dancers. The dance setting is usually outdoors or in a simulated outdoor setting in a courtyard, shrine, temple, or the imperial household. The fixed repertoire is composed of some 60 pieces handed down from ancient times. The works are divided into two categories according to basic style and assumed place of origin. The *Left Dance* (Samai) includes dances from China, India, and Indochina along with those from Japan in similar style. The movements are slow, gentle, and elegant. Dancers are costumed in robes of reddish color. The *Right Dance* (Umai) includes dances from Korea and compositions based on Korean dances. The movement is humorous and spirited. Dancers wear robes of a greenish color. In the Left Dance the dancers enter the stage from the left of a large drum located at the rear of the stage or stage right. The Right Dancer enters the stage from the right of the drum or stage left.

Bugaku dances are divided into four types based on content. They are ceremonial (hiramai), military (bumai), running (hashirimai), and children (dodu) dances. Ceremonial dances are performed by two to four unmasked dancers wearing court or ceremonial robes. Military dances are performed in pairs. Dancers wear elaborate warrior robes and simulate battle action with swords and lances. Running dances are performed by solo masked dancers displaying a strong character. Children dances are composed for and performed by children.

NOH

Noh is held to be the greatest dance–drama tradition in human history. After appreciating the visual beauty and traditional conventions of Noh, those who make the effort will experience a powerful expression of the universal nature of man's spirit. The training and aesthetics of Noh were formulated by the writings of the famous performer, playwright, and philosopher Zeami in the mid 12th and early 13th centuries. His writings are still read by students, performers, and connoisseurs of the art, and his plays still form the core of Noh repertory.

A combination of the elegant world of the imperial court, Zen in the form of Buddhist meditation, and the code of ethics and conduct of the samurai were the main influences on the content of Noh dance–dramas. These three influences are seen in Noh plays in which samurai, nobles of the court, and Buddhist priests appear as characters.

Noh plays draw on the etiquette of Shintoism, including the carrying of the fan, the use of flute and drum, and on Kagura for ceremony. From Bugaku it drew its structure, namely the use of an introduction, development, and conclusion. Variety came from Sarugaku in the form of magic tricks, humorous skits, and acrobatics. Field music elements came from rice cultivation festivals. Dances performed by Buddhist priests (Ennem) at New Year festivals and popular songs and dances of the period are all part of the background and content of Noh theater.

Set movement patterns, meaning a form either in time or space, are the basis for construction of Noh dances. The movement patterns are composed of position and progression. The basic position requires the torso to be inclined and held in place with no rotation. The back is held in a straight line, knees slightly bent, and arms curved down and forward of the body, elbows slightly lifted to create a line for the large sleeves of the costume. The dancer imagines lines of force coming out of the center of the body to project his energy. This effort can be characterized as a level of high tension without being rigid. Concentration produces the effect of freedom coming from self–control.

Walking is the most characteristic movement. It is the progression that integrates the dance. In addition, it is the element by which the overall skill of the dancer is determined. The walk gives the impression that the dancer is gliding in space without effort. Stamping is also used and the resulting pattern of sound is augmented by placing clay pots under the stage to give resonance to this part of the performance.

The mechanics of turning and locomotion to various parts of the stage are highly codified in Noh. These movements are important to convey traveling to shrines, battlefields, or places in nature. Locale or the place depicted in Noh text is expressed primarily in movement, seldom with the aid of stage properties. Movements such as the activity of looking are depicted by a forward move, raising and pointing the fan, then backing away to add perspective. Some pantomime depicts praying, holding a shield, or riding a horse.

Noh dancing is not verbose in that most movements are minimal and subtle. The goal is to express the highest ideals with the simplest means. Noh has been continued by generations of people who have a great sensitivity to all arts and a special talent for dance–dramas.

KABUKI

Kabuki is one of Japan's most traditional and popular theater arts. Its beginnings date back to the latter part of the 16th century, a time when there was a rigid distinction between the warrior class and the commoners. Kabuki was cultivated by merchants who has become economically powerful but who remained socially inferior. The art of Kabuki was a means for expressing their resentment against the feudal system of the times. Kabuki themes were thus those of fundamental conflicts between humanity and the feudal system. It was the thematic content of Kabuki that endeared it to the public in its early development and even today.

In the beginning the players were women but when they began to attract undue attention from their male audience, public officials banned their appearance in the theater. Male actors became the sole performers. During the 250 years that the ban on female dancers was enforced, male actors perfected the art of female impersonation or "onnagata." Onnagata became such an integral part of Kabuki that, if derived of this element, the traditional quality of Kabuki could be lost forever.

Kabuki has incorporated parts of all preceding theater forms in its extensive and continuous evolution since the 16th century. It drew stage technique and repertoire from Noh. It adopted a comic element from Kyogen plays, which were interludes in Noh performances. It also drew from the puppet theater, which was developing at the same time. And finally, in the 19th century it added literary realism.

Dance–drama constituted a segment of some 300 plays in the Kabuki repertoire. Actors danced to both vocal and instrumental music. Many of these dramas told complete stories; others were primarily dance. Historical dramas presenting accounts of warriors and nobles and domestic dramas depicting plebeian life constituted the remaining repertoire.

The aesthetic principle underlying Kabuki is formalized beauty. To prepare for their roles, actors study the style modeled by their predecessors. Over the years these model styles became highly formalized and symbolic even if they are intended to present realism. Thus in acting, gestures became more like dancing than acting, posture and poses placed more emphasis on statuesque beauty, vocal delivery became elocution accompanied by music and sets. Kabuki costumes and makeup are recognized as the most lavish and extravagant in the world. Audiences enjoy this spectacle of dazzling and superb color even if unconvinced by the plot of the story. Visual beauty sustains the popularity of Kabuki even today.

The modern Kabuki theaters are built largely in Western style but have retained some significant features of the traditional theater. Two of these are the flower–walk ramp and the revolving stage. The flower–walk ramp (Hanamichi) is a passageway connecting the left side of the stage with the back of the hall. The ramp passes over the seats at head level with the audience. Actors enter and exit along the passageway and at the right and left exits on the stage. The passageway is part of the stage and often actors give important scenes of the play on the flower–walk. The revolving stage was invented in Japan some 300 years ago and is a major contribution to theater around the world.

Kabuki's greatness is primarily due to its actors, many of whom come from families of Kabuki actors that date back to the feudal era. To acquire all the skills needed, an actor must begin in childhood. The family system not only allows for early development but has made it possible to preserve the art of Kabuki.

The Kabuki actor of today no longer specializes in a particular role but has become more versatile. This is true except in the role of onnagata or female impersonation. In this role, specialization is still the rule. Formerly actors were popular among the masses but considered to have low social status. Today actors are held in high esteem and many have been elected to the Academy of Art of Japan. Kabuki enjoys wide popularity in Japan today, although its content does not depict contemporary themes. The principle reason for its sustained popularity lies in the fact that it has become a crystallized art form and thus seems destined to retain the affection and pride of the nation.

■ *Bali*

The word *Bali* conjures up romantic associations such as South Sea islands, tropical beaches, coconut trees, and a world of magic and enchantment. The island of Bali is a 90–by–50–mile speck off the east coast of Java. Bali is a country of spectacularly gifted people of mixed race, endowed with a great sense of humor and united by an ancient oral tradition to their revered ancestors.

The wave of Hindu culture and religion that flowed through Java found its terminal point in Bali. Today, Bali is the only Hindu country in the world outside of India. The Balinese are the recipients of India's highly developed music, dance, and aesthetic philosophy.

Communal village–centered life is the norm in Balinese culture. Yet over the centuries villages have bound together to form a highly sophisticated and interdependent wet–rice agricultural system. The need for cooperation is emphasized in ancient Balinese teachings from manuscripts dating back to the eighth century. Religion and spirituality are integral parts of life and making offerings in the form of food and flowers is considered a continual act of devotion. Dance is considered as one very special form of communal offering, and it plays a vital part in all ceremonies.

Each village has three temples, the Ancestor Temple, the Community Temple, and the Temple of

Death. Within the most sacred inner temple court-yard the Wali or most sacred Balinese dances are performed. Both the temple and the dances are thought to be of indigenous origin; however, some Hindu–Japanese elements may be seen in the dances. Temple form and layout date back to the Neolithic culture of ancestor worshippers who migrated to Bali from Southeast Asia between 2500 and 1000 B.C.

The Balinese observe an elaborate schedule of festivals according to the Hindu–Balinese religious calendar or Odalan. The Wali or group of dances performed in connection with religious rituals involves going into a trance in which the dancers are possessed by divine or sometimes demonic spirits. These dances also require a strong element of village and audience participation. They are performed in the sacred inner temple courtyard before the shrine of the gods. Prominent in the Wali or most sacred category are *Berutuk, Sang Hyang Dedari, Rejang,* and *Baris Gedes.*

BERUTUK

The Berutuk rite is performed by young bachelors wearing sacred masks, dressed in large aprons made from dried banana leaves and carrying a long fiber whip. The whips are used to ward off the audience, who cheer and tease the dancing monsters, hoping to get a piece of the sacred banana leaf costume. The dance-drama lasts all day. It is a performance that combines aspects of a game, a ceremony, and a ritual drama.

SANG HYANG

Sang Hyang Dedari is an ancient dance in a group known as Sang Hyang. Dances in this group all involve putting one or more dancers in a trance by means of incense, prayers, and chanting to receive the gods. Once possessed, the dancers interact with the audience by dancing, mimicking animals, and sometimes speaking as oracles. Possession differs among the many varieties of Sang Hyang. There is an element of ritual purification and exorcism in most Sang Hyang dances. Sang Hyang Dedari is one of the best known of these possession rituals. It means "Honored Goddess Nymph" and is performed by selected preadolescent girls from the village. Sang Hyang Dedari is not on the calendar of festivals and is performed as needed in cases of epidemic or disaster. Once the dancers are possessed by the deities they speak to the villagers, giving the cure or remedy for whatever sickness or disaster has occurred.

In other trance dances an animal spirit enters the body of the dancer. In *Sang Hyang Jaran,* a horse spirit invests the body of a male dancer who, once possessed, runs barefooted through hot embers astride a straw hobby–horse. In *Sang Hyang Celing* a pig spirit has the dancer symbolically eat the filth or impurities responsible for the disaster.

REJANG

Rejang is an important category of Balinese religious dance in which the performance is given for the gods rather than by the gods, as in Sang Hyang and Berutuk. The gods descend into doll–like wooden effigies called pratima. They are brightly decorated with flowers and placed in a portable shrine for the festival. Rejang is an ancient formal and elegantly dignified processional group dance performed by 40 to 60 women of all ages in the village temple. It is performed in the daytime, and dancers are dressed in formal traditional Balinese costumes topped off with fresh flowers. Dancers form four rows in front of the shrines where the pratima are placed and in turn the dancer at the head of each row dances forward toward the shrine. Once they reach the shrine the lead dancers move off to each side and the next dancer in line moves forward, repeating the action. Once all have danced up to the shrine with the pratima in it, the dance is over.

BARIS

The Baris dance dates from the 16th century in Indonesia and is the most important ritual dance in Bali. Baris is essentially a warrior's drill dance that ancient Balinese soldiers used to protect their kingdom. Baris is derived from the word *bebarison*, which means line or file formation. Even today there are many of these martial dances, each distinguished by the weapon being carried by the soldier. Weapons commonly used are spears, lances, shields, daggers, or even, in some villages, rifles.

In Baris the dancer–soldier wears a triangular–shaped headdress or helmet and performs stylized military movements, attacking and defending in turn. The movements are done in unison. The dance is performed by men in groups of 4 to 60, accompanied by the traditional Balinese musical orchestra gamelan gong. Aside from the ritualistic formation the show of physical maturity in handling weapons adds a patriotic element.

Baris is based on the pokok stance, which has to do with the contact of the dancer's feet on and with the earth and the special alignment of the legs and torso. The pokok stance is the basic posture of all Balinese dance. It pays homage to Balinese origin and roots; foot contact with the earth is important because it symbolizes the flow from and the connection with the earth as the foundation. Pokok is the point of departure for all dance steps. It is the connection with ancestral origins and provides the spiritual nature to the dance. Baris, therefore, demonstrated the sacred postures of the warrior of Eastern traditions and the martial origins of the dance. It is the preparation for and introduction to the dances of Topeng, the masked theater of Bali.

Balinese actors are trained in the pokok stance as a foundation from which all dance movement springs.

The 19th century saw the emergence of professional dance groups that traveled from village to village performing for hire at Odalan and other festivals. It was, therefore, no major step for these dance companies to begin performing at hotels for the tourist trade in the early 1920s.

The 1930s saw tourism increase to a steady flow and an increased demand for dance performances. Repetitive performances in village settings and structured performances at hotels led to adapting traditional forms and creating dances in response to the tourist market. A revue-style presentation featuring short versions of several dances became common.

By the 1980s tourism reached the million mark. Balinese dance companies were in demand not only at home but also abroad. Revenue from dance performances coupled with mass production of handicrafts became important to the economic life of the villages. Although contemporary forces have been rapid and extensive, the age-old tradition of unity and cooperation has served to integrate all that is foreign in philosophy, culture, religion, and politics into distinct Balinese forms.

■ *Maori*

Polynesia is a collection of large and small islands in the south Pacific Ocean. It is best envisioned by imagining a triangle formed by Hawaii on the north, Easter Island on the east, New Zealand on the south, and the Society Islands in the center. Settlement of the area is theorized to have been from a gradual west to east population flow out of Southeast Asia. Traditions and archaeological evidence seem to support this theory. The area has been the home of Polynesians for more than 4,000 years. The Society Islands appear to have been the dispersing point for population movement to all parts of the area. In their sturdy longboats a hardy and courageous people took their common language, religion, myths, traditions, and cultural materials wherever they traveled. Wherever they settled, these elements united them and identified their kinship over the vast triangle. These are the ancestors of the Maori people of New Zealand.

New Zealand was settled, it is believed, in the mid 14th century as a result of a series of migrations. The last and largest was the Fleet. It is from the leaders and chiefly families of the Fleet of seven canoes that the Maori proudly trace their descent. The canoes were 70 or more feet in length and carried food, water, seed, and livestock. They landed at various points on the north island of New Zealand. Tradition among the Maori tells the story of each canoe, its landing place and settlement. And until modern historical findings indicate otherwise, these traditional accounts of the settlement of the Maori in New Zealand will stand.

Much of the pre-European picture of the Maori can be attributed to Captain James Cook and his keeping of a daily account of his observations of the Maori. He was known for his care for his own men and his humane dealings with the Maori. From these and other early accounts a picture of the lifestyles and activities of the Maori have come.

The European explorers' first encounter with a group of foot-stomping, finger-quivering, eye-rolling, and tongue-protruding dancers accompanied by a roaring chorus of rhythmic chants caused many captains and their crews to weigh anchor and sail away. To those who weathered the encounter, it appeared to be a war dance. To the Maori it was *Laka*, the vigorous posture dance that symbolized the vitality of Maori manhood. More careful reading of early accounts of the dance interpret it as a formalized pattern of challenge to a stranger to determine if his intentions were friendly or hostile. Since it was more often used to welcome guests, this theory is well supported.

Poi, not described until the 19th century, is a woman's dance unique to New Zealand and is considered to be the most graceful in all Polynesia. It consists of twirling a small ball made of dry leaves on a cord. Several variations exist including twirling the ball on a short cord with the right hand while beating it with the left hand and touching the head, shoulders, and hips between beats. The dance is performed sitting or standing, often accompanied by foot movements. It is a dance of precision, harmony, and beauty and is accompanied by a lilting song.

Maoritanga is a modern movement to revive and preserve Maori culture and foster cultural pride. To many Maori, the most real and tangible expressions of their culture are their songs, games, and dances.

■ Philippines

The Philippine archipelago lies some 500 miles off the southeast coast of Asia and is an integral part of the culture emanating from southeast India and China. Early inhabitants of the more than 7,000 islands came from south China and the Malay Peninsula. Some parts were occupied by the Indo-Malayan empire of Sri-Vishaya in the third century A.D. and later the Japanese empire of Madjapahit. In the 15th century Arabians and Indians moved into Mindanao bringing the Islamic and Hindu religions to this southernmost part of the country. The remote mountainous regions of the northern islands became the home of the earliest inhabitants, the pygmy tribes. These influences serve as a basis for a very diverse cultural beginning.

The colonial period began with the discovery of the islands by Ferdinand Magellan of Spain in 1521.

The Spaniards brought Christianity to the islands, which was a strong and lasting influence for some 400 years. Today, except for the Muslim south and pagan north, the Philippines is the only Christian country in the Asian sphere.

In 1898 the United States took control and the American influence lasted for some 50 years. The Philippines became an independent country in 1946. Filipinos refer to their cultural heritage as "400 years in a convent and 50 years in Hollywood." Nevertheless, the Philippines are a rich mixture of Asian, European, American, and native cultures.

Although subdued by the missionary zeal of Christians and Muslims, cultural dance and drama are derived from four elements: Spanish, residual Filipino, Igorat (Aboriginal), and Muslim. In most provinces local folk dance is Spanish in name as well as movement, for example, *Polkabal, Mananguete, Surtido,* and *Los Bailes de Ayers.* In the large city ballrooms Filipinos execute rumbas, tangos, sambas, and paso dobles in a characteristically graceful Filipino style.

Among some of the remaining most conservative and aristocratic families, formal balls are still opened with the stately quadrille *Regadon d'Honor.* For the Regadon d'Honor ladies wear ternow or mestiza dresses with the renowned butterfly sleeves made of pineapple cloth, silk, satin, or brocade. The men wear black pants, shoes, socks, and the barong tagalog shirt made of fine linen or pineapple cloth with hand embroidery or ruffles and frills down the front. The *Maria Clara,* a minuetlike dance full of bows and curtsies, is also a popular replica of the past. The Maria Clara, popular toward the end of the Spanish rule, is often performed for formal occasions and as a part of historical stage dramas. For the Maria Clara the characteristic costume consists of a light blue dress with starched white long frilly sleeves, wide collars, and fans for the ladies and a velvet jacket and tight-fitting trousers for the men.

Two of the most well-known dances representing the residual or Filipino-derived dances are the *Binusan Candle Dance* and the world-renowned *Tinikling.* The Binusan dance consists of a series of virtuoso feats including a rollover on the floor while balancing lighted candles in a glass tumbler on the head. Historically, this feat appears in many dances from various provinces. The *Pandaggo su Illaw,* or dance of the lights, is a couple dance from Mindoro in which lighted oil lamps are balanced on the head and back of both hands. Tinikling is undoubtedly the most widely known dance associated with the Philippines. Its popularity makes it almost a national pastime. An early version or sighting described the dance as having four long bamboo poles and danced in 4/4 time by four dancers. The version most widely used, however, uses two bamboo poles struck together in 3/4 time. The

latter version appears in *Philippine National Dances* by Francisca Reyes Tolentino, published in 1946.

Dances performed among the Igorat (aboriginal inhabitants or tribes of the northern Luzon) are authentically primitive. Dances occur during feasts, weddings, when conferring tribal title, at rice planting and harvest festivals, when headhunting, and at moon or star worshipping ceremonies.

During American times headhunting was discouraged, except briefly during the Japanese occupation. Now a nut from a fern tree or a carved wooden head serves the purpose. Headhunting dances are performed when a tribe member dies from an accident or lightning strike or as a cure for illness. If all other remedies fail, dance is certain to cure the sick and ailing.

Tribal dances are performed by both men and women. They generally move clockwise in a circle accompanied by songs and gongs. Shouting, clapping, and stamping make these tribal dances more energetic and vigorous than those found in the lowlands. Costumes and dances vary among mountain tribes but all are colorful. Elaborate headdresses of native flowers, beads, turbans, and crowns made of bamboo adorned with rooster feathers are common. Necklaces of dog or pig teeth, colored beads, or metalwork highlight the costumes.

Dances among the Christian Filipinos center around fiestas held to honor patron saints. The Black Nazarene festival in Manila, a nine-day celebration, begins the year-round calendar of festivals. St. John's Day and St. Augustine's Day include colorful processions of people often led by dancers. In the province of Bulucan the *Obando Dance* is performed during celebration of the feast of Saint Clare. The dance is a fertility dance performed by childless married women who believe the dance prayer will give them children.

Harvest festivals are a time for singing, dancing, and eating. Courtship and wedding dances are the highlights of these most beloved Philippine festivities. Formal occasions such as inaugural balls for state and provincial officials or to entertain official guests are traditions carried on in cities and provinces. So it seems that Christians do, indeed, dance.

Perhaps the most important dancing in the Philippines, artistically and visually, is found among the Muslims or Moro (Mohammedans) in the southern part of the Sulu archipelago, Mindanao, and Palowan. Dance among the Mohammedans is a curious phenomenon since traditionally their religion does not tolerate dance. The mix of cultures including Hindus, who foster dance, and perhaps the remoteness of the southern islands from the mainstream of Islam produces less antipathy and intolerance of dance. Regardless of the reasons, the Muslim area of south Philippines has more dance variety and quality than all other areas of the country. The dances are in fact vestigial remains of dances of India and Indonesia with flowing movements of the arms, facial expressions, and extreme flexibility and use of the fingers. Ankle bells and fan manipulation complete the inheritance from southeast Asia.

The legacy of folk dance of the Philippines is found in the survival of the manuscript of the book *Philippine National Dances* by Francisca Reyes Tolentino, published in 1946 by Silver Burdett Company of New York. The manuscript was received in New York in 1941 but was not published until after the liberation of the Philippines from the Japanese in 1945. After the war contact was reestablished with Mrs. Tolentino, who reported that all her resource materials, books and records, pictures, costumes, and musical instruments were burned or destroyed during the war.

The book contains 54 dances with brief historical notes, costume descriptions, and pictures along with full piano scores for each dance. The piano scores are themselves of unique historical value. Mrs. Tolentino, who was physical education director of women students at the University of Philippines, was encouraged and supported in her original research of dances of less-developed regions of the country by the farsightedness of Dr. Jerge Bocobo, then president of the university. The first materials gathered between 1924 and 1926 were used for her master's thesis, which was later published in book form as *Philippine Folk Dances and Games*. Interest in Philippine dances was stimulated by the University of Philippines and the Bureau of Education as a valuable part of the curriculum of physical education classes in public schools. The result was a revival of interest and soon dance exhibitions and competitions were an integral part of school programs. The effect was an awakening of national pride.

As a result of this impetus, additional research was officially carried on by Lt. Antonio Buenaventura, Ramon P. Tolentino, Jr., and Mrs. Tolentino under the auspices of the University of Philippines President's Committee on Folk Songs and Dances. Costumes, music, and musical instruments were collected along with songs and dances. This research produced the manuscript that was published in 1946 as *Philippine National Dances*.

Many of the native dances show unmistakable Spanish influence; others reflect French, English, and Malayan influences to a degree. Performances over a long period of time, however, have given them the unmistakable stamp of Filipino interpretation, execution, and expression.

■ *Hawaii*

Before European contact, music in Hawaii was a completely integrated system based on the use of poetry, rhythm, melody, and movement, which served the gamut of social needs from prayer to entertainment. Without a written history or literature to refer to, Hawaiians used musical poetry to call on the gods, honor their chiefs, lament the dead, tell of the creation, and perpetuate their history down through the generations. Poetry, therefore, was functional to their religious and social organization. Dance was an extension of poetry in the form of stylized visual accompaniment.

Traditional Hawaiian dance, unlike Asian and Indonesian forms, contained no theatrical or dramatic characterizations. Dance movement interpreted specific words of a poem or described a characteristic or thing mentioned in the poem. There was no dialogue or pantomime in indigenous poetry meant to be accompanied by dance. Poetry was divided into two main types: all poetry not intended to be used with dance (oli) and poetry meant to be accompanied by dance (mele hula). The former (oli) was done as a solo while the latter (mele hula) was performed by a group.

Performers were trained in hula schools (lalau) by a teacher (kumu lula), a priest (kahuna) under a strict religious system imposed by the patron goddess (Laka) of hula. Hulas were performed, therefore, only by dancers who had graduated from a hula school. Although there were a great many taboos and religious rites connected with the training, many were anxious to learn since training was an entree into the life of the courts of the chiefs. Schools were subsidized by the chiefs for reasons of prestige and entertainment. The primary functions of the hula dance at court were to honor the gods and sing praises of the chief and his ancestors.

The traditional hula was performed standing or seated. The seated version was more strenuous since the dancer raised and lowered as well as circled the torso from a kneeling position in which the dancer sat between the legs. In addition, the dancer often played an instrument. The standing hula was, as they are today, movements done while standing.

Mele hulas or name chants were composed to honor a person. They became the property of that person and were passed down through generations. They told the story of the honoree in terms of his or her high birth, genealogy, or something for which the person was noted. The general structure of a performance consisted of music, usually percussion; reciting the poem, which was a two-line couplet; and movement or dance. Movement described specific words of the poem such as hands forming a flower or arms indicating the flight of a bird. If the dancer played an instrument, the body movements were used to convey the meanings.

Hulas are generally classified according to their instrumental accompaniment. The hula pohu (drum) is an important type danced to honor chiefs of high distinction. The *hula pa ipu* is danced accompanied by a gourd instrument struck by the hand or on the ground. The *hula uli uli* is a seated dance accompanied by a feathered rattling gourd. There are many hulas and instrumental combinations, including the unique *hula pa'uimauna* in which the chest and thighs are struck to generate two different sounds.

The modern–day hula is the result of Hawaiian contact with Western civilization. Captain Cook's visit in 1778 set in motion the change from a Neolithic society to one that integrated the cultural traits and values of Western civilization. Music and dance were most affected by the arrival of Christian missionaries in 1820. For a period of time after the influx of missionaries, Western values were represented on the one hand by sailors and on the other by missionaries. The contrast was at once bewildering if not at times humorous. The influence of the missionaries won; the dancers were clothed and the dance movements damned as lustful and evil. The dances, missionaries declared, not only violated Protestant values but took the Hawaiians from their work in the fields. The result was that the hula went underground.

In 1874 Kalakaua came to the throne and called hula teachers to his court to revive the dance and court dance troupes. The success of his effort culminated in an invitation for a Hawaiian dance group to perform at the 1893 World Columbian Exposition in Chicago. This was the first time the dance of Hawaii, the hula, was treated with the respect due an art form.

The revival of the hula was not without loss of the old and emergence of the new. The costumes became the "ti leaf" hula skirt and the long white frilly dress with fitted sleeves. The dance lost its religious restrictions and became open to everyone, not just trained professionals. Kalakaua's court marked the end of the traditional hula and the beginning of acculturated dance and music.

For over half of the 19th century Hawaiian music and dance was persecuted but was saved by the tenacity of a few conservative families. Traditional dance and music thus made its way into the 20th century to be publicly recognized by a statewide program to study and teach the ancient hula. In 1970, some 200 years after Western contact, only five individuals were known to be hula experts. Statewide conferences have since been held to revive and preserve the knowledge held by the remaining experts and to reinstate this ancient art form.

AMERICAN PERSPECTIVE

Dance heritage in the United States is a matter of perspective. Historically, we Americans have alluded to "our heritage" as being from Europe. This perspective is true if, in fact, we view our heritage as consisting of all the facets of culture brought by explorers and settlers from Europe.

Is there another perspective? What about our heritage from the Western hemisphere, from North, Central, and South America? Was the New World only a vast undeveloped land mass waiting to be discovered by Europeans? A second perspective, one that views our heritage from the Americas, is long overdue.

The sounds of Native American drums echoed through the Americas long before the arrival of the first Europeans. Over untold centuries, immigrants traveled across the Bering Straits into North America, Mexico, Central America, and South America. These early arrivals, whom we refer to as Indians or Amerinds, were loosely organized into tribes that varied enormously in appearance, language, and culture. Even a cursory recounting of their progress and achievements is enough to warrant a second perspective, a view that includes our heritage from the Americas.

Just what were the accomplishments of these aboriginal Americans? It has been estimated that three-fifths of the modern world's agricultural wealth is derived from plants first domesticated by American Indians. They cultivated corn to its environmental limit long before the first Europeans arrived. In addition, they grew potatoes, sweet potatoes, manioc, varieties of beans, squash, pumpkins, peanuts, tomatoes, chocolate, rubber, long–staple cotton, and tobacco. Their domestication of these plants was the basis for their civilizations and a heritage we enjoy daily in modern American life.

In the 15th century, the most developed cultures, with histories that reach far into the mythical past, were the Aztecs in the Valley of Mexico, the Maya in the Yucatán Peninsula, and the great agrarian culture, the Inca Empire of the South American Andes. The height of their civilizations is evidenced by the cities they built with richly carved stone; their knowledge of mathematics and astronomy applied to the development of a calendar that required no leap year and predicted the eclipses of the sun; their construction of strong governments; and their recognition of the need for a division of labor. Although these were essentially Stone Age civilizations, astronomy, mathematics, writing, fine arts, and the ability to work gold, silver, copper, and various alloys with artistry flourished in them.

In the arts, there existed a rich culture of music, song, and dance used in sacred ceremonies and secular festivals. Aztec musical instruments included drums, hunting horns, whistles, flutes, pipes, and bells made of precious metals and gems. Early Spanish missionaries wrote of the Mayan "House of Song," in which professors of music, song, and dance trained the young to perform so that they could participate in the constant rituals and celebrations. From *Historia de las Indias* by Diego Duran, Giselle Freund quoted an early Spanish missionary:

> There were songs and dances of great solemnity, with a rhythm measured and austere; others, for less serious occasions, were lighter and sang of love and happiness. Most elaborate of all were those that accompanied the floral offerings of the gods. The richness of the dance costumes imitating fruits and flowers, birds, and animals; the grace of the dancers representing the gods and their worshippers; and the strange and stirring music; all made Duran declare that this was "the most beautiful and solemn dance this nation possessed,"

and he never expected to witness again anything more wondrous. (Bauer and Peyser 1967; p. 50)

The Aztec, Inca, and Mayan empires were the centers from which flowed the cultural stimuli to the more primitive regions in the Americas. Cultural artifacts, such as rattles, flutes, whistles, bull roarers, Apache fiddles, and the most revered of all instruments–the drum–offer evidence of this stimulus and the cultural link in music, song, and dance throughout the Americas. We must begin today to appreciate the scale, the complexity, the host of accomplishments, and the long cultural evolution that mark the cultures of the Americas. This, then, is our American perspective, a dance heritage yet to be claimed.

2

Effective Group Instruction

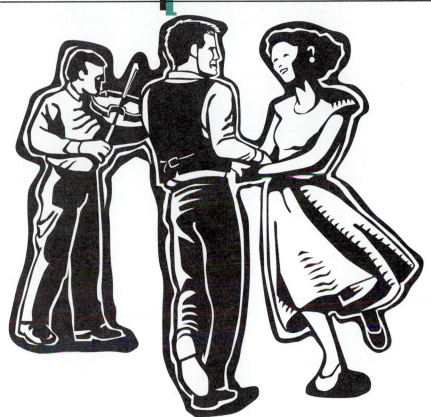

BEING AN EFFECTIVE DANCE teacher requires more than just knowing dance steps. You need to be a dancer, teacher, sound technician, facility manager, musician, event coordinator, and most importantly, you need to understand the purpose and value of dance in the curriculum. As an instructor, you must learn to relate to the learner, the learning process, the dance context, and the demands of the culture. For effective group instruction, the instructor must be able to analyze and cope with variable learning skills and thoroughly understand the resources and dance material. The purpose of this chapter is to explain the varied features of dance instruction as encountered in a learning environment.

WHY DANCE

When dance is part of the curriculum, students often ask: "Why do we have to dance?" To respond to this question, the instructor must understand the value of dancing and how it serves the students. The following points* describe the major benefits of dance education:

1. *Social interaction*: In the classroom, students interact as a group or with individual partners. At a dance, opportunities to meet new people are common.

2. *Aerobic exercise*: Dancing increases your heart rate, providing cardiovascular benefit. Research at the Miami Human Performance Laboratory has shown that even the "stop and go" effect of ballroom–dance sequences is not a deterrent to receiving aerobic and fat–burning benefits.

3. *Increased exposure to rhythm*: Moving in rhythm facilitates the student's understanding of music.

4. *Alternative to sports* (for nonathletes): Not many students are part of athletic teams, but all students can participate in dancing.

5. *Improved balance and coordination*: Dance training provides body awareness and stresses good posture.

6. *Artistic form of self expression*: Dance allows the incorporation of personal styling, making movement unique to each dancer.

7. *A lifelong activity*: Dance is easily adaptable to all age groups.

8. *FUN!*

PURPOSE OF DANCE

Classes in the community or at a school where dance is an elective attract students for many different reasons. The purpose can be learning to dance, improving dance skills, or understanding dance traditions. Once an individual demonstrates interest, the instructor has a unique responsibility to maintain and develop that interest.

Many dancers work to acquire dance skills that will enable them to join community dance groups, resulting in social relationships and an enjoyable pastime. Some dancers join groups for technical reasons, such as to acquire and/or increase their repertoire of dances, to develop a technical understanding of dance fundamentals, and to expand their performance skills. Either purpose is a viable reason for participating in a dance program, and both are important factors to be considered when preparing to teach dance.

---

*Refer to *Dance Education—What Is It? Why Is It Important?* Brochure, National Dance Association, 1991

FACILITIES

A well–ventilated room with good acoustics, adequate lighting and heating, and sufficient floor space is essential. An area too small may limit the freedom of movement and type of dance. An area too large may generate acoustical problems that can distort the music and verbal instructions and destroy the spirit of the occasion. Also, dancers may feel uncomfortable with too much space; it is better to be slightly crowded.

■ *Floor*

A preferred dance floor has a framed construction, known as a *sprung* floor, which provides dancers with a resilient surface. In contrast, an example of an inappropriate dance floor is concrete covered with wood or tile. Dancing for an hour on this surface is much more physically demanding. Avoid dancing on carpeted surfaces to prevent the transfer of static electricity.

Different dance forms require the surface (usually wood) of the floor to have varying degrees of slickness. This can be attained with different finishes and dance waxes.

For safety and facility maintenance, cleanliness is an essential. Changing into dance shoes (shoes for inside use only) at the perimeter of the floor or outside the class room will help keep dust and dirt off the floor. After each class, a quick sweep of the floor with a dust mop will also be beneficial.

■ *Acoustics*

Permanent acoustical treatment is very expensive and is seldom found in the variety of buildings used by dance groups. Poor acoustics is a handicap to a dance group. The following practical suggestions have proven useful in improving the sound in halls and gymnasiums adapted to use for dance.

1. Drapes of any material (burlap, flannel, rugs, blankets) suspended from the ceiling can improve sound.

2. Acoustics in an ordinary gymnasium can be improved by hanging mats around the walls.

3. Ceilings can be lowered with crêpe–paper streamers or similar decorations.

4. Human bodies absorb sound. The sound system adjusted to an empty room is not always adequate when the room is filled with dancers. This fact should be kept in mind when the sound system is set up for a large crowd.

EQUIPMENT

■ *Sound System*

A wide variety of electronic equipment is available to dance professionals. This section will assist you in making better choices for your program. A basic sound system consists of a cassette tape deck, CD player, microphone, amplifier or receiver and mixer, and speakers. The first three components plug into the amplifier, which sends the signal out to the speakers. This use of separate components is the most flexible approach: when one piece needs repair, the rest of the system is still functional. Also, upgrading and repair can be achieved one piece at a time. If a portable system is needed, several brands of reasonably priced karaoke machines (with a microphone jack) are available.

SPEAKERS

Good speakers are critical to a quality system. Placement should be in opposite corners of the room, at least **three feet above the dancers,** pointed toward their heads. If budget allows, having one speaker for each corner of the room creates an even distribution of sound. Speakers should be compatible with the amplifier output.

AMPLIFIER

A professional amplifier is equipped with several channels for individual volume controls. Each channel represents one component (tape deck, CD player, turntable, microphone). Two channels, or two components, can be operated at the same time: this allows the microphone to be used while playing music. Dance instruction is improved with this capability.

An amplifying device intended for home use is called a receiver, a combination of a radio receiver and an amplifier. In contrast to a professional amplifier, a receiver amplifies one component at a time. A mixer unit can be added to a receiver to use a microphone while playing music.

MICROPHONE

Microphones provide four distinct advantages for dance instructors: 1) vocal chord damage is minimized, 2) the learning environment is enhanced when the students can easily hear instructions, 3) professionalism is maintained when the instructor can talk rather than yell, and 4) regaining control of the class (when necessary) is facilitated. A couple of disadvantages should be noted: extra time is required to ensure that equipment is operational, and communicating through the microphone is not as personal.

Due to advances in technology, wireless mikes have become affordable. Sweat–resistant wireless microphones, developed for teaching aerobics, run about $150 more than typically used wireless microphones. A wireless system has two parts: the receiver that plugs into the amplifier and the microphone itself. The microphone is connected to a power pack that uses 9–volt batteries. Always be prepared with a belt or strap on which to clip the power pack. The newer models use a rechargeable battery that saves money and helps keep toxic trash out of the landfill.

Three styles are available: lapel, handheld, and headset. The headset is slightly more expensive than the other two styles, but provides increased freedom of movement while teaching. Most power packs have a mute switch that allows the instructor to mute the microphone without walking over to the amplifier. This muting capability is ideal for individual instruction, without the whole class hearing the comments. Also, when leaving the room wearing the microphone, sound will not be inadvertently transmitted.

Covering the mike is a piece of foam called a windscreen. This allows the user to get closer to the mike. Each instructor should have an individual windscreen for hygienic purposes.

To test a microphone, do not blow into it. The sound is not pleasant and transmitted moisture will eventually corrode the microphone. Counting "1, 2, 3, test, test" is a common way to adjust the volume. Standing in front of or in line with a speaker while wearing a microphone creates a squeal called *feedback*.

CD PLAYER AND TAPE DECK

Compact disc (CD) players and cassette tape decks are the most common components used for playing music. An essential feature of these components is pitch control* (variable speed control), which will adjust the speed of the music to the students' ability. CD players are equipped with real–time counters. This feature allows an instructor to start the music at a specific phrase. If the phrase is 27 seconds into the song, it is possible to fast forward 27 seconds and start the music. A real–time counter is not a standard feature on tape decks. If budget allows, purchasing a tape deck with a real–time counter is advantageous.

CD players have many advantages in teaching dance. Most important, you can go to the beginning of any song immediately–no fast forward or rewinding as with a cassette tape. CDs are more durable than cassette tapes; the machine will not "eat" or stretch the tape.

---

* These usually need to be ordered out of a specialty equipment catalog

The use of the remote is becoming an important skill for dance teachers. The remote allows instructors to operate the equipment from the middle of the classroom, without running back and forth. The remote also has a fade control which provides an excellent transition from dancing back to teaching.

Cassette tape decks are most useful for presenting music from multiple artists. Teaching a specific style (waltz, swing, etc.) can be facilitated through the use of a single tape versus multiple disks. When teaching individual dances, using "fast forward" to play two songs from different parts of the tape can be very distracting. Recording individual songs, one on each side of a short tape, alleviates this problem.

TURNTABLE

Turntables are no longer in common use, but occasionally, music for a specific dance can only be found on a vinyl record.

A turntable needs to be located for easy access for teaching and on a stand that will not be jarred by dancing feet. On gymnasium floors, needle bounce is common. The player may be located in a console. Seventy-eights are not being produced, but some distributors have some in stock and many schools/clubs have them. Therefore, a machine that has three speeds, 33, 45, and 78 rpm, is desirable. The quality of the music is extremely important in generating enthusiasm and style in dancers.

The essential features needed in a turntable are manual arm control, variable speed, volume and tone control, and microphone. The *variable speed* really facilitates teaching. The quality of the sound is directly related to the quality of the cartridge and needle. The magnetic cartridge gives a truer tone quality than the crystal type. A diamond needle will last longer than a sapphire needle.

CARE OF TURNTABLE AND RECORDS

Keeping the needle clean and changing it as needed are important. Taking care of the records will increase their longevity and maintain their sound quality. Store records in a vertical position in a case, dividers between each record. A thin foam cushion on the bottom protects rims, and a tight cover keeps dirt and dust out. The 45-rpm discs should be stored flat, in jackets.

■ *Camcorder/VCR*

The camcorder is a readily portable piece of equipment that records action and sound. A VCR and monitor are necessary for playback. In addition to providing the novelty of watching one's self, this instrument is especially helpful in developing style and working with performing groups.

MUSIC
■ *Recordings*

Recordings on discs and tapes are the primary sources of musical accompaniment for dance. The recording industry for dance is in a state of flux. Fewer companies are producing music for folk dancing. The most useful and practical recording type (record/tape) is not settled, but the cassette and CD are gaining. The availability of recordings to match one's equipment can be difficult to find. The problem of the ethics of copying music from someone and passing it along is increasing. It is driving dedicated companies out of business. Recorded music of superior quality and variety is available, making it possible to have colorful and authentic music for instruction and participation. The wide variety of domestic and foreign recordings available makes it necessary for the teacher or the leader to be discriminating in choosing musical accompaniment. The following suggestions may assist in making appropriate choices:

1. The music should include an introductory passage so that the dancers can begin in unison.

2. A steady tempo is desirable unless a change is appropriate to a particular dance.

3. The music should be authentic; that is, if a dance is traditionally done to a special tune and the recording is available, it should be used.

4. The phrasing should be clear and definite.

The following suggestions are appropriate to the selection of recordings for dance areas included in *Dance A While*.

FOLK DANCE

Several recordings are often available for the same Folk Dance. The version that corresponds in sequence to the direction for the dance should be selected. It is generally advisable to use the recording recommended by the dance reference. Since no list of suggested recordings can be kept completely up to date, it is advisable to ask the music shop or company to make a substitution when requested recordings are no longer available.

SQUARE DANCE

The problems of selection in Square Dance center on finding recordings that are suitable to the caller's voice and have the desired tempo and rhythm. Callers should make selections only after listening and practicing to a variety of recordings. There are several advantages to recordings with calls: They can be used as models for learning to call, as supplements to live calling for calls not in the musical key or vocal range of the teacher, and as opportunities for a group to dance to a wide variety of callers.

CONTRA DANCE

Only a few of the Contra Dances require special music; for instance, Rory O'More uses the tune by the same name. Therefore, it is the teacher's choice to select appropriate music for the specific flow of figures (storyline) in a given dance. Some dances suggest a Jig, others a Reel, others a March. Finding a recording that arouses the dancers and the caller is the next step. Eventually the teacher will rely on certain tunes for specific dances, because they "fit like a glove."

SOCIAL DANCE

The criteria for selecting Social Dance music include finding recordings that have a definite beat and a regular tempo and that are appropriate for listening. Longplay albums are advisable and economical for those who specialize or teach several classes in one type of dance, such as Latin or Jazz. Albums featuring a variety of dances on one record are recommended for those who teach few or occasional classes. The specialist needs greater variety in music. The radio is a continuous source of current and standard music. Jotting down the title and name of the recording artist aids in securing records from local shops and in keeping a current collection for teaching.

■ *Teaching with Recordings*

1. Before using a recording in class, know the music and be familiar with the phrasing and the dance sequence. Humming or whistling the tune can be advantageous.

2. Occasionally, students may bring their own music to dance class. Review this music in private, as it may not be appropriate for the class in tempo, style, or lyrics.

3. All recordings for a particular class should be preselected and arranged in order of use. When using cassette tapes, be sure your tape is cued, or set to start at the beginning of the selection (overcoming the common problem of "dead air"). The use of short tapes with one song per side is much more efficient than one tape with six songs on it. The class should not have to wait while the instructor fast forwards to a particular song.

4. Isolating a musical phrase on a recording to practice a certain movement is easily accomplished if your equipment has a real-time counter (e.g., the phrase starts 33 seconds into the song).

5. Play the music for the class to hear before presenting each part of the dance.

6. Practice ahead of time to give correct verbal cues synchronized to the music.

7. The starting signal (e.g., a hand movement) or cue (see page 35) should be matched to the introduction on the recording. Tell the class if the recording has no introduction.

8. An adjustable speed control (pitch control) allows practice at a variety of tempos. Without a pitch control, when you need to work with a specific recording, the dance should be practiced without music. The tempo of your verbal cues should be increased until reaching the tempo of the recording.

9. When teaching dances not associated with a single song and pitch control is not available, preselect recordings with several different tempos. This can be accomplished by varying the beats per minute (BPM) of each song. To establish the BPM of a song, count the number of beats that occur in a 6-second time frame and multiple by 10. As an example, with single time swing dancing, begin the music at 100 BPM and then gradually increase to 180 BPM. Dancing to the beat of a song is very difficult for many people. The problem is compounded if the tempo does not match their skill level.

■ *Live Music*

There is a resurgence of live music for dancing. A live band or orchestra accents the color, flavor, and festive atmosphere of the occasion. The opportunity for recreational musicians to play enhances country dances. Many ethnic groups, such as Scandinavian and Slavic groups, have developed musicians' groups playing native instruments for their dances. Even in Social Dance, Big-Band Sound, Country Western, and Salsa, musicians are available.

The best musicians, colorful as they may be, should blend with the group. The dancers are the focal point of the dance and, although musicians should enter into the spirit of the occasion, they should not become a distraction. They need to limit their solos and interpretive music.

The instruments commonly used for Square Dance and Contra Dance are the fiddle, piano, banjo, bass violin, and guitar. The fiddle is sufficient for small groups if the fiddler is good. A combination of three to five instruments is most desirable.

The instruments used for International Folk Dance vary. Accordions, horns, reed instruments, and foreign musical instruments native to a particular country are used with more common combinations of instruments.

■ Teaching with Live Music

Some dance teachers are very fortunate to have a fiddler, an accordion player, or a trio to work with, particularly for workshops. Very few institutions still have an accompanist. The primary advantage, in addition to the stimulation of live music, is the time saved by not having to attend to and adjust mechanical devices during the presentation of a lesson. Flexibility in applying music to the dance-teaching sequence is perhaps even more of an advantage than saving time. The accompanist can introduce music with the movement very early and make the rhythm clear and definite. The beginner can hear the beats of the music better. The introduction of accompaniment in the early stages trains dancers from the beginning to let the music help cue them in pattern and step changes, so counting is avoided. For Social Dance, a three- to seven-piece band is usually adequate, depending on the talent of the group. Keyboards are also available. Listening to an audition tape or attending a band rehearsal is usually advisable when an unknown band is being considered. Small bands or combos can sometimes be assembled from talent in the community or the school. In all cases, the band should be notified about the specific type and tempos of music planned. Rather than discussing how fast or slow a song is played, communicate with the musicians in terms of BPM. The type of music varies with the age and interest of the group to be entertained.

Dance musicians need an understanding of the dance itself and should realize that the character of the dance is influenced by the manner in which they play the tune. The tempo must be steady, and the length of the songs kept under three minutes. As they play, musicians need to watch the dancers, sometimes adjusting the tempo or emphasizing a phrase. Phrasing is extremely important for all dances. As the teacher and the accompanist work together, the accompanist will sense when to start playing while the group is practicing.

The working relationship between teacher and accompanist is important. They should begin by establishing certain vocal and hand signals. Most important, the teacher should stand at all times in view of the accompanist so that signals can be clearly seen or easily heard. Common vocal communications between the teacher and accompanist are "ready and" and "ready begin." Common hand signals are lowering the hand palm down to indicate a slow tempo, raising the hand palm up to indicate a faster tempo, nodding the head or raising the hand above dancers' heads to signal a stop at the end of the music, and waving the hand back and forth above the dancers' heads or saying "stop" to stop the music immediately.

The teacher can do a great deal to make the accompanist an integral part of the group. When the accompanist becomes a real part of the group, and not just a tool, everyone benefits because the involvement stimulates greater interest. The music should complement the activity; it should not dominate it.

Great care should be exercised in the selection of an accompanist. An accompanist should:

1. Have thorough musical training.

2. Play in a steady rhythm, accenting certain parts to help the dancers while they are learning a new dance.

3. Know the music well enough to be able to give attention to the group and the teacher during performance.

4. Rehearse all new music prior to the class.

5. Adjust the tempo to the dancers' ability or change the rhythm to accompany the teacher's analysis.

6. Know dance and be sensitive to ways in which cooperation between teacher, dancer, and accompanist can be enhanced.

7. Be able to develop and vary the music to make it interesting for the dancers because most folk music is noted simply.

PLANNING INSTRUCTION

■ Total Dance Program

PROGRAM CURRICULUM

In the formal school situation, the total dance program consists of a planned progressive sequence distributed throughout the entire school curriculum from first grade through graduation. The total dance program may be planned for six to eight grades in elementary school, middle school/junior high combinations that involves grades five to nine, and three to four in high school, depending on the numerical breakdown of the individual school system.

The year's program, at any school level, is further subdivided into units of instruction and daily lesson plans. Each subdivision is organized systematically, with specific objectives, content, learning experiences, and appraisals in the form of evaluations. Each part of the total program should combine with the others to form one sequentially related dance program.

Materials selected for a specific unit should be related to the overall plan. The overall program should be flexible enough to allow for adaptation of materials in smaller units to meet specific or unique needs of a particular group within the total system. Evaluation of the individual units in terms of stated objectives should provide information necessary for revision of the sequential program in relation to the changing needs of students.

EXTRACURRICULAR OPPORTUNITIES

The total dance program should not be an isolated experience to be participated in, in lockstep fashion, throughout the school curriculum. Ideally, the instructional phase of the total school program should be augmented by many extracurricular opportunities. Clubs, exhibition groups, festivals, and celebrations of special events and holidays are all opportunities for enriching formal learning sessions. In addition, dance may be integrated with other subject areas, for example, language courses or dramatic presentations such as operettas and musicals.

■ *Dance Unit*

A *dance unit* is a period of time during which a planned sequence of learning experiences concentrates on a specific form of dance. The dance unit is a segment of the total dance program. Units should be planned and linked together to offer progressive experience in each dance area included in the total program. The dance unit is not an isolated learning experience but rather one of many stepping stones that provide sequential learning experiences in each dance area included in the total dance program. The following factors should be considered in planning a dance unit: (1) general purposes or objectives of the unit; (2) age, gender, skill, and dance experience of the participants; (3) facilities and equipment; (4) time allotment (class periods per week, continuous or divided, number of weeks per unit); (5) relationship of unit to school curriculum; (6) leadership experience and background; (7) relationship to community recreational program; and (8) enrichment activities.

GOALS

Goals are statements in broad terms that indicate what activities will be accomplished over a long term. The statement, "The student will be able to perform six traditional dance steps," is an example of a goal for a dance unit.

■ *Daily Planning Instruction*

Planning for daily instruction must be planning with a purpose.

Prior to teaching a dance class, the instructor should be able to answer the following questions: Who does what, how, when, where, and for how long? In answering these questions, an instructor should include information about:

1. Equipment.
2. Arrangement of students, number of students in a class and their grouping (e.g., partners, individuals, small groups), location of students during instruction (line, circle).
3. Types and sequence of movements that will be taught. What will the instructor tell and demonstrate to students? (Plan to use complete, yet concise instruction to ensure the shortest time possible spent on instruction with a longer period of activity/practice.)
4. Ways to provide students with the greatest chance for success.

DAILY LESSON

A written outline of specific content and procedures to be presented in a given period of time is called a *lesson plan*. Using a lesson plan will ensure that activities are presented in a logical progression, which will allow for student success. A positive learning environment with fewer teacher frustrations and greater opportunities for student involvement will be created with the use of a lesson plan.*

The following sections explain the makeup of a lesson plan.

■ *Objectives / Student Outcome*

When planning to teach, the instructor should establish learning objectives. A learning objective is an act that the learner can do following observable and measurable instruction. An objective examines the potential outcome of the lesson. Objectives are implicit or explicit statements about what an instructor wants students to learn (in relationship to the three learning domains: psychomotor, cognitive, and affective). Well-stated objectives clearly identify what a student is to learn and/or perform as a result of instruction. An objective has three parts:

1. **Task:** What are students to accomplish?
2. **Situation:** What is "given"? (e.g., with a partner, individually, or practice versus putting all the steps of the dance together in a performance**)
3. **Criteria:** What does the instructor need to observe to measure attainment of this

---

*Refer to Dr. Barbara E. Cusimano, *Rhythmic Activities* p. 11, JOPERD, April 1989.

**In sports instruction, playing a game is referred to as the performance component of the class. This use of performance should not be confused with a "stage" performance.

objective? What are the critical elements or movements of the dance? Can students explain or demonstrate those elements?

The following statements illustrate how an objective is stated:

1. (Acceptable) "The student will be able to dance the Two–Step." This identifies the task but does not indicate the situation under which the demonstration occurs or the critical elements that are to be observed.

2. (Better) "The student will be able to dance the Two–Step with the beat of the music." The instructor can observe whether or not the student executes the Two–Step to the beat of the music (criteria), but there is still no description of the situation.

3. (Best) "The student will be able to dance the Two–Step (task) with a partner around the dance floor for two minutes (situation) and demonstrate the ability to execute the critical element of the foot work, step together step with the beat of the music (criteria)." This objective is measurable and observable with all three parts identified.

■ *Assessing Group Variables*

Assessing skills, knowledge, attitudes, and characteristics is an important first step in formulating objectives and selecting learning experiences. Some common group variations and suggested adaptations follow.

RANGE OF SKILL AND MOTOR ABILITY

Skill is seldom distributed evenly in a group. Although it may be clustered at one end or the other of a continuum, it will still represent a range. In an advanced group, the range is as apparent, although not as formidable, as in a beginning group. Materials should be selected to accommodate all skill levels and, at the same time, provide for sequential progression toward a minimum standard of accomplishment for all. Dances involving locomotor skills can keep the level of participation and incentive high until the skill range of a group is narrowed to a manageable range.

RANGE OF EXPERIENCE AND ASSOCIATION

Experience implies formal learning, such as a class or a club membership. Informal experiences like imitating dance movements without formal instruction and/or participation in rhythmic activities–such as marching in a band or a drill team, twirling a baton, or reacting to television or radio music–represent a type of association that constitutes a viable background for dance.

■ *Content Selection*

After diagnosing group needs and formulating objectives, the teacher must search dance literature for specific dance materials with which to build content. The search for dance content is more efficient and need serving when the teacher selects materials in terms of dance structure.

Dance structure refers to the component parts or basic elements that make up a dance. For most dance forms, these elements are basic step, position, formation, nationality, degree of difficulty, and musical meter. In Square Dance, these elements are patter, singing, basics, and figure type.

Refer to the classified dance indexes listing the structural parts of each dance in each section.

■ *Lesson Plan*

An average dance lesson plan will include five sections:

1. **Warm–up activities.** Have the music playing as the students enter the classroom, allowing them to begin dancing on their own. Start the class with as little instruction as possible, using simple (if applicable, non–partner) previously learned dances. A written prompt on a board close to the entrance may help to encourage students to start dancing. The primary purpose of the warm–up section is to give students immediate activity. At this time the instructor should move around the classroom and interact with students. Greet them, reinforce students' behavior, and generally set the tone for the class. In addition, the instructor may take roll quickly and efficiently.

2. **Review.** Review is a formal or informal coverage of previously learned materials. The review may be conducted as a formal part of the lesson by the instructor or it may be an informal student-participation session. The review serves two purposes: to refresh the students' memory of material from earlier classes, which often provides students with immediate success, and to help students who have been absent. Formal review does not necessarily have to be part of every lesson. Holding the review at the beginning of the class period is more of a tradition than a requirement. The review session may be integrated into the warm–up phases.

3. **New material.** This section of the lesson is for the introduction of material not covered in previous lessons. New materials may be in the form of a fundamental step (such as the polka), a new Square Dance figure, a Swing Dance variation, or an entire Folk Dance. New materials may also appear in the form of an adaptation of a dance, such as the conversion of an individual routine to a partner dance. The new material section may be presented in any part of a class period. Beginning the lesson with new material is a means of varying class procedure and providing a longer segment of the class time for presentation and practice. Ending with new material is possible, if the material is short, energetic, and especially designed as a fun ending to the class period.

4. **Activity.** This is the section of the lesson plan in which the new material is practiced in its entirety, emphasizing fun and enjoyment, which encourages student development in the affective learning domain. Dancing for fun will help to insure a feeling of success for both the student and teacher. This part usually takes place at the closing of the class. The students should leave with a sense of accomplishment and a feeling of anticipation for the next lesson. If the dance movement has been physically demanding (e.g., a fast swing or a high-paced Folk Dance) and the students are returning to other classes, ending with a calming dance (e.g., a slow waltz) is suggested.

5. **Closure/Evaluation.** The instructor should summarize the lesson and evaluate the objectives set for that class. Did the students understand and perform accordingly? Dance favorites or well-known dances can be an enjoyable conclusion for any class period.

This evaluation should consider both the students' and the instructor's actions.

A. *Students:* Clearly stated objectives include observable and measurable criteria for student performance (evaluation). Instructors may evaluate students' progress based on their ability to meet class objectives. The instructor might do an informal evaluation by scanning the class to see how the students are performing or a formative evaluation, where a checklist of movements is marked off for each student.

B. *Instructor:* If the students have met the planned objectives, this will be a good indication of the teacher's success or effectiveness. If a majority of students have not accomplished the objectives, the instructor needs to reflect on the content, programming, feedback given to the students, and practice opportunities of their lesson.

PROCEDURE AND ORGANIZATION

The material from the five activity sections of a lesson plan can each be divided into three subcategories.* Use columns to accomplish this task. The three subcategories are:

1. Movement Content/Experience: This section lists the movement that will be taught in the lesson, critical elements and specific verbal cues, and the sequence of instruction and practice scenarios.

2. Organization and Teaching Hints: This section provides points for efficient delivery of the content, including class structure and groupings. Any notes or recommendation for the teacher can be placed here.

3. Expected Student Objectives and Outcomes. (See Objectives, page 29.)

The following example is provided to illustrate this process of creating subcategories.

NEW MATERIAL (THIRD SECTION OF A LESSON PLAN)

Movement content	Organization/teaching hints	Objectives/ outcomes
Dance the Two-Step with a partner, using step-together-step footwork dancing to the beat of the music.	1. Arrange students in a circle. 2. Practice the steps without music. 3. Practice the steps with music. 4. Organize partners. 5. Practice with partner, no music. 6. Practice with partner with music.	*Psychomotor:* the student performed the footwork, step-together-step with the beat of the music.

ORIENTATION TO THE DANCE CLASS

■ *Setting the Stage*

Dance is typically and culturally consistent when taught with traditional male/female roles. Participation and promotion should be encouraged by both

---

* Refer to Robert P. Pangrazi, *Lesson Plans for Dynamic Physical Education for Elementary School Children,* p. iv, Allyn and Bacon, Twelfth Edition, 1998.

male and female faculty. Group participation in planning the dance unit enhances understanding and creates greater enthusiasm.

Several items should be discussed prior to beginning the dance unit. Good preparation elevates student interest and helps maintain the flow of the class.

1. Emphasize to the students that they will be able to use their new skills at the next dance event.

2. Try to relate dancing to current movies, dancing on TV, or famous people. If they have seen it somewhere else, it helps to validate their opinion of dancing.

3. Discuss personal hygiene with all age groups. Nothing is more uncomfortable than dancing with or next to someone who has an unpleasant odor.

4. Let the students know that nonparticipating students (sick students or those with specific religious beliefs against dancing) will be assigned to do other tasks. They should not be allowed strictly to observe. Bored spectators can be disruptive.

ETIQUETTE

Simple good manners and courtesy are part of helping everyone in a group have a good time. It is the teacher's responsibility to create the kind of atmosphere that contributes to easy social adjustment and relationships among members of the dance group. Assisting members in becoming acquainted with each other and learning to mix are the most important social responsibilities, and they add to the fun and pleasure of the occasion. Etiquette is everybody's responsibility.

The teacher's language (his or her choice of words and phrases) can remind group members of simple courtesies. Gentle admonitions are helpful; for example, "thank your partner for the dance and invite another lady to be your new partner," "get together with the couple nearest you, introduce your lady and exchange partners," "escort your lady off the floor and introduce her to someone who is sitting out," and "there are a few extra ladies (men), and so between dances will the ladies (men) who are dancing take turns trading out so that everyone will get a chance to dance." These simple pleasant directions set the tone for interpersonal relationships necessary in the dance group.

The following are a number of techniques for bringing about social intermixing to provide opportunities that gradually develop into pleasant habits.

SOCIAL AIDS

The use of an attractive name tag helps people to get acquainted and feel at ease. Square and Folk Dance clubs use them with tremendous success. They are equally welcomed by students in a class.

Still another successful idea has been the appointment of a host and hostess for each session. They have the responsibility of seeing that everyone has a chance to dance, that name tags are out and ready, that visitors are included in the activities, and that guests are met and made to feel welcome. In a large group, members can take turns playing host–hostess so that everyone has an equal opportunity to participate in the dancing.

FUN WITH CUTTING IN

In almost every mixer, there is a break during which an extra person can step in and steal a partner, which automatically puts someone out. This can be good fun if everyone gets into the spirit of it. If the leader shows the group how and encourages stealing partners during the mixers, the problem of extras in a group is reduced.

Cutting in is a fun technique also used in Square Dancing. However, it should be stressed that the skill of cutting in lies in the ability to cut the other person out and yourself in without breaking the continuity or rhythm of the figure.

Cutting in in Social Dance can also be made into a fun situation; for example, use one or two couples, give the girls a peach, the boys a lemon, and they cut in by passing the peach or lemon to another boy or girl.

UNEVEN NUMBERS: CREATING A "GHOST PARTNER"

For club and party dances, uneven numbers are a rather common occurrence and often are considered a problem. Event organizers need to be particularly alert and resourceful in handling this imbalance. An extensive repertoire of nonpartner dances, dances for threes, and simple partner-exchange mixers will allow everyone to participate.

During classroom instruction of traditional male/female partner dancing, people are commonly paired up with the same sex to balance out uneven numbers. This can be uncomfortable for some people and requires students to learn material that will not be used often. Using the concept of "Mr. or Ms. X" provides an efficient technique for working with uneven numbers. At the beginning of class, people without partners should be interspersed around the circle, and be assigned the "ghost partner" of Mr. or Ms. X. As the class proceeds, either males or females are selected to rotate (move around the circle to the next person, or "ghost partner") at intervals determined by the instructor. When a student encounters Mr. or Ms. X, they should be instructed to continue working on their own role. At the next rotation, they return to a real partner. Rotating partners fairly often insures that no one student is with a ghost partner for very long.

TEACHING STUDENTS WITH SPECIAL NEEDS

By Kristina Waller Golden, Laguna Hills, CA.

Nowadays the trend in education and in the community is for people with disabilities to participate in a full spectrum of school, family, work, and community activities alongside people without disabilities. To be sure, the segregation of individuals with disabilities into separate classrooms, separate schools, communities, or "sheltered workshops" is clearly on the decline, and in many regions has all but disappeared.

The prevailing philosophy in the consideration of individuals with disabilities in the United States is one of **inclusion,** the notion that all people have the right to be included with their peers in all age-appropriate activities throughout their lives. Educators may hear terms such as "mainstreaming," "integration," and "inclusion." Each term has its origins in the aim to bring individuals with disabilities into environments with their typical peers, and each accomplishes that end, though the means may vary. In any event, regardless of what this "bringing together of all people" is called where you live, there will be people with disabilities that will participate in dance, and will want to learn.

One needs to consider vision, hearing, physical abilities, cognitive abilities, and behaviors. However, one needn't be a trained "special educator" to include people with disabilities in dance activities and have success.

There are three key areas to consider: Physical Inclusion, Social Inclusion, and Instructional Inclusion. A teacher can ensure that inclusion will occur when planning addresses all three areas.

PHYSICAL INCLUSION: Is the learning environment physically accessible to everyone? Will a person with limited physical mobility need a helper? Are there safety issues for a person with limited vision, or, does everyone understand what a wheelchair can do when it spins around? Consider these kinds of points as you assess physical inclusion.

SOCIAL INCLUSION: Dance educators are often sensitive to this phenomena, as it is natural in our culture for dance learners to feel excluded (eg: those unsure of their physical abilities, those insecure with the opposite sex). Good dancers also tend to group or partner together, creating more exclusion of those less adept. Keep in mind that this may be compounded for a person with disabilities. Some peers may feel that a person with a disability is helpless or unapproachable. Of course this is not the case, and the teacher can be key in helping to promote interaction, even talking about the person's disabling condition in such a way to help everyone gain understanding, and thus opening the doors to social inclusion. Dance has a wonderful way of making people feel part of a group.

INSTRUCTIONAL INCLUSION: As with any group, choose material that is appropriate to the class members' skill level and adapt the teaching as necessary so that everyone can participate. This may involve use of an interpreter for a hearing-impaired student, a buddy for visually impaired, more copying the movements for those who are visual learners, pairing up with a student who has already caught-on. Let the students brainstorm ways to help include an individual in a dance. Allow for small successes and praise results. All participants experience a positive effect and benefit. It's a "win-win" for everyone. It is a helpful bridge to the real world in which we live.

■ First Class Meeting

The first class should be carefully planned to convey the feeling that the student will successfully learn to dance and have positive social interaction. This important first contact should give the student confidence and a desire to continue with the class. Significant factors to be considered for the first meeting include:

1. Select short and simple dances (e.g., a line dance) that the majority of students will be able to master.

2. Because younger students are reluctant to hold hands, make their dance experience positive with a contemporary line dance. The Electric Slide and Saturday Night Fever Hustle are beginning-level line dances. Moving into dances with little physical contact like the Virginia Reel and the Tennessee Wig Walk provides a good introduction to partner dancing. One thing leads to another, and suddenly they are ready to swing.

3. Use music that students will consider contemporary to facilitate their acceptance of dancing.

4. Use quick, easy sequences for forming set of three, four, six, and eight. Dances may be arranged in the order of numbers involved, thus making it easy to change from one formation to another.

5. During the first lesson with partners, use the grand march or a similar technique to organize the students. At any age, asking someone to dance can be a traumatic experience. Students are typically more comfortable when partner selection is made at the instructor's direction rather than their choice. As students gain confidence with partner dancing, the instructor should integrate social etiquette into the lesson. Both male and female students need to know how to ask a person for a dance and how to thank their partners after the dance. As the class progresses, they may be allowed or encouraged to choose their own partners.

6. Rotate partners often.

7. Emphasize activity. Long waits or lectures can test students' attention spans. Keep activity high by talking less.

8. Give individual instruction only after the rest of the class is dancing.

9. End the lesson with an exciting hint about something special in the next lesson.

CLASS PROCEDURE

■ *Strategies for Selecting Material and Presentation*

The suggestions that follow constitute rather specific guidelines for class procedures relevant to selecting materials, achieving variety within a class period, and using enrichment materials to make the class period a warm, friendly, and informative experience.

1. Materials should correspond to the skill level of the group.

2. Beginning activities should include the entire group. Nonpartner Circle Dances are recommended.

3. The warm–up dances should be simple and short.

4. Plan materials in progressive sequences so that each succeeding part relates and depends on the preceding part.

5. Mixers are a must, especially during the first few lessons. Include a generous number of nonpartner dances for uneven numbers of men and women. This eliminates the time for choosing partners and arranging formations and fosters more instruction and dancing.

6. Frequent partner changes should be used.

7. Plans should allow time and include opportunities for the group to be social.

8. Put new steps to use in the normal dance setting as soon as possible. Example: a Ballroom Dance step taught in a line or a circle formation should be danced in Ballroom fashion as soon as possible.

9. Include new and review material in each lesson after the first lesson.

10. Arrange the lesson content to provide for periods of activity and rest, contrast in style and steps, and variety in formation. Examples: circles, lines, sets, and so on.

11. To stimulate interest, presentation of material should include cultural information about the dance. This adds meaning to the dance and enhances understanding of style.

12. Discuss the unique features of a dance to help dancers distinguish one dance from another.

13. Allow ample time for practice, questions, requests, and suggestions, so that you can give individual assistance.

14. Encourage creative sequencing of moves; more experienced social dancers are often anxious to be free from set routines.

15. Visual aids supplement teaching. Pictures, diagrams, maps, cartoons, articles, movies, and special demonstrations stimulate interest. Costume dolls and other bits of folklore add to the cultural understanding of the dance. Learning is enhanced when dance titles are posted so that dancers can check their spelling and pronunciation.

■ *General Teaching Points*

In teaching any style of dance, the following concepts should be considered.

1. The instructor's top priority is to make dancing fun and nonthreatening. Students who have an unpleasant experience might not try dancing again.

2. The student's comfort/safety is also the instructor's responsibility. When students are crowded or close to a wall, the instructor, rather than a student, should tell them to move. With younger students, being close enough to intentionally bump into someone is

always a possibility. This "clowning" can disrupt the class and even cause injury.

3. The instructor should move around the class, allowing all students an opportunity to see the moves demonstrated.

4. Practice transitions from one move to another. The transition may be more difficult than the individual steps.

5. Reduce each move to its simplest form by "breaking down" each step. Once the basic step has been mastered, add more movement.

6. Build the movement sequence:

   Teach step A and practice.

   Teach step B and practice.

   Practice A and B together.

   Teach step C and practice.

   Practice A, B, and C together.

7. State directions as succinctly as possible, reducing the possibility of misinterpretation. (e.g., *Start by standing on your right foot*: Does that mean you start with your left foot free, or your left foot on top of your right foot?) Use proper grammar in your instructions. Beware of initiating your comments with phrases like: "OK," "UMM," "AND," and "SO."

8. Rotate partners often. This will:

   a. Provide students with an optimum learning experience by encountering students of varying skill levels.

   b. Ensure that no single student will be dancing the entire period with a (socially) less desirable classmate.

   c. Maximize student participation the majority of the time.

9. Emphasize *cueing*, which can be defined as verbal instruction, given "in rhythm" to aid the students with the movement or the beat. When a cue is not used, students are not sure what to do. When using introductory cueing with music, the cue should be given on count 5 of the previous measure. This will start the students on count 1 of the next measure.

   The use of these cueing techniques will enhance student learning:

   I. Introductory cueing, (while stationary), to help start a dance:
      Examples of cues starting on count 5:
      A. "1, 2, ready, go"
      B. "5–6–7–8"
      C. "ready and"

   Examples of a cue starting on count 1:
      A. "uh–one, uh–two, you know just what to do"

   II. Movement cueing, as a prompt while dancing:
      Examples of cueing a basic schottische step:
      A. Steps: "run, run, run, hop"
      B. Feet: "step right, left, right, hop left"
      C. Direction: "diagonal, 2, 3, hop"
      D. Counting: "1, 2, 3, hop "
      E. Sounds: "ba, ba, ba, boom"

   III. Lead cueing, to introduce the next move while dancing:
      Example of dancing a basic swing step and moving into an "Arch":

CUES	WHAT THE STUDENTS ARE DANCING
One, two, rock step	Basic swing step
do the arch (*next move*), go now	Basic swing step, hears the new move
lady goes under (*now the arch is executed*)	Arch

10. Make sure all students can hear the instructions. Use of a microphone can facilitate this requirement.

11. Dress the part. Teaching a basketball class wearing wing tips and a suit would not inspire the class anymore than basketball attire would motivate dance students.

12. This is the most important aspect of dance instruction: Make it FUN. Students should leave every class with a sense of accomplishment and enjoyment.

■ Teaching a Specific Dance

TEACHER PREPARATION

The teacher's preparation to teach a specific dance should include:

1. Knowledge of the basic steps.

2. An understanding of the sequence of the step patterns and their relation to the music.

3. A knowledge of the music (introduction, sequence, and tempo).

4. The ability to demonstrate the steps accurately, with or without music.

5. An organization of all materials that makes the best possible use of class time.

PRESENTATION OF THE DANCE

The analysis of each dance to be taught varies. However, many of the steps in the analysis are similar for all types of dance.

1. Give the name of the dance. Write it on the board. If it is unusual and uncommon, have the class pronounce the name.

2. Give the nationality of the dance and any background that will add interest and make the dance more meaningful. Such information need not be given all at once but can be interspersed here and there between steps.

3. Play a short part of the record, enough to give the class an idea of the character, the quality, and the speed of the music.

4. Arrange the group in the desired formation. It may be practical to do this first.

5. Teach the difficult steps or figures separately. Refer to the suggestions for teaching basic steps on pages 45–46.

   A. Teach basic step patterns, such as the Waltz or the Polka, independently of the dance. They should be mastered before being used in a dance.

   B. If the dance has steps that can be learned better in a line or a circle formation, isolate these and teach them before starting to teach the dance.

   C. If a specific step and pattern are involved, teach the isolated step first, then the figure. Talk the step through while demonstrating it and then direct the entire class in the pattern at the same time.

6. For dances with short sequences, demonstrate the entire dance and cue students as they do it. For dances with long sequences, analyze the part, try it without music first, and then with music. This process continues for the entire dance.

7. Give a starting signal or an introductory cue. This is helpful in getting everyone to start together.

8. Demonstrate with a partner as each part is explained to the group. It is not necessary to have a special partner. For many dances, the teacher can select an alert member of the class. As the teacher explains the step and demonstrates and leads the action, the partner should be able to follow easily. For a more difficult pattern, the teacher should practice with the student a few minutes before class begins. Do not use the same student all the time.

9. Correct errors in the whole group first. Give individual help as it is needed later.

10. Start the music slowly and gradually speed it up to normal tempo. When working with a machine without a speed–control mechanism, gradually speed up the dance with verbal cues until it is the same tempo as the record. For additional ideas refer to "Teaching with Recordings," p. 27, or "Teaching with Live Music," p. 28.

11. Use the blackboard to help explain and clarify rhythm patterns. Have the group clap difficult tempos and rhythms.

12. Teach first the repeated part of a dance. For example, teach the chorus and then the first verse. If the dance is long, it is not necessary to teach all the verses on the same day.

13. Give lead reminders to help the male student guide has partner into the figure or the pattern of steps.

14. Demonstrate and practice the style along with the step pattern. For example, the manner in which the foot is placed on the floor, the resultant body action, and the position of the arms is a total relationship that should be learned at one time. If it requires unusual coordination, style can be taught separately. For specific styling comments, refer to the directions given in Chapter 3, Dance Fundamentals.

15. Cue the dance steps on the microphone until the dancers have had sufficient practice to remember the routine.

16. Videotapes for instructional purposes are appearing on the market. Also, an instructor is sometimes able to make a video of a performing group. When a class is ready to perfect its style, a short video presentation gives the students a visual image for which to strive.

17. Change plans if a dance is too difficult or a poor choice for the group. Select another dance.

18. Be confident in correcting your own errors in teaching. All teachers make errors now and then. It is wise to correct them immediately. This can be done with a sense of humor or a light touch.

19. Be generous with praise and encouragement to the group.

20. Show personal enthusiasm and enjoyment for the dance. A teacher's enthusiasm and genuine interest in teaching does much to help others enjoy it.

■ *Review*

1. Review verbally, having the class tell the sequence of the dance. Then try the dance with the music while cueing the important changes.

2. Pick out the spots that need review and practice them. Point out the details of style and leading. Repeat the dance.

3. Announce the dance several days later, play the recording, and see how far the dancers can progress without a cue.

4. Avoid letting the class form the habit of depending on a cue to prompt them. Cueing is only a teaching device.

5. Make recordings or practice tapes available for those who wish to practice. Have the music playing when students come into class to encourage them to practice and to establish an appropriate atmosphere.

■ Evaluation

In the school situation where a final grade is required for each student in a dance class, some consideration must be given to a fair means of evaluating students. While some teachers feel that it destroys the recreational value of a class to conduct tests, most students are anxious to be graded if they feel that they have had a reasonable opportunity to show what they know.

Occasional tests serve to stimulate better learning, to show progression and accomplishment, and to serve as a booster to those who are slow or disinterested. From the teacher's point of view, they focus attention on the students who need special help or encouragement and on the material that needs review. Students are very interested in how grades are computed. They want to know the relationship (percentage of points) of written tests, practical tests, attendance, and improvement to the final grade. Students deserve a clear statement that coincides with the department's philosophy. There are two kinds of tests: the practical or skill test and the written test.

■ Practical Test

A *practical test* assesses the student's ability to perform a dance skill, such as a test on the Waltz, the Schottische, or the Polka; a test on the fundamentals of Square or Contra Dance; or a test on the basic steps in Social Dance. The following are types of practical tests that have been used for dance with reasonable efficiency and success.

1. *Subjective rating.* A subjective rating is determined from scores on a prepared checksheet. Five students at a time can be checked as they perform a skill individually or with partners. The sheet is given to the student so that he or she may benefit from comments; afterward, he or she signs it and turns it in.

2. *Systematic use of an achievement chart.* Each student can be checked off on an achievement chart as a few at a time are observed during the last ten minutes of a series of class periods.

3. *Cumulative grade system through use of name tags or numbers.* The teacher circulates and writes down a grade for each of the students as they dance. This should be done several times so that an average grade can be taken. If the students wear name tags throughout the course, the teacher can jot down grades at frequent intervals and thereby keep a progress chart on each student. Improvement may be quite evident with this system of checking.

4. *Colored tags used for grading.* The teacher circulates and gives each student a colored tag that represents the teacher's opinion of the student's ability (blue–excellent, red–good, yellow–fair, green–poor, and white–no opinion). At the end of the period, each student writes his or her name on the tag and turns it in. This method is effective in grading Ballroom Dance and can be used for each type of dance, including the Rumba, the Tango, and the Waltz.

5. *Student checklist.* Students check each other on a prepared checklist. For example: good rhythm, poor lead, inconsistent step, and so on. They can check five persons with whom they dance. The student should sign the checklist. The teacher can then draw up a summary of the opinions. This is very helpful in grading and also in knowing which students need extra help.

■ Written Test

The knowledge test gives every student a chance to show what he or she has learned, even though he or she may perform the skill poorly. More than one written test should be given, so that the student has a better understanding of how the questions will be phrased. For many, this is a different vocabulary. The student–teacher should respond to more information than a service student. Two kinds of written tests have proven most satisfactory for grading.

1. *The short quiz* is a five-minute test in which the student is asked to identify a fundamental step, a rhythm pattern, a specific style, a position, or a lead. It should require only a few words and should have a specific positive answer. These can be corrected in class.

2. *The objective test* is usually given as a final test. It should be given far enough in advance to get the papers corrected, returned, and discussed in class, with time allowed for questions and corrections. The objective test in dance should

be set up to include material on etiquette, fundamental steps, rhythm, position, style, and history. There should be several types of questions, including true or false, multiple choice, and identification. Directions should be clear so that students will not need to ask questions on procedures. The method of scoring should be indicated on the test paper.

A Model for Test Construction is presented in Appendix A. Sample questions illustrate how test questions are phrased in a variety of ways to gain the same knowledge. Some types are more difficult than others. The model is helpful to students in teacher training and service classes and to other teachers.

GRADING THE CLASS

Grading the class should be handled efficiently to avoid long periods of inactivity and subsequent loss of interest. All cards, tags, pencils, numbers, and other materials should be ready to use before class begins. A group that is prepared for the testing period in advance is usually cooperative and helpful. With proper motivation, the dancers should feel that they can have as much fun as usual even though they are aware of being graded.

Grading should not take up an entire period. Each class period should include some dancing just for fun, free from grading. This will restore the spirit and relieve the tension that is sometimes present during the grading time. Grading should be scheduled throughout the semester and not left until the end. All final grading should be finished before the last week so that the last two periods can be devoted to perfecting the dances and enjoying the activity as pure recreation.

■ *Enrichment Activities*

CLASS PROJECTS

Whether the class is oriented to teacher preparation or a regular "service" class, the opportunity for projects is rewarding. It recognizes the enthusiasm of those who want to do more and offers an opportunity for the student who may not perform well but excels in other skills related to the subject.

1. Make arrangements for a guest teacher to come and prepare written instructions.
2. Prepare a research paper related to a specific aspect of the dance or its country.
3. Prepare an audiovisual presentation (video, movie, or slides) of a specific dance or dance event.

4. Teach one dance in class.
5. Plan and execute a One-Night Stand event.

BULLETIN BOARDS

The class bulletin board is a place to share ideas and interests. It is a vital link between the teacher, the students, and the enrichment materials. It is an important teaching aid. The bulletin board can be used effectively in three ways: instructionally, promotionally, and creatively. A bulletin board theme can be developed around any of the following dance-related topics: basic skills, national background, region or geographic location, age groups, instruction, recreation, promotion, manners and customs, proper dress or costume, international politics, ethnic groups, seasons, holidays, states, female names, and many more. For example: take state names and symbols or slogans (state: Alabama; slogan: heart of Dixie; dance title: "Are You from Dixie"). Students could put up one bulletin board with all materials relating to this theme or make it a continuous project by putting up materials during the lesson before the lesson in which the dance is taught.

A teacher who maintains an informative and attractive bulletin board and brings interesting bits of information, pictures, clippings, and articles to the class is the teacher who turns the ordinary into the extraordinary and opens a whole new world of meaning and understanding.

CULMINATING ACTIVITIES

Interest and enthusiasm generated by a series of lessons or a season of dancing often culminate in the desire for a special event that appropriately celebrates the achievements in skills and fellowship attained by the group. The following suggestions assist in planning such an event.

1. Several beginning classes could be combined for a late afternoon or evening dance party.
2. A guest caller or teacher could be invited to make the last class session a special occasion.
3. The group could attend a festival or a jamboree together.
4. School groups could culminate their work by giving a demonstration for a school assembly, a parent-teacher association, or a service club group.
5. An exhibition team could be invited to put on a performance for the group. The exhibition group could teach and dance at least one simple dance with the group.
6. A list of community dance opportunities could be posted on the bulletin board. The list could

include classes, clubs, summer camps, workshops, clinics, festivals, and leadership training sessions.

COMMUNITY RESOURCES

Ethnic groups, foreign students attending local high schools or colleges, Square and Folk Dance clubs, museums, libraries, and art galleries are found in almost every community and can be involved in the school dance program in many ways.

Foreign students often can show regional or national costumes and musical instruments typical of their homelands and slides or movies of their homelands. Their presence in a community offers an obvious opportunity for cultural exchange.

Ethnic groups often carry on many of their former customs and can be invited to share and compare their culture in appropriate ways with the dance class. Many ethnic groups in the United States have forgotten specific dances but, because they retain their native language to a greater extent than other customs, they can share songs and music if not dances.

TEACHER RESOURCES

The teacher must bridge the gap between the daily task of teaching dance skills and the vast amount of dance-related information if the instructional experience is to be more than a social and psychomotor experience. Keeping current is a constant task in the teaching profession, and, if the dance teacher is to keep current, reviewing periodic literature in dance and dance-related periodicals is both a necessity and an efficient means of keeping abreast of the field. Current magazines carry information about other literature, including books, films, records, and costumes and so make it possible for the teacher to be more selective about the materials to be reviewed in depth.

A teacher who participates in the dance groups and the related activities in a community enriches and improves his or her instructional skill in an enjoyable and pleasant manner. Encouraging students to attend concerts, foreign films, festivals, art shows, exhibitions, plays, and selected television performances is important, but it is equally important that the teacher also participate in these cultural opportunities.

Traveling abroad has been a tradition with American school teachers, and it is a valuable professional and personal experience. Traveling at home is equally important. In fact, getting to know your state and region is important. Language, customs, dress, dances, songs, humor, and stories are different for every section of the United States. These regional differences are a rich part of our heritage and are the fabric of our culture. Visiting, talking, dancing, sightseeing, and sharing individual differences around a campfire, along a mountain trail, and across a tennis net are what learning and teaching are all about.

Refer to Appendix B p. 487–488, Organizations and Resources for specific addresses. Note *World Wide Web* sites.

ORGANIZING SPECIAL ACTIVITIES

■ *Family Dances*

Especially those who have had their children later in life yearn for a dance activity that involves the whole family. A sensitive leader and cooperative parents can make family dances work. Everyone looks forward to the occasion. *Coming on time* is important as the easiest dances come first. But the committee (leader) needs to have some activities ready to go–blowing up balloons, moving chairs, mixing lemonade, drawing with color markers on butcher paper attached to the wall with a theme, i.e., "spring green." Parents need to participate, too, even in some table games. Two activities are enough until a sufficient number of people are present to "circle up" and dance. These are called "ice-breakers." Start with simple dances to peppy music, circle left and right, and play party games like Skip to My Lou, Herr Schmidt, Ach Ja. Obviously the adults need to split up and dance with the children. Grand Marches are excellent. Families need to agree on a length of time for the very elementary dances. The program depends on the ages, ability, and flexibility of the group. *A good program does not just happen.* It takes thought and planning, reaching out to the dancers' level of ability and accommodating odd numbers. Singing, playing games, eating, and creating skits are other activities to have in addition to dance.

There needs to be a clear understanding of purpose and a group effort for success. Those with children may leave after the first hour; some may want to have another activity available after the first hour for the restless, so that the rest of the family can dance a while longer. Some children will prance on the side of the stage, perfectly happy, as the group moves on to more complicated dances. Family dances are very rewarding.

■ *One-Night Stand*

A class barn dance, church dance mixer, wedding, or special celebration is the occasion for a one-night dance party–thus the term **One-Night Stand.** An experienced leader is often brought in from outside the group to conduct party games and run the program. Many unknown factors make planning difficult: The number of participants is often indefinite; the range of ability may vary; and the balance of genders, more often than not, may be uneven. The one thing the group has in common is a desire to have a good time. An effective leader should be guided by these principles:

1. People enjoy group participation if they are allowed to join in willingly and are not forced to take part.

2. Plan a simple flexible program that can be quickly adjusted to the moods and the caprices of the situation.

3. Nonpartner dances, novelty activities, and mixers that are learned quickly are effective in these unpredictable groups.

4. Dances for threes or odd numbers are especially suitable when there are more of one gender than the other.

5. A high level of performance is not necessary. The group needs only to do the dances well enough to feel comfortable and have fun.

6. Careful planning includes getting the group active as soon as possible and moving from one activity to the next in well-planned transitions.

7. A dance or a mixer that has been particularly satisfying may be worth repeating. The group may even request a repeat. The leader can work request dances into the program when they are appropriate for the majority of the dancers.

8. A sensitive leader knows when to stop. Any single dance or mixer should not last more than five minutes. An hour of organized mixers and dances is generally sufficient. Square or Ballroom Dancing can be used to vary or extend the time. Other forms of social recreation—such as games, skits, stunts, and refreshments—can supplement the party.

9. Ballroom Dance is an all-time favorite dance activity for single sessions. An evening of Ballroom Dancing requires a minimum of planning, and leadership for program direction is not necessary. The primary objective is to create an evening of easy, pleasant activity during which old and new friends can meet and dance. A few mixers are appropriate and useful. Mixers should be of an informal partner-exchange type, carried out when couples are arranged informally around the floor. This is preferable to the circle-patterned step mixers associated with Square and Round Dance. The inclusion of a currently popular novelty dance provides a change of pace and adds to the fun of the evening. The planning committee should be cautioned to resist the temptation to turn this type of session into a grand mixer.

■ The Special Party

The program for a special party for members of a regular dance group should include familiar dance favorites. It is not an appropriate time to teach new dances or techniques. The general fun and enthusiasm can be enhanced with skits, novelty mixers, and exhibition numbers by special guest performers. Added festivity can be achieved by planning the program, decorations, and refreshments around a theme.

■ The Theme Party

Having a dance with a theme will add a special appeal to the event. Specific time periods, such as the fifties or sixties, swing or disco, Hawaiian or Latin are examples of popular themes for dances. An example of planning a circus theme party is provided below.

Occasion: Last club meeting.

Theme: Circus.

Promotion: Appropriate posters based on circus slogans: "Under the Big Top," "Greatest Show on Earth."

Costumes and decorations: Provide construction paper, wallpaper, and crêpe paper along with string, cellophane tape, and scissors, so that guests can construct clown hats to wear during the evening. Each guest can also make one item to hang on the wall for decoration.

Name tags: The guests' first names plus the name of a traditional circus animal organize the group into animal families for a special dance number, such as an animal Square Dance with each square made up of one type of animal. Examples: Gus Elephant, Diane Tiger, Willie Monkey, Jean Lion.

Master of ceremonies: The caller or the dance leader, depending on the type of dance group, leads the circus parade from outside in or around the dance floor. Followers mimic animal walks appropriate to their last names. Music should be a rousing circus-type march.

Program: Rename dances to fit the theme. For example: High-Wire Two-Step, Elephant Stomp, Trapeze Square, Tightrope Mambo, Tattoo Tango.

Last dance of the evening: All dancers gather in Square Dance sets or circles according to family name on name tag and, after the last dance, sit down on the floor in family groups.

Refreshments: A parade of animals, some juggling cookies or donuts and others carrying water pails of punch to fake dousing the guests, parade into the room led by the famous two-person horse. The horse is two dancers under a blanket or sheet, one as the head and the other as the rear end. A horse head can be made by simply drawing a likeness on a flat piece of posterboard. After the parade antics are over, the guests are served from the pails and the cookie platters brought in by the animals.

■ People with Physical Disabilities

Dance is a socially acceptable and rewarding activity for physically disabled persons. Therapeutic professionals use dance as one activity in the rehabilitation of certain disabilities. Three objectives of the rehabilitation program are to eliminate the physical disability; to reduce the physical disability; and to retrain the person to perform within his or her physical disability. Below are two sources for teaching dance to the physically disabled.*

■ Senior Dances

A variety of Senior Dances are scheduled to meet different needs and interests. In general the seniors thoroughly enjoy dances that they did in the 1940s, during World War II and immediately afterwards. Ballroom dancing, especially the jitterbug and Latin

dances, brings them to the floor along with the slow Fox Trots. They dance a smooth jitterbug. They like a few mixers and pattern dances–not too many sequences to remember. Seniors enjoy the comfort of the familiar, limited new challenges, and the opportunity to repeat every week the dances they know. If the seniors live in rural areas or in an ethnic community, they might like other dances. For instance, the Scandinavians smile and dance when the Schottische, Scandinavian Polka, or Hambo are played. If the seniors were especially active in Square Dance circles in the 1940s and 1950s, that's what they will seek out.

A leader needs to listen and be receptive to the seniors as they recall favorite dances. Find the music and include them. The chances are good that others know the dance or that the person would be willing to teach it. Seniors prefer to come to events scheduled in the daytime. They are reluctant to drive or take public transportation in the dark.

Senior or community centers will draw a regular following, even once a week. Sometimes a group of retired musicians form a band and delight in playing for the gang regularly. Sometimes the local musician's union will sponsor a monthly dance for seniors with live music.

Ethnic museums or lodges sponsor senior dances.

Retirement homes may sponsor two types: a regular dance or a very modified program for seniors with limited ability to move. Dances are modified considerably to meet their ability. Some enjoy sitting in a chair (wheelchair) and moving their arms to different dance rhythms. The leader has to be creative and use ingenuity to appeal to the residents. Even the adapted movement will bring joy as they remember other days.

---

*Hill, Kathleen. *Dance for Physically Disabled Persons. A Manual for Teaching Ballroom, Square, and Folk Dances to Users of Wheelchairs and Crutches*. Washington, D.C.: American Alliance for Health, Physical Education and Recreation, 1976.

Mason, Kathleen Criddle, editor. *Dance Therapy: Focus on Dance VII*. Washington, D.C.: American Alliance for Health, Physical Education, and Recreation, 1974.

3 Dance Fundamentals

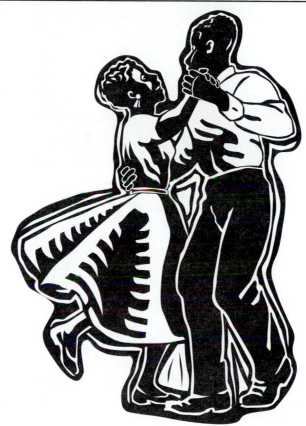

RHYTHM AND METER

■ Rhythm

Rhythm is the regular pattern of movement and/or sound. It is a relationship between time and force factors. It is felt, seen, or heard.

■ Beat

Beat is the basic unit that measures time. The duration of time becomes established by the beat, or the pulse, as it is repeated. It is referred to as the **underlying beat.**

■ Accent

Accent is the stress placed on a beat to make it stronger or louder than the others. The primary accent is on the first beat of the music. There may be a secondary accent.

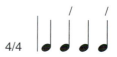

When the accent is placed on the unnatural beat (the off beat), the rhythm is *syncopated*.

■ Measure

A *measure* is one group of beats made by the regular occurrence of the heavy accent. It represents the underlying beat enclosed between two adjacent bars on a musical staff.

■ Meter

Meter is the metric division of a measure into parts of equal time value and regular accents. Meter can be recognized by listening for the accent on the first beat.

■ Time Signature

Time signature is a symbol (e.g., 2/4) that establishes the duration of time. The upper number indicates the number of beats per measure, and the lower number indicates the note value that receives one beat.

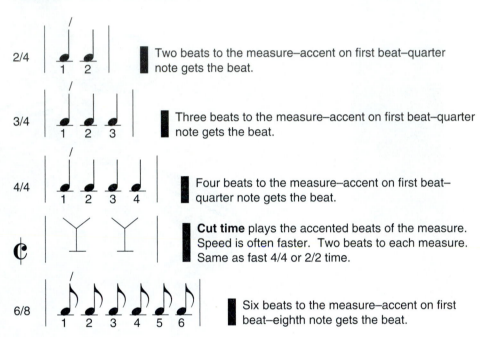

2/4 — Two beats to the measure–accent on first beat–quarter note gets the beat.

3/4 — Three beats to the measure–accent on first beat–quarter note gets the beat.

4/4 — Four beats to the measure–accent on first beat–quarter note gets the beat.

¢ — **Cut time** plays the accented beats of the measure. Speed is often faster. Two beats to each measure. Same as fast 4/4 or 2/2 time.

6/8 — Six beats to the measure–accent on first beat–eighth note gets the beat.

■ Note Values

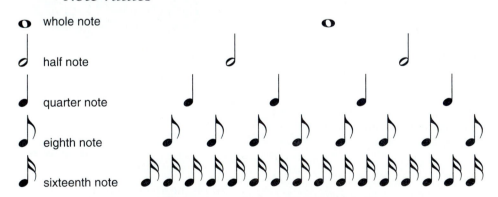

whole note

half note

quarter note

eighth note

sixteenth note

or

dotted quarter or dotted eighth notes
A *dotted note* increases the value by one half. Therefore the dotted note equals one and a half value of the original symbol. A dotted quarter note, then, is equal to a quarter plus an eighth; a dotted eighth is equal to an eighth plus a sixteenth.

triplet
A group of three notes played in the usual time of two similar notes. It would be counted *one-and-a* for one quarter note.

■ Line Values

Whereas the musical notation establishes the *relative value of beats,* these same relative values can be represented by lines:

one whole note	_____
two half notes	_____ _____
four quarter notes	_____ _____ _____ _____
eight eighth notes	__ __ __ __ __ __ __ __
sixteen sixteenth notes	_ _ _ _ _ _ _ _ _ _ _ _ _ _ _ _

■ Phrase

A musical sentence, or *phrase,* can be felt by listening for a complete thought. This can be a group of measures, generally four or eight measures. A group of phrases can express a group of complete thoughts that are related just as a group of sentences expresses a group of complete thoughts in a paragraph. Groups of phrases are generally 16 or 32 measures long.

■ Tempo

Tempo is the rate of speed at which music is played. Tempo influences the mood or the quality of music and movement. Sometimes at the beginning of the music or the dance, the tempo is established by a metronome reading. For example, metronome 128 means the equal recurrence of beats at the rate of 128 per minute.

■ Rhythm Pattern

The *rhythm pattern* is the grouping of beats that repeat for the pattern of a dance step, just as for the melody of a song. The rhythm pattern must correspond to the underlying beat. Example: meter or underlying beat 4/4.

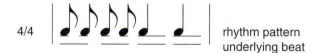

4/4 — rhythm pattern / underlying beat

■ Even Rhythm

When the beats in the rhythm pattern are all the same value (note or line value)–all long (slow) or all short (quick)–the rhythm is **even.** Examples: walk, run, hop, jump, leap, Waltz, Schottische.

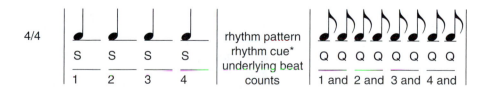

_____

*S = Slow; Q = Quick

■ *Uneven Rhythm*

When the beats in the rhythm pattern are not all the same value, but are any combination of slow and quick beats, the rhythm is **uneven.** Examples: Two–Step, Foxtrot.

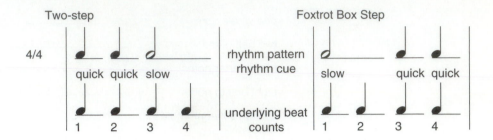

A *dotted beat* borrows half the value of itself again. Examples: skip, slide, gallop.

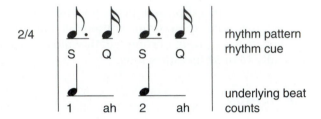

When the note comes before the bar, it is called a *pick-up beat.*

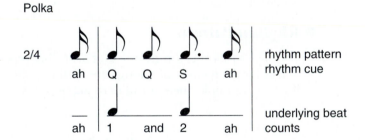

ANALYSIS OF A BASIC RHYTHM

A teacher should thoroughly understand the complete analysis of each basic dance step to be taught. The following example shows the eight related parts of an analysis. Each basic dance step has been analyzed in this manner (including the basic steps of Social Dance in Chapter 8).

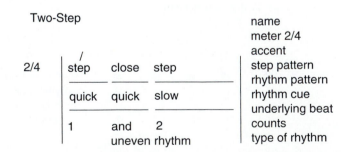

FUNDAMENTAL LOCOMOTOR MOVEMENTS

Easy movement has three variables: time, space, and force. **Time** involves the tempo or rate of speed, or duration (fast, moderate, or slow). **Space** involves the direction taken, distance covered, level, dimension (large, small), path (straight, twisted), and focus. **Force** involves the energy (power) expended, quality of movement; adjectives like brisk, quiet, hard, or gentle might apply.

Movement that travels through space is called **locomotor movement.** Movement that does not travel, like bending, twisting, pushing/pulling, is called **nonlocomotor movement.**

The following locomotor steps are simple ways to transfer weight in moving from one place to another. Combinations of locomotor movements form step patterns in Folk, Square, and Social Dance.

■ *Walk*

1. May be even or uneven rhythm.

2. A transfer of weight from one foot to the other, the weight rolling forward from the heel to the ball and toes on one foot, transferring to the heel, then the ball, toes of the other foot. In a **dance walk** the toes and ball of the foot strike first. **One foot is always in contact with the ground.**

```
        /
4/4   step   step   step   step
      R      L      R      L
      ___    ___    ___    ___

      ___    ___    ___    ___
      1      2      3      4
             even rhythm
```

■ *Run*

1. Fast, even rhythm.

2. A transfer of weight from the ball and toes of one foot to the other foot. During the weight transfer, both feet are off the ground.

```
        /
4/4   R L   R L   R L   R L
      _ _   _ _   _ _   _ _

      ___   ___   ___   ___
      1 and 2 and 3 and 4 and
             even rhythm
```

■ *Leap*

1. Even rhythm.

2. A transfer of weight from one foot to the other foot, pushing off with a spring and landing on the ball of the foot, letting the heel come down, and bending the knee to absorb the shock. At one point, both feet are off the ground.

3. A leap may be compared to a run with a greater period of suspension in the air.

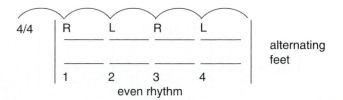

```
4/4   R      L      R      L
      ___    ___    ___    ___          alternating
                                        feet
      ___    ___    ___    ___
      1      2      3      4
             even rhythm
```

■ *Jump*

1. Even rhythm.
2. A transfer of weight with a springing action from both feet, lifting into the air and landing on both feet.
3. Feet push off floor with strong foot and knee extension, the heel coming off first and then the toe.
4. On landing, the ball of the foot touches the floor first and then the heel comes down and the knees bend to absorb the shock of landing.

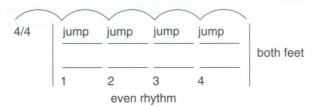

■ *Hop*

1. Even rhythm.
2. A transfer of weight by a springing action of the foot from one foot (push off from the heel/toe and land on ball then heel of foot) to the same foot.

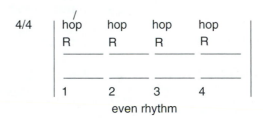

■ *Sissone*

1. Even rhythm.
2. A transfer of weight with a springing action from both feet, lifting into the air, and landing on one foot (a hop), sometimes referred to as a **JOP, J** for "jump," **OP** for "(h)**OP**."

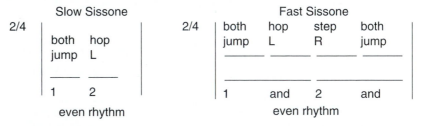

■ *Assemblé*

1. Even rhythm.
2. A transfer of weight with a spring from one foot, lifting into the air, and landing on both feet.

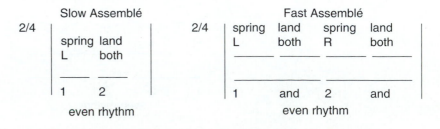

■ *Gallop*

1. A combination of a walk and a run.
2. Uneven rhythm (6/8 ♩ ♪ ♩ ♪ or 2/4 ♩♩♩♩♩) .
3. 2–1 ratio; long–short, long–short.
4. Movement forward, knee action, heel leading.
5. One foot maintains lead.

6/8	step	run		step	run		step	run		step	run
	R	L		R	L		R	L		R	L
	1	2	3	1	2	3	1	2	3	1	2	3

uneven rhythm

2/4	step	run		step	run		step	run		step	run
	R	L		R	L		R	L		R	L
	1	and	ah	2	and	ah	1	and	ah	2	and	ah

uneven rhythm

■ *Slide*

1. A gallop moving sidewards, right or left.
2. Uneven rhythm (6/8 ♩ ♪ ♩ ♪ or 2/4 ♩♩♩♩♩) .
3. 2–1 ratio; long–short, long–short.
4. Movement sideward can go right or left.
5. A step on the right foot, on the slow beat, close the left foot to right, shifting the weight quickly onto the left foot on the quick beat.
6. One foot maintains lead.

6/8	step	close		step	close		step	close		step	close
	R	L		R	L		R	L		R	L
	1	2	3	1	2	3	1	2	3	1	2	3

uneven rhythm

2/4	step	close		step	close		step	close		step	close
	R	L		R	L		R	L		R	L
	1	and	ah	2	and	ah	1	and	ah	2	and	ah

uneven rhythm

■ Skip

1. A combination of a walk and a hop.
2. Uneven rhythm. (6/8 ♩ ♪ ♩ ♪ or 2/4 ♫ ♫ ♫)
3. 1–2 ratio; short–long.
4. A step and a hop on the same foot. Alternate feet.
5. Timing: If the skip is high, the hop has two beats (the accent is on the hop while in the air); the step, one beat. If the skip is low, the step has two beats (the accent is on the step). The hop one beat.

6/8	step	hop	step	hop
	R	R	L	L
	1	2	3	1	2	3

uneven rhythm

2/4	step	hop	step	hop
	R	R	L	L
	1	and	ah	2	and	ah

uneven rhythm

■ Exercises for Fundamental Locomotor Movements

1. Practice each movement while clapping or playing rhythm instruments.
2. Vary the energy, space, direction, and style.
3. Put three different movements together and repeat the combination four times. For instance: run, run, leap, run, run, jump. Repeat four times. Write the rhythm pattern in counts and lines.
4. Compose a two–part dance (A, B) for 16 counts. Clap the rhythm or use rhythm instruments.

BASIC DANCE STEPS

■ Shuffle, Dance Walk, or Glide

1. An easy, light step, from one foot to the other, in even rhythm.
2. Different from a walk in that the weight is over the ball of the foot.
3. The feet remain lightly in contact with the floor.

■ Two-Step or Triple-Step

1. 2/4 or 4/4 meter.
2. Uneven rhythm.
3. Step forward on left foot, close right to left, take weight on right, step left again. Repeat, beginning with right.
4. The rhythm is quick, quick, slow.

2/4	step	close	step
	L	R	L
	Q	Q	S
	1	and	2

uneven rhythm

■ Polka

1. 2/4 meter.
2. An energetic, lively dance step in uneven rhythm.
3. Similar to a Two–Step with the addition of a hop so that it becomes hop, step, close, step. The hop comes on the pick–up beat.

2/4	hop	/ step	close	step	hop	/ step	close	step	hop
	L	R	L	R	R	L	R	L	L
	ah	Q	Q	S	ah	Q	Q	S	ah
	ah	1	and	2	ah	1	and	2	ah

uneven rhythm

■ Schottische

1. 4/4 meter.
2. Smooth, even rhythm.
3. Three running steps and a hop or a step, close, step, hop.

4/4	/ step	step	step	hop
	L	R	L	L
	Q	Q	Q	Q
	1	2	3	4

even rhythm

4. The Schottische dance form is four measures (step, step, step hop; step, step, step hop; step hop, step hop; step hop, step hop).
5. Common and popular variations are to hold, turn, or swing the free leg on the fourth count instead of hopping.

■ Waltz

1. 3/4 meter–accent first beat.
2. A smooth, graceful dance step in even rhythm.
3. Ladder step consists of three steps; step forward on the left, step to the side with the right, close left to right, take weight on left.

3/4	/ fwd	side	close	fwd	side	close
	L	R	L	R	L	R
	S	S	S	S	S	S
	1	2	3	1	2	3

even rhythm

4. The **Box Waltz** is the basic pattern for the Box Waltz turn. Step left forward, step right sideward, passing close to the left foot, close left to right, taking weight left; step right backward, step left sideward, passing close to the right foot, close right to left, take weight right. *Cue:* Forward side close, back side close.

3/4	fwd	side	close	back	side	close
	L	R	L	R	L	R
	S	S	S	S	S	S
	1	2	3	1	2	3

even rhythm

5. The **Running Waltz** used so often in European Folk Dances is a tiny three–beat running step with an accent on the first beat, three beats to each measure.

6. **Canter Waltz** rhythm is an uneven rhythm in Waltz time with the action taking place on beats one and three. The rhythm is slow, quick; slow, quick or long, short. (Refer to Canter rhythm, p. 507 and p. 426.)

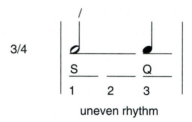

3/4			
	S		Q
	1	2	3

uneven rhythm

■ *Mazurka*

1. 3/4 meter.

2. Strong, vigorous, even three–beat rhythm–accent second beat.

3. Step left, bring right up to left with a cut–step displacing left, hop right while bending left knee so that left foot approaches the right ankle. Repeat, left foot leading.

3/4	step	cut	hop	step	cut	hop
	L	R	R	L	R	R
	S	S	S	S	S	S
	1	2	3	1	2	3

even rhythm

BASIC DANCE TURNS

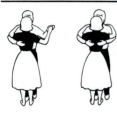

Using the fundamental dance steps, partners may turn clockwise or counterclockwise. Basically, if the man is leading with the left, the turn is counterclockwise; if he is lead–ing with the right, the turn is clockwise. But in Folk Dance, the majority of the partner turns are clockwise. A successful turn actually starts with the preceding step, the man's back to center and his body moving into the turn. The man steps left backward in the line of direction, which allows his right foot to lead on the second step.

■ *Schottische Turn Clockwise*

The Schottische rhythm is even 4/4 meter. The pattern is step, step, step hop; step, step, step hop; step hop, step hop, step hop, step hop. The last two measures of four are used for the partner turn. The starting position is generally a closed position or a shoulder–waist position. By turning gradually, the couple can make only one turn clockwise on the four step hops, or, by turning a half–turn clockwise on each step hop, they can make two full turns. They progress forward in the line of direction on each step hop.

■ *Two-Step Turn Clockwise*

The Two–Step rhythm is uneven 2/4 or 4/4 meter with a quick–quick–slow pattern. There is a half–turn on each measure (2/4 meter). The starting position is closed, with the man's back to center of the circle. *The turn is on the second count.*

LEFT-FOOT SEQUENCE (MAN)

Count 1	Step left sideward.
Count and	Close right to left, taking weight on right.
Count 2	Step left around partner, toeing in and pivoting clockwise on the ball of the foot a half-turn around.

RIGHT-FOOT SEQUENCE (WOMAN)

Count 1	Step right sideward.
Count and	Close left to right, taking weight on left.
Count 2	Step right forward between partner's feet and pivoting clockwise on the ball of the foot a half-turn around.

■ NOTE

The man starts with the left sequence, the woman starts with the right sequence. After a half–turn, the woman then starts with the left sequence and the man with the right sequence. They continue to alternate. By this process of *dovetailing with the feet,* man and woman can turn easily without stepping on each other's feet. Couple progresses in the line of direction as they turn.

■ STYLE

The steps should be small and close to partner. The body leans back and aids in the turn. The turn is on the ball of the foot. Each partner must give the impetus for the turn by pivoting on his or her own foot.

■ LEAD

Closed position, the man should have a firm right hand on the small of the woman's back so that she can lean back against it. His right arm guides her as he turns.

■ CUES

1. Left–Foot sequence: side close around.
   Right–Foot sequence: side close between.

2. Practicing together in closed position.
   Side close turn, side close turn.

■ *Polka Turn Clockwise*

The **clockwise turn** is used almost always for a Polka partner turn in Folk Dance. The Polka rhythm is uneven 2/4 meter. The pattern is hop, step, close, step. With the addition of a quick hop (pick–up beat) before each Two–Step, all the directions described for the Two–Step turn can be applied to the Polka turn. The starting position is generally a closed position or a shoulder–waist position.

▪ *Waltz Turn*

The Waltz rhythm is even 3/4 meter. Three patterns are presented: the Box Waltz, traditional step–side–close, and Running Waltz pattern.

▪ BOX WALTZ TURN—CLOCKWISE, COUNTERCLOCKWISE

The Box Waltz turn is used in social dancing and in some American Folk Dances and can go either to the left in a counterclockwise turn or to the right in a clockwise turn, depending on which foot leads the turn. (These turns are described under the Waltz box turn, pp. 428–429.)

▪ CLOCKWISE TURN

The clockwise turn is the turn most often used for Folk Dances. Two patterns are presented, the first based on the traditional step–side–close pattern and the second on the running Waltz pattern. It is in 3/4 meter.

▪ STEP-SIDE-CLOSE PATTERN (TRADITIONAL)

LEFT–FOOT SEQUENCE (MAN). Step left around partner, pivoting on the ball of the foot a half–turn clockwise (count 1). Step right sideward in line of direction (count 2). Close left to right, take weight left (count 3).

RIGHT–FOOT SEQUENCE (WOMAN). Step right forward between partner's feet, pivoting on the ball of the foot a half–turn clockwise (count 1). Step left sideward in the line of direction (count 2). Close right to left, take weight right (count 3).

▪ NOTE

The man starts with the left sequence, the woman with the right sequence. After a half–turn, the woman starts with the left sequence and the man with the right sequence. They continue to alternate. By this process of dovetailing the feet, dancers can turn easily without stepping on each other's feet.

▪ STYLE

The steps are small and close to partner. The pivot halfway around is on the ball of the foot on the first count. Each partner is responsible for supplying the impetus for the ball of the foot turn.

▪ LEAD

The man has a firm right hand at the woman's back. She leans back and is guided into the turn by his firm right hand and arm.

▪ CUES

1. Left-foot sequence: around side close. Right-foot sequence: between side close.
2. Practice together in closed position. Turn side close, turn side close.

▪ STEP-STEP-CLOSE PATTERN

LEFT–FOOT SEQUENCE (MAN). Step left in the line of direction (toeing in, heel leads), pivoting on the ball of the foot and starting a half–turn clockwise (count 1). Take two small steps, right, left, close to first step, completing half–turn (counts 2 and 3).

RIGHT–FOOT SEQUENCE (WOMAN). Step right in line of direction (toeing out *between partner's feet*, pivoting on the ball of the foot, starting a half–turn clockwise (count 1). Take two small steps, left, right, close to first step, completing half–turn (counts 2 and 3).

1. When the man steps backward left, the right foot leads the clockwise turn.

2. The man starts with the left sequence, the woman with the right sequence. After a half–turn, the woman starts with the left sequence and the man with the right sequence. They continue to alternate. When doing left–foot sequence, step backward in line of direction; when doing the right–foot sequence, step forward (but not as long a step as the first step in the other sequence). The dancers are turning on each count, but steps on counts 2 and 3 are almost in place. *Both feet are together on count 3.*

■ **LEAD**

The man has a firm right hand at the woman's back. She leans back and is guided into the turn by his firm right hand and arm.

■ **CUES**

Left–Foot sequence: Back turn turn.
Right–Foot sequence: Forward turn turn.

■ **REVERSE DIRECTION OF TURN**

If turning counterclockwise, the left foot leads. If turning clockwise, the right foot leads. To change leads from left to right or right to left, one measure (3 beats) is needed for transition. A balance step backward or one Waltz step forward facilitates the transition. Or turning counterclockwise, after a left Waltz step, immediately reverse direction with a right Waltz step, turning clockwise (a more difficult maneuver). Eventually the lead comes back to a left one, and another transition occurs.

SUGGESTIONS FOR TEACHING BASIC DANCE STEPS

The level of ability of the student and the degree of difficulty of the basic step will influence the manner in which a step is presented. The factors involved are interdependent and may be used in various combinations when the steps are being taught. The sequence of the factors and the starting point for teaching vary. Sometimes it is necessary to go back in the teaching process to an easier form. Several approaches may be necessary for everyone to learn the step.

■ *Analysis of Rhythm of Basic Step*

Explain and discuss accent, time signature, even or uneven rhythm, and foot pattern in relation to rhythm.

1. Listen to music.
2. Clap rhythm with students.
3. Write out on blackboard.
4. Demonstrate action.

■ *Method of Presentation*

1. Walk through with analysis and demonstration.
2. Practice.
3. Apply basic step in simple sequence.
4. Use basic step in simple dance.

■ *Interdependent Factors Influencing Procedure*

1. Position of teacher in relation to group. Ideally the teacher should be a part of the group, standing in the circle, two steps inside the circle, or facing the line. Avoid standing in the middle because the back is to part of the group. The dancers cannot hear, and the teacher is unaware of whether they understand. In large groups, the teacher is on a platform, slightly above the group so that he or she may be seen and heard. Otherwise, a mike is necessary. A wireless mike affords more flexibility of position.

2. Demonstrations. If facing lines, mirror demonstrate, rather than turn back on group. If demonstrating in the circle, give demonstration several times, moving to different locations, especially directly across the circle. Dancers tend to mirror what they see in a circle and forget to translate demonstration to the same foot and direction.

3. Formation of group for teaching.
   A. Line.
   B. Single circle.
   C. Double circle.

4. Position of people.
   A. Alone.
   B. With partner.
      1) Varsouvienne, couple, promenade, open, or conversation position.
      2) Closed or shoulder–waist position.

5. Accompaniment–with or without music.

6. Cue–with or without verbal cue.

7. Direction of movement.
   A. In place.
   B. Forward and backward.
   C. Sideward or diagonal.
   D. Turning.

PROCEDURE FOR TEACHING BASIC DANCE STEPS AND TURNS

■ *Schottische and Clockwise Turn*

Directions are for man; woman's part is reverse.

1. **Single circle,** facing line of direction.
   A. Beginning left, take two Schottische steps, moving forward in the line of direction. Rock forward on first step hop, rock backward on the second step hop, rock forward on the third step hop, and backward on the fourth step hop. Repeat.
   B. Beginning left, take two Schottische steps moving forward in the line of direction. Turn clockwise by rocking forward and backward twice to make one complete turn. Repeat. Discourage any body sway that may accompany the rock as soon as the pattern of turning is learned.

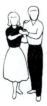

2. **Double circle,** take open position, facing the line of direction. Beginning left, take two Schottische steps, moving forward in the line of direction. Take closed or shoulder–waist position. Turn clockwise by rocking forward and backward twice to make one complete turn. Repeat. Emphasize the importance of turning to face partner on the last Schottische step so that the turn starts on the first step hop. Encourage more advanced dancers to make two turns.

3. Use a simple dance to practice Schottische step. For example: Schottische, p. 98, Road to the Isles, p. 273.

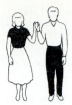

■ *Progressive Two-Step*

1. The forward Two–Step can be taught simply by moving forward on the cue **step, close, step,** alternately left, then right.
2. Take couple position. Take the Two–Step face to face and back to back, progressing in the line of direction.

■ *Two-Step Turn Clockwise*

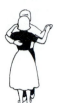

1. **Double circle formation,** man with his back to the center of the circle. Take closed position. Begin on man's left, woman's right.

   A. Moving toward the line of direction, take four slides, pivoting around clockwise on the last slide so that the man faces the center of the circle. Take four slides to the man's right still in the line of direction, pivoting on the last slide clockwise so that the man is back in original position. Repeat. Emphasize that the last slide is the pivot clockwise and that the man must lead the woman with his right arm as he goes around so that they can turn together.

   B. Moving to the man's left (line of direction), take two slides and pivot clockwise halfway around on the last slide. Then, reaching in the line of direction, take two slides to the man's right and pivot clockwise to original position. Repeat.

2. Use a simple dance to practice Two–Step turn. For example: Boston Two–Step, p. 105.

■ *Polka*

1. Step by step rhythm approach.

   A. **Single circle,** all facing line of direction.

      1) Analyze the Polka very slowly and have class walk through the steps together in even rhythm (hop, step close step).

      2) Gradually adapt the rhythm until there is a quick hop and a slower step close step.

      3) Gradually accelerate the tempo to normal Polka time. Add the accompaniment.

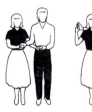

   B. **Double circle,** take promenade, Varsouvienne, or couple position, facing line of direction. Polka forward with partner.

   C. Use a simple dance to practice Polka step. For example: Klumpakojis, p. 320.

2. Two–Step approach

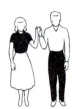

   A. **Single circle,** facing the line of direction. Beginning left, Two–Step with music, moving forward in the line of direction. Gradually accelerate the tempo to a fast Two–Step and take smaller steps. Without stopping, change the music to Polka rhythm and precede each Two–Step with a hop. If musician is available, this rhythm change can be made with music. Otherwise, cue without music until step is learned and then use Polka recording.

   B. **Double circle,** take promenade, Varsouvienne, or couple position, facing the line of direction. Polka forward with partner.

   C. Use a simple dance to practice Polka step. For example: Klumpakojis, p. 320.

3. Slide approach

   A. **Single circle,** all facing center, hands joined.

      1) Take eight slides to the left and eight slides to the right. Take four slides to the left and four slides to the right. Take two slides to the left and two

---

slides to the right. Repeat the last group of two slides over and over. *Emphasize that in order to change direction each time, a hop is added.* This last series of slides with the hop is a Polka step.

2) Repeat this last series of slides, moving forward toward the center of the circle and then moving backward away from the center.

B. **Double circle,** take promenade, Varsouvienne, or couple position, facing the line of direction. Polka forward with partner.

C. Use simple dance to practice Polka step. For example: Klumpakojis, p. 320; Heel and Toe Polka, p. 106.

■ *Polka Turn Clockwise*

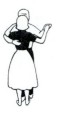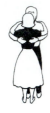

1. Learn the basic Polka step forward.

2. Repeat the process, describing how to learn the Two–Step turn clockwise, p. 53.

   A. When a change of direction is made on the fourth slide or on the second slide, *add a hop.*

   B. When a change of direction is made on a pivot, *add a hop,* as the pivot is made.

   C. *Cue:* Slide and step hop, slide and step hop.

   D. Then put the hop first and *cue:* Hop, slide and step, hop, slide and step.

3. Practice individually and then with a partner. Dovetail feet as in two–step turn.

4. Use a simple dance to practice Polka turn. For example: Doudlebska Polka, p. 286.

■ *Running Waltz*

Single circle, hands joined. Move one step with each beat of music. Accent first step of measure slightly.

■ *Box Waltz and Turn*

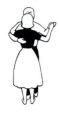

1. Learn box pattern individually.

2. Take closed dance position with partner. The man steps forward on the left and the woman backward on the right.

3. Practice turning left and right. *Cue:* Turn side close, back side close.

■ *Waltz Turn Clockwise*

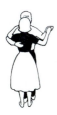

1. Learn step pattern, turning clockwise individually. Sometimes to establish a complete half–turn, it is helpful to travel the length of the hall and indicate one wall to be faced on the first measure and the other wall to be faced on the second measure. The dancers try harder to complete one turn and always face the correct direction.

2. Partners take closed position and practice turn together.

3. Use a simple dance with a clockwise turn. For example: Swedish Waltz, p. 361.

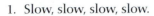

■ *Pivot Turn*

The continuous pivot turn, used in Folk Dance and Social Dance, is a series of steps turning clockwise as many beats as desired and to different rhythms.

1. Slow, slow, slow, slow.
2. Quick, quick, quick, quick.
3. Slow, slow, quick, quick.
4. Slow, slow, quick, quick, quick, quick.

The man should be careful that he has room to turn, as the pivot turn progresses forward in the line of direction if done properly, and he should not turn so many steps as to make his partner dizzy. The principle involved in the footwork is the dovetailing of the feet, which means that the right foot always steps between partner's feet and the left foot always steps around the outside of partner's feet.

■ ANALYSIS OF PIVOT TURN

Take closed or shoulder–waist position. Preparation to start clockwise turn is the **preceding beat** of the pivot turn.

RHYTHM CUES	STEPS
Slow	**Preliminary step.** Man steps right between partner's feet and leads into the turn by bringing his left shoulder toward his partner, increasing the body tension; shoulders become parallel and remain in that position for entire pivot.
Slow	Step left, toeing in across the line of direction and rolling clockwise, three–quarters of the way around the ball of the left foot.
Slow	Step right, between partner's feet forward in the line of direction, completing one turn.

Last two steps repeat alternately.

■ WOMAN

The woman receives the lead as the man increases body tension. She does the same. She places her right foot forward in between his feet on the line of direction, left foot across the line of direction, right foot between, left across, and so forth.

■ STYLE

The hips and legs are closer together than most steps. They both must lean away, pressing outward like "the water trying to stay in the bucket." The concept of stepping each time in relation to the line of direction is what makes it possible to progress while turning as a true pivot turn should do.

■ NOTE

1. In Scandinavian pivots, some have found it helpful to step on the right heel, transferring the weight to the sole of the foot; step left on the sole of foot, in effect pivoting on the right heel, left sole.
2. For further analysis, see Pivot Turn, Social Dance, pp. 388–390.

■ *Spin or Twirl*

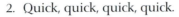

Whenever the woman is turned under her arm one or more turns (spins or twirls), it is important for the man to hold his left hand over the apex of her head; joined hands should be loose to allow turn.

DANCE POSITIONS

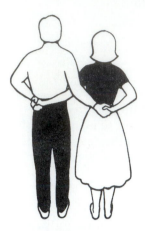

1. Back Cross

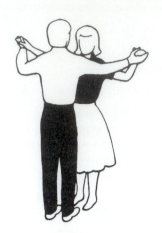

2. Butterfly

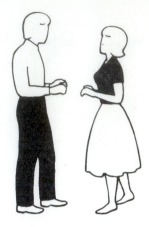

3. Challenge Shine

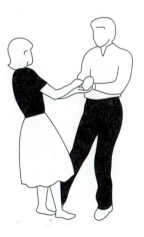

4. Cross

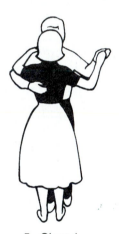

5. Closed

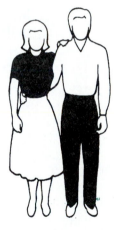

6. Conversation Open

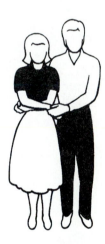

7. Cuddle

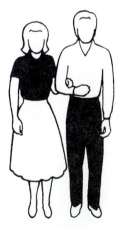

8. Escort

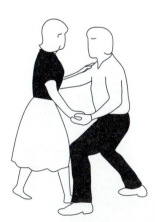

9. Face Off

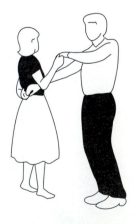

10. Hammerlock

Detailed description for each position is given in the Glossary.

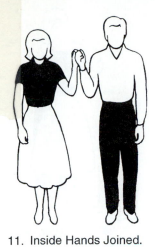

11. Inside Hands Joined.
    Side by Side. Couple

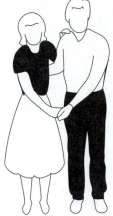

12. Jockey

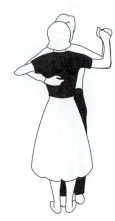

13. Latin Social

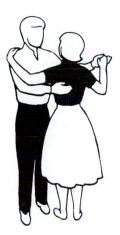

14. Left Parallel.
    Side Car

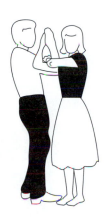

15. Little Window

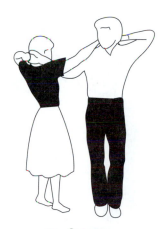

16. Octopus

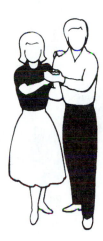

17. Open

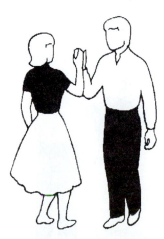

18. Pigeon Wing
    Right Hand Start

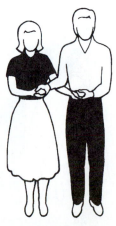

19. Promenade

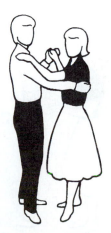

20. Reverse Open

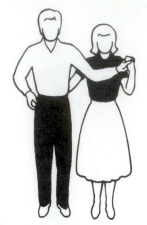

21. Reverse Varsouvienne

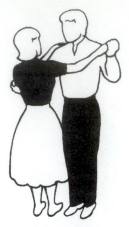

22. Right Parallel. Swing, Banjo

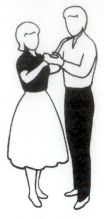

23. Semiopen

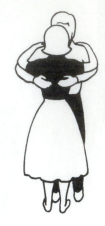

24. Shoulder-Waist

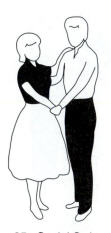

25. Social Swing

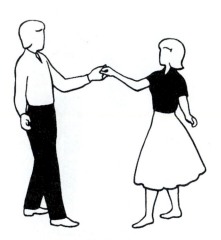

26a. Swing Out. Flirtation

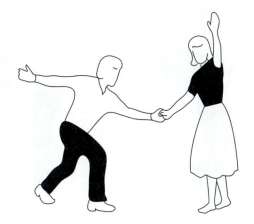

26b. Swing Out– Lindy Style

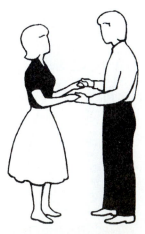

27. Two Hands Joined. Facing

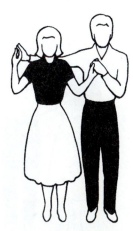

28. Varsouvienne (Traditional) Sweetheart (Modern)

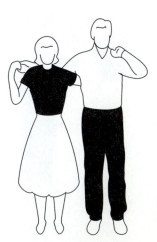

29. Yoke, Bridge

DANCE FORMATIONS

The dance formations are representative of the dances in this book. There are many other variations.

1. NO PARTNERS

   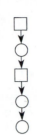

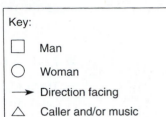

Key:

☐   Man

○   Woman

→   Direction facing

△   Caller and/or music

Head couple is nearest to the caller and/or music.

Single circle   Broken circle   Line, side by side   File, one behind each other

2. COUPLES IN A CIRCLE

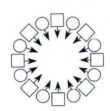 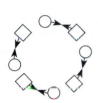 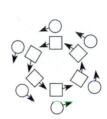 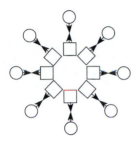

Single circle, facing center   Single circle, man facing the line of direction, woman facing the reverse line of direction   Double circle, couples facing the line of direction   Double circle, partners facing, man's back to center

3. THREE PEOPLE

 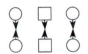

Set of three in a line, side by side   Set of three, facing set of three   Single circle, facing center

4. TWO COUPLES

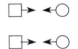 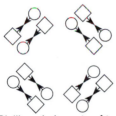

Set of two couples, partners facing   Sicilian circle, sets of two couples, couples facing

5. COUPLES IN A FILE DOUBLE FILE

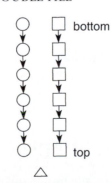

Longway or contra set, couples facing head

6. COUPLES IN A LINE

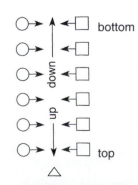

Longway or contra set, partners facing

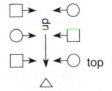

Couples 1, 3, 5 cross over Contra Set

7. FOUR COUPLES

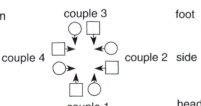

Set of four couples

MUSIC IN RELATION TO DANCE

One problem that plagues the dance teacher more than any other is how to teach a student to hear and move to the beat of the music. A person who cannot hear the beat and constantly fumbles with all the relationships in movement that depend on being on the beat has a psychological handicap. Perhaps there are some basic understandings that can be learned and explored.

■ *Listen to the Beat*

The underlying beat is usually carried by the string bass, the piano, and the drums. In Latin rhythms, the beat is carried by the bongo drum, the clavs (sticks), or the wood block.

■ THE BEGINNER

The beginner should try to pick out a steady beat that is most dominant and synchronize his or her step with this downbeat. Quite often, people who think they have no sense of rhythm can clap a consistent pattern of beats but do not know what to listen for. If an individual can clap accurately to the basic beat and can depend on this beat to be consistent throughout a piece of music, he or she usually has the major problem solved. Regular practice moving with the beat brings confidence for dancing.

When an individual cannot clap to a regular beat and cannot hear a beat, the only way for him or her to learn is to:

1. Visually follow the clapping of the teacher or someone else in class.
2. Try to relate this with listening for the basic beat of a very obvious piece of Square Dance or march music. Mark time in place with feet and then try to walk to this beat alone.
3. Gradually progress to other music that has a less obvious beat.
4. Walk with a good partner and try to feel the relationship of the movement to the beat until the individual can move with the beat.

The melody or the vocal can be very distracting to the individual who has difficulty with rhythm, and he or she tends to speed up or slow down. The more a dancer is concentrating on a dance step pattern, style, or lead, the easier it is to forget about listening to the music. A teacher can help in this case by calling attention to listening for the music. Thorough understanding and practice of the difficult step without music also permits greater freedom to listen to the music.

■ THE DANCER

When one has accomplished the hurdle of being able to dance to the beat of the music, the next step is to learn to listen to the rhythmic changes in the music.

1. The dancer should be able to recognize the beginning and the end of a phrase and anticipate this in his or her movement or call.
2. He or she should be able to recognize and adjust the movement to changes of tempo.
3. He or she should be able to identify the parts of a dance by the melodic changes in the music and therefore be able to make smooth transitions in movement or position.
4. He or she should be able to note the quality of the various parts of the music and be better able to interpret the appropriate style.
5. He or she should learn from experience with different types of rhythm to identify correctly one basic rhythm from another.
6. Finally, with experience, he or she should be able to interpret the music and in combining dance steps feel the relationship of the step to the music.

■ How to Recognize Music for Dance

Certain facts must be learned to recognize music for specific dances.

1. Each dance rhythm is in a definite meter. For example, the dancer learns to recognize Waltz music if he or she knows to listen to 3/4 meter with an accent on the first beat.

2. Each dance has a pattern of movement, the quality or feeling of which should identify with the quality of the music. For example, the dancer needs to know the Rumba has a smooth, rolling Latin quality; the Samba has a faster, bouncy, rocking quality; and the Mambo has an offbeat, heavy, sultry quality. By trying to recognize this quality in the music, the dancer can usually identify the appropriate music.

3. Some types of dances have particular instruments that carry the base or the melody. For example, the Latin American dances have the bongo drums, the sticks, the wood blocks, and the maracas, one or two of which carry the basic beat and another the rhythm pattern.

4. In Folk Dance, the music, the pattern of steps, and the style often relate to the meaning or the origin of the dance, and this association helps the dancer to remember and identify the music.

■ Rhythm Training and Appreciation

There are different approaches for understanding rhythm. The Orff–Schulwerk process is one that is meeting success. It is a sequential approach to music education that uses all the elements of music (rhythm, melody, form, timbre, and harmony) in the development of conceptual understandings. Movement is one aspect. Teachers should explore a variety of approaches to this subject.

The teacher can contribute to rhythm training and appreciation through dance by following these guidelines:

1. Be thoroughly familiar with the music used for any specific dance, in order to
   A. Give verbal cues in the correct rhythm.
   B. Give the starting cue at the appropriate time.
   C. Cue the group with regard to the length of the musical introduction before the dance begins.

2. Direct the group to clap out difficult rhythms.

3. Point out rhythmic changes in the music and allow time for listening to the transitions from one part to another.

4. Point out and allow the class to listen to particular instruments or qualities in the music that help them remember the dance.

5. Provide frequent opportunities for student identification of music rather than announcing the dance.

6. Plan the program to include interesting cultural contrasts in music and dance.

7. Use words and meanings to folk songs that accompany dance.

8. Add significant authentic sounds to the recorded music, such as:
   A. Appropriate shouts or claps.
   B. Appropriate percussion instruments, such as tambourine or drum.
   C. Appropriate words or yodeling.

9. Explain meanings of music or dance and add highlights of folklore or background information.

10. Allow sufficient practice and review of dances so that the group can know dances well.

The Beautiful Dancer

A beautiful dancer is one of the most satisfying sights to watch. It is really not the intricate steps or figures that are noticed, but rather the rhythmical way the dancer seems to glide around the floor. There is an alertness, a vitality, a strength, and a beauty that transmits the feeling of complete control over the entire body.

The dancer receives more pleasure by continuously striving for the special style that makes each dance–Square, Tango, Country Western, Scottish Reel–different. It is as important to execute the style and mannerisms inherent in the dance of any country as it is to be able to dance the steps and pattern sequences. If twirls, whoops, and yells are added to every dance, the dances lose their individuality and become uninteresting. Without care, a fast clogging routine blurs into the intricate Slavic Kolos.

Ear and Ankle Alignment

The subtle thought of maintaining ear and ankle alignment in an easy, natural way gives a person the poise and confidence so rightfully desired by all. The dancer who practices this secret of body balance will not tire as easily. Dancers who adopt the "ear to ankle lineup" as a slogan, whether dancing a favorite Folk Dance, in a Square Dance set, or on the ballroom floor, will have more assurance of what to do and how to do it, will wear their dress (costume) with greater charm and distinction, and will have a great deal more fun. The body carriage adds style to the dance pattern performed and gives the dancer that "finished look."

Good Posture—Key to Body Balance and Control

1. Keep yourself upright–do not lean forward or backward. Do not stick out in the rear.
2. Keep your weight up–not dragging over your feet. This cultivates that "light on your feet" feeling.
3. Keep yourself a moving weight–alert all the way through your body–not planted on every spot you take.
4. Transfer weight smoothly and evenly from foot to foot without unnecessary motion of the hips from side to side or of the body up and down.
5. Move on a narrow base with the feet and legs close together.
6. Practice walking backward–the woman must learn to keep her balance when taking long, gliding steps backward.
7. Keep your eyes off the floor and the feet.
8. Bend the ankles, the knees, and the hips when executing a dip–not the back and head. The trunk is held erect.
9. Be at ease but in complete control of all parts of the body.
10. Relax, listen to the music, and *enjoy* dancing!

Achieving Appropriate Style

One needs to make a conscious effort to develop style. Observation of dancers who have good style is a starting point; careful analysis and application must follow.

1. The expression on the dancer's face should reflect enthusiasm and a friendly, relaxed attitude. Dance with joy and pride.
2. Proper body mechanics are influenced by optimum posture. Age, body type, and personality influence the style, but still the goal is the same: smoothness, graceful carriage, and appropriate action for the dance. The position (contact) of

the arms and hands for the different positions influence the style. *Resistance,* or "weight," is essential in partner dances. The tendency to stare at one's partner is uncomfortable for both, but occasional eye contact and focus toward partner or over partner's shoulder is important. Refer to dance walk, leading and following, and closed position in Chapter 8, Social Dance, for specific details as they are fundamental to style.

3. The blending of one step or figure to the next is important. The body position adjusts in preparation for a different step, figure, or direction. Smaller footsteps frequently solve some basic problems.

4. A study of different nationalities, their culture, and their way of life all give the dancer a broader understanding of the movement itself. Consider the influence of the costumes on the dance movement. For instance, tight jeans and large silver buckles have an influence on Country Western dance style.

5. Consider the movement of a particular ethnic group and look carefully at their method of walking and their body movement. Is the upper body flexible or rigid above the waist? Basic body movements tend to reflect basic feelings and attitudes. Do they move quickly or slowly? Are they "happy go lucky," temperamental, quiet, or reserved?

■ *Teaching Style*

Some already have an innate sense of how to achieve style or have had a fair amount of dance training. Here the focus is making the dance style unique.

The average dancer has difficulty developing style and may feel that style is a nebulous thing or that the dance is for "fun" and is an end in itself.

1. The teacher must consciously incorporate the element of good style in his or her teaching, whether it's for a one-night stand, a class, or a performance.

2. The teacher, by virtue of his or her own posture, style of movement, and exemplification of different styles, sets an example—a visual one—that stimulates the dancer in an indirect way. A teacher should take every opportunity to attend workshops given by ethnic dance teachers to learn style firsthand. A live experience surpasses every written description.

3. The careful selection of music for each dance is important. A recording with native instruments, quality live music, and arrangements that are versatile and interesting all add flavor to the dance and encourage the dancer to aspire to better dancing.

4. In an atmosphere of gym shorts and tennis shoes, the teacher is challenged to promote appropriate style. All teachers know how much they may request students to bring shoes that will slide more easily and clothing that would be worn for informal dancing.

5. Special clothing frequently enhances the dance. Full skirts are very much a part of Mexican dances and Square Dances. The opanci—a soft, leather, moccasin-type shoe worn in Slavic dancing—allows for the rolling forward and backward action of the feet. This is a specific type of footwear that allows the feet to respond closely to the Slavic style. The movement pattern of the dance frequently relates to the costumes of the period and nationality.

6. The teacher should experience greater success in developing style among dancers when only a few specific suggestions are made for each dance presented.

7. The teacher should point out the exact position of hands in relation to the waist and clothing; the action of hands and arms as in the manipulation of a skirt; any unusual body position, as in arching the upper torso in a draw step; the position and interaction of the individual in relation to partner and group; the details of footwork in terms of length of step, foot mechanics, and quality of step; the

amount of energy expended in a movement; and the facial expression, including the focus of the eyes and the direction of the head.

8. The teacher should invite dance studio professionals, club dancers, foreign students, or community ethnic groups to dance with the students on special occasions or show films or videotapes of special styles. A visual experience with the real flavor of a dance often encourages dancers.

9. The use of mirrors and/or videotapes gives dancers an opportunity to see themselves and study specific movements.

10. Sometimes, if the teacher actually *moves* the dancers' arms or heads in the desired pattern, a kinesthetic sense of the movement is established, which is more meaningful than a verbal or a visual explanation.

11. The discipline that results from polishing a specific dance for an audience has a carry-over value for individual dancers as, subconsciously, they tend to apply better body control, precision, focus, and projection in their future dancing. Their attitudes and emotional responses are also different. To perform for others stimulates dancers to accept the demands of repetitive practice and achieve at a higher level. Even costuming excites and brings pleasure to the dancer.

4 American Dance Sampler

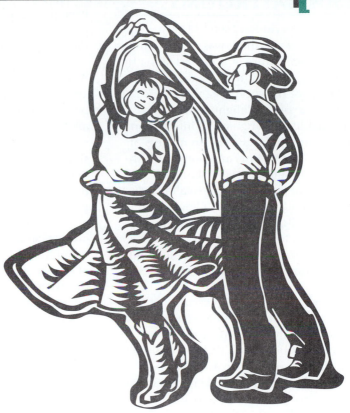

THE DANCES COVERED IN this chapter are those that the people–"the plain folk," "society," "young folk," "old folk," and "breadwinners"– enjoyed in the past for their own pleasure. Yesterday's Social Dances are today's Folk Dances.

Our dances come from several sources: the Country Dance tradition of England and Scotland, as evidenced by the Contra Dances; the Square and Circle Dances of New England; the Kentucky Running Sets of Appalachia; the Play Party Games; the dances of the French court; the Spanish–Mexican dances in the Southwest and early California; and the syncopated rhythms of the African Americans.

The dance scene in western Europe in the 1600s and 1700s was the foundation of our Social Dance tradition. English country dances were the rage in England and France. The French called them *contree-danse*.* The settlers brought these dances, the progressive longways for "as many as will" and the square formation, to the New World. There are records of Morris and Court dances, too.

---

*Contree-danse was shortened through usage to *Contre*. *Contre* dances were square and longways. In those days a "contre dance" (country dance) could be either formation. In 1918 Elizabeth Burchenal's *American Country Dances* book reflects "twenty–eight Contra Dances," quadrille, longways, and Sicilian Circle formation. Almost all the dances were from New England and reflected the notion that the terms "country dance" and "contra dance" were synonymous. At some point "contra dance" came to be applied only to progressive longway dances.

Country dancing in the United States was the primary recreation for all classes. The majority of the settlers in the North were lower and middle class. In the South some had more money and also had the assistance of the slaves to work the land, which meant they had more time for amusements. During the colonial period the upper class eventually began to dance the dances of the European courts.

DANCES FROM THE EUROPEAN COURTS TO THE AMERICAN BALLROOMS

Historians refer to the period of 1600 to 1700 as the Age of Enlightenment. Everything was ordered: the architecture, the nomenclature of flora and fauna by Linnaeus, the box hedges and the formal gardens, and even the dances of the courts. France was usually thought of as the base of the Enlightenment, and French was the established language of international diplomacy, culture, and polite society. In matters of dress, literature, art, architecture, and home furnishings, London set cultural models and standards that were accepted by all the colonies. The wealthy colonists sent their children "home" to England to be educated. With this cultural flow, it was natural for the latest Court dances to be very much a part of American society balls. Through mimicry, the bonded servants and slaves transplanted the court dances into their culture.

The sophisticated, polished group dances with set figures, such as the Minuet and Cotillon (sometimes referred to as the German dance), were the most popular dances at the balls before the Waltz. It was common to use European music in the American ballroom. The *Minuet* is based on triple meter, and it appeared in many formations: two men and a woman, longway sets (Ford 1943; p. 96), quadrille sets (Ford 1941; p. 35), and later as a couple dance (Ford 1943; p. 112). Every action was studied. The stately, stylized posturing, promenading, deep bows, and curtseys of the Minuet are an excellent example of a dance being influenced by the dress of the day; the elaborate headdresses, the heavy panniered skirts, and the powdered wigs of the women and the lace cuffs falling below the wrist and the brocade knee britches of the men reflected the style and the pattern of the Minuet. The Oxford Minuet is one of the variations of the Minuet still danced today. The *Gavotte*, closely related to the Minuet, preceded such familiar American round dances as the Badgers Gavotte and Glowworm Gavotte.

The Waltz, the Polka, and the Varsouvienne arrived on the Social Dance scene and sent couples whirling around the dance floor. The dancing master established his trade and traveled from town to town to teach the finer points of dance. Americans began to publish books such as *The Art of Dancing*, written by Edward Ferrero and published by Dick Fitzgerald in 1859.

THE UNIQUE CONTRIBUTIONS OF AFRICAN AMERICANS

In the history of European dance, the Spanish–Moorish dances express African characteristics, as do the musical rhythms of tambourines, castanets, and stringed instruments. Some Catholic fiesta dances from the Middle Ages have links with Africa. Indirectly the African influence was brought to the New World by the Europeans.

As a direct influence, consider the eight million Africans who were imported as slaves during the 17th and 18th centuries. African Americans in the South brought with them the most primitive instrument of all–the human body. Bare feet stomped, hands clapped, and voices sang songs, albeit aboard a slave ship, on the auction block, or on their white master's plantation. Dancing, whether by command or choice, furnished a meaningful link with the past and a temporary escape from the present.

Dancing depended on the whims of the white owners. Some encouraged dancing and even provided the fiddle, thus recognizing dance as a means of entertainment for both the African Americans and their owners. A good fiddler was prized by his owner not only for his ability to play for plantation balls, but also for the higher price he brought at auction. It was common for African American musicians to furnish music for dancing at the Big House, and many times they also called out the dance figures.

Whereas Europeans traditionally accent the first beat of a measure, African Americans accent the second beat, the upbeat. Soon beats were skipped and the accent was placed on unexpected counts. This different accent is now labeled syncopation. As the result of an uprising in 1739, the slaves were forbidden to use drums, so they transferred their rhythm to their feet, shook tambourines (perhaps acquired from the Spanish Creoles of the South), clacked bones (like castanets), and changed the African bonja (gourd with strings) to the banjo.

African American dancing was generally of two kinds: dance movements that pantomimed animals and highly acrobatic movements that required endurance and skill. The *Pigeon Wing*, *Buzzard Lope*, and *Turkey Trot* mimed animal movement and, as in the case of the Buzzard Lope, acted out the story of a buzzard seeking and finding food. The *Buck* and the *Jig* dances were of the individual acrobatic type and were the objects of dance contests sponsored by the white owners. The *Cake Walk*, although used in contests, was mostly a festival dance common at harvest or crop-over times. Many of the dances were done with a container of water placed on the head–a continuation of the African custom of carrying burdens in this manner.

The house servants were the link between the Big House and the field hands in matters of manners and fashions. It was through them that the field hands learned the fashionable quadrilles, cotillon, reels, and big circles of the day. In the latter days of slavery, white influence was very apparent in black dance.

African Americans enjoyed dancing on special occasions such as Christmas, corn shucking, quilting bees, weddings, and funerals, but most of all on Saturday nights. Saturday night was a celebration of the end of the work week and was looked forward to and sung about in the fields all week in anticipation. Dancing included set dances (squares), quadrilles, Jigs, cutting the Pigeon Wings, Cake Walks, and Virginia Reels.

From the days before the American Civil War came such folk dances as Juba, Ole Aunt Kate, Jimmie Rose, Brother Eprum, Got Corn, and Gone On. Juba was quite famous in Georgia and the Carolinas. It was considered a simplified version of the African *Giouba*. The *Shout* and *Ring Shout* were sacred dances that remained on the plantations and in the Protestant churches. Shuffling, clapping, and singing in a ring that circled around and around was a way of retaining some vestige of their African heritage.

New dances continue to appear from the African American culture's never-ending creativity. African Americans have made a major contribution to American music and dance.

THE SPANISH-MEXICAN INFLUENCE

The explorers and colonizers from Spain came across the Caribbean to Mexico and Central and South America and eventually to the American Southwest and California. Although they tried to colonize New Mexico during the 1500s, the Spanish rule and culture were not established there until 1692. The New Mexican colonial dances, Spanish in origin, also reflect the influence of the native Pueblo Indians of the area. Although both the Spanish and English claimed California, the first settlement, in San Diego in 1769, was Spanish and the Franciscan fathers soon began to establish some 21 missions along the coast.

Two types of Spanish dance were brought to America: the classical dance by the Spanish artists who set up schools in the East and the dances of the people brought along by the colonists, which were later influenced by the native Mexicans. The second type is seen mostly in the Southwest and California. The early isolation of the territories resulted in the dances becoming well established, thus retaining their European characteristics. The music and dance forms were the social dances of the settlers during this era. El Jarabe, El Fandango, La Bamba, and the Minuet were some of the oldest dances. Song games such as El Burro and El Caballo, and the Fandangos, Bailes, and Fiestas were all a part of this early tradition.

DANCES OF THE PEOPLE

It is important to remember that the social dances traveled from the court to the middle-class drawing-room to the dance hall just as the dances of the common people moved upward to elite society. This phenomenon occurred in the 1600s just as it does today, the dances taking on the flavor of local traditions and the manners of a given lifestyle.

■ *Square Dances*

The American Square Dance is truly a product of American culture, although it originated with the Quadrilles of the French court and the Country Dances of England and Scotland. The prompter became the caller who cued the dancers and established the rhythm of the dance with a running pattern of rhymes along with figure commands. Refer to Chapter 5, Square Dance, History, for further elaboration.

■ *Play Party Games*

Play Party Games, sometimes referred to as Folk Games, are actually dances. They were developed mostly by the early settlers in Tennessee, Kentucky, West Virginia, and Ohio, and traveled westward with the pioneers. The dancers made their own music by singing the verses and the people on the sidelines joined in the song, clapping their hands and stamping their feet to add to the jollity of the occasion.

American Play Party Games were definitely courtship dances that were eagerly endorsed by the young people. Although many religious groups opposed dancing and thought the fiddle was an instrument of the devil, Play Party Games (as opposed to the Hoedowns*) were approved by the elders, because even they remembered playing the same games when they were courting. The simplicity, the social interchange, and the opportunity for young

---

*Although *Hoedown* is a dance step (a clog dance step or heel and toe), the term eventually was used to refer to rural dancing with instrumental music, usually fiddlers.

people to "kick up their heels" all contributed to the spread of Play Party Games, particularly in rural America where people had to rely on their own resourcefulness for their amusements.

The songs and figures of many Play Party Games came originally from Scotland, England, Ireland, and Germany, where they were among the customs and the traditions that the early settlers brought with them from the Old Country.** Similar types of dances, such as Old Dan Tucker, Paw Paw Patch, Bingo, Yankee Doodle, and Shoo Fly, are as American as apple pie. They were passed from one generation to the next by word of mouth, and, of course, many versions of a song or a dance appeared for the same tune. Today, many of these same Play Party Games are kept alive as children's dances in elementary schools or by fun-loving recreational leaders who incorporate them into one-night stands and parties for young people, suggesting some of the charm and dramatics that accompany the dance. With this spirit, modern dancers enjoy them just as much as the pioneers did.

■ *Round and Novelty Dances*

The American dancing public quickly adopted the Waltz, the Polka, the Schottische, and the Varsouvienne as their favorites. From these couple dances, the popular round dance movement was born. Newly arranged dances done to popular tunes based on basic steps appeared regularly. After World War II, this practice mushroomed. A similar situation occurred in the 1600s: when John Playford's *English Dancing Master* first appeared, it contained 104 dances; 17 editions later, 918 dances were included. With the mass of newly composed American Round Dances, the prompter has again appeared on the scene to cue the dancers through the sequence. The old favorites persist and are referred to as old-time dances or pattern dances. The newly composed ones are here today, gone tomorrow.

Nonpartner dances like Ten Pretty Girls have mushroomed since World War II, and even more so in the '80s and '90s. Today the trend for set patterns to peppy tunes like Twelfth Street Rag, or dances like Amos Moses, the Hustle, and Achy Breaky all become a part of the scene.

■ *Contra Dances*

The English Longway Dances, Irish Cross-Road Dances, and Scottish Reels are the backbone of American Contra dancing. Contra dancing was best known in New England. It is currently enjoying a surge of

popularity all over the United States and the world. Refer to Contra Dance History in Chapter 6.

■ *Appalachian Clog Dances*

The popularity of the *Appalachian Clog Dance* has continued to grow throughout the United States since the mid-1960s. Clogging is believed to have originated in the Appalachian Mountains. There are three styles of clogging: freestyle clogging (which evolved from buck dancing), square dance clogging, and precision clogging. Refer to History of Clogging on page 88.

■ *Cajun Dance*

Cajun dance is an excellent example of a dance tradition whose roots go back to France. In 1604 the French colony of Acadie was established in Nova Scotia. Eventually the colonists were deported and a large number migrated to Louisiana. Cajun music and dance is a live tradition that has evolved from contact with the French, Spanish, English, black Creoles, East Texans, even rock and roll. Only a few dances remain, but they are very popular. Refer to Cajun Dance, page 367.

MUSIC

The tunes for dance came from the Old World, dance patterns blending with the new environment, variants and new dances arising with westward expansion, and transmission from generation to generation. The Ballroom Dances used the European melodies. Eventually, new tunes were created for dance.

The violin (fiddle) has long been the traditional instrument for dance accompaniment. In New England the transverse or German flute was also used along with the violin in the late 18th century. The banjo, the guitar, the bass, and the harmonica are frequently parts of the musical group. Different sections of the country favored special instruments, usually developed from the settlers' own creativity, for they were long accustomed to "makin' out" with whatever they had and using substitutes. The mountain folk of Appalachia made a cornstock fiddle for their children; a long-necked gourd became a "banjer"; the mouth harp, a small whistle imitating a recorder; and the dulcimer. But the fiddle was their favorite. In the absence of musicians, the hand clapping and feet stomping of spectators and/or the patter rhymes of the caller established a rhythm and excitement for square dancers. Play Party Games illustrate a group of courting dances that move to the joyous singing of the dancers. Military brass bands were popular in America in the mid-1800s for fancy balls, but for the parlor or drawing-room a piano or a violin alone was

---

**For example: "Ach Ja," Germany; "Ja Saa," Norway; "A Hunting We Will Go," England; "Pop Goes the Weasel," England.

preferred. A combination of two violins, flute, clarinet, cornet, and bass was used, however, in larger rooms.

One way or another, if the people wanted to dance, they made their own music even when a musician was not present. Although live music is always vibrant and stimulating, the record player and tape recorder make it possible for more people to dance to good authentic recordings. True music for recreational folk dancing is growing.

DRESS

The clothing that a particular class of people wore during a particular era is the clue to what they wore for dancing. The lower classes and the working classes have traditionally worn garments that fit more loosely and allow greater freedom of movement. The construction and the material of shoes determined the action of the feet (for example, the boots of a cowboy). Fancy ball gowns represent just one class of American society. Wigs and panniers were worn in colonial times, hoops in antebellum and Civil War times, and bustles in the 1870s and 1880s. The garments definitely restricted the movement of the dancers. Probably one of the greatest changes in style for women occurred when Irene Castle wore clothing of lightweight material and full skirts, thus setting a casual style.

Almost anything goes as long as the dancer is comfortable. Whether a woman wears a dress, slacks, Levis, or shorts, she is more concerned about dancing for fun and is likely to wear what her peers do. But, without a doubt, the graceful movement of a full skirt enhances many a dance.

A SOCIAL OCCASION

Dancing is a social occasion. It is a time to visit, to greet, to meet new people, to court, and to celebrate. Whenever people gathered together for barn raisings or quilting parties, the dancing began when the work was accomplished. Different parts of the country had their traditions, but, from the beginning, pushing back the furniture in the kitchen (New England) or dancing on the porch (Appalachia) was a common practice. Eventually, the school house, the Grange, the barn, and, in the warmer climates of California and the Southwest, the courtyards, allowed for more couples on the floor. To be sure, the upper level of society had their ballrooms and others had their dance halls and saloons. But, for a large segment of America, dancing was a family affair. The stories of bundling children down at Square Dances on the frontier are common. With the advent of nightclubs, children were no longer part of the adult dance scene. Granges, community clubs, some churches, and some ethnic groups sponsor dances where children are welcome.

Although the dancing masters helped to establish the etiquette of the period for the upper class, the plain folk were also concerned with courtesy in dance. It is interesting to note the presence of the "address, honor, and salute" in the dances of the court (Minuet, Lancers, Quadrilles) and the absence of them in the Kentucky Running Set and Play Party Games. "Honor your partner" is part of the Square Dance tradition; yet it is absent in the Big Circle, Contra, and Sicilian Circle.

The social dances of a particular era reflect the social customs of that era. At Contra Dances in the 1990s the practice of changing partners after each Contra leads to a scramble for the next partner of choice, leaving the last partner in the middle of the floor; either person may ask another for the next dance. From the disco period, two or more people of the same sex might dance together or even one dance alone. Country Western dancers follow the older tradition of always escorting their partner back to the side.

The social dances are a vital part of the school recreational program. More churches today incorporate dancing activities into their recreational programs. And dance clubs and dance halls specialize in different kinds of social dance.

REVIVAL OF FOLK TRADITIONS

Prior to the First World War, folk traditions began to be revived. Folk dance was introduced in public schools and was encouraged by the efforts of Henry Ford and the activities of the WPA during the Depression. After World War II another surge of interest came, particularly in square dancing. Ballroom dancing has returned, especially Swing. In the '90s Contra and Country Western are extremely popular.

Country dancing is a term that has returned to common usage. The cornerstone to the revival of old-time country dancing is live music. Contras and Squares dominate the program with a few Round Dances, ranging from a Waltz to a lively Polka, with Mixers sprinkled in. Because dancing is definitely a social occasion, dancers change partners after every Contra or after two Squares. The dancers enjoy variety but do not care to remember sequences from one week to the next. The caller gives a quick walk-thru and away they go.

More opportunities for the family to dance together are created. Dance programs and family camps consider the range of abilities. Adults who have had their children later like having the family dance together. More dances are scheduled for seniors. They enjoy the dances of the '40s and also pattern dances.

THE MELTING POT VERSUS ETHNIC IDENTITY

The colonists, the immigrants, the explorers, the slaves–each brought their culture and their dance with them, blending their ways with the New World as they established roots. Many were anxious to lose their Old World identity and their old languages and traditions and take on the new ways quickly. Yet others clung together, still holding fast to their traditions and continuing to pass these down to their children even while they learned the American way of life. The Greek communities illustrate this point well, particularly at their weddings and baptisms.

The concept of the melting pot dominated American thinking until around 1940. Then interest in ethnic identity, particularly among the minorities, began to grow. Native Americans, Hispanics, and African Americans have received in recent years considerable federal assistance to reinforce their ethnic heritages. As a result, other ethnic groups have found a rekindled interest in keeping their traditions alive and meaningful, including music, dance, dress, and art.

All Americans have benefited from this movement. Each group has greater pride and all Americans have gained a greater understanding and appreciation for the contributions that each group has made to society.

CONCLUSION

The sampler of the dances of the American people was presented to illustrate the cultural patterns, beginning in 1620 and continuing to the present. The dances that have been included in this chapter are viable in that they trace a dance tradition, are still danced today in the communities (in schools, recreational groups, and dance halls), and represent various dance formations and basic dance steps. At different times in history, each type has enjoyed great popularity in a particular area and with a special segment of society.

This chapter also includes contemporary folk dances, recently composed. Some follow a pattern from long ago; many are composed to popular tunes; some are line dances, which not only accommodates situations where there is an unequal number of men and women, but allows for individuals "to do their own thing." Many are mixer–type dances, which allows for changing partners. In the past many of these dances would be considered "ice breakers." Most of these dances are *pattern dances*, set sequences (the exceptions would be the Waltz, Polka, Schottische, and Two–Steps) and therefore are placed in the folk dance section as opposed to the Social Dance chapter.

The diversity of American traditional folk dance continues to flourish as a means of understanding our heterogenous heritage. And it allows for countless opportunities of social exchange and recreation. Yes, American dance is alive and doing well!

TEACHING SUGGESTIONS

■ *Various Approaches*

1. **American Dance Sampler.** The Big Circle Square dances include examples of the following: Quadrille, Square Dance, Contra, Play Party Games, Round Dances, and Mixers. A sampling of these types reinforces the history of our dance.

2. **Basic steps and formations:** Select dances that include walk, Schottische, Two–Step, Polka, Waltz, Mazurka, and nonpartner, couples, Square, set of three, Longway, and Circle with sets of two couples.

3. **Old–time dances, novelty dances, mixers.**

4. **Exhibition dances:** Prepare for a program and/or incorporate customs, dances, and costumes with a theme illustrating an American tradition, such as a kitchen junket, fiesta, quilting bee, or barn raising.

5. **Party time or special fun dance:** Plan a class period or a special event to dance the favorites of the group with a theme, a few traditions, maybe a game, a song, or a skit. Encourage dancers to dress specially for the event, and plan refreshments to relate to the era or the theme.

6. **Local community identity:** Relate choice of material to local community, particularly local ethnic groups, and invite local citizens to share their talents with the group.

7. **Related curriculum:** Wherever possible, relate American dances to other subjects in the school curriculum or to local events.

Grand March

Let the dance begin! The *Grand March* has long been a part of American dance tradition. At ceremonial occasions and balls, the instrumental groups would play a short concert prior to the dancing. Then the floor managers of the ball would signal for the dance to begin: The instrumentalists would play a march and the couples would begin a grand promenade around the room for the Grand March. Today, for special occasions, dance festivals, and one–night stand dance parties, the Grand March is part of the program. It may not be first but perhaps after the intermission. Dancers look forward to that moment of everyone dancing together, winding in and out from one pattern to the next.

The Grand March may be used as an end in itself, since it is impressive and stimulates group feeling, or it may be used as a means for organizing a group quickly for another activity. A Grand March is most effective when many people participate. Since guests do not always arrive punctually, this fact should always be considered in scheduling a Grand March.

Dance A While CD: #5 "Grand March."

Music: Any lively March, Two–Step, or Square Dance tune.

Position: Escort.

Formation: Double circle, couples facing the line of direction, or two single files, men in one and women in the other.

DIRECTIONS FOR THE GRAND MARCH

■ Leadership

The leader stands at either the front or the rear of the room. A change in pattern is indicated as the group nears the leader. It is helpful if the first two or three couples are familiar with the various figures to be used in the Grand March. Experienced couples will follow the leader's cues more easily and set the pattern for the others to follow. An assistant standing at the opposite end from the leader facilitates the flow.

■ Beginning

A Grand March may be started either in couples or from two single files of individuals. The latter is particularly suited for groups not already acquainted.

1. **Two single files:** Men line up on one side of the room and women on the other. Both files face either the front or the rear of the room as indicated by the leader. **Note:** The leader must be careful to indicate the proper direction for the two files to face so that the women will be on the right side of the men when couples are formed. Each line marches toward the end of the room, turns, and marches toward the opposite line. The files meet, forming couples in escort position, ladies to the right of the men, and march down the center of the room.

2. **Couples in a double circle:** Couples in escort position form a double circle and march counterclockwise. One couple is selected as the leader and that couple, followed by the others, moves down the center of the room.

Grand March (continued)

■ Figures

These figures may be used in any order as long as they flow from one to the other.

1. **Single files**

    A. **Inner and outer circle.** When each couple reaches the front of the room, partners separate, men left and women right, and travel down the side of the room until they meet at the opposite end. Then the lines pass each other. The women travel on the inside, men on the outside, and down the side of the room until they meet again at the front of the room. They pass again, the men traveling on the inside, women on the outside, and down the sides of the room.

    B. **The Cross (X).** When each file reaches the rear corner, the leader of each file makes an abrupt turn and travels diagonally toward the front corner on the opposite side. Both files cross in the center of the room, lady crossing in front of partner. The files travel down the side of the room toward the rear corners. The diagonal cross is repeated, the man crossing in front of his partner.

    C. **Virginia Reel.** Couples move down the center in double file. When each couple reaches the front of the room, partners separate, men left, women right, and travel down the sides of the room to form two files about 10 to 15 feet apart. Both lines face each other. The head woman and the foot man meet in the middle and dance away. Then the head man and foot woman meet in the middle in like manner and dance away. This process is repeated until all have partners and are dancing.

2. **Couples**

    A. **Four, eight, or sixteen abreast.** When the couples marching down the center arrive at the front of the room, the lead couple turns to the right, marches to the side of the room, and back toward the rear of the room. The second couple turns left, the third right, and so on, and march to the side and back to the rear of the room. When they meet at the rear of the room, the two approaching couples march down the center of the room together, thus forming a group of four abreast. At the front of the room each group of four marches alternately to the right and left, down the sides and at the rear of the room they form a line eight abreast. The same procedure is followed to form lines of 16 or more abreast. After the group has formed lines of 16 abreast they may be instructed to mark time in place.

    B. **"Ring up" for squares.** If groups of eight are desired for the next activity, for example, a Square Dance, the couples mark time when they are eight abreast. Each line of eight then "rings up," or makes a circle.

    C. **Over and under.** When the couples are four abreast, the two couples separate at the front of the room, one turning right, the other left. When the couples meet at the rear of the room, the first couple of the double file on the right side of the room makes an arch. The first couple of the other double file goes under the arch and quickly makes an arch for the second couple they meet. All couples in both double files are alternately making an arch or traveling under an arch.

    D. **Snake out.** When the couples are 8 or 16 abreast, the person on the right end of the front line leads that line in single file to the right of the column of dancers and in between lines two and three. As the person on the left end of the first line passes the person on the right end of the second line, they join hands and line two then follows line one. The leader then leads the line between lines three and four and again as the last person in the moving line passes the right end of the third line, they join hands and line three joins with lines one and two. The moving line weaves in and out of the remaining lines and each time the person on the end of the moving line passes the right end of the next line they join hands and continue weaving in and out. After all lines have been "snaked out," the leader may lead the line in serpentine fashion around the room and eventually circles the room clockwise in a single circle, all facing the center.

E. **Danish march.** When the couples are in a double circle or double file, partners face and stand about 4 feet apart. The first couple joins hands holding arms out shoulder height and slides the length of the formation used. The second couple follows, and so on. When couples reach the end, they join the group. This may be repeated with partners standing back to back as they slide.

F. **Grand right and left.** When couples are in a single circle, partners face and start a grand right and left. This may continue until partners meet or until the leader signals for new partners to be taken for a promenade or other figure.

G. **Paul Jones.** When couples are in a single circle, any of the figures for a Paul Jones may be used. See p. 80.

■ *Ending*

There is no set ending for a Grand March. However, the ending should be definite so that there is a feeling of completion and satisfaction. It may end with people in groups for the next activity or in a circle with everyone joining in a song or dancers may swing into a Waltz, a Polka, or some other planned activity.

Virginia Reel

THE *VIRGINIA REEL*, KNOWN as Sir Roger de Coverley in England, was first published about 1685. This was one of many dances the colonists brought to America, and the name eventually changed to Virginia Reel. It was danced in the ballrooms and on the village greens, by all. The Virginia Reel is a Contra Dance that children today learn in school and fondly remember as part of their American heritage of dance. Adults enjoy the dance at one–night stands and family gatherings.

Virginia Reel is a traditional Contra. It is a longways dance and there is progression (the top couple moves to the bottom at the end of the dance). The directions presented are for one of the common ways that recreational groups dance the Virginia Reel today because everyone is dancing most of the time.

Dance A While CD: #17 "Irish Washerwoman."

Records: "Irish Washerwoman" or any good Hoedown. DC 162303; EZ 706, 728; FD LP 3; Grenn 16016; High/Scope RM3; Mac 7345; MAV Album 3; MH 74; WT 10023.

Cassettes: DC 162303, 487; MH C74; High/Scope RM3.

Music: Irish Jig tune such as "Irish Washerwoman."

Meter: 6/8

Formation: Contra Dance formation. Four to eight couples, partners facing.

Virginia Reel (continued)

A1   **Forward and bow** (8 counts). Lines walk forward, curtsey and bow to partners, and walk backward to place.

      Forward and right hand 'round (8 counts). Lines walk forward, partners join right hands, turn clockwise once around, and move backward to place.

A2   **Forward and left hand 'round** (8 counts). Lines walk forward, partners join left hands, turn counterclockwise once around, and move backward to place.

      Forward and two hands 'round (8 counts). Lines walk forward, partners join two hands, turn clockwise once around, and move backward to place.

B1   **Forward and do–si–do** (8 counts). Lines walk forward, partners do–si–do, and move backward to place.

      Head couple sashays down the center and back (8 counts).

B2   **Head couple, right arm to partner and reels** (sequences of 8 counts). To reel, partners hook right elbows in middle of set and turn clockwise once and a half, separate; head man turns next woman counterclockwise in line, with left elbows hooked once around as head woman turns next man in line with left elbows hooked once around; head couple meets in middle of set, partners hook right elbows, turn clockwise once around. Head couple moves down set turning alternately next person in line with left elbow and then each other with right elbow, until they reach foot of set.

      Head couple sashays back. Partners turn each other a half–turn (now on original side), join two hands, slide to head of set.

      Head couple casts off, forms an arch. Partners separate and walk down outside of set, man left, woman right, to foot of set. Each person in line follows the head person, single file. Head couple join two hands to form an arch at foot of set.

      Pass through and form your sets. Partners join inside hands as they go through arch and promenade to head of set. Head couple is now at foot; original second couple is now head couple.

Continue to repeat dance until couples are back to original positions. Wait for the beginning of a new phrase to repeat the dance.

■ **NOTE**

Although most figures are based on 8 counts, the number of couples in a set influences the length of the music for one complete round of the dance.

Grand Square Quadrille

THE QUADRILLES ORIGINATED IN the French court ballet, became established in the British Isles, and were very popular among the colonists in America. Quadrilles are still danced today, particularly in New England. The Quadrille originally had six parts (Czarnowski 1950; p. 141), but later was shortened to five parts. A different piece of music is played for each figure, with a pause between figures for the dancers to catch their breath and an introduction of music before each figure. Eventually the

Quadrille was reduced to three parts. The numbering of couples differs from Square Dances in that the head couples are 1 and 2, side couples, 3 and 4. Quadrilles are traditionally **prompted;** that is, the caller gives the name of the figure.

Grand Square Quadrille is still danced today, particularly in New England. This version is based on a call by Bob Osgood of Sets In Order American Square Dance Society. Although the call **grand square** is known today by square dancers as one of the basics and is used as a break in Square Dance, the figure as such was part of many of the Lancers, namely the fourth figure (Czarnowski 1950; p. 145).

> **Records:** Any march music may be used. Suggested records: Folkraft 102; EZ 717, 730; LS E–34; E 34.

> **Formation:** Set of four couples in Square Dance formation. Couples are numbered as in square dancing today.

DIRECTIONS FOR THE DANCE

Meter 4/4

■ *Measures*

1–2	Introduction (8 counts): no action.
1–4	**Grand square** (16 counts). See Square Dance section, grand square, pp. 144–145, for directions.
5–8	**Reverse grand square** (16 counts).

Figure I

9–12	**Head couples right and left through and back** (16 counts).
13–16	**Side couples right and left through and back** (16 counts).
9–12	**Head couples to the right, right and left through and back** (16 counts).
13–16	**Side couples to the right, right and left through and back** (16 counts).

Chorus

1–4	**Grand square** (16 counts).
5–8	**Reverse grand square** (16 counts).

Figure II

9–12	**Head women chain over and back** (16 counts).
13–16	**Side women chain over and back** (16 counts).
9–12	**Head women to the right, chain over and back** (16 counts).
13–16	**Side women to the right, chain over and back** (16 counts).

Chorus

1–4	**Grand square** (16 counts).
5–8	**Reverse grand square** (16 counts).

Figure III

9–12	**Head couples half–promenade and right and left home** (16 counts).
13–16	**Side couples half–promenade and right and left home** (16 counts).
9–12	**Head couples half–promenade right and right and left home** (16 counts). Couples 1 and 2 (couples 3 and 4) half–promenade with each other and right and left home.
13–16	**Side couples half–promenade right and right and left home** (16 counts). Couples 2 and 3 (couples 4 and 1) half–promenade with each other and right and left home.

Grand Square Quadrille (continued)

Chorus

1–4   **Grand square** (16 counts).

5–8   **Reverse grand square** (16 counts).

■ **NOTES**

1. The caller prompts by giving the directions for the next maneuver on the last two to four counts of the preceding eight–count phrase.

2. Dancers dance to the music, using the exact number of beats to execute each maneuver, with action flowing from one pattern to the next.

Paul Jones Your Lady

During the 19th century, the group dances with set figures, like the Quadrille, the Lancers, and the *Paul Jones*, allowed for the interchange of partners. Paul Jones, formerly danced in the ballroom and frequently used as the first dance at a party, is still danced today as a lively mixer. In some parts of the West, the same dance is called *Circle Two-Step* or *Brownee*.

Music: Any lively two-step.

Position: Promenade.

Formation: Double circle, couples facing line of direction.

Steps: Shuffle, Two–Step.

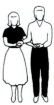

DIRECTIONS FOR THE MIXER

The leader calls out each figure and signals clearly. Each figure is danced briefly as it is merely a method of changing partners.

  I. Paul Jones Your Lady or Promenade

     Couples promenade around room in one large circle.

  II. Figures

    A. **Single circle.** Couples form a single circle, hands joined. Slide left, right, and/or shuffle to center and back. Each man takes his corner woman for a new partner.

    B. **The basket.** Women form an inner circle, hands joined and slide left. Men form an outer circle, hands joined, and slide right. Both circles stop. Men raise joined hands. Women move backward through arches made by men and stand beside a man. Men lower arms. Everyone slides left, then right. Each man takes woman on right for a new partner.

    C. **Across the circle.** Couples form a single circle, hands joined. Slide left, right, and shuffle to center, back, and center. Each man takes woman across the circle as a new partner.

    D. **Grand right and left.** Couples form a single circle, hands joined. Slide left, right, and shuffle to center and back. Face partner and grand right and left around the circle. Each man takes woman facing him or lady whose hand he holds when leader signals for new partners.

E. **Gentlemen kneel.** Couples form single circle and face partners. Men kneel, women move in reverse line of direction, weaving in and out between kneeling men. Each man takes woman facing him when leader signals for new partners.

F. **Count off.** Double circle, couples facing counterclockwise. Women stand still and men move forward, counting off as many women as indicated by leader. Men may stand still while women move forward and count off in like manner.

III. Two–Step

Couples in closed position, Two–Step about the room. Upon signal "Paul Jones Your Lady," they again fall into a double circle and promenade counterclockwise around room until the signal for a new figure action is given.

Ninepin Reel

Ninepin REEL IS DANCED traditionally in America and England and was formerly known in Scotland. There are variations of figures but all have the common figure of five men circling in the center of the square and suddenly a break occurs; all choose a new partner; obviously, one is not able to claim a partner, and thus there's a new "ninepin." Some American versions have a caller who calls various Square Dance figures and when the call "ninepin" occurs, each man changes partners and once again there is a new "ninepin."

Elizabeth Burchenal in *American Country Dance* (1918; pp. 61–62) has recorded two Quadrille dances from New England with an extra man in the center: John Brown and Old Dan Tucker. There are dances for nine in Scotland, England, America, Germany, Sweden, and Finland with different names and many variations, from simple musical game types to very complicated figures.

This particular version was presented to Skandia Folkdance Society about 1952 by a Canadian couple attending summer school in Seattle, Washington. The pattern is similar to the English dance, Cumberland Square Eight.

Records: Any reel music. E2 5008.

Formation: Set of four couples in Square Dance formation. Extra man or woman stands in middle of set and is referred to as "ninepin." In this case, directions assume "ninepin" is a man. If more than one set, arrange sets in file and line formation.

Steps: Slide, buzz step, Polka, shuffle.

Ninepin Reel (continued)

DIRECTIONS FOR THE DANCE

Meter 2/4 • Directions are the same for both woman and man, except when specially noted.

■ *Measures*

Figure I. Slides

1–4   In closed position, head couples take eight slides (man beginning left, woman right) across set, exchanging places. Couples pass to the **right** of the "ninepin." If more than one set, couples may travel through other sets in a straight line, always passing to the right of "ninepin." Couples **do not** turn at end of eight slides.

5–8   Head couples take eight slides (man beginning right, woman left) to return home, passing to **left** of "ninepin" (women's backs to "ninepin").

9–16   Side couples repeat action of measures 1–8.

Figure II. Circle left and right

17–24   Head couples join hands in circle ("ninepin" in middle) and circle left, taking eight slides or four Polka steps; circle right, taking eight slides or four Polka steps.

25–32   Side couples repeat action of Figure II, measures 17–24.

Figure III. Swing

1–16   "Ninepin" swings (waist swing, buzz step) woman of couple 1 (8–count swing). While "ninepin" swings, displaced partner moves to center of set and waits for each displaced partner to join him. At completion of swing, woman returns home; "ninepin" travels around set to each couple (2, 3, 4), swinging each woman and each displaced partner moves to center; women remain in home position.

Figure IV. Circle

16–23   At conclusion of last swing, "ninepin" travels to center to join the four men. All men join hands, circle left and right, taking Polka steps or slides. **At any point, "ninepin," as he takes woman of his choice, calls "break."** Other men hurry to take new partner. Everyone swings to completion of musical phrase. Obviously, there is a new "ninepin." Couples take home position of woman to swing and to repeat dance.

Figure V. Swing

24–32   All couples swing (see note 3).

■ NOTES

1. Ninepin Reel is obviously a rollicking, fun-loving mixer that absorbs extra people. Remember the "ninepin" can be a man or a woman and each set can differ.

2. Everyone enjoys sliding (galloping) through more than one set, sometimes the length of the hall. Dance etiquette implies that one couple does not pass a preceding couple while galloping.

3. In Figures IV and V, if the "ninepin" is a real "swinger," he might call "break" after a couple measures of circling; whereupon there is a longer swing. On the other hand, the "ninepin" may prefer to complete the circling figure and call "break" at measure 24. The element of suspense created by the "ninepin" deliberately waiting until the last minute to indicate his choice of partner adds to the spirit of the dance.

4. Extra dancers on the sideline have been known to cut in when the "ninepin" calls "break," by casually waiting behind a couple. Someone from the original set must retreat to the sidelines or cut in on someone else at the earliest opportunity.

Portland Fancy

Portland Fancy IS A traditional Contra.

Records: "Portland Fancy," Folkraft 1131, 1243; EZ 4004, 5003; Fretless FR203; or similar Jig.

Cassette: New England Chestnuts ACL 203/4.

Music: "Portland Fancy," Ford, Henry, *Good Morning*, 4th edition, p. 52; "Portland Fancy" and "Blackberry Quadrille," Page, Ralph, *An Elegant Collection of Contras and Squares*, pp. 78, 79.

Formation: Sets of four couples, Contra formation, two couples facing two couples. Sets may be in a circle.

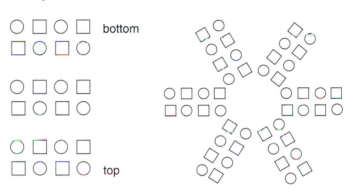

Line formation   Circle formation

DIRECTIONS FOR THE DANCE

A1 **Circle left eight hands around** (16 counts).

A2 **Right and left thru, right and left back** (16 counts). Opposite couples, right and left.

B1 **Ladies chain over and back** (16 counts).

B2 **Forward and back** (8 counts). Join hands in line, take four steps forward and four steps back. **Forward again and pass thru and face a new foursome** (8 counts).

■ *Variation*

Pass through two groups and face a new foursome.

Big Circle Square Dance

VERY MUCH ALIVE TODAY in the southern Appalachian region and a variant of the Running Set is *Big Circle Square Dance*, a dance known by many names, such as the Mountain Square Dance, Appalachian Big Circle, and Great Circle.

It is interesting to note that the concept of the Big Circle with sets of two couples (active and inactive couples, or odds and evens) is known throughout the United States. New England does a version referred to as the Circle, Sicilian Circle, or Cirassian Circle, which has traveled to the four corners of our country. In 1945, when the authors were teaching at the University of Texas, the Big Circle was a common dance, both as a traditional form in the community and as a teaching method for Square Dance.

The Big Circle Square Dance has much in common with the Kentucky Running Set. At this time, there is an effort to differentiate between the two. Glenn Bannerman, pro–fessor of recreation and outdoor education, Presbyterian School of Christian Education, Richmond, Virginia, has researched and assisted in keeping the western North Carolina style alive. The ideas presented follow this style.

The Big Circle Square Dance is a social occasion. The dancers come to see their friends, and during the Big Circle, friends greet one another and quiet exchanges of news may go on during the dance. It differs from the Kentucky Running Set as follows: A walking step is danced even on the swing and is referred to as "smooth dancing," or single– and double–clog steps, by the spirited dancers; the Varsouvienne position is used for the promenade; and there are more people involved, maybe as many as 50 in a circle, all couples dancing and the figures changing frequently.

Records: Many tunes available. Appalachian Clog Dancing & Big Circle Mountain Square Dancing AR53C; Big Circle Mountain Dance Music LP 36L; Big Circle Mountain Square Dancing AR 52L; "Boil Them Cabbages Down," MacGregor 1100; Country Dance Album CLR 16L; Dances from Appalachia II BER 2L; Mountain Dance Music Comes Alive AR 82L; Old–Time Music Dance Party FF 415L; "Old Joe Clark," Folkraft 1071.

Cassettes: Appalachian Clog Dancing & Big Circle Mountain Square Dancing AR53C; Country Dance Album CLR 16C; Dances from Appalachia I BER 1C; Mountain Dance Music Comes Alive AR 82C; Old–Time Music Dance Party FF 415C.

Formation: Couples, woman on partner's right, in large single circle. Even–numbered couples. Prior to dancing, determine head couple and number couples 1, 2, 1, 2, and so forth, so that at the call "odd couple out to the even couple," couple 1 moves into the circle (backs to center) to face couple 2 (face center). Couple 1 always progresses on the inside in the line of direction (counterclockwise) to the next couple; couple 2 progresses on the outside in the reverse line of direction (clockwise).

Steps and Style: A walking step, even on the swing, swing position. When moving in one large circle or in small circles, joined hands are held at shoulder height. Promenade in Varsouvienne position.

The Caller: Preferably the caller (lead man or lady of head couple) calls from the floor while dancing. If the group is large, then he or she stands by the musicians and uses a microphone.

DIRECTIONS FOR THE DANCE

The caller uses a variety of figures, one pattern leading to the next. The basic structure includes: an introduction (with the whole group in a large circle), a series of figures (with the group in small circles), and a closing (with the group in a large circle again).

■ INTRODUCTION

Large–circle figures are called involving the whole group in a large circle. Any of the following large–circle figures may be called: circle left and right, promenade, swing partner, swing corner, promenade single file, grand and left, queen's highway, king's highway, shoo fly swing, and Georgia rang tang.

■ *Georgia Rang Tang*

Circle left
The other way back
With the Georgia rang tang. The leader releases his left hand with his corner and travels through the arch made by his partner and her corner; then he continues to weave in and out through the arches made by each succeeding two dancers, his partner and other dancers following in and out. Do not let go of hands. The circle continues to move right until everyone has completed the figure. The leader may go on with endless rhyme such as:
Make your feet go whickety whack.
Hurry, hurry, hurry.

■ *King's Highway*

Promenade.
Gents turn back on the king's highway. The head man steps behind his partner, turns right, and travels in the reverse line of direction around the circle, followed in succession by the men behind; the women continue to travel forward.
Promenade. When each man meets his partner, he crosses to the inside of the circle, **behind** his partner, and they promenade in the line of direction.

■ *Queen's Highway*

Promenade.
Ladies turn back on the queen's highway. The head woman turns right and travels in the reverse line of direction around the circle, followed in succession by the women behind; the men continue to travel forward.
Promenade. When each woman meets her partner, they promenade.

■ *Shoo Fly Swing*

Shoo fly swing around the ring. The man of the head couple faces his partner (man's back to center of circle).
Right to your own. He swings his partner by the right hand.
Left on the side. She swings the man of the next couple (to the woman's right) by the left hand. Now back to own partner with the right, left to the next man (second couple to right), and so on around the circle. Her partner follows on the inside of the circle. After the first couple has passed three couples, the next couple starts the same pattern. Each couple continues until they are back home.

■ FIGURES

Odd couples out to the even couples. They join hands, circle four to the left until a small circle figure is called. Any of the following small–circle figures may be called: circle left and right, right- and left-hand star, ladies chain, right and left thru, butterfly twirl, bird in the cage, take a little peek, lady 'round the lady, dive for the oyster, and

Circle Square Dance! (continued)

shoot the owl. At the call "odds on to the next," the active couple moves forward on the inside to the next couple and circles four.

■ The Basket

Circle four hands around.
Ladies join your hands.
The men the same. Women join two hands across, men join two hands above the women.
Ladies bow the gents know how. The men raise their arms over the heads of the women (women bow under) and lower them behind women's backs.
The gents bow, the ladies know how. The women raise their arms over the heads of the men and lower them behind men's backs.
Circle left. With right foot forward, scoot to the left with a modified buzz step.
Break and swing your corner. And now your own. And on to the next.

■ Bird in the Cage

Circle four hands around.
Cage the bird with three hands 'round. Active woman steps in center. Inactive couple and active man join hands and circle around active woman.
Bird flies out, crow hops in. Active man steps in center as active woman joins circle with inactive couple.
Ring up three and you're gone again.
Crow hops out and make a ring.
Swing your partner and on to the next.

■ Box the Gnat and Box the Flea

Circle four.
With your opposite box the gnat.
Now box the flea. Same person.
Do–si–do. Same person.
Now swing that gal high and low.
And circle four.
Repeat call with own partner.
And lead onto the next.

■ Butterfly Twirl

Ladies twirl. Women turn in place.
Gents twirl. Men turn in place.
Everybody twirl a butterfly twirl. Everybody turns in place.
Now swing your corner girl.
And swing your own.

■ Dive for the Oyster

Circle four.
Dive for the oyster. Without releasing hands, active couple moves forward through an arch made by the inactive man and back to face the inactive couple; the active man stands in place.
Now circle four once around and on to the next.

■ Lady 'round the Lady

Lady 'round the lady and the gent solo. The active woman leads, her partner following, and goes between the inactive couple; the woman goes behind the inactive woman, around her and in front while her partner goes behind the inactive man, around him and back to face the couple.

Lady 'round the gent and the gent don't go. The active woman goes between the inactive couple, travels behind and around the inactive man and back to face the inactive couple; the active man stands in place.

Now circle four once around and on to the next.

■ *Mountaineer Loop*

Circle four.

Mountaineer Loop. The even couple raise their arms for the odd couple to pass through. The odd couple releases man's right, woman's left, as they go through the arch; man turns left, woman right and travel back home, the even couple turning under their arch. Odd couple rejoins hands.

And circle left.

■ *Pop them Thru*

Circle four.

Back with a left–hand star.

Then gents reach back and Pop them through to a right–hand star. Men reach across their chests with right hands (under left arm) for their opposites' right hand. All release star as men turn their opposite under their right arms and all form right–hand star.

Gents reach back and Pop them back. Men repeat above action using left hand to form left–hand star.

Swing your opposite on the same old track. Men turn to swing the woman following them in the star.

Swing your partner

And onto the next.

■ *Shoot the Owl*

Three hands 'round if you know how. Active man circles three with inactive couple.

When you get right, shoot the owl.

Two hands up, the gents shoot under. Circle three once and a half. Inactive couple "shoots" active man under arch to partner.

Grab your partner and swing like thunder. Active couple swings.

Circle four and on to the next.

■ *Take a Little Peek*

Around that couple and take a little peek. Active couple separates, woman peeks right, man peeks left around behind inactive couple.

Back to the center and swing your sweet. Active couple swings.

Around that couple and peek once more. Couple repeats "peeking" action.

Back to the center and circle four.

Lead to the next.

■ ENDING

Large–circle figures are called involving the whole group in a large circle.

■ NOTES

1. When determining the active and inactive couples, always count around the circle counter-clockwise. Also, do not let the couple to the left of the head couple start counting clockwise; it adds to the confusion, especially if there is an uneven number of couples present.

2. During the small circle figures, at the call "odds on to the next," the active couple moves forward to the next couple. They join hands and circle four to the left until a new figure is called.

Circle Square Dance (continued)

3. If dancers become mixed up, call "find your partner, and everybody swing."

4. There is no end of figures that may be used, once the format of the Big Circle Square Dance is learned. The figures presented are just a few.

Clogging

By Dr. Sandra L. Gallemore, Georgia Southern University, Statesboro, GA.

HISTORY

Clogging is a dance of sound. An American folk dance form enjoyed by people of all ages and all ability levels, clogging is primarily a combination of the rhythms, motions, and steps of the English, Scottish, and Irish immigrants who settled in the Appalachian area of the South during the 1700s and 1800s. Clogging is sometimes called Appalachian Mountain Style Dancing because the Appalachian area between southern Pennsylvania and northern Georgia is the primary area where this dance form has been preserved.

Historically, the style that generally today is simply called "clogging" included such terms/styles as clog dance, foot stomping, dancing, hoedowning, jigging, surefooting, flatfooting, little chugging, buck and wing, shuffling, heel and toe, buck dancing, and old English stepdancing.

■ Buck Dancing

The style of clogging called buck dancing originated in the Appalachian mountain area. Although the origin of buck dancing is not clear, generally it was considered a solo dance form. Some cloggers today view buck dancing as solo clogging; others view it as a unique form of dance separate from traditional clogging.

In buck dancing, the feet remain very close to the floor. With the exception of the legs, little body movement is used. The accompaniment is simple (perhaps only a fid–dle). The steps used in buck dancing were learned from the slaves brought to this country from Africa. Added to these steps were some of the ceremonial dance steps of the Cherokee Indians.

■ Step Dancing

Step dancing, a predecessor of clogging and a popular dance form in Canada, came to Ontario via early Irish settlers. The movements in step dancing are performed on the balls of the feet with the heels rarely touching the floor, a style distinctly different from the flat–footed action of buck dancing. Like traditional buck dancing, however, the movements originally were restricted to the legs and feet. Today, clogging taps are used on the shoes and the steps use more total body movement.

■ The Term Clogging

In 1939 the Soco Gap Dancers from western North Carolina performed for King George VI and Queen Elizabeth of England when they visited the White House. The queen commented that the dance looked like the English clogging. Thereafter, the term *clog-ging* began to be used for all styles of clogging.

■ *Three Styles*

Three main types or styles of clogging popular today are freestyle clogging (which evolved from buck dancing), square dance clogging, and precision clogging. Freestyle clogging is a solo dance. It includes a wide variety of step variations and combinations that use lively foot stomping, leg swinging, and considerable body action.

From early times, in addition to the freestyle solo clogging, dancers clogged in a square dance formation using traditional square dance movements. Originally, people danced using simple fast walking steps, adding clogging steps only occasionally. Clogging during the entire square dance did not become common until the 1930s. The steps performed in square dance clogging generally are freestyle in nature, with individual cloggers using steps of their own choosing. Such freestyle clogging is also performed in Big Circle Mountain dance.

Precision clogging, which began in the late 1950s, uses the same types of steps as freestyle clogging, but the dancers perform prescribed routines. James Kesterson's Blue Ridge Mountain Dancers in western North Carolina were possibly the first dancers to perform using this style. Of these three styles, precision clogging is the most spectator-oriented. Clogging routines in which individual dancers, partners, and groups perform a set sequence of dance steps have become popular with education and recreation groups, as well as with exhibition groups.

■ *Clogging Competitions*

Clogging competitions exist for advanced dancers who wish to exhibit their skill. The first recorded clogging team competition occurred in 1938 in Asheville, North Carolina, at Bascom Lamar Lunsford's annual Mountain Dance and Folk Festival, the oldest folk festival in the country. The winners of the competition, Sam Queen's Soco Gap Dancers, performed a combination of freestyle clogging and mountain–style square dance figures. Queen was well known for his own dance ability, as well as for his leadership of dance teams in the western North Carolina area.

In the 1940s, interest in clogging increased and, as a result, wearing special costumes and shoes became customary. Clogging began to attract spectators as a popular form of entertainment, making the activity more performance–oriented than had been the case in earlier years.

■ *Clogging in Early Physical Education Programs*

During the 1920s and 1930s, clogging, frequently called clog dance, was taught in public school and university physical education departments. These dances (frequently referred to as character dances) often had a dramatic quality not evident in today's clogging. These early clog dances appear to be related more closely to tap dance than what today is called clogging.

■ NATIONAL ORGANIZATION

Originated in 1976, the National Clogging and Hoedown Council (NCHC)* was formed to help preserve traditional clogging by collecting information about clogging styles and steps, as well as assembling historical material on clogging. In addition, to assist with communication among cloggers about more current dance routines and the historical materials, NCHC has established a written vocabulary of basic terminology.

Clogging (continued)

---

*National Clogging and Hoedown Council (NCHC), 507 Angie Way, Lilburn, GA 30247.

■ Costumes and Shoes

Although recreational cloggers wear any comfortable clothing, exhibition cloggers traditionally wear costumes very similar to those used in square dance. The major difference between exhibition square dance attire and exhibition clogging attire is the length of the women's skirts; cloggers usually wear shorter skirts than do square dancers.

■ SHOES

The clogging shoes of today, quite different from the practical and comfortable dancing shoes of earlier times, hold a special fascination for both dancers and spectators. Clogging shoes are low-heeled shoes. Clogging (or "jingle" or "staccato") taps are attached to the heels and toes of the soles. This type of tap creates a louder tapping sound than regular taps because the clogging tap has a loose two-part construction that allows metal to flap against metal and produce a jingle or rattle sound. Popular styles include square dance or tap dance shoes and lace-up shoes. It is critical that the shoe stays securely on the foot.

Taps on the shoes are not essential for participating in clogging. Many individuals clog successfully in shoes with a smooth sole (leather preferred). The main advantage of taps on the shoes when learning to clog is the feedback the learner receives from the sound produced.

■ Music

Traditional clogging music, sometimes termed "old-time" folk music, used primarily fiddle and/or banjo and on occasion another instrument, such as a guitar. It was the music of the 19th century and earlier.

Fiddle/banjo bluegrass or hoedown music is the accepted traditional form of clogging music today. Clogging instructors find the same hoedown musical selections with a definite repetitive beat and little melody that the square dance caller uses for patter calls appropriate for clogging.

The use of more current country and pop music is gaining in popularity for modern cloggers. Cloggers of today dance to almost any kind of music with a strong 2/4 time signature and an appropriate tempo for the skill level of the participants.

■ Style

Clogging style and steps, as they have been since early times, frequently are regional in nature.

Traditional clogging style calls for a torso that is almost motionless, even though the footwork consists of quick-moving intricate steps. Characteristic of the footwork is the use of the flat-foot action. When performing various steps and step patterns, both legs are straight (but not stiff) or both are slightly bent. The arms are relaxed and used only for balance, although in some modern exhibition clogging arm movement or claps may be included in the choreography.

■ LEG ACTION

When the heel is sounded against the floor, the legs are flexed. They straighten on count "and" of the music. The result is the customary up-and-down body movement identified with clogging. This up-and-down movement is combined with the forward-and-backward sliding motion of the feet to achieve the characteristic body action associated with skillful cloggers.

Most step patterns in clogging are designed so that when one foot has taken the weight the opposite foot is lifted from the floor (the lift may be very low to the ground or moderately high, depending on the steps involved). Although the legs bend and straighten to produce the appropriate style, looseness in the legs is needed for smoothness in the up-and-down bounce and also for the dancer to be ready to perform the following step.

■ *Basic Clogging Steps*

Eight basic steps or movements adopted by the National Clogging and Hoedown Council in 1978 are the basis for a wide variety of steps and combinations of steps used in clogging. Generally, the steps are performed in place. These basic movements are divided into two categories: heel movements and toe movements.

■ HEEL MOVEMENTS

The heel movements (step, slide, heel) take place on the downbeat (accent) of the music. Both legs are slightly bent. Heel movements are accented as the weight is trans–ferred to the entire sole of the foot.

2/4	/		/		/		/	
	heel		heel		heel		heel	
	movt		movt		movt		movt	
	L		R		L		R	
Q	Q	Q	Q	Q	Q	Q	Q	Q
&	1	&	2	&	1	&	2	&

■ TOE MOVEMENTS

The toe movements (rock, drag, toe, double–toe, brush) occur on the upbeat (count "and") of the music. Both legs are straight (but not stiff).

2/4		/		/		/		/
toe		toe		toe		toe		toe
movt		movt		movt		movt		movt
R		L		R		L		R
Q	Q	Q	Q	Q	Q	Q	Q	Q
&	1	&	2	&	1	&	2	&

The basic clogging steps are presented in the order taught. The usual abbreviation for the movement found on clogging cue sheets is included, i.e., Step (S), Rock (R).

■ STEP (S)

1. 2/4 meter.
2. A flat–footed **heel** movement on the downbeat (accent); a weight–bearing movement.
3. Both knees are slightly bent on STEP left, on the following upbeat (count "and") both knees straighten; repeat beginning right.
4. Both feet remain close to the floor, alternating left and right.

2/4		/		/		/		/	
		Step		Step		Step		Step	
		L		R		L		R	
Q		Q	Q	Q	Q	Q	Q	Q	Q
&		1	&	2	&	1	&	2	&

Clogging (continued)

- ## ROCK (R)

  1. 2/4 meter.
  2. A **toe** movement on the upbeat (count "and").
  3. A weight–bearing movement in which the weight is taken on the ball of the foot, which usually is placed directly under or slightly behind the center of gravity.
  4. Both knees are straight (not stiff) on the ROCK; on the following downbeat (accent) of the music, both knees bend slightly while performing the next movement.
  5. Both feet remain close to the floor.

  2/4

	/		/		/		/	
Rock	Step	Rock	Step	Rock	Step	Rock	Step	Rock
L	R	L	R	L	L	R	L	R
Q	Q	Q	Q	Q	Q	Q	Q	Q
&	1	&	2	&	1	&	2	&

  even rhythm

- ## DRAG (DR)

  1. 2/4 meter.
  2. A **toe** movement on the upbeat (count "and").
  3. A weight–bearing movement, which may be performed on one foot or on both feet simultaneously.
  4. Similar to a chug step, the DRAG is a movement that scoots **backward** a few inches as the weight is shifted to the balls of the feet. Heels skim the floor during the movement.
  5. Both knees are straight (not stiff) on the DRAG; on the following downbeat (accent), both knees bend slightly while performing the next movement.
  6. In the analysis below, one may start on the **and** with a DRAG or on the **accent** with a STEP.

  2/4

	/		/		/		/	
Drag	Step	Drag	Step	Drag	Step	Drag	Step	Drag
L	R	R	L	L	R	R	L	L
Q	Q	Q	Q	Q	Q	Q	Q	Q
&	1	&	2	&	1	&	2	&

  even rhythm

■ **SLIDE (SL)**

1. 2/4 meter.
2. A **heel** movement on the downbeat (accent).
3. A weight–bearing movement, which may be performed on one foot or on both feet simultaneously.
4. Feet scoot **forward** a few inches as weight is shifted from balls of feet to heels. Heels skim along the floor.
5. Both knees are slightly bent on the SLIDE; on the following upbeat (count "and"), both knees straighten while performing the next movement.
6. The combination DRAG SLIDE performed on one foot is much more difficult than performing the combination on both feet simultaneously. In the analysis below, during the first measure the left foot remains in contact with the ground while the right foot/leg is off the ground; the style of both knees bent on the SLIDE and both straight on the DRAG refers to performing this movement on one–leg combination as well as on both simultaneously.

2/4

Drag	/ Slide	Drag	/ Slide	Drag	/ Slide	Drag	/ Slide	Drag
L	L	L	L	L	both	both	both	both
Q	Q	Q	Q	Q	Q	Q	Q	Q
&	1	&	2	&	1	&	2	&

even rhythm

■ **TOE (T), HEEL (H), TOUCH (TCH)**

1. 2/4 meter.
2. The TOE step is a weight–bearing **toe** movement on the upbeat (count "and"). It must be followed by a HEEL step.
3. The HEEL step is a weight–bearing **heel** movement on the downbeat (accent).
4. A variation of the TOE is the TOUCH, which involves no change of weight. The ball of the foot touches the floor on the upbeat (count "and") and lifts on the downbeat (accent) as another movement is performed.
5. The weight is shifted to the ball of the foot for the TOE step; this leg is very slightly bent and the opposite leg is straight.
6. The weight then shifts to the entire sole of the foot for the HEEL step as the heel slaps the floor; legs bend slightly.

2/4

Toe	/ Heel	Toe	/ Heel	Toe	/ Heel	Toe	/ Heel	Toe
L	L	R	R	L	L	R	R	L
Q	Q	Q	Q	Q	Q	Q	Q	Q
&	1	&	2	&	1	&	2	&

even rhythm

2/4

Touch	/ Heel	Touch	/ Heel	Touch	/ Slide	Touch	/ Slide	Touch
L	R	L	R	L	R	L	R	L
Q	Q	Q	Q	Q	Q	Q	Q	Q
&	1	&	2	&	1	&	2	&

even rhythm

Clogging (continued)

▪ DOUBLE-TOE (DT)

1. 2/4 meter.

2. A **toe** movement on the upbeat (count "and").

3. No weight change occurs in the DOUBLE-TOE. The foot performing the movement makes two clicking sounds with the ball of that foot. A small brushing movement of the ball of the foot forward and a small brushing movement backward occur during the "and–ah" count.

4. The DOUBLE–TOE action generally occurs slightly in front of the center of gravity.

5. The knee of the supporting leg is straight; the knee of the leg performing the movement straightens on the small brushing movement of the ball of the foot forward and relaxes on the small brushing action backward. On the following downbeat (accent), both knees bend slightly while performing the next movement.

2/4		/			/		
Brush	Brush		Brush	Brush		Brush	Brush
Fwd	Bkwd	Step	Fwd	Bkwd	Step	Fwd	Bkwd
L	L	L	R	R	R	L	L
Q	Q	S	Q	Q	S	Q	Q
& – ah		1	& – ah		2	& – ah	

uneven rhythm

▪ BRUSH (BR)

1. 2/4 meter.

2. A **toe** movement on the upbeat (count "and").

3. No weight change in the BRUSH. The leg performing the movement swings forward as the ball of the foot brushes the floor. Generally the brush and following action is within a few inches of the floor.

4. Brushes also may cross in front of the body or swing out to the side. Less frequently they are performed brushing backward.

5. Both legs are straight; on the following downbeat (accent), both knees bend slightly while performing the next movement.

2/4	/			/	/			/
Brush	Slide	Toe	Heel	Brush	Slide	Toe	Heel	Brush
L	R	L	L	R	L	R	R	L
Q	Q	Q	Q	Q	Q	Q	Q	Q
&	1	&	2	&	1	&	2	&

even rhythm

■ *Teaching Clogging*

■ PROGRESSION

The following order for teaching the basic steps is suggested: Step, Rock, Drag and Slide, Step, Rock, Toe and Heel, Double–Toe, Touch, Brush.

The instructor should develop sequences in phrasing with the music for practicing and learning to combine step patterns. For most musical selections routines should use the same step or step pattern for four or eight measures.

■ EVALUATION

Students may be evaluated for the purpose of assigning a grade on clogging performance and clogging knowledge. Appropriate competencies for performance evaluation include the following:

1. Students will demonstrate each of the basic steps in clogging.
2. Students will demonstrate a variety of step combinations.
3. Students will demonstrate appropriate clogging style.
4. Students will combine steps in a manner that compliments the phrasing of the music.
5. Students will perform dance routines accurately and skillfully.

Appropriate competencies for knowledge evaluation include the following:

1. Students will exhibit knowledge about the proper techniques of performing the basic steps.
2. Students will exhibit knowledge about clogging style.
3. Students will exhibit knowledge about the relationship of music to the steps and the step combinations used in routines.
4. Students will exhibit knowledge about the history and background of clogging.

EXAMPLE OF STEP COMBINATIONS

Music: Any 2/4 music; bluegrass or hoedown suggested.

Formation: Scattered, all facing music.

Steps: Double–toe, step, rock, toe, heel, touch, brush, drag, slide.

DIRECTIONS FOR THE DANCE

Meter 2/4

■ *Measures*

1–4   Beginning right, double–toe step (right), rock step (left, right); double–toe step (left), rock step (right, left); double–toe step (right), rock step (left, right); double–toe step (left), rock step (right, left).

5–8   Beginning right, double–toe step (right), double–toe step (left); double–toe step (right), rock step (left, right); repeat sequence beginning left foot.

9–16   Repeat action of measures 1–8.

Alabama Gal

Alabama Gal, a Play Party Game, was taught by Jane Farwell at the Oglebay Folk Dance Camp, Wheeling, West Virginia, in 1948.

Record: World of Fun M112.

Formation: Longway sets, men on left, ladies on right, partners facing. Large groups should be divided into sets of 16 couples or less.

■ *Singing Call*

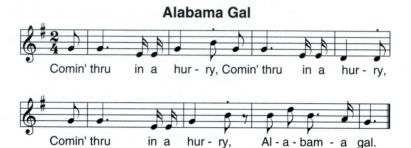

Alabama Gal

Comin' thru in a hur - ry, Comin' thru in a hur - ry,

Comin' thru in a hur - ry, Al - a - bam - a gal.

Verse 2
You don't know how how
You don't know how how
You don't know how how
Alabama Gal.

Verse 3
I'll show you how how
I'll show you how how
I'll show you how how
Alabama Gal.

Verse 4
Ain't I rock candy
Ain't I rock candy
Ain't I rock candy
Alabama Gal.

DIRECTIONS FOR THE DANCE

1. Everyone or just the caller sings the verses.
2. Head couple joins two hands, extending arms shoulder height. Slides down and back between two lines.
3. Head couple reels down the set by starting with a right–hand swing, once and a half. When the active couples reach the foot of the set, they join the lines.
4. As soon as all four verses have been sung, next couple starts to slide down center and back and reel. Therefore, each time the first verse is sung, a new couple starts "comin' thru in a hurry." The fun comes when a new couple begins to slide through the set while the reeling continues!

Nobody's Business

NOBODY'S BUSINESS IS A FUN–LOVING American Play Party Game. The tune is catchy and it is an excellent mixer.

Dance A While CD: #5 "Nobody's Business."
Record: Folk Dancer MH1107.
Cassette: Play Party Dances for Early Childhood, Can–Ed Media Ltd.
Formation: Single circle, couples facing center, lady to right of partner, hands joined.

■ *Singing Call*

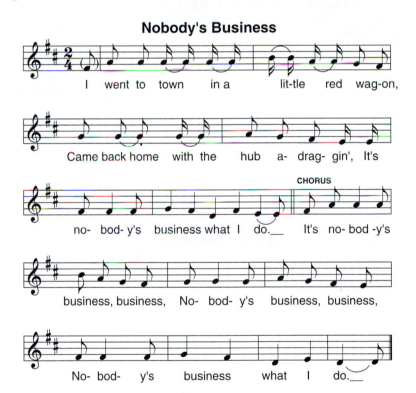

Nobody's Business

I went to town in a lit-tle red wag-on,

Came back home with the hub a- drag- gin', It's

no- bod- y's business what I do.__ It's no- bod -y's

business, business, No- bod- y's business, business,

No- bod- y's business what I do.__

Verse 2
Way down yonder about a mile and a quarter,
Some old man's going to lose his daughter,
It's nobody's business what I do.

Verse 3
Butterbeans has killed my baby
Popcorn has killed the old lady,
It's nobody's business what I do.

Verse 4
I've got a wife and she's a daisy,
She won't work and I'm too lazy,
It's nobody's business what I do.

Nobody's Business (continued)

DIRECTIONS FOR THE DANCE

1. Everyone sings the verses with the chorus between each verse.

2. For each verse, all join hands and circle to the left, walking briskly.

3. For the chorus, release hands, partners face, ready for a grand right and left with an elbow swing. Partners hook right elbows and make one complete turn (each turn lasts one line of the chorus). Each meets the next person, men always progressing counterclockwise, women clockwise, with a left elbow swing; then the next with a right elbow swing. There are three elbow swings. Complete the last swing, men taking this one for their new partners.

4. For the next verse, all join hands and circle left. Continue alternating the action with each verse and chorus.

Schottische

Dance A While CD: #14 "Schottische."

Music: Any Schottische. Schottische melodies and styles of arrangements relate to the quality of movement: a lively, bouncy one for step–hops; a smooth one for Ballroom variations and Texas Schottische variations.

Position: Open, couple, or conversation.

Steps: Schottische.

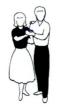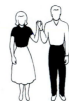

DIRECTIONS FOR THE DANCE

Meter 4/4 • Directions are for man; woman's part reverse.

■ *Measures*

	Basic
1–2	Open dance position. Beginning left, move forward in line of direction with two Schottische steps.
3–4	Closed position or waist position. Turn clockwise with four step–hops. Progress in line of direction.

Variations

I. Woman's Turn

1–2	Repeat action of measures 1–2 in basic Schottische.
3–4	Four step–hops, man moves forward, while the woman turns clockwise under upraised left arm of partner. Woman may make one or two complete turns. Progress in the line of direction.

II. Man's Turn

1–4	Directions are the same as for the woman's turn, except man turns clockwise under upraised right arm of woman.

III. Both Turn

1–2   Repeat action of measures 1–2 in basic Schottische.

Four step–hops, partners turn away from each other, man to his left, woman to her right.

Partners may make one or two complete turns.

IV. Diamond

1–2   Man and woman take one Schottische step diagonally forward away from each other.

Man and woman take one Schottische step diagonally forward toward each other.

Progress in the line of direction.

3–4   Repeat action of measures 3–4 in basic Schottische.

V. Wring the Dish Rag

1–2   Repeat action of measures 1–2 in basic Schottische.

3–4   Partners face, join two hands and with four step–hops turn back to back (turning to man's left, woman's right) and continue roll until face to face. Join hands and swing through between couple, below waist, and quickly overhead. The couple may make one or two turns.

VI. Rock

1–2   Repeat action of measures 1–2 in basic Schottische.

3   Step forward on left, take weight (counts 1–2). Step backward on right, take weight (counts 3–4). Rocking effect is produced by swaying body forward and backward.

4   Repeat action of measure 3.

VII. Ballroom Schottische

1–2   Repeat action of measures 1–2 in basic Schottische. On count 4, the hop is omitted and the free leg swings forward, toe pointed close to floor.

3–4   Closed position. Beginning left, pivot turn clockwise four steps, progressing in line of direction.

VIII. Schottische for Four–Horse and Buggy Schottische

Two couples stand one behind the other, both facing the line of direction. Join inside hands with partner. The outside hands joined link the two couples together. The front couple is number one, the back couple is number two.

1–2   Repeat action of measures 1–2 in basic Schottische.

3–4   Four step–hops. No. 1 couple releases partner's hand and turning away from each other, man left, woman right, they move around couple No. 2 on the outside and come in behind them. Joining hands with partner, they therefore become the back couple and No. 2 couple, the front couple. Or No. 1 couple may take step–hops backward through the upraised arms of No. 2 couple. This action will cause No. 2 couple to turn the dish rag in order to become straightened out. After turning No. 2 couple becomes the front couple. These variations, if repeated, will return couples to starting position.

1–4   Repeat the entire action of measures 1–4 with No. 2 couple turning out or moving backward with step–hops, to return couples to original positions.

Schottische (continued)

■ Mixer

Double circle, couples facing line of direction. Dance basic Schottische. The woman moves forward to a new partner on the second Schottische step.

■ Style

Three styles are used in this Schottische: Traditional–the Schottische step is danced as a step, close, step, hop. Barn dance–the Schottische step is danced as a step, step, step, hop or run, run, run, hop. Ballroom dance–step, close, step, lift. The hop is replaced by a slight lift of the body. Point toe of the free foot. The step–hops are replaced by a step-lift, with a rocking action forward and back.

   The American style is to swing the free leg forward on the hop and the pattern is very smooth. The European style keeps the leg under the body and the hop has a bouncy action.

Ping-Pong Schottische

Position: Varsouvienne.

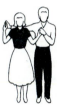

DIRECTIONS FOR THE DANCE

Meter 4/4 • Directions are same for man and woman.

■ Measures

1	Beginning right, place heel, then toe by left foot.
2	Take one two–step, moving forward.
3–4	Beginning left, repeat action of measures 1–2.
5–6	Beginning right, take eight count grapevine, traveling sideways to right; stepping to right side (count 1), then left behind right (count 2), step side right (count 3), cross left in front of right (count 4), step side right (count 5), cross left behind right (count 6), step right (count 7), bring left to right but do not take weight (count 8).
7–8	Beginning left, repeat action of measures 5–6, traveling sideways to left.

Texas Schottische Variations

THE *TEXAS SCHOTTISCHE WAS FIRST* seen by the authors as part of an exhibition danced and taught by Herb and Pauline Greggerson. The Texas Schottische was also referred to as the El Paso Schottische, because El Paso was home base for the Greggersons in those days. There are many Texas Schottische variations such as Douglas, Belen, and Scotch. As originally danced, these steps were not done in any special sequence.

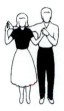

Dance A While CD: #14 "Schottische."

Records: FD LP 4; MAV Album 4; Shaw E 23, or any smooth Schottische.

Position: Varsouvienne.

Steps: Variations of grapevine, Schottische and Two-Step.

DIRECTIONS FOR THE DANCE

Meter 4/4 • Directions are same for man and woman.

■ Measures

I. Military Schottische

1	Point left toe in front of right foot (counts 1–2). Point left toe sideways to left (counts 3–4).
2	Step left foot behind right (count 1). Step right foot to right (count 2). Close left to right (count 3). Hold (count 4).
3–4	Beginning right, repeat action of measures 1–2.
5–6	Beginning left, two walking steps forward followed by one Two–Step.
7–8	Beginning right, repeat action of measures 5–6.

II. Peter Pan Schottische

1	Step forward left (counts 1–2). Step forward right (counts 3–4).
2	Step forward left, right, (counts 1–2), step left and pivot to own right (count 3), swing or lift right leg (count 4). Couple now faces in the reverse line of direction.
3	Moving backward, step right, lift left (counts 1–2). Step left, lift right (counts 3–4).

Texas Schottische Variations (continued)

4	Step right, left, right, pivoting to own left (counts 1, 2, 3, 4). Couple now faces line of direction.

III. McGinty Schottische

1–2	Step forward, slightly to left, with left foot, close right to left, step left, and swing right across left with a slight kick. Repeat stepping forward, slightly to right, with right foot. (Right, close, right, swing left across right with slight kick.)
3–4	Beginning left, take four step swings (kicks), moving forward in line of direction: step left and swing right across in front of left, step right in front of left and swing left across in front of right; repeat action. Body sways with a roll during the step swings.

IV. Blue Bonnet

1	Beginning left, take one Schottische step to left, sideways, stepping left, step right behind left, step left, swing right in front of left as body rises and lowers on left foot.
2	Take one Schottische step to right, sideways, woman rising and lowering on step swing.
3–4	Partners release left hands. Man and woman take 12 small steps in a quick quick slow rhythm (four times). Woman, beginning left, takes three small steps (quick, quick, slow), turns right face to face partner, and moves so right arms are almost extended; woman travels around her partner, to man's right, behind him, to his left side, and back to original Varsouvienne position while taking three more series of small steps to the rhythm of quick, quick, slow. On the last quick, quick, slow, the woman turns clockwise under her right arm as she moves into her original position. As the woman is sweeping around the man, the man guides her raising his right arm and circling his right hand above his head (lariat fashion); and the man takes 12 steps to the rhythm of quick, quick, slow, four times almost in place, moving slightly to assist the movement of his partner. See Note 2.

■ NOTES

1. In El Paso, Texas, McGinty is the name for a "big beer." In Lloyd Shaw's *The Round Dance Book* (1948), under Texas Schottisches, this variation is listed as Drunken Schottische.

2. Although **quick quick slow** is a Two–Step rhythm, the Greggersons did not Two–Step this figure; rather, they used a smooth travel of steps.

Texas Schottische for Three*

URING WORLD WAR II, the Texas Schottische and Put Your Little Foot were the two round dances most frequently danced between squares in the Southwest. Following the folk–transmission process, set patterns known as the *California Schottische* and *Oklahoma Mixer* have come from variations of the Texas Schottische. Jane Farwell adapted the Oklahoma Mixer and named it *Texas Schottische for Three*, partly to compensate for the man shortage during the war.

Dance A While CD: #14 "Schottische."

Records: Any smooth Schottische. MAV Album 4; Shaw E23; World of Fun MH 130.

Formation: Line of three, man between two woman, facing line of direction; man reaching back holds outside hand of each woman, woman join inside hands behind man.

Steps: Two–Step, walk, heel toe.

DIRECTIONS FOR THE DANCE

Meter 4/4 • Directions are same for man and woman.

■ Measures

1–2   Beginning left, take two Two–Steps, moving diagonally left, then right.

3–4   Beginning left, four walking steps forward.

5–6   Place left heel forward, place left toe close to right instep (counts 1–4). Women release, inside hand. Man backs up three steps, pulling women around in front, as women take three steps (left, right, left) in line of direction, turning back to face reverse line of direction. Man faces line of direction, women face reverse line of direction. Beginning right, repeat heel, toe. Man gives a slight pull of hands, then releases hands as all take three steps (right, left, right) forward. Man passes between the two women, and joins hands with new partners; women turn toward each other, pivoting on third step to face line of direction.

■ NOTES

1. A marvelous mixer for extra men to cut in, and, in Jane Farwell's words, "snatch two women" leaving another man to become one of the "thieves."

2. An excellent dance to teach the Schottische steps.

---

*Texas Schottische for Three included by permission of the late Jane Farwell, Folklore Village Farm, Dodgeville, WI.

Salty Dog Rag

T HE *SALTY DOG RAG* IS A novelty dance composed to a popular tune, based on the Schottische rhythm.

Records: DC 73304; High/Scope RM 9; MCA 60090; Nama LP 2.

Position: Promenade.

Steps: Grapevine Schottische, step–hop

DIRECTIONS FOR THE DANCE

Meter 4/4 • Directions are same for man and woman.

■ *Measures*

1–8   Introduction: no action.

Part I

1–2   Beginning right, take two grapevine Schottische steps, moving diagonally forward right (step right, step left behind right, step right hop) diagonally forward left (step left, step right behind left, step left hop).

3–4   Moving forward, take four step–hops (or step swings).

5–8   Repeat action of measures 1–4.

Part II

1   Dropping right hands, left hands remain joined, woman turns to face partner on her first step. Beginning right, take one grapevine Schottische step sideways to own right (partners move away from each other).

2   Beginning left, each takes a three–step turn, turning left, toward partner. Begin impetus for turn by each pulling joined hands slightly, then drop hands to complete solo turn.

3–4   Catch right hands, shoulder height, elbows bent. Beginning right, take four step–hops (or struts), making one complete turn clockwise.

5–8   Repeat action of part II, measures 1–4. On last step–hop, take promenade position and face line of direction.

Part III

1–2   Beginning right, place heel forward, step right in place; place left heel forward, step left in place; rise on both toes swinging heels out (pigeon–toed); click heels together; stamp right, stamp left.

3–4   Take four step–hops forward.

5–8   Repeat action of part III, measures 3–4.

■ NOTE

Many people dance parts I and II alternately, omitting part III.

Boston Two-Step

THE *BOSTON TWO-STEP*, OF English origin, has become part of the American fabric of dance and is an old–time favorite still danced at the Grange halls and dance halls, where social dances (Foxtrot, Waltz) prevail. The dance programs feature occasional pattern dances like the Boston Two–Step.

Records: RPT LP106; Shaw E 46.

Position: Partners face, man joins woman's right hand with his left or join two hands.

Steps: Step swing, three–step turn, Two–Step.

DIRECTIONS FOR THE DANCE

Meter 2/4 • Directions are for man; woman's part reverse.

■ Measures

Part I

1	Beginning left, step in place, swing right over left.
2	Step right in place, swing left over right.
3–4	Release hands. Traveling in the line of direction, take one three–step turn (man turning counterclockwise; woman clockwise) and swing right over left.
5–8	Join hands. Beginning right, repeat action of measures 1–4, three–step turn, moving forward in the reverse line of direction.
9–12	Join hands. Beginning left, repeat action of measures 1–4, three–step turn moving forward in the line of direction, **stamp right** (instead of last swing). Place weight on right foot.

Part II

13–16	Closed position. Beginning left, take four Two–Steps, turning clockwise, progressing in the line of direction.

■ Variation

In Part II, a pivot may be substituted for the last two Two–Steps or for all four Two–Steps.

Heel and Toe Polka

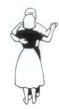
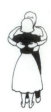

Dance A While CD: #19 "Polka."
Music: Any lively polka.
Position: Closed or shoulder–waist.
Steps: Heel and Toe Polka, Polka.

DIRECTIONS FOR THE DANCE

Meter 2/4 • Directions are for the man; woman's part reverse.

■ *Measures*

I.   Heel and Toe Polka

1–2   Moving to the left, hop right (count **and**), place left heel close to right instep (count 1), hop right (count **and**), place left toe close to right instep (count 2), take one Polka step to the left (counts 1 **and** 2).

3–4   Moving to the right, repeat action of measures 1–2, hopping on right.

5–8   Repeat action of measures 1–4.

II.   Polka

9–16   Take eight Polka steps, turning clockwise, progressing in the line of direction.

■ *Polka Variations*

1. **Crossover Polka:** Varsouvienne position. Man and woman both begin Heel and Toe Polka by hopping right. Without releasing hands, woman crosses over to man's left on the hop step, close, step, man dancing almost in place. Woman crosses back to original position on second Heel and Toe Polka. This action repeats. Second part, couple takes eight Polka steps, moving forward in the line of direction.

2. **Crossover Polka with Three–Step Turn:** During the Crossover Polka, part I, woman makes a three–step turn to cross over and back. Heel toe, heel toe, release right hands and turn under left arm, stepping left, right, left; rejoin right hands. Repeat to right, releasing left hands for turn. Part II, Polka forward.

3. **Slide Polka:** Closed position, man's back to center of circle. Heel toe, heel toe, take four slides, traveling in the line of direction (the last slide is not completed in order to change direction). Repeat traveling in the reverse line of direction. Take eight Polka steps, turning clockwise, progressing in the line of direction.

4. **Falcon Hop:** In 1950, at the after–parties of the National Folk Festival in St. Louis, it was fun to dance with the Polish–American dancers. To sprightly Polka tunes, especially the Polish ones, in closed or shoulder–waist position, they danced the Falcon Hop. The Falcon Hop is a small Polka step, turning clockwise as they progressed forward, but actually not traveling very far. The dancers appeared to "jiggle" as they hopped.

Cotton-Eyed Joe

Dorothy Scarborough identifies *Cotton-Eyed Joe* as an authentic slavery tunesong in her book *On the Trail of Negro Folksongs*. One song antebellum blacks played and sang dealt with Cotton–Eyed Joe. Judging by the many verses–all in the same vein–he was a tantalizing, intriguing, and devilish character.

> Hadn't been for Cotton–Eyed Joe
> I'd ` a' been married twenty years ago
> With an old gourd fiddle and a cornstalk bow
> None could play like Cotton–Eyed Joe.

The fiddle tune, written in 2/4 meter, may be found in several references, one being Ira W. Ford's *Traditional Music of America*. Some references present the same tune in 4/4 meter.

According to Uncle Dave Dillingham of Austin, Texas, who learned the dance in Williamson County in the early 1880s, Cotton–Eyed Joe is nothing but a Heel and Toe "Poker," with fringes added. For the most part, the fringes, or variations, over and above the Heel and Toe Polka were originally clog steps, which required skill and extroversion on the part of the dancer.

Uncle Dave, at age 81 (1947), recalled the visits of Professor Whitehead, the visiting dancing master, who dealt with the finer points of ballroom dancing. The dancing master taught the Heel and Toe Polka in every community he visited, along with the Waltz, and so forth. But the short duration of his visit, the scarcity of students, and the ability of dancers no doubt contributed to the fact that the Heel and Toe Polka was not mastered by the majority of the dancers. In addition to these difficulties, the fringes that really make the dance were for the most part made up of clog steps, which not only require skill but also require an extroversion that is not a common trait attributed to the average dancer but is easy for the "Fancy Dan" who was, and still is, an exception on the dance floor. The dance as described is a simple version, commonly danced in Texas.

Records: Belco 257; Express 405; EZ 715, 6003, LP 506; FD LP 5; MAV Album 5; HM 35, 74; LS E 35; World of Fun MH 130.

Cassettes: DC 162105; MH 35, C 74.

Music: Dave, Red River, "Cotton–Eyed Joe," Southern Music Co., San Antonio, TX.

Position: Closed.

Steps: Polka, Two–Step, push step.

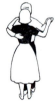

Cotton-Eyed Joe (continued)

DIRECTIONS FOR THE COUPLE DANCE

Meter 2/4 • Directions are for man; woman's part reverse.

■ *Measures*

I. Heel and Toe Polka

1–2   Hop right, touch left heel out to the left (count *and* 1). Hop right, touch left toe behind right foot (count *and* 2). Polka to left (counts *and* 1, *and* 2), in the line of direction.

3–4   Repeat beginning with hop on left foot and travel in the reverse line of direction.

II. Individual Turn

5–8   Three Two–Steps left turning in a small circle. The man turns counterclockwise, the woman turns clockwise. Finish with three alternating quick stamps in place, facing partner.

III. Push Step

9–10   Step left sideward in line of direction (count 1), place the weight momentarily on the right (count *and*), push back onto left foot, chugging left sideward again and flip right heel out to the side (count 2). Push with the right (count *and*), chug left (count 1), push with right (count *and*), chug left (count 2). Weight remains on left.

11–12   Repeat action of measures 9–10, starting with the right foot, and moving to the right.

IV. Two–Step or Polka

13–16   Four Two–Steps in closed dance position, turning clockwise, progressing in the line of direction. These may be Polka steps.

■ *Variations*

The dancers perform the variations at random, measures 9–16. After the variation, the Heel and Toe Polka and the individual turn are repeated.

1. **Two–Step Away and Toward Partner:** Moving away from partner, takes four small Two–Steps; step left directly behind right (count 1), step right in place (count **and**), step left in place (count 2); step right directly behind left (count 1), step left in place (count **and**), step right in place (count 2); repeat. Moving toward partner, take four small Two–Steps.

2. **Hooking:** Partners grasp right hands, free left arm curved and raised shoulder height as each dancer hops on left, extending right foot to meet partner's right foot, hooking foot just back of partner's right ankle. Take eight hops, couple turning clockwise in place. Reverse direction, grasping left hands, hooking left ankles, and taking eight hops, beginning left. Couple turns counterclockwise. Partners lean away from each other, slightly offering resistance or counterbalance as they turn; hooked leg is straight.

3. **Jig Steps:** These Jig and Clog steps are listed for historical significance and for the advanced dancer to pursue. They are not analyzed. Partners face each other and do Jig or Clog Dance steps such as shifting sands, seven steps, grapevine twist, pigeon wing, double shuffle, buzzard loop, triple step, and rock the cradle. Uncle Dave Dillingham at 80 would dance these steps, doing a solo, while his partner marked the rhythm, moving ever so lightly in place, perhaps working her skirt "à la Square or Mexican" dance styling.

DIRECTIONS FOR THE LINE DANCE

Formation: Lines of three, four, six, or as many as desired, arms around neighbor's waist, facing line of direction. Lines move like spokes in a wheel. Or lines of two in Varsouvienne or Promenade position.

Steps: Kick, Two–Step.

Meter 2/4 • Directions are same for man and woman.

■ Measures

I. Kicker

1	Beginning left, cross left foot and knee in front of right knee; kick left foot forward.
2	Back up, taking one Two–Step.
3–4	Beginning right, repeat action of measures 1–2.
5–8	Repeat action of measures 1–4.

II. Two–Step

9–16	Beginning left, take eight Two–Steps in line of direction.

Improvisation may take place in part II, such as turning, backing up, or walking around.

Blue Pacific Waltz

THE *BLUE PACIFIC WALTZ* WAS composed by Henry "Buzz" Glass of Oakland, California.

Records: LS E 48; Windsor 7609.
Music: *Over the Waves.*
Position: Inside hands joined.
Steps: Waltz, three–step turn.

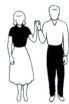

DIRECTIONS FOR THE DANCE

Meter 3/4 • Directions are for man; woman's part reverse.

■ Measures

I. Three–Step Turn and Swing

1	Beginning left, step left and swing right across left, turning slightly away from partner.
2–3	Beginning right, take a three–step turn clockwise (woman counter-clockwise) exchanging places with partner (holding count 2, move on counts 1, 3, 1). Swing left across right, turning slightly away from partner

Blue Pacific Waltz (continued)

(counts 2–3). The rhythm of this figure is known as the Canter. Lead: Man draws woman across in front of him into the turn with his joined hand, releasing just in time to make the turn, and then catches the opposite hand after the turn.

4–5	Beginning left, repeat action of measures 2–3, swinging right across.
6	Step right, turning to face partner. Touch left to right, keep weight on right. Take closed position.
7–8	Two Waltz steps turning clockwise, progressing in line of direction.
9–16	Repeat action of measures 1–8.

II. Twinkle Step

17	Semi–open position, facing line of direction. Step left forward, swing right forward.
18	Step right forward, step left in place facing partner, step right in place facing reverse line of direction (counts 1, 2, 3). This movement is called the twinkle step (Waltz time).
19	Step left across right in reverse line of direction, step right in place, facing partner. Step left in place to face line of direction in open position.
20	Step forward right, touch left to right, keep weight on right.
21–28	Repeat action of measures 17–20 twice.
29	Step left forward, swing right forward.
30	Man: Step right across left, close to left toe (count 1). Pirouette on toes turning one–half counterclockwise (counts 2–3). Woman: Three little steps (right, left, right) and follow man's turn counterclockwise, walking around him.
31–32	Closed position. Two Waltz steps turning counterclockwise. Open into couple position to repeat dance from beginning.

■ **NOTE**

For simplification of measures 30–32, step right forward, touch left to right, keep weight on right and take closed position. Two Waltz steps turning clockwise.

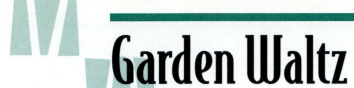

Garden Waltz

THE *GARDEN WALTZ* IS A German–American Waltz for three dancers. It originated in New Braunfels, Texas. There are two rhythms, Waltz and Polka. It is also known as the *Butterfly*.

Ancestors of the Butterfly are: German, Schmetterlingtanz ("Butterfly Dance"); Czech, Zahradniček ("The Gardener," from "Zahrada" = "Garden"); Polish (Silesian), and Zasiale Górale ("The Mountaineers sowed oats").

Record: Bellaire 5031.

Formation: Set of three, man between two women, facing line of direction. Man's arms around women's waist, women's inside arm around man's waist, or hook elbows.

Steps: Hesitation Waltz, Waltz, Polka, or Two-Step.

DIRECTIONS FOR THE DANCE

■ *Measures*

Meter 3/4 • Directions are same for man and women.

I. Waltz Forward

1–16   Beginning left, take 16 Hesitation Waltz steps forward. Hesitation Waltz step: Step forward left, knee slightly bent (count 1), bring right to left, rising on balls of both feet (count 2), end weight on left (count 3). Repeat beginning right. Styling: body falls count 1, body lifts counts 2 and 3, similar to body action in a step–swing.

Meter 2/4

II. Polka Turns

1–16   Release hold. Beginning left, man takes 16 Polka or Two–Steps, first hooking right elbows with right-hand woman, turning clockwise with four Polka steps; then hooking left elbows with left-hand woman, turning counterclockwise with four Polka steps. Turn right-hand woman, then left-hand woman again. If quick, turn each four times alternately.

■ *Variation*

Meter 3/4

Waltz Turns

1–8   Beginning left, take eight Hesitation Waltz steps forward.

9–16   Inside hands joined with man, raise arms. As man takes eight Waltz steps forward, two women spin under raised arms away from man, right-hand woman counterclockwise, left-hand woman clockwise. Women may take eight Waltz steps turning.

Meter 2/4

Polka Turns

1–8   **Elbow Turns:** All dance eight Polka steps as man hooks right elbows with right-hand woman, turn with four Polka steps, then hooks left elbows with left-hand woman, turn with four Polka steps.

9–16   **Arches:** All take eight Polka steps: right-hand woman travels under arch made by man and left-hand woman, then back to place; man turns under his left arm; left-hand woman repeats.

Varsouvienne

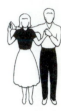

THE *VARSOUVIENNE* IS ALSO KNOWN, especially in Texas, as *Put Your Little Foot*.

Records: Folkraft 1165; Windsor 4615; LS E 45; EZ 715; World of Fun MH 130.

Music: Lloyd Shaw, *Cowboy Dances*, p. 392.

Position: Varsouvienne.

Steps: Mazurka.

DIRECTIONS FOR THE DANCE

Meter 3/4 • Directions are same for both woman and man.

■ *Measures*

I. Long Phrase

1	Swing left heel across in front of right instep (count 3, pick up beat). Step left, close right to left, weight ends on right (counts 1–2).
2	Repeat action of measure 1.
3–4	Swing left heel across in front of right instep (count 3, pick up beat). Step left, right, left (counts 1, 2, 3) and point right foot to right (counts 1–2).
5–8	Beginning right, repeat action of measures 1–4.

II. Short Phrase

9–10	Repeat action of measures 3–4.
11–16	Beginning right, repeat action of measures 9–10 through three times.

■ *Variations for Measures 3–8 (Part I)*

1. **Crossover:** Beginning left, the man moves the woman across in front of him to his left side with three steps. Beginning right, he moves her back to his right side.

2. **Turnback:** During the three steps, make half–turn clockwise and point in opposite direction. Beginning right, turn counterclockwise. **Note:** Forward or backward movements with a pivot on first or third step may be used.

■ *Variation for Measures 9–16 (Part II)*

Swing In and Out: Beginning left, repeat action of measures 3–4 as follows: Man: Take steps in place. Woman: Release man's right hand and take three steps toward center of circle to face reverse line of direction, out to the left and slightly in front of man. Beginning right, take three steps turning counterclockwise under man's upraised left arm and finish in original position. Repeat action toward center and back to original position.

- **Mixer**

  On measures 15–16 in the swing in and out variation, woman may move in reverse line of direction to a new partner and turn counterclockwise into place beside him in Varsouvienne position.

- **NOTE**

  Since parts I and II of the music vary on different records, the repetition of the action should vary accordingly.

Oh Johnny

OH JOHNNY IS A POPULAR SINGING call that may be done as a Square Dance or large Circle Mixer.

Records: Blue Star 1690; EZ 718, 721; Folkraft 1037, 2042; MacGregor 2042.
Formation: Single circle, couples facing center, woman to right of partner, hands joined.
Steps: Shuffle.

DIRECTIONS FOR THE MIXER

- **Singing call**

  Oh, you all join hands and circle the ring. Circle moves clockwise.
  Stop where you are and you give her a swing. Gents swing partners.
  Now swing that girl behind you. Swing corner woman.
  Go back home and
  Swing your own if you have time. Swing with partners.
  Allemande left with your corner girl. Allemande left with corner.
  Do–sa 'round your own. Do–sa–do (sashay) around partner.
  Now you all run away with your sweet corner maid. Promenade counterclock-wise with corner woman for a new partner.
  Singing, oh, Johnny, oh, Johnny, oh! Repeat call to end of recorded music.

Amos Moses

AMOS MOSES IS A novelty dance with no partner.
Meter 4/4 • Directions presented in beats.

Records: High/Scope RM8; RCA 447 0896.

Cassette: High/Scope RM8.

Formation: Scattered, all facing music.

Steps: Grapevine, stamp.

DIRECTIONS FOR THE DANCE

■ *Beats*

1–4	Beginning right, place right heel forward, step right in place; place left heel forward, step left in place.
5	Grapevine in direction of music: pivoting a quarter turn left, step sideward right.
6	Step left behind right.
7	Step sideward right.
8–9	Turning right one–half turn, step left, right in place.
10	Stamp left foot, taking weight, and at the same time clap hands.

■ NOTE

After each sequence all will face one–quarter turn to the right.

Popcorn

POPCORN IS A NOVELTY DANCE with no partner. It is also known as *Alley Cat*.
Meter 4/4 • Directions presented in beats.

Records: "Popcorn," (fast) Eric 4009; High/Scope RM 3, 7; Musicor 1458, 1959;
"Alley Cat," DC 687, 73304; (moderate) Atlantic 13113.

Cassette: High/Scope RM 3, 7.

Formation: Scattered, all facing music.

Steps: Touch, kick, jump.

DIRECTIONS FOR THE DANCE

■ *Beats*

	Introduction: no action.
1–4	Beginning right, touch right toe in front, then touch along side left. Repeat.
5–8	Beginning left, repeat action of beats 1–4.
9–12	Beginning right, touch right toe backward, then touch alongside left. Repeat.
13–16	Beginning left, repeat action of beats 9–12.
17–20	Kick right, knee up in front of left knee and return. Repeat.
21–24	Kick left, knee up in front of right knee and return. Repeat.
25–28	Repeat action of beats 17–24. Action is double time.
29–30	Clap both hands together once.
31–32	Jump and turn a quarter turn to right.
	Repeat dance from beginning making a quarter turn to right at end of each sequence.

■ NOTE

Introduction: "Popcorn" 24 beats; "Alley Cat" 1 beat.

Twelfth Street Rag

*T*WELFTH *S*TREET *R*AG IS A novelty dance composed to a popular tune.

Records: DC 74505; High/Scope RM5.

Cassettes: DC 15X; High/Scope RM5.

Formation: Single circle, hands joined; scattered; or lines of four to five, hands joined, facing line of direction.

Steps: Strut, Charleston, grapevine.

DIRECTIONS FOR THE DANCE

Meter 4/4

■ *Measures*

1	Beginning left, strut four steps forward.
2	Point left toe forward, then to side. Beginning left, take three steps backward.
3–4	Beginning right, repeat action of measures 1–2.
5	Beginning left, take seven quick steps sideward to left. Type of step options could be shuffle, step close, grapevine, and swivel steps.
6	Beginning right, take seven quick steps sideward to right.
7–8	Beginning left, take two Charleston steps in place.
	Repeat dance.

Interlude

1	Jump forward on both feet, throwing hands up in air. Jump backwards on both feet, throwing hands back, turn and face the other way.
2	Turn individually to own right, taking three steps (strut right, left, right) and clap own hands on fourth count. Improvise during interlude.

Plain and Novelty Mixers

GAIN OR EXCHANGE PARTNERS

1. **Upset the Cherry Basket:** When the music stops, the leader requests that everyone change partners. If couples are asked to change with the couple nearest them, everyone is involved, and no one walks to the side for the lack of a partner.

2. **Snowball, Whistle Dance, Pony Express, or Multiplication Dance:** One to three couples start to dance. When the music stops, each couple separates and goes to the sidelines and gets a new partner. This is repeated until everyone is dancing.

3. **Line Up:** The men line up on one side of the room, facing the wall; the women on the other side, facing the wall. When the signal is given, each line backs up until they gain a new partner.

4. **Arches:** All the dancers form a single circle and walk counterclockwise around the circle. Two couples form arches on opposite sides of the circle. When the music stops, the arch is lowered. Those caught in the arch go to the center of the circle, gain a partner, and go back to the circle to form new arches. Eventually, just a few dancers will be walking through the tunnel of arches. When all have partners, the dancing proceeds.

5. **Star by the Right:** Six men form a right-hand star in the center of a single circle formed by the group. The star moves clockwise, and the circle counterclockwise. As the leader gives the signal, six women hook onto the star; alternate genders are called out until all have hooked onto the star. A little spice is added if the last person on each spoke winks or beckons a specific person from the ring to join his or her spoke. When the star is completed the woman dances with the man on her right.

6. **Matching:** Advertising slogans (Ivory Soap–99.9 percent pure, it floats), split proverbs (a rolling stone–gathers no moss), famous couples (Romeo–Juliet), pairs of words that belong together (ham–eggs), playing cards (spades match with hearts for each number, clubs with diamonds), pictures cut in half (cartoons), or songs may be used for this mixer. Half of the slips of paper are given to the men, and the corresponding halves are distributed to the women. As the people circulate, they try to find the person with the corresponding half of their slogan, proverb, cartoon, or whatever has been selected to be matched. When everyone has found his or her partner, the dancing proceeds. If songs are used, each person sings his or her song until he or she finds the person singing the same song.

7. **Musical Chairs:** Set up a double row of chairs, back to back, almost the length of the room. Leave space between every group of four chairs so that partners can get together. The group marches around the chairs. When the music stops, each person tries to gain a seat. A man must sit back to back with a woman. These two become partners and proceed to dance while all the others continue to play the game until all have partners. When all are dancing, the next signal is given and partners separate and rush for a chair, thus providing a change of partners. **Musical knees:** Played like musical chairs, except that on a signal, the men get down on one knee and the women rush to sit on a knee. Those left out go to the side.

Plain and Novelty Mixers (continued)

8. **Ice Cube Pass:** Double circle, men on the outside, women on inside. Pass an orange around men's circle; an ice cube around the women's circle. When the music stops, the man with the orange and woman with the ice cube step to center of circle or its outside and become partners. Repeat over and over, until all have partners. Several oranges and ice cubes may be passed simultaneously.

9. **Mexican Broom Dance.*** As couples are dancing, an extra man with a broom knocks the broom handle on the floor several times. Partners separate, women line up on left side of man with the broom and men on right side. The two lines are about five feet apart. All clap their hands while lining up and until they get a new partner. After everyone is in line, the man with the broom goes up and down the line and decides with which woman he wants to dance. When he has made his choice, he drops the broom and grabs his partner, while everyone else takes a partner, too, and dancing resumes. Then the extra man picks up the broom and the procedure starts all over again. More fun is added to the mixer if the man in going up and down the line pretends to drop the broom but actually keeps on looking for a different partner.

TRADE DANCES

1. **Are You on the Beam?** While everyone is dancing, a spotlight is suddenly focused on a specific area. Those people standing in the rays of the light are requested to give a yell, sing a song, or trade partners.

2. **Hats Off!** Four hats are distributed among four couples. Each couple with a hat places it on one member of another couple. When the music stops, the couples with the hats must change partners.

TAGS

1. **Women's Tag or Men's Tag:** Certain dances may be designated as women's tag or men's tag.

2. **Similarity Tag:** Either a man or a woman may tag, but the person tagging can only tag someone who has a similar color of hair, eyes, shirt, shoes, and so on.

3. **"You Take the Lemon, I'll Take the Peach":** A few lemons or other designated articles are distributed among the men or the women. Anyone who holds the article may tag. Additional fun may be had by stopping the music periodically and anyone holding the article pays a forfeit. Later the forfeits are redeemed by performing a humorous stunt.

ELIMINATION DANCES

1. **Number Please?** Each couple is given a number. Each time the music stops, a number is called out and the couple or couples having the numbers called sit down. Numbers are called out until only one couple remains.

2. **Lemon Dance:** An object—for example, a lemon—is passed from couple to couple. When the music stops, the couple with the object sits down. Eventually one couple is left.

---

*Herb Greggerson, author of *Herb's Blue Bonnet Calls*, saw this mixer danced in Mexico and presented it for the first time at a Square Dance Institute at the University of Texas, April 1948. Directions were first printed in *Foot 'n' Fiddle*, Editors, Anne Pittman, Marlys Swenson, and Olcutt Sanders, May 1948, p. 4.

3. **Dance Contest:** Determine the type of dancing for the contest, for example, Waltz or Jitterbug. It should be conducted in a casual manner with qualified judges. Gradually, the contestants are eliminated until one or two couples remain. Choosing two couples, instead of one, for the winners keeps competition from becoming too keen.

4. **Orange Dance:** Each couple balances an orange or a tennis ball between their foreheads and proceeds to dance. Slow music like a Tango allows the dancers to concentrate on keeping the orange in position and still move to the music. When a couple drops the orange, they go to the sidelines. Eventually one couple is left and the rest have enjoyed the antics of those trying to keep the orange in position. Change the rhythm of the music to match the ability of the dancers.

Jiffy Mixer

JIFFY MIXER WAS COMPOSED BY Jerry and Kathy Helt, Cincinnati, Ohio.

Records: Windsor 4684; LS E 35; DC 74506.
Position: Butterfly.
Formation: Double circle, man's back to center of circle.
Steps: Balance, walk, chug, step–close–step, heel and toe.

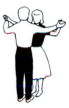

DIRECTIONS FOR THE MIXER

Meter 2/4 • Directions are for man; woman part reverse.

■ Measures

1–4	Introduction: Wait 2 measures. Beginning left, balance away from partner (step touch), balance together (step touch).
1–4	Beginning left, heel, toe, heel, toe, step side in line of direction, close right to left, step side left, touch right toe to left.
5–8	Beginning right, repeat the action of measures 1–4, moving in the reverse line of direction.
9–12	Release hands. Take four chug steps away from partner (both are backing away from each other), clapping between each chug. Chug (count 1), clap (count 2). The clap is on the upbeat of the music.
13–16	Beginning left, take four slow, swaggering steps, diagonally right, each progressing to a new partner. The women move forward in the line of direction; men in the reverse line of direction. Take Butterfly position to begin dance over.

■ Variation

An easier version, no partners, single circle, hands joined, all facing the center. Everyone begins the dance on the left foot, doing the same foot work. After the chug step, rejoin hands and travel in the reverse line of direction four slow steps *or* turn left, making a small circle, solo, four slow steps, to face center. Join hands and repeat dance.

Patty-Cake Polka

Records: Folkraft 1260; Windsor 4624; EZ 3008, 6002; LS 228, E 24.

Cassette: DC 887.

Position: Partners face, two hands joined.

Formation: Double circle, man's back to center.

Steps: Heel and Toe Polka, slide, walk.

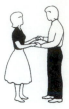

DIRECTIONS FOR THE MIXER

Meter 2/4 • Directions are for man; woman's part reverse.

■ *Measures*

I.	**Heel and Toe Polka and Slide**
1–2	Beginning left, place left heel to left, place left toe to right instep. Repeat.
3–4	Take four slides in line of direction.
5–8	Beginning right, repeat the action of measures 1–4, moving in reverse line of direction.
II.	**Claps**
9	Clap own hands, clap partner's right hand.
10	Clap own hands, clap partner's left hand.
11	Clap own hands, clap partner's hands (both).
12	Clap own hands, slap own knees.
13–14	Hook right elbows and walk around partner and back to place.
15–16	Man moves forward in line of direction to new partner. Woman spins clockwise twice, as she moves in reverse line of direction to new partner.
	Variation
9	Clap partner's right hand three times.
10	Clap partner's left hand three times.
11	Clap partner's hands (both) three times.
12	Slap own knees three times.

Mexican Mixer

T HE *MEXICAN MIXER* IS A popular Texas–Mexican Mixer dating from the French influence in Mexico. According to the noted Mexican dance authority Nelda Drury, San Antonio, Texas, the dance was introduced into Mexico during Maximilian's time and was danced to Viennese music.

Records: "Atotonilco," Musart 1154; MAV Album 7, FD LP7; Folkraft 1516; DOM 8102; High/Scope RM3; or any good Mexican Polka.

Cassette: High/Scope RM3.

Music: "Trompeta Magica," Werner, Robert, *The Folklore Village Saturday Night Book*, p. 24.

Formation: Double circle, couples facing line of direction.

Position: Promenade position.

Steps: Walk, balance, step swing.

DIRECTIONS FOR THE MIXER

Meter 4/4 • Directions are for man, woman's part reverse.

■ *Measures*

Walk and Grapevine

1–2   Beginning man's left, walk forward four steps. Face partner, give eye contact, hold right hands; man steps left to side, right behind left, steps left to side, swing right across left or stamp right lightly, no weight.

3–4   Moving forward in the reverse line of direction, repeat action of measures 1–2. Man begins right.

Balance and Turn

5   Single circle, man's back to center, woman faces center, partners' right hands joined, left hand to dancer on the left (corner). Beginning left, balance forward and back.

6   Release left hands. Turn partner with right–hand hold halfway around with four steps. Now men face center, ladies face out.

7   With partners' right hands joined, man joins left hands with dancer on his left. Beginning left, balance forward and back.

8   Release right–hand hold, turn with left–hand hold half around counterclockwise with four steps. End with new partner in promenade position facing line of direction.

Show enthusiasm by occasionally yelling or put tongue against upper teeth and make a continuous sound.

Tennessee Wig Walk

THIS DANCE WAS COMPOSED by Harry and Dia Trygg, Tucson, Arizona, in 1954.

Records: "Tennessee Wig Walk," MCA 60051; "Hey Good Looking," Wagon Wheel 824.

Formation: Double circle, couples, right–hand star position, men face line of direction, women face reverse line of direction.

Steps: Grapevine, walk.

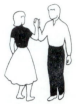

DIRECTIONS FOR THE MIXER

Meter 4/4 • Directions are for man; woman's part reverse.

■ *Measures*

1–2	Introduction: no action.
1–2	Beginning left, point left toe across in front of right, point left toe to left side (slow, slow); exchanging places, grapevine, step left behind right, step right, cross left in front of right, hold (quick, quick, slow, slow). Man now on outside, woman inside, both facing original direction. Change to left hand star.
3–4	Beginning right, repeat action of measures 1–2 with opposite feet, returning to original position.
5–6	Right hand star position. Turning clockwise, make one full turn, stepping left, right, left, brush right; right, left, right, brush left. End facing original direction.
7–8	Release hands. Leave partner and move forward with step, step, step, brush step, step, step, brush. Man progresses in line of direction, woman reverse line of direction, passing first person on first "brush"; meeting next person on second "brush." Join right hands.

Repeat dance from beginning with new partner.

Red River Valley

Records: Can–Ed A783; EZ 3003, 6015; Folkraft 1269; Pioneer 3007; Windsor 753; World of Fun Vol. I.

Position: Set of three, man between two women, arms linked.

Formation: Two sets of three, facing each other in large circle. Each set alternately faces line of direction and reverse line of direction.

DIRECTIONS FOR THE MIXER

■ *Swinging Call*

Verse 1
Now you lead right down to the valley. Walk diagonally forward to right and pass opposite set to meet new set.
Circle to the left, then to the right. All join hands and circle left, then right.
Now you swing with the gal in the valley. Man swings (elbow or waist swing) right–hand woman.
And you swing with your red river gal. Man swings left–hand woman.

Verse 2
Now you lead right on down the valley. Each set links arms. Walk diagonally forward to right and pass opposite set to meet new set.
Circle to the left, then to the right. All join hands and circle left, then right.
Now the girls make a wheel in the valley. Four women make right–hand star, walking clockwise once around and return to place.
And the boys do–sa–do so polite. Two men do–sa–do, passing right shoulders.

Verse 3
Now you lead right on down the valley. Each set links arms and passes opposite set as before to meet new set.
Circle to the left, then to the right. All join hands and circle left, then right.
Now you lose your gal in the valley. Two right–hand women change places crossing diagonally.
And you lose your red river gal. Two left–hand women change places in same manner. Each man now has two new partners for repeat of dance.

Levi Jackson Rag*

THE *LEVI JACKSON RAG* IS AN Anglo–American Mixer for a five–couple set. It is a sprightly dance and ragtime–style tune by the late Pat Shaw; it was commissioned by the Mountain Folk Festival, Adult Section, of Berea College in 1975. The Adult Festival is held annually at Levi Jackson State Park near London, Kentucky.

Pat Shaw had a passionate interest in music and kept his interest in both folk song and dance centered in his life. He contributed significantly in the research, publication, and composition of music and dance and in the leadership of the folk dance movement.

Records: Country Dance Album CLR 16L; Festival 801; LS E 28; Folklore Village FLV 103; Shaw E 28.

Cassette: Country Dance Album CLR 16C.

Music: "Levi Jackson Rag," Werner, Robert, *The Folklore Village Saturday Night Book*, p. 35.

Formation: Five–couple set, one head couple and four side couples.

Steps: Walk, swing.

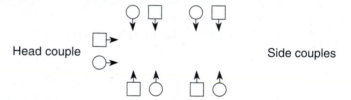

Head couple   Side couples

DIRECTIONS FOR THE MIXER

Meter 2/4

■ *Measures*

	1–4	Introduction: no action (8 counts).
A	1–18	Side couples right and left through and back with opposite side couple. For measures 3–4, head couple, inside hands joined, walk halfway down center of set; for measures 7–8, continue to foot of set.
	9–12	Side couples join hands with opposites to circle four left once around, while head couple separates, casts back to home place.
	13–16	All partners do–si–do.
B	1–4	All five ladies chain to third man: right–hand star past partner and next man to third man, who turns woman with a courtesy turn. Head man should chain his partner around fairly fast, so that she may get back into the star that follows.
	5–8	All five ladies chain on two more places as above where they meet their new partners (their original corners).
	9–10	Promenade new partner in line of direction to next place, taking four steps.
	11–12	Balance partner right and left.
	13–16	All swing new partners in new places.

Repeat whole dance four more times, ending in original position.

*Levi Jackson Rag included by permission of Mountain Folk Festival, Berea College, Berea, KY.

5
Square Dance

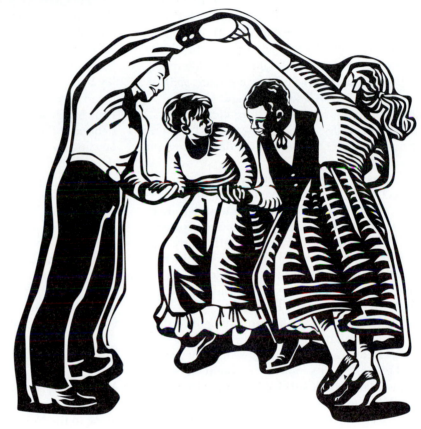

HISTORY

■ *Antecedents*

The antecedents of modern American *Square Dance* are the English Country Dances and the French Contredanse–Cotillon and Quadrille. The English Country Dances–the *Rounds, Longways,* and *Square Eight*–were introduced into France in the late 17th century. The Round and Square Eight forms were transformed by the French into the *Contredanse Francaise* and a later form called the *Cotillon.* The Contredanse and the Cotillon were dances for two and four couples in a square formation.

The word *Cotillon* means "underpetticoat" and comes from a French peasant song to which it was danced. The Cotillon was strictly a square in formation. Writers of the time used the terms *Contredanse*

and *Cotillon* interchangeably, making it difficult to clarify the early development of these dance forms. Historians, however, agree that these forms were the antecedent of the Quadrille and thus of our modern Square Dance.

The Quadrille was a five–figure dance done by four couples in a four–sided figure or square. In its early form, the Quadrille consisted of four of the most popular Contredanses of the time. A fifth figure derived from the Cotillon–*Le Final*–was added at a later date to make the traditional five figures of the dance. The five figures were *Le Pantalon, L'Ete, La Poule, La Frenis,* and *Le Final.* French Quadrilles were for two, four, or any number of couples, and each remained vis-à-vis, dancing only with each other. In England, the Quadrille was danced with only four couples. Quadrille music was as exciting as the many and varied dance figures. The French used semiclassical music, light opera tunes, and music composed especially for the Quadrilles by well-known composers of the time.

Couple dances were also gaining in popularity at the same time the Quadrilles were in vogue. The Waltz, Polka, Mazurka, and Redowa were exciting new dances featuring daring dance positions and flying feet! The coexistence of the two resulted in combining Quadrilles with couple-dance steps. Waltz Quadrilles were especially numerous and popular.

The *Lancers* was a very elegant and elaborate form of the Quadrille. It must, therefore, be counted among the antecedents of our modern Square Dance. The Lancers consisted of four couples arranged vis-à-vis, and the five figures were danced with the opposite couple. In reality, the Lancers was a sequence of five Square Dances, each part danced to a different tempo. The fifth figure was usually a rousing military style 4/4 tempo. The well-known Grand March is actually the fifth figure of a long-forgotten Lancers. Although a Quadrille, the Lancers was listed and thus distinguished from Quadrilles on the dance program of the day.

Lancer music was usually written by well-known composers of the time and played by live full orchestras. Many American Lancers were danced to Gilbert and Sullivan melodies and some to Stephen Foster songs. Although known and danced in the early 1800s, Lancers did not become popular until the mid to late 19th century. In America, the French Quadrilles were cast aside in favor of Lancers in all the major urban areas of the time.

These were the dance forms flourishing in western Europe. And like all other parts of the culture brought by immigrants to the New World, they were subjected to the test of a radically different environment. Those dances that survived emerged irrevocably altered. Just as the individual identities of colonial Americans were being molded from, for example, Scotch-Irish to New York citizen to loyal American, so were dance forms being molded and shaped into new forms with new identities.

Colonial America inherited a rich dance tradition. It is no wonder that dance was one of the most significant features of colonial life. Indeed, dance was reported to be the chief amusement. Dance was not limited by social class or ethnic group, but was enjoyed by people of all stations. The dance map was becoming clear. Dances of English and French origin were being done throughout the colonies from north to south. Pockets of Scotch-Irish, Germans, Dutch, and others were maintaining the Old World dance traditions wherever they settled. African Americans in the middle and southern colonies brought their own dance traditions. American Indians continued their dance heritage despite colonial intrusion. It

seems clear that colonial America enjoyed a healthy and heterogeneous dance repertoire.

■ New England

The early part of the 19th century saw America becoming a dancing nation. Dancing masters were everywhere for hire; the new minister was welcomed at an Ordination Ball; even teachers and ministers doubled as dancing masters to augment their salaries. Plain folks danced everywhere and on all occasions, in taverns, town halls, and kitchens; at barn raisings, husking bees, and roof raisings.

New Englanders cast aside the five-part Quadrille for a simpler, free-flowing adaptation—the *Singing Quadrille*. These "modern Quadrilles" were set to such dashing American folk tunes as "Darling Nellie Gray," "The Girl I Left Behind Me," and "Hinkey Dinkey Parley Voo." The latter was perhaps a salute to the French Quadrille, its forerunner, and to the predominance of French dancing masters. In any case, the tunes, the dances, and the rhyming caller became widely popular. Singing calls by the hundreds were invented and flourished from New York to Maine. The French-Canadian populace of New England were especially enthusiastic participants, and they are credited with embellishing these modern Quadrilles with the long count swing and buzz step.

Nineteenth-century Singing Quadrilles settled comfortably along beside the New England Contra to become widely known as New England–type dancing. Little did the average New Englander of the time suspect that this new American hybrid would be the basis for 20th-century Square Dance.

■ The South

The *Running Set* is a dance form of the people of Kentucky and the southern Appalachian Mountains who came to the New World from northern England and the lowlands of Scotland. They found, in the hills and valleys, an isolation that for many years permitted them to practice and thus preserve almost unchanged the customs and traditions of their homelands. It was this isolation that allowed the vigorous folk strain of rounds and chain dances to ferment and later to flow over the trails of the western frontier.

Cecil J. Sharp, the noted English folklorist, came to the Appalachian Mountains in 1917 in search of early English ballads and songs. While there, he observed the dance form known as the *Running Set*. His scholarly observations and inquiries led him to conclude that it was, indeed, the earliest form of the English Country Dance. The absence of courtesies such as bowing, saluting, and honors indicated to him that the dances were uninfluenced by court manners and thus predated dances found in Playford's first dance book of 1650. He further suggested that the history of the Running Set might date back to 17th-century England and Scotland or even earlier to the May Day Rounds, a pagan quasireligious ceremonial of which the Maypole Dance is the best example.

The Running Set was more in the tradition of the Round Eight than the Square Eight. The dance action moved around the square as opposed to across it. The Running Set was danced in either a big set or circle for as many couples as desired or, as was more typical, in a square or set for four couples. The typical dance action consisted of the first couple leading to the right, dancing a figure, then to couple three repeating the figure, and then couple four repeating it. As the action began with couple four, couple two began the "follow up" action with couple three. The do-si-do, a staple of Western Square Dance, was used to finish off the figures. The "follow up" action allowed for 12 repeats of a figure in a square and as many repeats as there are couples in a "big set or circle." The dance done in either form was long and very vigorous!

The characteristics of the Running Set as danced in Kentucky and the southern Appalachian Mountains make it the most immediate antecedent of the Western brand of Square Dance. The two most enduring characteristics are the use of a caller and the figure action of moving or visiting around the square.

In the Running Set, the caller either called from within the set, prompting the dancers, or from outside the set. If calling from outside the set, the caller would add folksy, rhythmic lines of "patter" to the directions for executing the figure. This was the forerunner of the colorful Western patter calls of the early 20th century. The caller is truly an American innovation whose role particularly in the early days, was to keep the dance alive by passing along calls and figures from generation to generation solely by oral tradition.

The step used was a bouncing run that beat out the rhythm against the dance floor. Dancers appeared erect with loose jigging action of the arms and limber disjointed action of the legs and feet. This style, or clogging action, is the trademark of the Running Set. In early times, the sound of the rhythm of the feet was the music for the dance. Play Party Games, or dancing without fiddle music, was then an offspring of the Running Set. Play Party Games allowed dancing to continue and thus endure times of fanatical religious disapproval. (Refer to Play Party Games, p. 71)

■ Texas Square Dance

Texas Square Dance heritage came largely from the South with the settlers who moved to the frontier after the Civil War. Before the war, East Texas settlers developed the area into a replica of Southern plantation life with an economy based on cotton farming and slaves. A festive social life soon developed. Balls and parties attracted guests to around-the-clock dancing from as far as 20 miles away. Settlers brought with them not only their love of dancing, but also their dance traditions–the visiting couple figures, do-si-do, and Square Dance caller.

The Civil War and Indian depredations retarded settlement in west Texas. Once the vast area was opened, social life was patterned around ranching and the demands of ranch life rather than cotton farming. The sparseness of settlements and the distances to be traveled made social gathering rare but highly prized. In west Texas, the two most important ingredients of social life, women and fiddlers, were as scarce as "hen's teeth."

Fiddlers were so rare that many callers began the dance with "Honor the Fiddler!" Although honored at dances, expressions such as "lazy enough to be a good fiddler" and "thick as fiddlers in Hell" attest to their general personality types. Regardless of their shortcomings, pioneer fiddlers enjoyed their art and would often get together for an evening of straight fiddling. When an itinerant fiddler showed up in ranch country, a dance was arranged regardless of the day of the week. The first band to play in the Texas Panhandle came from Fort Worth, some 277 miles away, to play for a ball held in 1889. Fiddlers and their music were in short supply in west Texas, but the enthusiasm for dancing to the sounds of the "fisky fiddle" was not.

The sparseness of settlements and the scarcity of women made any kind of social gathering of the two sexes as rare as a "fiddler beyond the Pearly Gates!" Usually there were three times as many men, even counting all the females from the youngest to the oldest. At dances in the early days, wall-flowers were nonexistent. Women prided themselves on being able to dance all night without missing a set, and, more often than not, they would easily wear out their shoe soles in one evening. Cowboys were said to have noticed that "slabsided," or fat, women were often more durable than "scantlings," or skinny, women as dance partners. Social gatherings were so important to the cowboy that he thought nothing of riding a great distance to "squire" a woman to a dance. One cowboy is reputed to have ridden 10 miles to hire a buggy, 15 miles to get the woman, 15 miles to the dance, 15 miles back to the woman's home, 15 miles to return the buggy, and, finally, 10 miles on horseback to reach home–a total of 80 miles. Square Dancing was serious business in Texas, and the conditions of frontier life made it possible for the Square Dance to become firmly embedded in Southwestern culture before the region began to suffer from the inroads of urban civilization.

Texas became the home and stronghold of the colorful patter call and the intricate dance figures that were created by the uninhibited imagination of the callers. Texas Square Dancing was the product of the oral rather than the written tradition. Calls were passed along and repeated as remembered. Unaware of the more traditional spelling of Square Dance terms, cowboy callers called them as they sounded; thus "dos–a–dos" became "do–see–do," "chassez" became "sashay," and "allemande" became variously "al–a–man" or "alamand."

■ *Early Leaders*

In the early 20th century, when Square Dancing was at a low ebb in other parts of the United States, folks in west Texas were working hard all day and dancing harder all night. One of the most important pioneers of this period was H. F. Greggerson, Jr., of El Paso, Texas, better known as Herb. Greggerson was a dancer, caller, and writer who used his feet as a mail carrier during the day and, in his leisure moments, as a dancer at a faster tempo at night. He was a strong force in helping El Paso build its reputation as the center of Western cowboy Square Dancing. Before World War II, dancers by the hundreds attended Herb's "barn" to learn and dance to his directions, which were embellished by colorful patter and delivered with a twinkle in his eye.

Greggerson and his wife Pauline traveled and danced throughout west Texas and New Mexico collecting old–time calls and dances. The resulting collections were published in two books, *West Texas Square Dances* and *Herb's Blue Bonnet Calls*, the latter copyrighted in 1937.

In 1939 the Greggersons traveled with their exhibition group, The Blue Bonnet Set, as guests of the Highway 80 Association to the World's Fair in New York. The occasion was a showcase for different dance groups from all parts of the United States. The opportunity for fellowship and exchange between dancers and callers led to a greater appreciation and awareness of the status of Square Dance in America. Exhibitions at the Roosevelt Hotel in New York and at the Edgewater Beach Hotel in Chicago earned them the title of World Champion Square Dancers. The authors of *Dance A While* recognize the work of Herb Greggerson in collecting, teaching, and calling the traditional dances of the Western cowboy as a major contribution to the history of Square Dance in America.

Lloyd Shaw and his wife Dorothy were two giants among the few of their kind in the early development of Square Dancing in the West. In addition to his talent as a teacher and writer, Shaw was more importantly an innovative and creative leader. Early in pursuit of his interest in Square Dancing, he envisioned a future in which all Americans would be

Square Dancing. His Cheyenne Mountain Dance Group showed America the joy and spirit of the dance. He further ensured his vision by spending his summers instructing hundreds from all walks of life how to teach Square Dancing.

As principal of the Cheyenne School in Colorado Springs, Colorado, Shaw's first interest in dance came from searching for an adjunct to the school's athletic program. He began teaching European folk dance and, after winning over the football team, the dancers became an official group. The Cheyenne Mountain Dancers' first performing tour found them doing all European dance. Later they added some American dances from the Henry Ford "Good Morning" collection of New England Contras and Quadrilles. It was not until Shaw became interested in the dances that were indigenous to the Colorado Mountains in which he lived that the Cheyenne Mountain Dancers became an all–cowboy dance group.

The Shaws' love of the mountains and the indigenous activities made it a labor of love to research and collect from old–timers the dances of miners, prospectors, and cowboys in the Rocky Mountain West. The dances they found had come along with settlers migrating West and were the offsprings of the Southern mountain Running Set, four–couple squares with patter calls and figures reflecting western ways in their titles. In 1939, Shaw published *Cowboy Dances*, his collection of calls and figures gathered in Colorado and the surrounding mountain area. This was followed in 1948 by the *Round Dance Book*. Important as his writings and teachings were, it was his high-school exhibition team, the Cheyenne Mountain Dancers, performing cowboy dances for the American public in the 1930s and 1940s that aroused a spirited and widespread interest in American dance. Getting America interested in American dance was his vision, and it happened!

The Lloyd Shaw Foundation is an incorporated, nonprofit organization founded by former summer-class members to perpetuate his memory, his work, and his special philosophy. The foundation trains teachers and dance leaders, produces records and teaching materials, sponsors recreational dance weeks, publishes books and pamphlets, and collects and disperses dance material of historical interest.

■ *Post-World War II*

The rapid growth and expansion of Square Dance after World War II was largely the outgrowth of population movements and technical advances in sound equipment. Population movements were of two kinds: movement to urban areas because of continued industrialization and population displacement associated with service in the armed forces and employment in defense-related industries. The technical improvements in the quality and availability of sound equipment made teaching and calling to groups of all sizes possible and effective. Portable equipment made ownership by schools, families, teachers, and callers a reality, thus multiplying the opportunities for dance experience. In addition, the durability and availability of properly recorded music provided the correct dance tempo and authentic sounds for dancing.

The American penchant for following the latest fad was also a factor. In the 1940s and 1950s, Square Dance hobbyists contributed greatly to the popularity of Square Dance through public performances and exhibitions that introduced nonparticipants to the dance. The precision and style of these exhibitions became a standard for performance for other dancers to emulate, thus raising the skill level of the dance. As an added bonus, the massive effort to serve the social needs of wartime America created a rich opportunity for developing leadership in Square Dance for the future. These are the factors that made it possible for thousands of Americans to be introduced to their own heritage, the American Square Dance.

The postwar years were characterized by mass participation in Square Dance. Classes for over a hundred at a time were common. Communities vied to host the largest and best jamborees, festivals, or Square Dance contests. The major special events, such as inaugurations, patriotic celebrations, and civic anniversaries, featured Square Dance as a main social event. Crowd estimates at these early dance events ranged from 5,000 to 10,000 people. This formerly quiet, predominantly rural form of recreation had suddenly become the mass mania of urban living.

The fast-growing Square Dance population became the target market for a host of goods and services. Among the services were Square Dance publications. The first such publication, *Foot 'n' Fiddle*, a Texas Square Dance magazine, began publication in November 1946. The editors were Anne Pittman and Marlys Swenson Waller, physical education instructors at the University of Texas, and Olcutt Sanders, head of the American Friends Service committee. The headquarters was in Austin, Texas. The magazine chronicled the early years of the Square Dance movement in the southwest from the mid-1940s to the late 1950s.

A second publication, *Sets In Order*, appeared in November 1948, in response to the growing population of dancers in southern California. The editor, Bob Osgood, combined his enthusiasm for Square Dancing with considerable journalistic skills to launch what became the number-one Square Dance magazine in America. *Sets In Order*, later known as *Square Dancing Magazine*, chronicled the Square Dance movement in the United States and points overseas from 1948 until it ceased publication in December 1985.

Other commercial ventures included merchandising of current dress styles for men and women. Recording companies flourished by providing a wide assortment of recordings and sound equipment. Teaching materials in the form of books, pamphlets, and recorded teaching progressions became available. Former part-time teachers and callers became full-time professionals. Summer calendars began to be filled with institutes, workshops, and vacation-oriented opportunities to dance in exotic places. In 1970, a group known as Legacy was formed to provide a vehicle for communication between manufacturers, producers, publications, and Square Dance associations. Square Dancing had arrived in the marketplace.

As dance skill and experience increased, dance moved from a mass activity into smaller organized units. The dance club became the heart of Square Dancing. Club calendars included classes, interclub exchanges, and travel to major special events. Associations were the outgrowth of club activities. Today there are over 300 Square Dance publications and associations in the United States.

Solid growth in regional organization in various parts of the country made the step to a national-level organization easy and logical. Annual national Square Dance conventions began in 1952, at a time when interest in the movement was on the upswing. Since the first convention, cities from North to South and coast to coast have hosted the national convention. Attendance figures for early conventions were between 15,000 and 20,000. Attendance figures for the 1970s exploded to between 40,000 and 50,000. It is estimated that at present more than 6 million people square dance. American Square Dance is in vogue as an international form of recreation in Canada, Japan, Australia, England, Germany, and many other countries. A world Square Dance directory is available for those who wish to become international square dancers.

Square Dance is no longer a quaint cowboy or country hillbilly activity. Media coverage, movies, and television have been instrumental in making Square Dance a familiar activity to an extensive American audience. A commemorative stamp issued by the United States Postal Service in 1970 increased the visibility of Square Dance. The third week in September has been set aside as Square Dance Week and has been officially proclaimed by mayors and governors across the country. The spirit of Square Dancing is found in the simple cooperative effort dancers engender by dancing. Square Dance is truly America's folk dance.

■ *Standardization of Basic Movements*

The picture of Square Dance in its formative years was a mosaic of regional dance differences. The two dominant types were the singing calls of the eastern states and the patter calls of the western states. The upsurge of interest in Square Dance led to a natural flow of dances from one section of the country to the other. Western Square Dance became popular in the East while at the same time singing calls became popular in the West. Although the skilled and experienced dancer could travel and dance comfortably in any area, the regional differences in basic steps, promenade positions, dance tempos, type and duration of swings, balance steps, and stylings gave the Square Dance movement a "Tower of Babel" effect. There was no common vocabulary of dance terms understood and used by teachers, callers, or dancers. In effect, there was your way and my way, but no common or right way to perform basics. The increased number and mobility of square dancers within and between regions made this a major problem.

The widespread enjoyment of Square Dancing is largely due to the fact that dancers from coast to coast and overseas execute the same fundamental movements, called basics. The dance movements and steps, and the styling of hands, arms, and positions, are all taught and executed in the same manner. The rationale behind this standardization of basics and learning progressions is to make it possible for dancers to learn calls in any given area and thus be skilled enough to dance to calls anywhere, across the country or overseas.

The guiding force behind the movement to standardize Square Dance movements and teaching procedures has been Bob Osgood of Los Angeles, a teacher, caller, and long-time editor of *Sets In Order*, later known as *Square Dancing Magazine*, the official publication of the Sets In Order American Square Dance Society. As early as 1960, a booklet describing 30 basics was available from *Sets In Order*. The work was the result of a cooperative study Osgood made with the help of prominent callers across the country. The success and acceptance of this early work led Osgood to head a larger study in 1969, which resulted in organizational changes to facilitate the work of standardization. The work of standardization, adoptions, and changes was carried on by *Callerlab*, an arm of the International Association of Square Dance Callers. All standardized movements and plateaus, or ability levels, were published in *Square Dancing Magazine* as a joint venture with Callerlab. Over 30 years of study and experimentation have gone into developing the following plateaus and movement basics.

The Basic plateau covers 1 to 50 movements. Additional basics bring the total to 59 and with the addition of the Mainstream movements, the total is 78 for this edition. The more advanced levels such as Plus, Advanced, Challenge, C–1, and C–2 serve the interest of highly skilled and dedicated dancers. The terms attached to the various levels are also used by clubs to identify their dance skill level. This allows dancers of similar skill the opportunity to visit and enjoy dancing whereever they travel at home or abroad.

■ *Contemporary Notes*

The waning days of the 20th century find a dramatic drop in the number of square dancers and an even greater reduction in the number taking lessons. Two reasons seem apparent. The post World War II generation that so enthusiastically embraced the dance and helped propel it to a worldwide audience also took it with them to the recreational vehicle parks and senior centers. The present generation see square dance as an "old folks" activity. Secondly, the standardization of calls into various levels increased the learning period from a minimum of six months to a year. That time commitment greatly delayed club participation and any anticipated enjoyment and sociability.

In an effort to counter this downward trend, leadership in the field has made it a top priority to define an entry–level program that has worldwide acceptance and that can be taught in one season. At present, the Mainstream and Plus level clubs are, in fact, acting as entry–level programs. If a community has a predominance of Mainstream clubs, lessons teach Mainstream movements. The same is true where there is a preponderance of Plus clubs.

It is estimated that the Mainstream and Plus levels account for 90 percent of all square dancers. At the present time, the Plus level takes more than one season, or approximately a year, to learn all the movements. The Mainstream level takes about one half that time but cannot cover all possible movements. Frequency studies of movements used indicate that it is possible to shorten an entry level list of movements and teaching order. Such a move would shorten the learning period, increase dancer participation, keep mobility of dancers viable, and not pose a problem to Plus dancers since they already know Mainstream movements.

SQUARE YOUR SETS

The caller is a teacher and a group leader and, in like manner, the teacher is a caller and a group leader. The success of a series of Square Dance lessons depends upon creating a pleasant, friendly, and fun–filled atmosphere in a class or club setting. The caller–teacher must first be a trained teacher to select and present materials in an orderly progression. The caller–teacher must also be an accomplished dancer to demonstrate the movements and dance style effectively.

■ Calling

Patter and singing calls have historically been the mainstay methods of moving dancers through their paces. Patter calling featured colorful rhyming phrases accompanying the call directions used in Western cowboy dance figures. The additional phrases allowed time to execute the movements. With the advent of basic movements, the additional lines of patter were curtailed in favor of more directions and less color. The patter caller was still, however, free to call extemporaneously, thus retaining the competitive aspect of this method of calling.

The present-day singing calls are largely done in the same mode as in the past. The calls follow a set sequence and are arranged to the melody of a song. The usual sequence is an opener, main figure, break, main figure, and ending. Often the opener, break, and ending are the same. As in the past, dancers tend to memorize the dance action and are not wholly dependent upon the caller. Singing calls follow popular musical trends and are continually being choreographed to the latest hit tunes. This feature makes singing calls current in each succeeding generation of dancers.

Calling is far more demanding today than in the past due to the sheer volume of movements and the intricate and varied choreography. In addition, dancers are more sophisticated and the competition between callers on the national and local levels is keener. Callers must, therefore, find and develop their own method.

There are a variety of methods for moving dancers through a sequence of calls and returning them to home positions in the set. The easiest method is the use of *cue cards*, or prearranged written sequences. The caller's emphasis on notes, however, negates his role as an attractive and entertaining caller. The *pure memory* caller must commit to memory volumes or materials. Although it overcomes the lack of eye contact between dancer and caller, as when using cue cards, calling from memory is inflexible and lacks variety in presentation. The *module caller* uses certain sequences of a few basics that are more or less rigidly learned. However, they can be put together rather spontaneously to provide fairly interesting sequences. *Sight calling* is much like patter calling. It gives the caller complete freedom to "ad lib" and move dancers around with interesting combinations without attention to where any one individual dancer is during a call sequence. However, once the sequence is to be terminated, the caller must find four predetermined dancers and assess their positions to get them back to original home positions. This is due to the fact that most basic movements and all of the Mainstream movements are danced symmetrically in lines. Dancers need to be in the proper order so that an "allemande left" call will return them to home positions. Should this not be the case, callers must know several "get-outs" to get dancers in position for an allemande left. The *image system* of calling requires the caller to have an affective mental image of the entire square while following a key dancer around the pattern as it changes. The caller thinks of himself as the key dancer. A good metaphor for this system is that the caller is in the "footprints" of the key man or that he is the "ghost" or "image" of that dancer.

■ Sight Calling

The ultimate objective of Square Dance calling, regardless of method, is to call sequences that are possible to execute, are logically linked and flow smoothly one to the other, stimulate the interest and enthusiasm of the dancers, and finally, return dancers to their partners and home positions at the end of a sequence.

Sight calling is the method most used by contemporary callers. It allows the caller to "ad lib" freely and to use advanced and challenge level calls where appropriate. This method removes any restrictions from the callers' choreographic designs.

There are three steps to sight calling:

1. Establish primary and secondary couples. The primary couple should be easily recognizable. The secondary couple should be the couple to the left of the primary couple. For insurance, select two couples in more than one square to offset the possibility of a break down during a call.

2. Call any sequence moving dancers around freely but be aware of formations.

3. Terminate the call sequence by matching up the primary and secondary couples and putting the square in lines with their original partners. The square is thus ready for the call "allemande left," which moves dancers back to home positions.

■ Tips for Sight Calling

1. The primary couple should be the one couple easiest to remember. They may be friends or acquaintances or simply have on colorful outfits. Tall couples are more prominent and visible and thus make good primary couples.

2. Establish primary and secondary couples in at least three squares. The odds of three squares breaking down are in the caller's favor.

3. Use squares in the front of the hall. The better dancers tend to gather there and are less likely to make mistakes.

4. Call several quick left allemandes watching a different square each time to reinforce the identity of the primary and secondary couples.

5. The sight calling system always works as long as the calls are symmetrical, so that the whole square moves to the call. It does not work when only half of the square is active.

■ *Keys to Good Calling*

Clarity: Enunciate clearly and emphasize the "action words" and short directive phrases: "*Ladies* star left," "Allemande left."

Rhythm: Keep an active "patting foot" call on the beat of the music. Call the next movement while dancers are executing the last call. Be aware of musical phrases. Begin the call on the phrase or downbeat.

Command: Project calls out; do not swallow or mumble the calls. Call within the framework of dancers' knowledge and ability level.

Judgment: Adjust dance progressions and practice time to the ability level of the dancers. Review often and in interesting combinations of basics. Avoid endless walk- and talk-throughs without music.

Enthusiasm: Approach each lesson in a natural, sincere, and friendly manner. Display humor, reward progress, and encourage the better dancers to dance with and help upgrade the skills of other dancers.

■ *Calling Sequence*

The movements of the Basic and Mainstream level are simply called one after the other without additional colorful rhymes or phrases. The calls sound similar to those of an auctioneer in that they are announced in rapid and clipped fashion. In putting together a sequence of calls or when calling ad lib, several rules need to apply. First, the movements must be possible to execute in the order called; that is, they must be linked and flow one from the other. Second, the first call must get the square into the formation needed to begin executing the sequence. Mainstream and Plus calls are executed from several line type formations such as eight chain thru, two faced lines, and ocean wave. Line formations begin and end all sequences. The ending line formation should put the dancers in position to execute an allemande left, thus allowing the dancers to move to home position with their original partner.

Two general rules to remember. Mainstream calls or movements work in lines and the allemande left is the key call for resolving or terminating the

sequence. Callers should have in mind several "get-out" calls that do indeed get dancers into the proper position should the free-wheeling calls they use not do so. The "get-out" is a short call that rescues the caller from an improper sequence to a proper one.

■ *Use of Prerecorded Calls*

In public schools and recreational groups the use of calls on cassettes, CDs, and videos serves to keep the class dance materials current, provides an opportunity to dance to professional calling, and serves as a model to upgrade the teacher–caller's live calling ability.

Overuse of recorded calls can restrict the class to one type of call and thus distract from the spontaneity and challenge of live calling. It can also contribute to poor preparation by the teacher–caller. Live calling reinforces knowledge of the call pattern and increases the teacher–caller's understanding and acquisitions of the many Basic movements to be taught.

Using prerecorded calls presumes that the teacher knows and has danced the call and that all basics have been taught and used in other dances. A suggested teaching progression follows.

1. Play the new material to accustom the class to the sound of the caller's voice and the tempo. This also gives the class a preview of the basics involved in the dance.

2. Analyse and walk the class through the first segment of the call.

3. Call it live and up to tempo, no music.

4. Dance to recorded call and music.

5. Repeat steps 2 and 4 for the remainder of the dance. Note: Modern equipment allows user to stop and start recordings at any point. This aids and reinforces instruction.

STYLING

Dancing style begins with the dance step. The step should be a gliding shuffle with each step on the beat of the music. The result is a smooth, flowing movement enjoyable to the individual and the dance group. From the first musical note, dancers should begin to respond to the rhythm by taking three small steps and a touch forward then backward. Dancers not involved in the call should maintain this rhythmic action to be ready to move into the call.

Styling results from executing basics in the proper number of counts or beats of music. Timing varies, but it is an important part of learning the basics. Women's chain over and back, including the courtesy turn, takes 16 counts. Women move across and courtesy turn in eight counts and repeat to home position in eight counts. Hand clasps, arm holds, wrist holds, swing and turn positions are all part of the style, comfort, and logic of dance movement. Dancing the basics in the proper counts gives style and elegance to the dance action. Teach styling and timing techniques with each Basic movement. Dancers will enjoy and take pride in making the right moves.

TEACHING APPROACHES

Teachers may choose one of two approaches for teaching the beginning Square Dance basics. The Big Circle Approach makes use of the single circle, double circle, and Sicilian circle for teaching and practicing basics that can be done without reference to the square formation. The Set approach begins with the dancers in the square formation and teaches the basics in reference to positions and movement directions as they evolve from the use of a simple Square Dance call.

The Big Circle approach is immediately attractive in that it allows all class members to be active at once; since the teacher makes the class "odd or even" in numbers, there can be no extras. The single circle is particularly useful for demonstration. Dancers can see the mechanics and style of a Basic move. Basics appropriate to the single circle are the shuffle (circling left, right, forward and back), do-sa-do, swing, allemande left, honor, twirl, single-file promenade, grand right and left, and forearm turns. The double circle is appropriate and useful in teaching promenade, California Twirl, you turn back, box the gnat, and wheel around. The Sicilian circle is a formation in which two couples face, one facing clockwise and the other counterclockwise. It is useful in teaching ladies chain, right and left thru, pass thru, box star position, square thru, star thru, or any Basic movement requiring this set-up.

The Big Circle approach is useful for class warm-up and review. It allows all class members to be active, including the teacher, who may fill in if there is an extra dancer. It may also be used as a part of a lesson to present and demonstrate new basics. The Big Circle approach is versatile and should be used throughout a series of lessons whenever appropriate and needed.

The Set approach combines maneuvering in the square with learning the Basic movements as they occur in a given dance sequence. After all, the set is only a "square" in concept. Once dancers respond to a call, the set can become a single circle, double circle, or parallel lines. This is an exciting approach because it plunges the dancers into full Square Dance action. Their objective to learn to square dance, happens in the first lesson and is not delayed by practice and drill on style and technique. In a short series of lessons, getting to the heart of the dancing motivates the dancer to listen and learn.

■ Planning Units and Lessons

The basics in this text provide materials for beginners and intermediates. The Mainstream movements are more suitable for those who wish to join in club level dancing. Beginning materials are covered in levels 1, 2, and 3. Intermediate materials are covered in levels 4 and 5. Mainstream movements provide more advanced techniques and formations. In addition, there are ample dance call (figures) sequences and singing calls to provide practice in learning and combining movements for all levels.

Public schools and recreation groups may find it advantageous to divide the materials into a series of five or six lesson units progressively linked and scheduled throughout the year. Recreation groups and after-school clubs can easily cover the first 50 Basic moves in one year. The additional Basic and Mainstream movements will need to be progressively distributed over a period of a year.

A rule of thumb suggests that instruction should go slowly enough for dancer to learn and enjoy each lesson and fast enough to hold their interest and provide a challenge. Planning in relation to a specific "on the job" situation provides the best estimate of content and length of intructional period. The overall objective should be to provide a sound skill basis in an atmosphere of fun and fellowship and challenge enough for dancers to choose Square Dance as a lifetime recreational pursuit.

A daily lesson plan is a systematic checklist of progress toward the overall goal of learning the Square Dance. Mastering a few skills during each lesson may include:

1. Warm-up and review of Basic movements in a circle to include all class members. Or dance a figure using previously learned basics.

2. Presentation of new Basics. Isolate each one from any specific dance and include a walk-though and practice call.

3. Call and dance of one or more dances containing new Basics with combinations of several previously learned dances. Or allow the class to request favorites.

MIXERS FOR SQUARE DANCE

Frequent changes of partners and sets are needed to help class members get acquainted and to establish a good rapport within the group. Mixers are of prime importance in dealing with extras and with groups in which the number of men and women is uneven.

Random changes can serve to mix ability groupings and upgrade the overall dance–skill level. Meeting a variety of class members adds to the fun, sociability, and feeling of fellowship.

Mixing can also be seemingly unintentional means of breaking up cliques and getting the attention of inattentive class members. Mixers can work as a gentle and even pleasant way to apply discipline, particularly when working with school and recreation groups. In any event, it is always wise to have a "pocket full of miracles" in the form of mixers when teaching dance.

Mixers to meet the demands of a variety of circumstances can be found in Chapter 4 under Plain and Novelty Mixers and Paul Jones Your Lady. The following are samples of the kind that would accomplish the uses suggested in the foregoing discussion. All mixers should be done to musical accompaniment. Square Dance mixers should be called as illustrated by the following samples.

■ *Big Circle Mixers*

1. Couples promenade counterclockwise. Men turn left and roll back to promenade their partner in the trailing couple.

    Promenade go two by two

    Gents roll back and promenade that gal behind you.

2. Couples promenade counterclockwise. Men move forward to the next woman and promenade.

    Promenade this little pal

    Now move up one and take a new gal

    And all promenade

    Promenade a little bit more

    Move up one as you did before

    And all promenade.

■ *Methods for Squaring Up*

1. **Grand March:** The Grand March is a traditional way of squaring sets. It serves chiefly as a mixer of couples rather than individuals. It is a particularly good and efficient way of organizing a large crowd into sets. Refer to p. 75 for a detailed description of the procedure.

2. **Paul Jones:** This procedure will enable a group to get partners for forming sets. Women form a single circle facing out, circle to the left. Men form a single circle around the women,

facing in, circle to the left. The larger group usually forms the outside circle. When the music stops, the men take the women directly opposite or nearest them for partners. Refer to Paul Jones Your Lady, p. 80 for additional variations.

3. **Circle Two–Step:** Once partners are secured, the leader may call out "circle four," "circle six," "circle ten," or any even number so that partners are not separated. Eventually "circle eight" may be called and sets arranged for dancing. Younger groups may enjoy this procedure: The leader blows a whistle or claps hands to indicate the number of couples he or she wishes to have form a circle.

4. **Grand Promenade:** After partners are secured, the leader may use following call to organize the group into sets.

    Promenade go two by two

    Now promenade a little bit more

    Pick up two and make it four

    Promenade and don't be late

    Grab a four and make it eight

    Line up now and keep it straight

    Spread that line way out wide

    And circle up eight on all four sides.

5. **Promenade Around the Hall:** This call may be used at the beginning of the dance or at the end of any one call during the dance to arrange couples in different sets for the next call.

    Promenade one and promenade all

    Promenade around the great big hall

    Circle up four with any old two

    Go 'round and 'round like you used to do

    Now break that four and circle up eight

    Hurry up gents now don't be late

    Find your place right in that set

    Stand right there, we ain't through yet.

    Variation: The following variation of the preceding call may be used to break up the sets and arrange the dancers in formation for a round dance.

    Break up your sets and promenade all

    Promenade, go around the hall

    Around the great big beautiful hall

    Now stand right there upon the floor

    Stand right there, we'll dance some more.

■ Methods for Changing Partners or Moving to a New Square

1. **Promenade Out of the Square:** During a call, usually where a trim or break is in order, the caller may change a couple or couples from one set to another and finish the call with new couples in every set. The following call indicates how this may be done.

> One and three–promenade
>
> Right out of that square
>
> And find yourself a brand new square
>
> Promenade, go anywhere
>
> Just find yourself a brand new square
>
> Look for hands around the floor
>
> Fill in there–they need two more
>
> There's a spot–go over there
>
> They need two more to make a square
>
> One for the money, two for the show
>
> All get set–'cause here we go!

Variation: While the promenading couples are relocating, the caller may keep the other couples dancing by calling a ladies chain, right and left thru, or do-sa-do. The following call indicates how this may be done.

> One and three–promenade
>
> Right out of that square
>
> And find yourself a brand new square
>
> Now two and four–while they are gone
>
> Circle up four and carry on
>
> Do–sa–do in the middle of the set
>
> 'Cause one and three ain't ready yet
>
> Two and four go home to your places
>
> And take a look at the brand new faces.

2. **New Partner Calls:** The following may be used to secure new partners at the end of a call.

> Honor your partner and thank her too
>
> Now swing the gal to the left of you
>
> Swing your corner, that pretty little maid
>
> Keep this gal and all promenade
>
> Honor your partner, corners too
>
> Swing that gal across from you
>
> Swing that gal but not too hard
>
> Stand right there with a brand new pard!

3. **Directed Changes:** The leader may direct dancers to change places as follows.
   a. All women move one position to the right in the set.
   b. Each gentleman takes his opposite, corner, or right-hand woman for a new partner.
   c. All the women or gentlemen move to the adjacent square and take the same positions in the new set.
   d. Women (gents) leave the set and move anywhere around the room to a new square. Dancers should be in new square before the next dance call begins.

> Gents (ladies) to the center
>
> And stand right there
>
> Ladies (gents) run away to a brand new square
>
> Sides (heads) to the center
>
> And hold on there
>
> Now the heads (sides) promenade right out of that square
>
> Go anywhere I don't care
>
> And find yourself a brand new square.

4. **Scoot and Scat:** Scoot is the cue for the men and scat is the cue for the women. In general, the leader must explain the action to the group so that they will respond in the desired manner. The women or men may be directed to form a star in the center of the set; while the star is rotating, the leader calls "scoot" and the men leave the square and go to another one to form a star. If women are directed into a star figure, on the call "scat," they leave the square and get into another to form a star.

   Scoot and Scat may also be called as part of Texas Star. If the men are on the outside spokes of the star, "scoot" is called. The women continue to star and the men hook onto the spoke of the women's star in another set. When all squares have eight people, the caller continues the Texas Star. New partners promenade to the home position of the woman.

5. **Birdies in the Cage:** The following variation of the regular Bird in the Cage–Seven Hands 'Round (refer to p. 166) may be used as a mixer.

> All four gents swing your right-hand lady
>
> With a right hand around
>
> Partner left with a left hand around

Corner lady with a right hand around

Now swing your partner with two hands around

And cage those birds as you come around

Now four hands up and away we go

The birds fly away through that open door!

All four women are placed in the center of the set back to back. The men join hands and circle left around the women (birds). The men hold their hands up high, forming arches through which the women (birds) fly on the call, "The birds fly away through that open door." The call may be repeated with the "crows," the men, in the center and the women circling around with joined hands raised high. The "crows" fly away on the call, "The crows fly away through that open door." The "birds" or "crows" simply go to any new set and take a new partner for a repeat of the call.

BASIC MOVEMENTS

The Square Dance basics included in this text are aimed at the beginning, intermediate, and club dancer and teacher–caller. The levels included are Basic Movements, Additional Basics, and Mainstream.

Level 1A: Beginner Basics 1–8

1. Shuffle
2. Honors
3. Do-sa-do
4. Promenade
5. Twirl
6. Single–File Promenade
7. Waist Swing
8. Allemande Left

Level 1B: Orientation to the Square

a. Forming the Square
b. Maneuvering in the Square
c. Practice Basics 1–8

Level 2: Beginner Basics 9–20

9. Grand Right and Left
10. Split the Ring
11. Pass Thru
12. Separate Go Around One
13. Texas Star Basics
14. Forearm Turns
15. Courtesy Turn
16. Ladies Chain
17. Circle to a Line–Lines of Four

18. Bend the Line
19. Right and Left Thru
20. Weave the Ring

Level 3: Beginner Basics 21–33

21. Four Ladies Chain
22. Do Paso
23. All Around Your Left–Hand Lady–Seesaw
24. California Twirl
25. Dive Thru
26. Ends Turn In
27. Roll Away to a Half–Sashay
28. U–Turn Back
29. Cross Trail Thru
30. Grand Square
31. Box the Gnat
32. Allemande Thar
33. Rip and Snort

Level 4: Intermediate Basics 34–44

34. Buzz Swing
35. Single–File Turn Back
36. Square Thru
37. Star Thru
38. Double Turn Back from Grand Right and Left
39. Three–Quarter Chain
40. Box the Flea
41. Alamo Style
42. Wheel Around
43. Slip the Clutch
44. Double Pass Thru

Level 5: Intermediate Basics 45–50

45. Wheel and Deal
46. Eight Chain Thru
47. Turn Thru
48. Ocean Wave
49. Swing Thru
50. Circulate

■ *Teaching Progression and Analysis for Basic Movements of Square Dance*

The basic movements of Square Dance have been arranged from simple to complex in a recommended teaching progression. Basics may be combined and called to practice interrelated movement patterns within the overall progression. The progression is designed to give the teacher–caller full information germane to each basic. The information includes: analysis or description of movement, specific teaching suggestions for each movement, diagrams for visual aid, calls for practicing basics as used in a dance, and recommended singing and/or patter calls using the basics in a dance figure.

■ Level 1A: Beginner Basics 1–8

The beginning basics 1–8 should be practiced in a single circle to provide opportunity for all class members to participate regardless of class size. The single–circle formation allows for easy demonstration and viewing of class progress from the center of the circle. The teacher-caller may also "dance and call" from this formation or simply call out basics from the center of the circle.

1. SHUFFLE

An easy, light, walking action in even rhythm, with the ball of the foot kept lightly in contact with the floor. The action should be in time with the music. The body is held upright.

> **Teaching aids:** (a) Practice in a single circle moving left, right, forward, and back.
> (b) Styling of hand clasp: man's palm up, woman's palm down. (c) Move with small steps, synchronize with partner, and step to the beat of the music.

2. HONORS

Partners turn slightly to face each other while shifting the weight to the outside foot and pointing the inside foot toward partner. Often called Bow to Partner.

> **Teaching aids:** (a) One may dip slightly, keeping the back straight and the weight over the outside foot (man's left, woman's right.) (b) The action can take four counts in all: shift weight and dip (count 1), hold (2), and recover facing the set (counts 3 and 4).

3. DO–SA–DO

Partners face, pass each other right shoulder to right shoulder, move around each other back to back and return to original position facing partner.

> **Teaching aids:** (a) Dancers should learn to keep hands and arms down to the sides and slightly behind. (b) Dancers can turn slightly on a diagonal in passing so as to make it easier to get around without bumping.

PRACTICE CALL [1] (using first three basics)
All join hands and circle left
Everybody go forward and back
Face your partner, do–sa–do
Bow to your partner.

4. PROMENADE

Partners take promenade position (see Glossary) and move counterclockwise around the circle.

> **Teaching aids:** (a) The joined right hands are on top. (b) The hands are joined (man's palm up, woman's palm down) at about waist level. (c) The man may take the initiative to lead slightly as they move forward. (d) A clockwise direction is called a **wrong–way promenade.**

5. TWIRL

Partners face, join right hands. Man lifts right hand, turning woman under man's right arm once clockwise. As lady completes turn, man takes her left hand. Couples resume promenade position or as directed by caller.

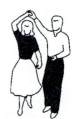

> **Teaching aids:** (a) Woman must move along line of direction while turning to stay slightly ahead of man who is following woman's turn. (b) A good demonstration helps dancers style the twirl. (c) Twirl is not always called. It is a styling movement done automatically. **Note:** In practice call 2 the twirl may be done twice, once after each call "right to your partner, promenade."

PRACTICE CALL [2] (using the first five basics)
All join hands and circle to the left
Now circle to the right
Everybody go forward and back
Do–sa–do your partner
Right to partner, promenade
All join hands to forward and back
Do–sa–do your corner
All join hands and circle to the left
Now circle to the right
Face partner, do–sa–do
Right to partner and promenade.

6. SINGLE-FILE PROMENADE

Dancers turn to face counterclockwise and shuffle one behind the other single–file around the circle.

PRACTICE CALL [3]
All join hands, circle left
Break, promenade single file
The other way back
Face the center, go forward and back
Honor your partner.

Bow to partner, promenade
Promenade single file
Home you go and do-sa-do.

> **Teaching aid:** Dancers may go into single–file
> promenade from a promenade. The woman steps
> in front of the man, and they move one behind
> the other counterclockwise around the circle.

7. WAIST SWING

Partners take swing position (see Glossary). Dancers shuffle (gliding walk)
around each other, turning twice
around clockwise in four or eight
counts.

> **Teaching aids:** (a) Body erect,
> lean back from waist and look at
> each other. (b). Woman rolls off man's right
> arm to next position called or may twirl to a
> promenade position. (c) More advanced styling
> may be added later (i.e., buzz step swing and
> twirl).

8. ALLEMANDE LEFT

Corners take a left forearm grasp and turn each other
once around and go back home.

> **Teaching aids:** (a) Left elbow is bent, dancers
> pull away slightly on the turn. (b) Grasp
> forearm with palm of hand rather than fingers.

PRACTICE CALL ☐5 (using basics 1–8)
Honor your partner, swing your partner
All join hands and circle left
All to the center and back
Now swing your partner round and round
Promenade her single file
Join hands and circle left
All to the center and back
Allemande left your corner
Do-sa-do your partner, do-sa-do corner
Swing your partner
Bow your partner and stand right there.

■ *Level 1B: Orientation to the Square*

Dancers need to learn how to form a square and to
understand and practice the movement possibilities
based on its structure.

A. FORMING THE SQUARE

1. Four couples form a square. Each couple forms
   one side of the square. All couples face the
   center of the square, each man with his partner
   on his right. This is **home position** for each
   couple.

2. Couples are numbered counterclockwise or to
   the right around the square. Couple 1 always
   has their backs to the caller and music; couple
   2 is to the right of couple 1; couple 3 is across
   from couple 1 and to the right of couple 2;
   couple 4 is across from couple 2 and to the left
   of couple 1.

3. Couples 1 and 3 are called **head couples** and
   are numbered 1 and 3 in most of the calls.
   Couples 2 and 4 are called **side couples** and
   are numbered 2 and 4. □ = man, ○ = woman.

4. The woman to the left of each man is the
   corner lady. The woman in the couple to the
   right of each man is the **right–hand lady.** The
   woman directly across from each man is the
   opposite lady.

5. Couples are called **active couples** when their
   number is called for an action. **Inactive
   couples** are those not called for an action, but
   they may be involved in an action by the
   active couples. The active couple is also called
   the **lead–off couple.**

Practice call 7 is designed to provide practice in
learning home positions, couple numbers, individual
numbers, and interaction with partner and corner.
Basics 1–8 are used as they relate to the square formation. For full and complete practice the call
sequence should be: opener, main figure for women,
break, repeat main figure for gents, repeat break
(gives extra allemande left practice), and add the
ending.

PRACTICE CALL ☐6
OPENER
Honor your partner, honor your corner
All join hands and circle left
Circle right the other way back
Into the center and give a little yell
Back right out and circle left
And home you go.

MAIN FIGURE
Two little sisters form a ring
   (Women 1 and 2 join hands in center of square)
Circle left don't be slow
   (Women 1 and 2 circle once around)
Home you go and do-sa-do (or swing)
Three little sisters form a ring
   (Women 1, 2, 3)
Circle left don't be slow
   (Circle once around)
Home you go and do-sa-do (or swing)
Now four little sisters form a ring
   (Women 1, 2, 3, and 4)
Circle left don't be slow
Home you go and do-sa-do (or swing).

BREAK

Allemande left that pretty maid
Back to your partner and promenade
Once around the square you go
Home you go there is more.

Repeat figure for gents

ENDING

Honor your partner, corner too
Thank you folks, I'm all through.

> **Note:** Teachers may wish to teach Basic 14 "forearm turn" and use it as a "single arm swing" rather than using the waist swing at this early stage of learning. This would be a good choice in classes that have more women than men. More important, there is less style and technique in the "forearm turn" used as a "single arm swing," thus allowing the class to go through the first eight basics and get to a whole Square Dance in the very first lesson.

B. MANEUVERING IN THE SQUARE

Maneuvering in the square means learning to move in relation to eight dancers. It is a group action and therefore requires group timing to achieve smooth interaction and transitions. The following "traffic" rules will help dancers move as a group more efficiently.

> *Rule 1:* Standard practice is to dance forward and back with three small steps and a touch on the fourth count.

> *Rule 2:* While dancers are executing the first call, they should listen for the next call. The caller will overlap the action of the first call with the second. Remember calls can be ad lib, or extemporaneous; dancers must listen!

> *Rule 3:* The size of the square may be kept compact by the men promenading with left shoulders pulled in toward the center of the square. Distance to home is shortened and movement is better timed.

> *Rule 4:* When a couple or individual dancers moves around the outside of the square, dancers should move to center as they pass.

> *Rule 5:* Promenading around the square: Men should always promenade partners (own or new one) to the man's home position. A promenade may be called for less than once around. These fractional promenade distances may be danced outside or inside the square.

> *Rule 6:* Dancers are always in home position with original partner at the end of a call sequence. It is the responsibility of the caller to make this happen.

> *Rule 7:* The best solution to a breakdown in executing the call is to go to home position. This will allow the figure to become untangled and dancers may "pick up the call" and continue dancing in good order.

> *Rule 8:* How far to promenade: The rule of thumb is to promenade home if the distance is one quarter or more to go. If the distance is less than one quarter (you are almost home), you should go full around to home position.

> *Rule 9:* Lead to the right simply means couples move to the right of the square and stand in front of the appropriate couple. Example: Couple 1 and 3 move to the right and stand in front of couple 2 and 4.

> *Rule 10:* Dancers should react to the various positions in the square rather than to "a person" who is supposed to be there. Example: Allemande left, dancer should move to the corner position and react with whomever is there.

> *Rule 11:* Dancers are in sequence when they are in the original order in the square (i.e., as numbered 1 to 4 counterclockwise). Dancers are out of sequence when any two have changed places (i.e., couples 1 and 3 pass through or all couples pass through or as individuals change in a two ladies chain.

> *Rule 12:* Swing the opposite lady: Men swing opposite by moving simultaneously, allowing the man on the left to pass across in front before reaching opposite woman. Or they may make a brief right–hand star in the center to reach the opposite in more orderly fashion. Men move right across in front of partner to swing right–hand lady, face center, and wait for next call.

C. PRACTICE BASICS 1–8

Refer to 1A: Beginner Basics 1–8
Practice Basics 1–8 in square formation.

■ Level 2: Beginner Basics 9–20

9. GRAND RIGHT AND LEFT

Partners face and join right hands, move forward, pass partner, extend left hand to the next dancer, right to the next, and so forth, until dancers meet original partner. Men move counterclockwise; women move clockwise.

> **Teaching aids:** (a) Dancers release hand grasps quickly as they pass. (b) Dancers meet partner or person with whom they began the figure. Listen for next call; it could be "swing

(continued)

partner," "do-sa-do" or "promenade home." (c) To promenade, man should take woman's right in his right and turn woman clockwise into promenade position.

PRACTICE CALL 7
Face your partner
Grand right and left
Meet partner, promenade.

PRACTICE CALL 8
Allemande left with your left hand
Right to partner, keep going
Right and left grand
Meet partner, promenade.

10. SPLIT THE RING

The lead-off couple moves between the man and woman of the opposite couple.

> **Teaching aids:** (a) Couple being "split" moves sideways and apart to let lead couple through. (b) After moving through, lead couple must listen for next call. **Example:** "Separate go around the outside ring, home you go and swing."

PRACTICE CALL 9
First couple go down the center
Split the ring, separate,
Go back home
Everybody do-sa-do.

Repeat for each couple.

PRACTICE CALL 10
1 and 3 go forward and back
Forward again, face the sides
Split the ring, separate
Go back home, do-sa-do.

Repeat for 2 and 4.

11. PASS THRU

Two couples face. Dancers move forward passing opposite dancer's right shoulder to right shoulder.

> **Teaching aid:** Dancers pass thru and listen for next call.

PRACTICE CALL 11
1 and 3 pass thru
Separate, come around two
Right back home
2 and 4 go forward and back
Everybody do-sa-do.

Repeat for 2 and 4.

12. SEPARATE GO AROUND ONE

Men move left, women right to separate. Dancers then move around the nearest inactive dancer to face partner in center of square. Wait for next call.

PRACTICE CALL 12
1 and 3 pass thru
Separate, go around one
Come in between the sides
Go into the middle
Pass thru, split the next two
Separate, go around one
Come down the middle
Pass thru face partner
Swing and square set.

Repeat for 2 and 4.

> **Square dance:** Split the Ring, Go Around One.

PRACTICE CALL 13
1 and 3 pass thru
Separate, go around one
Line up four, go forward and back
Center four join hands
Circle four halfway 'round
Pass thru, split two
Separate, go around one
Line up four, go forward and back
Allemande left.

Repeat for 2 and 4.

13. TEXAS STAR BASICS

The following basics are used in the dance figure Texas Star. However, they may be used separately in other combination.

> **Four Gents Star:** Men go to the center, touch hands, fingers up, and move around the center of the ring.

> **Teaching aids:** (a) The men make a right-hand star, turning clockwise, and a left-hand star, turning counterclockwise. (b) When changing from a right-hand star to a left-hand star, the men release with the right hand, make a right face turn, and form the star with the left hand. (c) The four women may form the star in the same manner.

> **Star Promenade:** Four couples move in same direction. Men star with left hand moving counterclockwise. Women star with right hand moving clockwise.

> **Teaching aids:** (a) Each man put right arm around partner's waist, woman's left arm should rest on man's upper right arm. (b) Woman needs

to move toward man to be picked up to begin the star. Remember, men are holding hands in a left-hand star as they start the pickup.

Gents Swing Out Ladies Swing In: Men break the star and back up, turning as a couple counterclockwise. Women move into center to form a right-hand star. The "swing out and in" may be a half turn or a turn and a half to put the women in the star.

Box Star Position: Dancer (man or woman) places right or left hand on the wrist of the dancer in front. This wrist hold is also called a *packsaddle*.

Square dances: Texas Star and Gents Star Right.

14. FOREARM TURNS

A means of turning in place with the use of a forearm grasp. This basic may be used instead of or along with the waist swing as a "single arm swing." It is easy to learn and is useful in classes where there are more women than men, or vice versa.

> **Teaching aid:** Dancers should pull away slightly, keeping the elbow bent, the arm firm, and palm against the partner's arm.

PRACTICE CALL 14

All face your partner
Turn partner right arm round
Men star left in the center
Meet your partner, do-sa-do
All join hands and circle left
Go once around and get back home
Now gents star right, one time around
Pass your partner, allemande left
Come back to partner and swing.

> **Square dances:** Arkansas Traveler and Mañana.

15. COURTESY TURN

Couple face in same direction. Man takes woman's left hand in his left, places right arm around waist. Couple turns as a unit, man backing up as couple turns counterclockwise to face original direction or as caller indicates.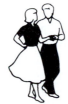

> **Teaching aids:** Woman's right palm should rest lightly on her right hip over man's hand.

16. LADIES CHAIN

Two couples are facing each other. The two women take right hands and pull by and then give a left hand to the opposite man. The man takes her left hand in

his left and does a courtesy turn, turning once around to face the other couple. The two women have changed partners. Repeat to home position.

> **Teaching aids:** (a) Couples 1 and 3 execute ladies chain across in the square formation. This acts as a demonstration for other couples. Repeat for couples 2 and 4. (b) Men should take Two-Step to the right after releasing women and reach out with left hand to receive new partner for courtesy turn. (c) Dancers may also practice all at once in a diagonal formation (i.e., couples 1 and 2 chain as couples 3 and 4 chain). (d) Use practice call 16 for all four couples to practice on the diagonal (i.e., couple 1 with 2 and couple 3 with 4). (e) Use practice call 17 in the set or square formation. (f) Use practice calls 18 and 19 to teach and practice four ladies chain or grand chain.

PRACTICE CALL 15

Bow to your partner
Bow to your opposite
Two ladies chain across
Chain right back
All four go forward and back
Two ladies chain
Now chain 'em back.

PRACTICE CALL 16

Bow to your partner
Couples 1 and 3 promenade outside
Go all the way around
Couples 2 and 4 ladies chain
2 and 4 chain back
Couples 2 and 4 promenade outside
Go all the way around
1 and 3 ladies chain
1 and 3 chain back
All join hands and circle left
Break and promenade single file
Home you go, everybody swing.

> **Square dance:** Hurry Hurry Hurry.

17. CIRCLE TO A LINE

Couples 1 and 3 (or 2 and 4) lead to the right, circle two-thirds around; active man drops left hand grasp and pulls the line out straight.

> **Teaching aids:** (a) To get the notion of couple positions in the line, simply have couples 1 and 3 (or 2 and 4) move over and stand beside couples 2 and 4. Men 1 and 3 will be opposite their home position. (b) Practice having 1 and 3 (or 2 and 4) move from home position, circle with 2 and 4 into position as in (a). The inactive women should turn counterclockwise under partner's right arm to move comfortably into position at end of line.

18. BEND THE LINE

From any line of an even number (usually four people), the line breaks in the middle, the centers of the line back up, and the ends of the line move forward until both halves of the line are facing.

Teaching aids: (a) The center two people release hands and back up at the same time that the two end people move forward so that each half of the line pivots to face the other. (b) When two lines of four face each other, bend the line; the result is that two new lines of four are formed, facing each other in the new direction.

PRACTICE CALL 17
1 and 3 lead to the right
Circle, break and make a line
Go forward up and back
Bend the line
Go forward up and back
Bend the line
Join hands and circle right
Home you go and do–sa–do.

Repeat for 2 and 4.

PRACTICE CALL 18
1 and 3 lead to the right
Circle, break and form a line
Go forward up and back
Pass thru and bend the line
Go forward up and back
Pass thru and bend the line
Go forward up and back
Pass thru and bend the line
Go forward up and back
Pass thru and bend the line
Now all join hands and circle eight.

Repeat for 2 and 4.

Square dances: Easy Bend the Line and Bend It Tight.

19. RIGHT AND LEFT THRU

Two couples face each other. Dancers join right hands and pull past opposite, passing right shoulder to right shoulder. Couples have backs to each other. Courtesy turn to face again and repeat to original place.

Teaching aids: (a) Practice in square formation or on the diagonal as suggested for ladies chain. (b) The call is not necessarily followed by a "right and left back" call. Dancers must listen to caller for directions. (c) Use practice call 19 on the diagonal and calls 20 and 21 in the square formation.

PRACTICE CALL 19
Honor your partner
Honor your opposite
Go right and left thru
Right and left back
Do–sa–do your opposite gal
Go right and left thru turn your pal
Now do–sa–do opposite, don't be slow
Right and left thru and back you go.

PRACTICE CALL 20
Bow to your partner
1 and 3 go right and left thru across the set
Right and left back
2 and 4 go right and left thru
Right and left back
1 and 3 ladies chain across
2 and 4 ladies chain
All 4 ladies chain back
Join hands, circle left
Home you go.

PRACTICE CALL 21
Couples 1 and 3 go right and left thru
Couples 2 and 4 go right and left thru
Couples 1 and 3 go right and left back
2 and 4 go right and left back
Head ladies chain across
Side ladies chain across
All 4 ladies chain back.

Square dances: The Route, Promenade the Outside Ring, Split the Ring Variations, and Old-Fashioned Girl.

20. WEAVE THE RING

Same as grand right and left except that dancers do not touch hands when passing each other.

Teaching aid: Dancers may turn slightly on a diagonal when passing so as to pass each other closely without bumping.

PRACTICE CALL 22
All join hands and circle left
Break, reverse, go single file
When you get home, swing your partner
Allemande left and weave the ring
In and out 'til you meet your maid
Take the little girl and promenade.

■ *Level 3: Beginner Basics 21–33*

21. FOUR LADIES CHAIN

All four women move to the center, touch right hands, and move clockwise to opposite man. Opposite man and woman courtesy turn, women move back into center, touch right hands clockwise to home position, and courtesy turn. Basic also called grand chain.

Teaching aid: The four women need to keep track of where they are so they will only pass one man and be turned by the opposite. Use practice calls 20, 21.

Square dances: Tie Me Kangaroo Down.

22. DO PASO

Starting position is a circle of two or more couples. Partners face, take a left forearm grasp, and turn each other counterclockwise until facing the corner. Turn corner with right forearm grasp until facing partner. Take partner with the left hand, and man turns woman with courtesy turn.

Teaching aid: Practice first in circle of four or more couples, then practice in circle of two couples.

PRACTICE CALL 23
All join hands, circle left
And around you go
Break into a do paso
Partner by the left, corner by the right
Now turn your own if it takes all night
Join hands, circle.

Repeat all.

23. ALL AROUND YOUR LEFT-HAND LADY

Often used with seesaw your taw. Corners move one time around each other in a loop pattern, the man starting behind the corner, on around her and back to place, the woman starting in front of him and around him back to place. This completes half of the loop. Seesaw your partner is a similar action that completes the other half of the loop.

Teaching aid: Dancers learn that these are companion figures, but the second loop does not always follow the first loop; it depends on the call.

PRACTICE CALL 24
Walk all around your left-hand lady
Oh boy, what a daisy
Seesaw your pretty little taw
She's the best you ever saw.

Square dance: Goodbye My Lady Love.

24. CALIFORNIA TWIRL

The same as the frontier twirl. This basic is used by a couple to reverse the direction they are facing. If they are facing out, they turn to face in, and vice

versa. Partners join inside hands (man's right, woman's left). The man walks around the woman clockwise as he turns her counterclockwise under his right arm.

Teaching aids: (a) The woman begins and ends on the man's right side. (b) They must let the hands slip easily around each other so as not to twist the wrist. (c) Both actually turn a half-turn.

PRACTICE CALL 25
Head couples pass thru
California twirl
Side couples pass thru
California twirl.

Repeat all.

25. DIVE THRU

Two couples are facing each other. The couple whose back is to the center of the square makes an arch by joining inside hands. The couple facing them ducks under the arch and moves forward. The arching couple now facing out turns a California twirl.

Teaching aid: The California twirl is done automatically from this position. The caller does not call it.

PRACTICE CALL 26
Head ladies chain across
But don't chain back
1 and 3 lead to the right
Circle halfway 'round
Now dive thru pass thru
There's your corner
Allemande left.

Repeat for 2 and 4.

26. ENDS TURN IN

Starting position is when two lines of four are facing out. The two persons in the center of the line form an arch, and the two persons on the ends of the line drop hands, walk forward, and go together under the arch, moving into the center of the square. The arching couple California twirls.

Teaching aid: To practice, direct 1 and 3 men to stand next to corner women and 1 and 3 women stand next to corner men. The two facing lines move forward, pass thru and join hands, lines are facing out. Repeat practice for 2 and 4.

Square dances: Ends Turn In and Inside Arch Outside Under.

27. ROLL AWAY TO A HALF-SASHAY

Partners are side by side, facing same direction, woman on the man's right. The woman rolls across in front of the man to his left side. As she rolls, she makes one complete turn counterclockwise.

Teaching aids: (a) The man guides the woman across with his right hand and simultaneously steps to his right so that they end up having exchanged places. (b) He will release her left hand and take her right in his left. (c) In star promenade position, the man will have his right arm around the woman's waist and will help her roll across in front of him to the other side. (d) Dancers learn to respond to this basic as half–sashay, roll away, or whirl away (synonymous terms).

PRACTICE CALL 27

All join hands and circle left
Roll away with a half–sashay
Circle left in the same old way
Ring, ring, ring, I say
Roll away with a half–sashay
All you gents listen to my call
Swing the girl across the hall.

28. U TURN BACK

An individual turn or about–face to move in opposite direction.

PRACTICE CALL 28

1 and 3 pass thru
U–turn back
2 and 4 pass thru
U–turn back.

Repeat all.

PRACTICE CALL 29

1 and 3 roll away with a half–sashay
Up to the center and back that way
Pass thru and U–turn back
Right and left thru on the same old track.

Repeat for 2 and 4.

Square dances: Roll Away Combo #1 and Gentle on My Mind.

29. CROSS TRAIL THRU

Two couples are facing each other. Each person passes by the opposite right shoulder to right shoulder and then the woman crosses to the left in front of the man. The man crosses to the right behind the woman. They all stop facing out, side by side, woman on left of man, and follow the next call.

Teaching aids: (a) Next call may be "go around two." (b) May be done from line formation; couples end up facing out. When facing out in a line, the two in the middle of the line are corners and will turn to face for allemande left. End dancers will find corners behind them on the end of the opposite line.

PRACTICE CALL 30

1 and 3 cross trail thru
Separate and go around two
Home you go, pass by your own
Allemande left
Honor your partner at home.

Repeat for 2 and 4.

PRACTICE CALL 31

1 and 3 promenade the outside ring
Go just halfway round
Same two cross trail thru
Now allemande left with your left hand
Right to partner, shake her by the hand
And there you stand.

Repeat for 2 and 4.

PRACTICE CALL 32

1 and 3 lead to the right
Circle, break, and make a line
Go forward up and back
Right and left thru
Now ladies chain on the same old track
Turn 'em boys and chain 'em back
Now pass thru and bend the line
Go right and left thru
Now cross trail thru, you're facing out
Allemande left.

Repeat for 2 and 4.

Square dances: Another Trail, Roll Away Combo #2, Arkansas Traveler with Cross Trail, and Split the Ring Variation #2.

30. GRAND SQUARE

A no–patter call. Dancers walk individually around a square pattern on the floor. Each side of square is four counts. Dancers move along each side with three steps and turn or hold as indicated.

Teaching aids: (a) All dancers should practice action from the head and side couple position. (b) Caller may cue with word cues as in practice call.

PRACTICE CALL 33

Honor your partner–the lady fair } A
All get set for grand square

Walk 2 3 turn ⎫
Walk 2 3 turn ⎪
Walk 2 3 turn ⎪
Walk 2 3 reverse ⎬ B
Walk 2 3 turn ⎪
Walk 2 3 turn ⎪
Walk 2 3 turn ⎪
Walk 2 3 hold. ⎭

A. Introduction to music *on* last eight counts of phrase.

B. First 32 counts of music. Start figure with new phrase.

Grand square figure:

Heads

1. Go forward three steps and turn on fourth count to face partner.

2. Take opposite's hand beside you and back up three steps, turning on fourth count to face the person by your side.

3. Drop hands, back away from this person three steps, turning one-quarter on fourth count to face partner.

4. Move forward three steps toward partner and hold the fourth count (do not turn).

Reverse

5. Move backward away from partner three steps, turn one-quarter on fourth count to face the opposite person.

6. Move forward toward opposite three steps, turn one-quarter on the fourth count to face partner.

7. Take opposite's hand beside you and move forward three steps, turning on the fourth count to face opposite.

8. Drop hands, take partner's hands, back up three steps into home place, and hold the fourth count.

Sides
Start with 5, 6, 7, 8, 1, 2, 3, 4.

Square dances: Gentle On My Mind using grand square for opener, middle break, and closer, or any previous Square Dance, using grand square as trim.

31. BOX THE GNAT

Partners face, join right hands, and exchange places, as the woman turns counterclockwise under the man's right arm, man walks around woman clockwise. Partners end facing having exchanged places.

Teaching aids: (a) The hands are allowed to slip easily around each other so as not to twist the wrists. (b) Dancers should learn to listen for "box the gnat, pull by," in which they hold on with the right hand after box the gnat and use that hand to pull by that person. (c) Practice this first with partner, then with corner, and then use practice calls 34 and 35.

PRACTICE CALL 34
1 and 3
Roll away to a half-sashay
Box the gnat across the way
Pull by for a right and left thru.

Repeat for 2 and 4.

PRACTICE CALL 35
1 and 3 go forward and back
Right to opposite, box the gnat
Pull her thru and U-turn back.

Repeat for 2 and 4.

32. ALLEMANDE THAR

A star formation for all four couples in square. Dancers allemande left, back to partner with right, pull by to next with left forearm grasp. Men turn this woman a half-turn counterclockwise until men can make a box star (packsaddle) in center. Men travel backward in the star, women travel forward. On call "shoot the star," men release box-star position, turn woman on left arms halfway around; women are facing clockwise, men counterclockwise. Dancers release arm position, move forward to the next with right hand, pull by, a left forearm grasp to the next, men turn as before into box star backing up. "Shoot the star" again and turn the woman halfway around, move forward to meet original partner and follow the next call.

Teaching aids: (a) The key word to this basic is *thar.* (b) Men should let women set movement pace in box star. (c) Allemande thar star is used as a trim and as part of a patter call any time from a left-arm turn.

PRACTICE CALL 36
Allemande left and allemande thar
It's right and left and form a star
Gents back up in a right-hand star
Now shoot that star to the heavens whirl
Go right and left to a brand new girl
And form that star again
Back 'em up boys but not too far
Shoot that star and find your own
Promenade, go right on home.

33. RIP AND SNORT

Basic use in a circle of eight. The designated couple, without releasing hands, lead across the center and under arch formed by opposite couple, pulling the whole circle under arch. Once under, lead couple drops inside hands. Woman pulls her line round to the right as the man pulls his line left and back to place. The arching couples turn under their own joined hands without releasing hands to face center of circle.

(continued)

First couple rip and snort
Down the center, cut 'em short
Lady go right, gent go left
Pull 'em through
Join hands, circle eight.

■ Level 4: Intermediate Basics 34–44

34. BUZZ SWING

A more advanced swinging technique. Dancers are in the same position as they were for the shuffle swing. They turn twice around as before and open up facing the center of the square. The difference in the buzz swing is that the rhythm is uneven. Instead of being an even beat shuffle (♪♪), it is a long–short–long–short (♩.♪) rhythm.

Teaching aids: (a) Each person places the outside of the right foot close to partner's right foot and turns the foot a little each time, pivoting around a center point between the two dancers. The right foot takes the long beat, and the left foot takes the short beat and acts in a pushing motion to propel the turn around. (b) Dancers should lean away from each other and take advantage of the centrifugal force. (c) Momentum must be stopped near the end of the turn so that they can make a controlled stop in place. (d) The buzz swing should be very smooth. Avoid bobbing up and down.

35. SINGLE-FILE TURN BACK

From a single-file promenade, traveling counter-clockwise, either man or woman may be designated by the caller to step out of the circle, about face to the right, and go the other way, making another circle traveling clockwise.

Teaching aid: The designated person who steps out and goes in the opposite direction will go all the way around. Since the inside circle is also traveling forward, partners pass each other halfway around and meet the next time to go into the next call.

PRACTICE CALL 38
Promenade single file
Gents turn back on the outside track
Go once around
Meet partner, right
Go all the way around
Allemande left.

36. SQUARE THRU

Two couples are facing each other. Right square thru, starting with the right hand, will be described here. The square thru may be full-square thru (four hands), three-quarters-square thru (three hands), half-square

thru (two hands), or square thru five hands, as described below.

Full–Square Thru: Face opposite, take right hand, pull by, turn one-quarter to face partner, give left hand, pull by, turn one-quarter to face opposite, give right hand, pull by, turn one-quarter to face partner, give left hand, pull by, and stop.

Teaching aids: (a) Take four hands, R, L, R, L, hand over hand; the women travel counter-clockwise around the center of the square; the men travel clockwise. (b) Drop the hand after pulling by. (c) Do *not* turn the last time. (d) Each person ends facing his or her corner.

Three–Quarters–Square Thru: Take three hands, R, L, R.

Teaching aids: (a) Do *not* turn the third time. (b) Each person ends facing out.

Half–Square Thru: Take two hands, R, L.

Teaching aid: Do not turn the *second* time.

Square Thru Five Hands: Take five hands, R, L, R, L, R.

Teaching aids: (a) Do not turn the *fifth* time. (b) Will end facing out.

Note: A left-square thru is executed in the same manner, beginning with the left hand.

PRACTICE CALL 39 (full-square thru)
1 and 3 square thru
Count four hands, R, L, R, L.
Then split the outside two
Go around one and come back home.

Repeat for 2 and 4.

PRACTICE CALL 40 (full-square thru)
1 and 3 promenade halfway 'round
Same two square thru
Split the outside two
Come around one to the middle
Cross trail thru
Allemande left.

Repeat for 2 and 4.

PRACTICE CALL 41 (three-quarters-square thru)
1 and 3 up and back
Square thru three hands 'round
Then separate, go 'round one
Into the middle
Square thru three-quarters 'round
That's what you do
Split the sides, go 'round one
Into the middle, cross trail
To a left allemande.

Repeat for 2 and 4.

PRACTICE CALL 42 (half-square thru)
1 and 3 half-square thru
Right and left thru with the outside two
Dive thru, pass thru
Allemande left.

Repeat for 2 and 4.

> **Square dances:** Easy Square Thru, Pitt's Patter #3, Half-Square Thru Combo, Half-Square Thru and Then Three–Quarters, Five Hands, Just a Breeze, A Fooler A Faker, and Don't Let the Good Life Pass You By.

37. STAR THRU

When two couples are facing, each person works with the opposite. The man takes the woman's left hand in his right hand and turns her one-quarter counterclockwise as he walks around her one-quarter clockwise. They end up side by side. This woman is now his new partner on his right.

> **Teaching aids:** (a) The new couple has made a quarter-turn and ends up facing the other couple who were their original partners. (b) The fingers need to slip around each other's easily in order to feel comfortable.

PRACTICE CALL 43
1 and 3 go forward and back
Star thru, star thru again
Cross trail back and find the corner
Allemande left.

Repeat for 2 and 4.

> **Square dances:** Star Thru–California Twirl, Star Thru Square Thru Combo, New Star Thru, Go the Route, and Chime Bells.

38. DOUBLE TURN BACK FROM GRAND RIGHT AND LEFT

While doing grand right and left, dancers meet partner, take a forearm grasp, and turn each other halfway around to face back the way they came. They grand right and left the wrong way 'round until they meet partner and with a forearm grasp turn one-half again to face the original grand right and left direction. They grand right and left and meet partner the third time and promenade or follow the call.

> **Teaching aids:** (a) The cue is "meet partner and turn right back, go the other way." (b) The turn back may also be done with box the gnat and pull by.

PRACTICE CALL 44
Allemande left, grand right and left
Corn in the crib, wheat in the stack
Meet your honey and turn right back

Up the river and around the bend
Meet your honey turn back again
Meet your partner and promenade.

39. THREE-QUARTER CHAIN

The designated women make a right–hand star in the center and pass two positions, or three–quarters of the way around the ring and meet the man in the third position, who will turn her with a courtesy turn.

> **Teaching aids:** (a) If starting from home position, the women will travel three-quarters of the way around the ring and be courtesy turned by their original corner. (b) The man may do this same maneuver, called three-quarter star, and the call will indicate some other move when the men get three-quarters of the way around in place of the courtesy turn.

PRACTICE CALL 45
Four ladies chain three-quarters 'round
Roll away with a half-sashay
Circle left in the same old way
Home you go.

> **Square dances:** Sail Away, Mucho Combo.

40. BOX THE FLEA

Similar to box the gnat except that both man and woman use the left hand instead of the right. The lady is turned clockwise under the man's right arm; the man walks around her counterclockwise. They end up facing each other but have changed places.

> **Teaching aids:** (a) The hands slip easily. (b) Dancers should listen for a pull by to follow.

PRACTICE CALL 46
Allemande left your corner
Meet partner, box the gnat
Pull by and with your corner
Box the flea, pull by
Swing your partner.

> **Square dance:** Gnat and Flea Combo #1.

41. ALAMO STYLE

A variation of grand right and left. All eight dancers do an allemande left, hold on to the corner, but shift to a hands–up position and take partner right with a hands–up position, making a complete circle with the men facing in and the ladies facing out (diagram a). Dancers balance a short step forward and a short step back. Release the left hand and turn partner with a right hand halfway around so that the men now face

(continued)

out, the women face in. Join hands in the circle (diagram b). Repeat balance forward and back. Release with the right hand and turn with the left hand halfway around. Rejoin hands in the circle. Repeat balance and right–hand turn. Repeat balance and left–hand turn. There is your partner, follow the call.

Teaching aids

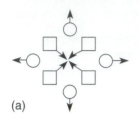 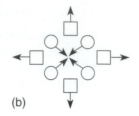

(a) (b)

PRACTICE CALL [47]
Allemande left, Alamo style
Right to your own, balance a while
Turn with the right half about
Balance in and balance out
Turn with the left and balance Joe
Balance again and don't be slow
Turn with the right on the same old track
Balance forward, balance back
Turn with the left—one more time
Find your own, you're doing fine
Swing.

42. WHEEL AROUND

From a promenade, a couple will turn half-way around counterclockwise to face the couple behind them.

> **Teaching aids:** (a) Keeping the promenade position, the man will back up and the woman will move forward so that the move is a pivot in place. (b) The man who was on the inside for the promenade is now on the outside. (c) The dancers should learn to listen for the cue "promenade but don't slow down." (d) The caller may call "all four couples wheel around," in which case they will all be promenading the wrong way around with the woman on the inside. (e) The caller may call "1 and 3 wheel around," in which case 1 turns to face couple 4 and 3 turns to face couple 2. All should adjust slightly so that couples 1 and 2 are in line facing couples 3 and 4. If the caller calls "2 and 4 wheel around," then couples 2 and 3 are in line facing couples 4 and 1. (f) The next call might be "pass thru go on to the next," and couples will pass through the couple they are facing and proceed as a couple around the circle of couples in the direction they are facing, to meet the couple coming toward them.

PRACTICE CALL [48]
Promenade but don't slow down
First and third wheel around
Go right and left thru

Cross trail to an
Allemande left.

Repeat for 2 and 4.

PRACTICE CALL [49]
Promenade but don't slow down
First and third wheel around
Go right and left thru
Pass thru to a brand new two
Right and left thru
Cross trail, there's your corner
Allemande left.

Repeat for 2 and 4.

PRACTICE CALL [50]
All promenade don't slow down
Couples 1 and 3 wheel around
Star thru, dive thru
Pass thru right and left thru with the outside two
Then dive thru and pass thru
Right and left thru with outside two
Then star thru and cross trail
Find your corner, allemande left.

Repeat for 2 and 4.

> **Square dance:** Duck and Wheel Around.

43. SLIP THE CLUTCH

Start from the allemande thar star. Man will release partner on his left arm, move forward one place to the corner for an allemande left, and follow the call.

PRACTICE CALL [51]
Ladies to the center, back to the bar
Gents center, right–hand star
All the way 'round
Turn partner left, corner right
Partner left to an allemande thar
Slip the clutch to an allemande left.

> **Square dance:** Pitt's Patter #2.

44. DOUBLE PASS THRU

A simple pass thru done by four couples instead of two.

Teaching aids

(a) Starting position facing in:

(b) Finish position after both couples passed thru facing out:

PRACTICE CALL 52

2 and 4 right and left thru, same ladies chain
Now 1 and 3 promenade outside halfway 'round
2 and 4 star thru, double pass thru, first couple left
Next couple go right, right and left thru, turn this girl
Cross trail thru to an allemande left.

Repeat starting with 1 and 3.

    Square dance: Four in the Middle.

■ Level 5: Intermediate Basics 45–50

45. WHEEL AND DEAL

From a line of four, the right couple in line pivots counterclockwise halfway around the person nearest the center. The left couple moves forward two steps and then pivots clockwise halfway around the person nearest the center and comes in behind the right–hand couple. Starting formation: two lines of four facing out.

    Teaching aid: When the couples have completed the figure, they are lined up in double file, left–hand couple behind the right–hand couple. Both are facing the same direction.

PRACTICE CALL 53

Side ladies chain
1 and 3 lead to the right
Circle to a line
Pass thru
Wheel and deal
Center four star thru
Cross trail
Left allemande.

Repeat for 2 and 4.

PRACTICE CALL 54 (combine with double pass thru)

1 and 3 lead to the right and form a line
Forward up and back you reel
Pass thru wheel and deal
Double pass thru
First couple left, second couple right
Meet the next two
Go right and left thru
Cross trail to an allemande left.

Repeat for 2 and 4.

    Square dances: Sides Break to a Line, Now Hear This, and Hello Dolly.

46. EIGHT CHAIN THRU

For starting position, 1 and 3 take the opposite and face the sides as shown in the diagram. Four couples are lined up across the floor, two are on the outside facing in while two couples on the inside are facing the couples on the outside.

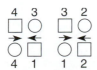

The action is like grand right and left across the set and back, using a right and left thru when facing out.

    Teaching aid: Inside couples start with a right and left thru; outside couples give a right hand, pass by to inside, give a left to the inside couple, pass by, and then do a right and left thru to turn around. The process is repeated to get them back to starting position.

PRACTICE CALL 55

1 and 3 go forward and back
Take your opposite, face the sides
Now everybody eight chain thru
All the way over and back
Meet that couple, right and left thru
Allemande left.

Repeat for 2 and 4.

    Square dances: Eight Chain Combo 1 and Combo 2 and A Long Way Over.

47. TURN THRU

Two dancers are facing each other. They take a right forearm grasp and turn each other around clockwise 180 degrees, so as to end up facing the direction they had their backs to when they started.

Teaching aids

(a) Start facing   (b) Turning clockwise   (c)

(d) When dancers are turning, they are actually side by side because of the forearm grasp. (e) After turning halfway around, pull past each other and release grasp.

(e)

PRACTICE CALL 56

Partners face
Turn thru
Now allemande left the corner
Go back and bow to partner.

PRACTICE CALL 57

Head couples turn thru
Separate, go around one
Come into the middle
Turn thru, meet your corner
Allemande left.

Repeat for side couples.   *(continued)*

PRACTICE CALL 58

Heads square thru, four hands
Split the outsides, around one
Line up four
Turn thru, bend the line
Turn thru
Allemande left.

Repeat for side couples.

PRACTICE CALL 59

Head ladies chain
Heads roll away to a half-sashay
Star thru, circle four
Head men break to a line
Turn thru, bend the line
Turn thru, cross trail
Allemande left.

Repeat for side couples.

PRACTICE CALL 60

Promenade but don't slow down
1 and 3 wheel around
Right and left thru
Turn thru, bend the line
Turn thru, bend the line
Cross trail thru to the corner
Allemande left.

Repeat for 2 and 4.

Square dance: Turn Thru Combo 1.

48. OCEAN WAVE

A line of dancers, usually four, facing in alternate directions.

Teaching aids: (a) The call usually is "do–sa–do to an ocean wave." Two couples facing each other do-sa-do with opposite all the way around and step forward as if to pass thru and stop when they get four in line. (b) Note diagram. Man and lady of couple 1 face one direction and man and lady of couple 3 face opposite direction. (c) All join hands in line, hands up, elbows down.

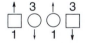

(d) All four balance forward (step touch) and backward (step touch). On the backward balance, dancers should reestablish relationships with their own partners by noting which one is facing the same direction as they are. (e) If the next call is right and left thru, they pull by the person who has their right hand and reach for partner with left for courtesy

turn. (f) If the next call is box the gnat, it is done with the person who has their right hand in the line. (g) If next call is pass thru, release hands and move straight ahead. Same action for starting cross trail thru.

PRACTICE CALL 61

1 and 3 go forward and back
Now do-sa-do, go all the way 'round
To an ocean wave
Rock it up and back
Do right and left thru
And cross trail
To an allemande left.

Repeat for 2 and 4.

PRACTICE CALL 62

1 and 3 bow and swing
2 and 4 promenade half the outside ring
Come into the middle and do–sa–do
All the way 'round to an ocean wave
Rock it up and back
Box the gnat across the track
Change girls, box the flea
Join hands and circle left
Allemande left.

Repeat for 2 and 4.

Square dance: Easy Wave.

49. SWING THRU

From an ocean–wave position, the two on each end of the line turn each other with a right arm halfway around. Then the two in the center turn each other with a left arm halfway around. All balance forward and back and follow next call.

Teaching aids: (a) Dancers must have joined hands in the up position, palm to palm. A firm grasp when turning permits the turn to be quick and controlled.

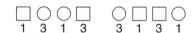

(b) Swing thru may be repeated before adding anything else. (c) The figure ends with woman 3 and man 1 facing the same direction, and man 3 and woman 1 facing the same direction. They would be partners if the next call were right and left thru, pass thru, cross trail, and so on. Box the gnat would be done with person holding the right hand.

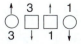

PRACTICE CALL 63

1 and 3 go forward
Swing thru in the middle of the set
Right hand first, then centers left
Go forward and back
  (here note, each has a new partner)
Swing thru one more time
Balance forward, back, you're doing fine
  (here note, each has original partner)
Cross trail, find your corner
Left allemande.

Repeat for 2 and 4.

PRACTICE CALL 64

1 and 3 half–square thru
Count two hands, then U–turn back
Box the gnat
Swing thru
Swing thru
Pull by to your corner
Left allemande.

Repeat for 2 and 4.

PRACTICE CALL 65

1 and 3 star thru
Swing thru
Swing thru
Pass thru, allemande left.

Repeat for 2 and 4.

> **Square dances:** Ocean Wave and Swing Thru Combo #1, Happiness Is, and Ocean Wave and Swing Thru Combo #2.

50. CIRCULATE

From two ocean–wave lines, dancers on the outside or the inside of the line may circulate by moving for–ward to the next end position in a circle.

Teaching aids

(a) If men are circulating, they move clockwise one place.

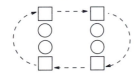

(b) If women are circulating they move counterclockwise one place.

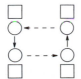

(c) If all circulate, they have moved up two places.
(d) After bend the line, the men may be on the inside and the women on the outside. The same situation may develop with swing thru.

PRACTICE CALL 66

1 and 3 go forward to the center
Face the sides
Do–sa–do to an ocean wave
Go forward and back
Men circulate
Girls circulate
Men circulate
Girls circulate
Right and left thru
Dive thru, star thru
Cross trail thru
Allemande left.

Repeat for 2 and 4.

> **Square dances:** Ocean Wave and Circulate and Circulate Sue.

■ *Additional Basics 51–59*

51. RUN

The directed active dancer, such as Boys, Girls, Ends, or Centers, run around inactive dancers 180 degrees to face opposite direction. Inactive dancer side steps to become either the center or end.

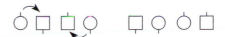

52. TRADE

Any two dancers–Partners, Boys, Girls, Ends, or couples–trade by moving in a semi–circle pass right shoulders to exchange places ending facing opposite direction.

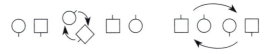

Partners Trade   Couples Trade

53. ZOOM

Two couples, one behind the other, exchange places. The lead couple separates moving away from partner to end in trailing couples position. The trailing couple move forward to allow the exchange.

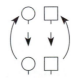

■ 54. FLUTTERWHEEL

Couples facing. Women move toward center to join right forearms then move to extend their left hand to the opposite man's right. The line of four moves around to the women's original position. Men and new partners end in opposite positions couples facing.

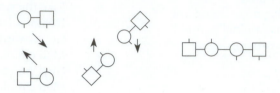

■ 55. SWEEP A QUARTER

Couples move left or right one quarter in direction of the call. Couples end facing.

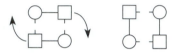

■ 56. VEER LEFT OR RIGHT

Couples facing move diagonally left or right and forward to end in a two-faced line or mini wave. Couples may veer right from the line and end back to back.

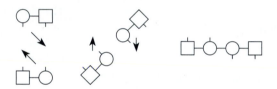

■ 57. TRADE BY

Formation may be a Pass Thru Eight Chain Thru or a Square. Couples facing do a pass thru, couples facing out do a partner trade to face in.

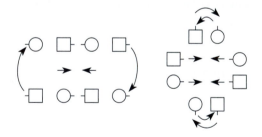

■ 58. TOUCH ONE QUARTER

Couples face, touch right hands, and turn one–quarter by the right.

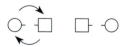

■ 59. FERRIS WHEEL

Two face parallel lines, couples facing center move to the center. As women touch hands, couples wheel and deal to face center. Outside couples wheel and deal to face in to form a double pass thru formation.

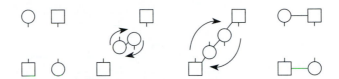

■ *Mainstream Movements 60–78*

■ 60. CLOVERLEAF

Begin from a completed double pass thru. Dancers follow the dancer in front ending in a double pass thru down the center.

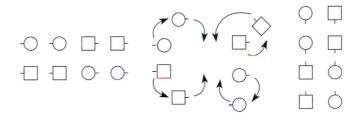

From a square, heads pass thru, then do a cloverleaf while sides do a right and left thru in the center or a square thru.

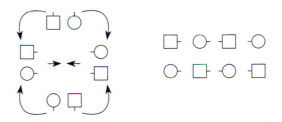

■ 61. TURN THRU

Couples face, join right forearms, turn halfway around, release arms, and move forward to stand back to back.

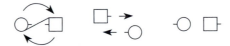

■ 62. EIGHT CHAIN THRU

Facing dancers join right hands and pass thru courtesy turn while center dancers join right hands and pass thru. Repeat to chain 1–8 hands.

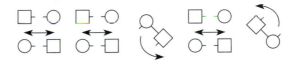

■ 63. PASS TO CENTER

Begin in eight chain thru or parallel waves formation. All dancers pass through and as they do, the outside dancers trade partners. End in double pass thru formation. The movement is the same as pass thru and partner trade.

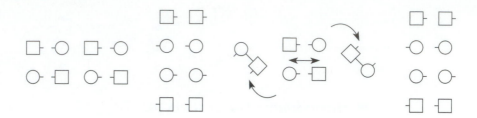

■ 64. SPIN THE TOP

Begin in ocean wave formation. Ends and centers turn one half, new center (man) turns three quarters, outside dancers move forward a quarter circle to meet original partner.

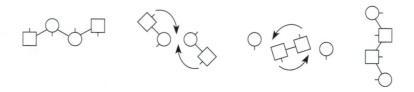

■ 65. CENTERS IN-OUT

When there is a couple with back to center of set standing behind another couple (eight chain thru or double pass thru), on the call "centers in" the outside couple moves sideways apart as the center couple moves up to form a line. On the call "centers out" the center couple steps apart to move up to form a line.

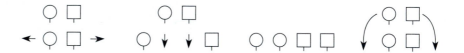

■ 66. CAST OFF THREE-QUARTERS

Begin in any wave or line. Each couple in line pivots three-quarters. End dancers are the pivot points for each couple.

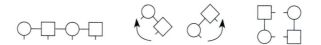

■ 67. WALK AND DODGE

Begin couples facing or box circulate. Dancers facing into box walk forward to take the place of dancers in front. Dancers facing out of box step sideways (dodges) to position left by walkers. The call must indicate the move, i.e., "men walk, ladies dodge."

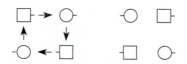

■ 68. SLIDE THRU

Dancers face, pass thru, man turns right one–quarter, woman turns left one–quarter. Dancers end side by side.

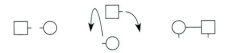

■ 69. FOLD

Any two dancer formation. Call may be "Boys fold," "Ends fold," "Centers fold," or "Cross fold." Active dancers fold toward inactive dancers.

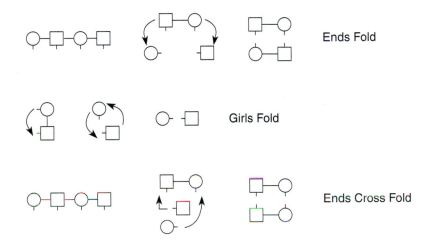

Ends Fold

Girls Fold

Ends Cross Fold

■ 70. DIXIE STYLE TO AN OCEAN WAVE

Couples facing. Women step forward, join right hands, pull by and join left hands with opposite man and turn one–half around. New centers join right hand to form left–hand ocean wave.

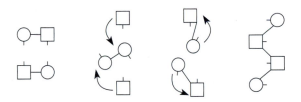

■ 71. SPIN CHAIN THRU

Begin with parallel waves. Ends and adjacent center dancer turn one–half. New center of each wave turn three–quarters to make wave across set. Centers of new wave turn half to reform wave across set. The two outside pairs or the center wave turn three–quarters to join the waiting end to form parallel ocean waves.

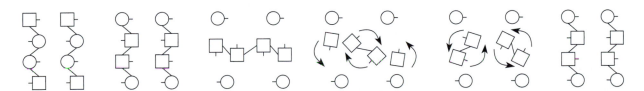

■ 72. PEEL OFF

Two couples facing the same direction one behind the other. Couple in front separates and moves in a semi-circle to become the end or the line. Rear couple steps forward and does a U-turn back individually to become the center of the line.

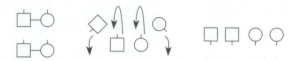

■ 73. TAG

Any line with an even number of dancers. *Full Tag:* dancers face center of line, take a short step to the side left and walk forward passing right shoulders with all dancers from the other half of the line. The call following may be "In" "Out" "Right" or "Left." Dancers turn in direction or call. *Half Tag:* dancers stop moving forward when original center from each side or line meets the original end from the other side. Form a four-person line ending in a right-hand box circulate. *Partner Tag:* Two dancers turn to face each other and pass thru.

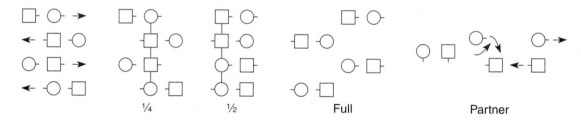

¼   ½   Full   Partner

■ 74. CURLIQUE

Dancers face, join raised right hands to form an arch. Woman turns left face under arch three-quarters. Man walks forward around woman turning right one-quarter. End in a right-hand mini wave.

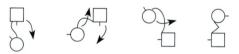

■ 75. SCOOT BACK

Begin in a box circulate formation. Dancers facing in (men) move forward, join right forearms and turn half, step forward to end in position vacated by the dancer who was facing out. Dancers facing out move into the position vacated by dancers doing the forearm turn.

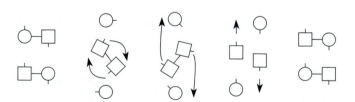

▪ 76. FAN THE TOP

Begin in an ocean wave or two-faced line. Centers of the line turn three-quarters, outside dancers move forward a half circle. End line is at right angles to beginning line.

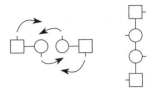

▪ 77. HINGES

Begin in a line or two-faced line. *Couple Hinge:* Each couple executes a couple trade to end in a two-faced line at right angle to the original line. *Single Hinge:* Begin in a mini wave formation. Dancers do a half trade with each other to end in a mini wave at right angle to the original wave. *Partner Hinge:* Couple does a half partner trade to end in a right-hand mini wave at right angles to original starting position.

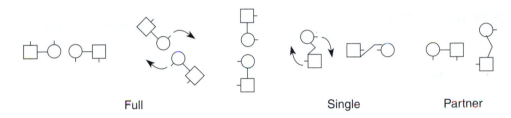

Full   Single   Partner

▪ 78. RECYCLE

Begin in an ocean wave formation. Ends of wave fold as centers of wave fold in behind and follow them around and face in to end in as couples facing.

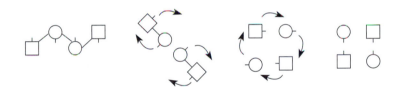

PATTER CALLS NOTES ON THE DANCE FIGURES

Only the basic figures are presented in these dances. The caller must select an opener, break, and ending to choreograph a full Square Dance call. The basics used in these dances are fully explained for teaching and calling purposes under Teaching Progression and Analysis for Basic Movements of Square Dance, earlier in this chapter. Each basic in the teaching progression is accompanied by an analysis or a description of the movement, teaching aids, diagrams, and suggested dance figures using the basic. Basics are also analyzed in the Glossary.

Each call brings the dancers back to a promenade or an allemande left position. If the dance ends with "promenade" or "allemande left," the caller must make up a continuity line to direct the dancers to home positions. When there are exceptions, a note will indicate to the caller where the dancers end up and how to repeat the call to bring them to home position. When the call is given for couples 1 and 3, it should be repeated for couples 2 and 4. When the call is given for couple 1, it should be repeated for all couples.

The calling sequence for singing calls will be noted at the end of the call when necessary.

■ *Dances*

PROMENADE THE RING

Basics: Preliminary basics.

Bow to your partner
Heads promenade go halfway 'round the outside ring
Sides up to the middle and back
Sides promenade go halfway 'round
Heads up to the middle and back
All join hands circle left
Go halfway 'round
When you get home face your own
Do–sa–do your partner
Same lady swing and promenade
Promenade single file
Go back home, face your own
Bow to your partner, corner too
Wave at the girl across from you.

GENTS STAR RIGHT

Basics: Star halfway 'round, preliminary basics.

Gents star right, just halfway 'round
Turn your opposite left
Now star back home and here we go
Meet your partner do–sa–do
Now gents star left go all the way 'round
Meet your partner right, right arm 'round
To the corner, allemande left
Back to your partner, right and left grand
Hand over hand till you
Find your own, promenade
Come right on home.

BEND IT TIGHT

Basics: Split the ring, pass thru, bend the line.

1 and 3 do a pass through
Split the ring and go around two
Hang on tight form two lines
Go forward and back keep in time
Pass thru and bend the line
Pass thru now and bend it tight
Circle up eight and keep it right.

TEXAS STAR

Basics: Four gents star, star promenade.

Ladies to the center and back to the bar
Gents to the center and form a star
Right hand crossed
Back with the left and don't get lost
Meet your pretty girl, pass her by
Hook the next gal on the fly (Star promenade)
The gent swing out, ladies swing in
Form that Texas Star again
Break that star and everybody swing

Promenade home with the new little thing.
(Men have new partners)

Repeat three times until women are back to original partners.

ARKANSAS TRAVELER

Basics: Forearm turns.

1 and 3 go forward and back
Forward again
Turn your opposite right arm 'round
Partner left, left arm 'round
Corners right, right arm 'round
Partner left, left arm 'round
Promenade your corner as she comes around.

Note: Gent promenades the corner each time until he gets his original partner back. Called four times.

EASY BEND THE LINE

Basics: Do–sa–do, bend the line.

1 and 3 promenade three–quarters outside
Go 'round the ring
Line up four with 2 and 4
It's forward up and back
Do–sa–do across the way
Bend the line, that's what I say
Now do–sa–do in the center once more
Then circle eight, go 'round the floor.

Note: Two lines face each other on the diagonal.

SPLIT THE RING AND AROUND JUST ONE

Basics: Pass thru, split the ring.

1 and 3 bow and swing
Up to the center and back to the ring
Pass through, separate
Come around just one
Go down the middle, pass thru
Split the ring, separate
Go around one down the middle
Pass thru, separate
Come around one, pass thru
Meet your corner, left allemande
Right to partner, right and left grand.

ARKANSAS TRAVELER WITH A CROSS TRAIL THRU

Basics: Forearm turns, cross trail thru.

1 and 3 go forward and back
Sides do cross trail thru, separate
Go around the outside track
Heads go forward
Turn your opposite, right arm around

Partner left, left arm 'round
Corner right, right arm 'round
Partner left, left arm 'round
Promenade your corner as she comes around.

> **Note:** Couples 1 and 3 are doing the Arkansas Traveler figure, while 2 and 4 cross trail, separate, and go around the outside. At home, they must pass by partner to be ready to meet corner with right arm around.

THE ROUTE

> **Basics:** Ladies chain, right and left thru.

1 and 3 bow and swing
Lead to the right
Circle, break, and form a line
Forward eight and back you go
Forward again do–sa–do
Go right and left thru across the set
Right and left back, you're not thru yet
Chain those ladies across the hall
Turn and chain them down the line
Chain those ladies across the hall
Chain those ladies down the line
All join hands and circle left
And home you go.

Repeat for 2 and 4.

> **Note:** When ladies chain across hall and down the line, not all couples have the same amount of turn on the courtesy turn, so all need to adjust so that the timing works out right.

PROMENADE THE OUTSIDE RING

> **Basics:** Right and left thru, ladies chain, bend the line, promenade three–quarters, pass thru.

1 and 3 promenade three–quarters 'round the outside ring
While the roosters crow and the birdies sing
Line up four with the sides
Diagonally now go forward and back
Go right and left thru
Right and left back
Two ladies chain, chain back
Forward eight and back in time
Pass thru and bend the line
Now right and left thru, you're doing fine
Forward eight and back once more
Pass thru and bend the line
Go right and left thru to your own land
Allemande left, go right and left grand.

> **Note:** "Line up four with the sides" means to go to the far side of the line nearest home.

SPLIT THE RING VARIATION 1

> **Basics:** Split the ring, pass thru, ladies chain, right and left thru.

Four ladies chain across the hall
Chain them back and don't you fall
1 and 3 pass thru, go round one
Into the middle, right and left thru
Turn on around right and left back
Pass thru, split the ring
Come 'round one, go down the middle
Pass thru, 'round one into the middle
Right and left thru
Turn on 'round right and left back
Pass thru
Watch out man there's your corner
Left allemande.

ROLL AWAY COMBO 2

> **Basics:** Roll away to a half–sashay, right and left thru, bend the line, cross trail thru, U–turn.

1 and 3 lead to the right
Circle, break, form a line
Roll away to a half–sashay
Pass thru, U–turn back
Right and left thru, turn your girl
Pass thru bend the line
Right and left thru
Pass thru bend the line
Do–sa–do
Cross trail thru
Allemande left.

ENDS TURN IN

> **Basics:** Split the ring, pass thru, California twirl, dive thru, ends turn in.

1 and 3 go forward and back
Pass thru split the ring
Go around two and line up four
Forward eight and back with you
Pass thru, join your hands
Arch in the middle, the ends turn in
Circle four in the middle of the floor
Go one time around, same two
Pass thru, split the ring
Go around one and line up four
Forward eight and back with you
Pass thru, join your hands
Arch in the middle, ends turn in
Circle four in the middle of the floor
Go one time 'round, same two
Pass thru, watch out man
Left to your corner left allemande
Right to partner, right and left grand.

ROLL AWAY COMBO 1

Basics: Roll away to a half–sashay, pass thru, split the ring, U–turn back.

1 and 3 roll away to a half–sashay
Pass thru separate come around one
Into the middle, pass thru, split two
Go around 1, down the middle
Pass thru, U–turn back
Allemande left.

BOX THE GNAT—PULL BY

Basics: Roll away to a half–sashay, box the gnat, right and left thru, ladies chain.

Head 2 couples do a half–sashay
Come up to the middle and back that way
Right to opposite and box the gnat
Pull by for a right and left thru
Same two pass thru and separate go 'round one
Meet in the middle for a right and left thru
Same two pass thru and split the outside
Go around one to a line of four
Forward eight and back like that
Right to opposite box the gnat, pull by
Right and left thru
Ladies chain across the track
Chain back in the usual way
Roll away to a half–sashay
Join hands circle eight
Allemande left.

SPLIT THE RING VARIATION 2

Basics: Promenade halfway, right and left thru, pass thru, cross trail.

1 and 3 promenade halfway 'round
Go forward up and back
Pass thru, separate, go 'round one
Into the middle, pass thru
Split the ring, go 'round one
Into the middle, right and left thru
Cross trail thru
Left allemande.

ANOTHER TRAIL

Basics: Roll away to a half–sashay, right and left thru, cross trail thru.

1 and 3 do a half–sashay
Up to the middle and back that way
Pass thru and U–turn back
Go forward and back on the same old track
Pass thru separate come into the middle
Pass thru split the ring, go 'round one
Come into the middle, right and left thru
Now cross trail thru, find your corner
Left allemande.

THERE'S YOUR CORNER

Basics: Roll away to a half–sashay, pass thru, box the gnat, cross trail thru.

1 and 3 roll away to a half–sashay
Up to the middle and back that way
Pass thru, split the ring, go 'round one
Come into the middle, box the gnat
Right and left thru the other way back
Turn on around and pass thru
Split the ring and around just one
Come down the middle, right and left thru
Turn your girl and cross trail back
Separate, come around one into the middle
Box the gnat, pull her by
There's your corner, allemande left.

EASY SQUARE THRU

Basics: Right and left thru, dive thru, square thru.

1 and 3 square thru
Right left right left
Right and left thru with the outside two
Dive thru, pass thru
Right and left thru with the outside two
Dive thru, pass thru
Allemande left.

PITT'S PATTER 3

Basics: Cross trail thru, square thru, box the gnat.

1 and 3 do cross trail thru
Go 'round one, that's what you do
Down the middle, pass thru
Split two, go 'round one
Cross trail in the center once more
Round just one, into the middle
Full square thru to the tune of the fiddle
Face your partner, box the gnat
And swing–she's your own.

HALF-SQUARE THRU COMBO

Basics: Right and left thru, dive thru, box the gnat, U–turn back, half–square thru.

1 and 3 half–square thru
Right and left thru, outside two
Dive thru, pass thru
Right and left thru with outside two
Dive thru, half–square thru
Separate, go 'round one
Come into the middle, box the gnat
U–turn back
Left allemande.

JUST A BREEZE

Basics: Square thru three-quarters, half-square thru, bend the line.

1 and 3 lead to the right circle four
Go once around and a quarter more
Now pass thru, on to the next around the ring
Right and left thru, turn on around
Square thru three-quarters, hear me shout
Two lines of four facing out
Now bend the line and pass thru
On to the next right and left thru
Square thru three-quarters 'round
Then bend the line when you come down
Do a half-square thru, look out man
There's your corner, left allemande.

FIVE HANDS

Basics: Square thru one-half, three-quarters, five hands.

1 and 3 square thru, four hands
Right and left thru, outside two
Dive thru, square thru three-quarters 'round
Split the sides, go 'round one
Into the middle, half-square thru
Right and left thru, outside two
Dive thru, square thru five hands
Allemande left.

HALF-SQUARE THRU AND THEN THREE-QUARTERS

Basics: Half-square thru, three-quarter square thru.

1 and 3 forward and back
Half-square thru, two hands 'round
Right and left thru with outside two
Turn on around dive thru
Square thru three-quarters, three hands 'round
Then split thru, separate, go 'round one
Right and left thru, go down the middle
Allemande left.

SAIL AWAY

Basics: Three-quarter chain, roll away with a half-sashay, bend the line, cross trail, U-turn back.

Four ladies chain three-quarters 'round
Turn her left then settle down
1 and 3 will swing and sway
2 and 4 roll away with a half-sashay
Heads pass thru go 'round just one
Line up four, let's have some fun
Forward eight and back you sail
Bend the line, then cross trail
U-turn back and join hands circle left

Then roll away to a half-sashay, circle left in the same old way
Allemande left.

STAR THRU SQUARE THRU COMBO

Basics: Cross trail thru, star thru, square thru.

Heads promenade just halfway 'round
Go down the middle, right and left thru
Then heads lead right—circle break
And make a line
Go forward and back—star thru
Square thru, four hands 'round
Now bend the line, then
Cross trail thru to allemande left.

STAR THRU—CALIFORNIA TWIRL

Basics: U-turn back, box the gnat, California twirl, half-square thru, star thru.

1 and 3 star thru
California twirl
Star thru
Right and left thru
Half-square thru
U-turn back
Box the gnat
Change hands
Allemande left.

GNAT AND FLEA COMBO 1

Basics: Box the gnat, box the flea.

1 and 3 go forward and back
Right to opposite, box the gnat
Pull 'em thru and separate go 'round just one
Down the center, pass thru
Split the ring to 'round one
Come down the middle, left to opposite
Box the flea, pull 'em thru
Separate, go 'round one—come into middle
Swing your own right there at home.

NEW STAR THRU

Basics: Star thru, cross trail thru, box the gnat, roll away to a half-sashay.

1 and 3 go forward and back
Pass thru U-turn back
Now star thru
Right and left thru the outside two
Now dive thru, star thru
Right and left thru
Same ladies roll away to a half-sashay
New star thru across the way
Right and left thru with the outside two
Turn your girl

(continued)

Dive thru, star thru
Right and left thru
Now cross trail thru go 'round one
Come into the middle
Box the gnat, pull her by
Allemande left.

GO THE ROUTE

Basics: Star thru, square thru, dive thru, bend the line.

Head two ladies chain to the right
New side ladies chain across
Turn this girl is what you do
Now face the middle, star thru
Right and left thru and turn your Sue
Then pass thru, star thru to lines of four
Forward eight and back with you
Forward again, star thru
Then dive thru, pass thru
Square thru with the outside two
Four hands 'round, you go the route
Two lines of four, facing out
Now bend the line and star thru
Right and left thru and turn your Sue
Then dive thru and pass thru
Square thru with the outside two
Count four hands, you go the route
Two lines of four, you're facing out
Bend the line, go right and left thru
Allemande left.

MUCHO COMBO

Basics: Three-quarter chain, half-sashay, star thru, square thru three-quarters.

Four ladies chain
Turn 'em boys and don't get sore
Ladies chain three-quarters 'round
Take her by the left, turn her around
1 and 3 do half-sashay
Up to the middle, back that way
Go forward again and star thru, face the sides
Right and left thru the outside two
Then dive thru and pass thru
Star thru the outside two
Right and left thru, turn this girl
Pass thru, on to the next, star thru
Square thru three-quarters
Find the corner, left allemande.

PITT'S PATTER 2

Basics: Allemande thar, slip the clutch.

1 and 3 bow and swing
Promenade the outside ring
Sides pass thru
Step in behind the old head two (2 behind 3, and 4 behind 1)

Gents turn back in a right-hand star
Gals progress just as you are
Pass your honey and turn the next
To an allemande thar
Back up boys, not too far
Slip the clutch to an allemande left
Back to your partner, pass her by
Swing the next girl on the fly
Promenade.

SIDES BREAK TO A LINE

Basics: Wheel and deal, double pass thru, cross trail thru.

1 and 3 lead right, circle four
Head gents break, line up four
Forward eight and back you reel
Pass thru, wheel and deal
Inside two pass thru, right and left thru outside two
Turn your girl and circle four
Side gents break and line up four
Forward eight and back you reel
Pass thru, wheel and deal
Double pass thru, first couple left, second couple right
Pass thru the first two, meet the next
Cross trail thru
To a left allemande.

DUCK THEN WHEEL AROUND

Basics: Roll away with a half-sashay, star thru, wheel around, ends turn in, cross trail.

First and third go forward and back
Do a right and left thru across the track
Roll away with a half-sashay
Star thru and hear me say
Split the sides
Go 'round one and make a line of four
Forward eight and back you do
Forward again and pass thru
Join hands centers arch
Ends turn in
Go into the middle
Wheel around in the middle of the square
Do a right and left thru
With the outside pair
Dive thru
Right and left thru in the middle of the set
Pass thru
Split two go around to a line of four
Forward eight and back once more
Pass thru and join hands
Ends turn in–go into the middle
Wheel around in the middle of the square
Do a right and left thru
With the outside pair
Dive thru, pass thru

Split two and around one
Down the middle
Cross trail and find the corner
Left allemande.

FOUR IN THE MIDDLE

Basics: Ladies chain, roll away to a half–sashay, bend the line, California twirl, double pass thru.

Four ladies chain across the way
1 and 3 roll away to a half–sashay
Couple 1 down the middle
Split couple 3, around 1 to a line of 4
Forward 4 to the middle of the ring
Bend the line and face those two
Double pass thru that's what you do
First couple California twirl
Guess who, the corner girl
Left allemande.

NOW HEAR THIS

Basics: Star thru, double pass thru, wheel and deal, square thru three–quarters.

1 and 3 go forward up and back
Cross trail thru, separate go 'round two
Line up four, forward up and back
Star thru, double pass thru
First two left
Next two right
Meet two, pass thru
Wheel and deal
Inside two square thru three–quarters
Left allemande.

EIGHT CHAIN COMBO 1

Basics: Square thru, eight chain thru.

Heads to the center and back you do
Forward again do a full square thru
Count four hands don't get mixed
Right and left thru the outside two
Eight chain thru
All the way over and back you bet
Meet that couple right and left thru
To a left allemande in front of you.

A LONG WAY OVER

Basics: Star thru, square thru, eight chain thru, wheel around.

Promenade, don't slow down
1 and 3 wheel around
Right and left thru the couple you've found
Star thru, eight chain thru
It's a long way over and then right back
Right and left go along the track
Square thru with the same two

Go all the way 'round make two lines
You're facing out, bend those lines
Star thru across from you
Square thru three–quarters, right left right
Allemande left.

TURN THRU COMBO

Basics: Ladies chain, bend the line, turn thru, ends turn in, square thru, star thru.

Head ladies chain
Heads star thru, pass thru
Split those two, go around one
Lines of four go forward and back
Turn thru, bend the line
Pass thru, bend the line
Turn thru
Centers arch, ends turn in
Square thru, four hands
Separate around one
Into the middle, star thru
All four to your corner
Allemande left.

INSIDE ARCH AND OUTSIDE UNDER

Basics: Dive thru.

Couple one bow and swing
Lead to the right and circle half
Inside arch and outside under
Cross the hall and go like thunder
Some will arch, some dive under
Hurry up boys, don't you blunder
Lead to the next, circle half
Dive thru, lead to the next
Circle half and here we go
Inside arch and outside low
Dive thru, don't you blunder
Inside arch, outside under
Home you go and everybody swing.

Note: Inside arch and outside under is continuous until the lead couple is in the middle of the set and can lead to couple 3. The side couples are opposite home. The repeat will take everybody home.

EASY WAVE

Basics: Square thru, ocean wave.

1 and 3 square thru
Count four hands that's what you do
Do–sa–do to an ocean wave
Balance forward up and back
Right and left thru turn your girl
Dive thru, pass thru
Do–sa–do to an ocean wave
Balance forward up and back

(continued)

Right and left thru, turn your girl
Dive thru, pass thru
Allemande left.

OCEAN WAVE—SWING THRU COMBO 2

Basics: Wheel around, ocean wave, swing thru, box the gnat, star thru.

Four men do a right–hand star
Back by the left not too far
Meet your own and
Promenade, but don't slow down
1 and 3 wheel around
Do–sa–do to an ocean wave
Swing thru, balance back
Box the gnat, go right and left thru
Star thru, dive thru
Pass thru, do–sa–do to an ocean wave
Swing thru, balance back
Box the gnat, go right and left thru
Star thru, cross trail thru to an
Allemande left.

OCEAN WAVE—CIRCULATE

Basics: Square thru, ocean wave, circulate.

1 and 3 square thru
Count four hands
Do–sa–do to an ocean wave
Balance forward and back
Men circulate
Go right and left thru
Turn your girl, dive thru
Pass thru
Do–sa–do to an ocean wave
Balance forward and back
Men circulate
Right and left thru
Turn your girl and dive thru
Pass thru to an allemande left

Repeat for 2 and 4, women circulate.

OCEAN WAVE—SWING THRU COMBO 1

Basics: Box the gnat, star thru, swing thru, box the flea, ocean wave.

Heads star thru, pass thru, do–sa–do
All the way round to an ocean wave
Forward up and back then swing thru, go up and back
Box the gnat, pull by for right and left thru
Now dive thru, pass thru
Do–sa–do the outside two
Make an ocean wave with the same pair
Go forward and back, swing thru
Box the gnat, now listen to me
Pull on by, face partner
Everybody swat the flea
Change hands to right and left grand.

CIRCULATE SUE

Basics: Square thru, ocean wave, circulate.

1 and 3 square thru
Four hands 'round in the middle you do
Now do–sa–do to an ocean wave
Go forward up and back
Men circulate
Girls circulate
All circulate
There's your corner, allemande left.

■ *Supplementary Square Dance Patter*

OPENERS

Honor your partner, lady by your side
All join hands and circle wide
Break and trail along that line
The lady in the lead, the gent behind
Now you're home and now you swing.
Clap your hands
Now slap your knees [twice]
Bump-si-daisy if you please [partners bump hips together].
Hi diddle, diddle
All eight to the middle
Back right out and swing your own
To the tune of the fiddle.
Honor your partner, lady by your side
All join hands and circle wide
Break and trail along that line
Lady in front and the gent behind
Home you go, you're doing fine.
All jump up and never come down
Swing your partner 'round and 'round
And promenade, boys, promenade.

ENDINGS

Honor your partner, corners all
Honor your opposite across the hall
And that is all.

Promenade–you know where
And I don't care
Take her out and give her air.

All you folks listen to the call
Thank you, ladies–that will be all.

Honor your partner and your corner too
Now wave at the gal across from you
Thank you folks, I'm all through.

BREAKS

Allemande left, say what do you know
Back to your own and do–sa–do.

Allemande left as pretty as you can
Right to your honey
And a right and left grand.

Promenade around the ring
While the roosters crow and the birdies sing.

Here we go in a little red wagon
Rear wheel's broke and the axle's draggin'
Promenade, boys, promenade.

With your big foot up
And your little foot down
Promenade, go 'round and 'round.

Promenade, go 'round and 'round
Like a jaybird hoppin' on the frozen ground.

Allemande left with your left hand
Right to your partner
And a right and left grand
Promenade eight when you come straight.

Ace of diamonds, jack of spades
Meet your honey and all promenade.

Two, four, six, and eight
All promenade when you get straight.

Swing the girl across the hall
Go back home and swing your own.

Alamo style

Allemande left in Alamo style
Right to your honey and balance awhile
Balance in and balance out
Turn with the right hand half about
Balance out and balance in
Turn with the left hand half about
Balance in and balance out
Turn with the right hand half about
Balance out and balance in
Turn with the left hand half again
Swing your partner and promenade.

BREAKS FOR FOURS

Half–square thru

1 and 3 go forward and back
Now half–square thru around the track
Right and left thru with the outside two
Dive thru, pass thru to an allemande left.

Square thru

Heads go forward and back you do
Forward again and full–square thru
Now count four hands is what you do.
Head two couples go square thru
Right, left, right, and pass a few
Partner left and now you're thru.

Star thru

Heads go forward, back with you
Go forward again and pass thru
Around just one is what you do
Into the center and star thru
Cross trail thru, look out, man
There's your corner, left allemande.

BREAKS FOR EIGHTS

Wheel and deal

Head two couples swing and sway
Side ladies chain across the way
Heads go right and circle four
Head gents break to a line of four
Forward eight and back you peel
Pass thru, wheel and deal
Inside two square thru three–quarters
Don't stand, left allemande.

1 and 3 right and left thru
Lead to the right, circle to a line
Ladies chain
Pass thru
Wheel and deal
Centers pass thru
Box the gnat
Right and left grand.

Wheel around

1 and 3 wheel around
Square thru three–quarters 'round
Go on to the next
Left square thru all the way 'round
Allemande left.

Promenade and don't slow down
Keep on walking that girl around
Heads back track and pass thru
Sides back track and follow those two
Lead two couples wheel around

Box the gnat with the two you found
Do a right and left thru

The other way back
Turn this girl, and
Cross trail thru.

Promenade, but don't slow down
First and third, wheel around
Right and left thru
Cross trail back to an allemande left.

Promenade, but don't be slow
1 and 3 wheel around
Star thru, square thru
Four hands count 'em too.

Gimmick for bend the line

Fourth couple bow and swing
Couple 1 promenade three–quarters to the right of number 4
Forward 4 and back
Couple 2 bow and swing
Up to the middle and split those four
Separate, go around two and line up six
Couple 3 promenade around one
Crowd into the line and make it eight.

Red Hot

Promenade red hot
Turn the right–hand lady, right arm 'round
Partner left, go all the way 'round
To your corner right, right arm 'round
Partner left, go once around
Promenade your corner as she comes 'round.

Do paso

Eight hands up and away we go
Circle left and don't be slow
Break right out with a do paso
Partner left, corner right
Back to your partner
Turn that gal if it takes all night.

Rip and snort

First couple go down the center with a rip and snort
Down the center and cut 'em short
Lady to gee and the gent go haw
Circle eight as you come straight

Double back track

Corn in the crib, wheat in the stack
Meet your honey and turn right back
Up the river and around the bend
Meet your honey turn back again
Meet your partner and promenade.

Listen folks to what I say
Meet your gal and go the other way
Whirl the rope and jerk the slack
Meet your partner and turn right back
Promenade, boys, promenade.

Meet your honey and sing a little song
Turn right back you done gone wrong
Meet your honey and sing once more
Turn right back as you did before
Meet your partner and promenade.

WESTERN COWBOY SQUARE DANCE

The figure is the dominant characteristic of the *Western Square Dance*. The caller follows the figure but may change and use any opener, break, or ending. If the figure is long, the breaks should be short. If the figure is short, the breaks can be longer and more complicated. Breaks should be chosen to complement the formation the dancers are in at the time it is to be used. When dancers are circling four, use a break-form four.

The dances included in this section are representative of the following figure types: symmetrical, Forward Up Six, Catch All Eight, Sides Divide, Bird in the Cage–Seven Hands 'Round, and Tea Cup Chain; double lead out, Forward Up and Back, and Milagro

Square; single visiting, Sally Good'in; accumulative, Cowboy Loop. Chapter 4 lists several "visiting couple" figures–such as Shoot the Owl, Take a Little Peek, and Lady 'Round the Lady–under the title Big Circle Square Dance. These figures may also be done in the square formation. So now "Buckle up your belly bands, loosen up your traces, all to your place with a smile on your face and let's do some old time square dancin'."

BIRD IN THE CAGE—SEVEN HANDS 'ROUND

First couple bow, first couple swing
First get out to the right of the ring
Turn the right–hand lady right arm around
Back to your partner, left arm around
Opposite lady, right arm around
Partner left and left arm around
Corner lady right arm around
Swing your partner with two–hand swing
Cage that bird in the middle of the ring
    Lady 1 whirls into center.
Seven hands up and circle left
    All remaining dancers circle around bird.
The bird hops out and the crow hops in with bird
    Gent 1 exchanges places with bird in the center.
Seven hands up we're gone again.
Crow hops out with an allemande left
    All dancers allemande left.
Meet your partner and right and left grand.

Repeat for gents 2, 3, and 4.

CATCH ALL EIGHT

First couple balance and swing
Down the center and split the ring
    Couple 1 goes across set and walks between (splits)
    couple 3.
Lady go gee, gent go haw
    Lady goes right, gent goes left.
Meet your honey in the hall
    Couple 1 meets in home position.
Catch all eight with the right, go half way around
    All swing partner half turn around clockwise with
    right forearm grasp.
Back with the left go all the way around
    All swing partner one full turn counterclockwise
    with left forearm grasp.
Swing your corner with a two–hand swing
    Join both hands with corner, turn once around
    clockwise.
Meet your partner pass her by
    Pass partner's right shoulder.
Pick up the next girl on the fly and promenade.
    Promenade new partner (right hand lady) to gents'
    home position.

Repeat for couples 2, 3, and 4.

COWBOY LOOP

First couple out to the couple on the right
Circle four with all your might
Break and trail that line to the next
> Gent 1 breaks circle by unclasping left hand, leads line of four to couple 3.

Two hands up and four trail thru
> Couple 3 raises joined inside hands, line of four passes under arch.
> Couple 3 walks forward over line to position 1 in set.

Turn right around and come back thru
> Gent 1 pulls line around toward center of set and prepares to go under arch the second time. Couple 3 does California Twirl, walks back to position as line of four passes under arch to center of set.

And tie that knot like the cowboys do
> Gent 1 turns right and pulls the line through arch formed by last couple in line.

Circle up four and away we go
Pick up two and make it six
Circle left till all get fixed
> Gent 1 breaks circle with left hand and picks up couple 3 on left side.

Break and trail that line to the next
> Gent 1 breaks circle with left hand, leads line of six through arch formed by couple 4.

Two hands up and six go thru
> Couple 4 raises joined inside hands, line of six passes under arch.
> Couple 4 walks forward over line to position 2 in set.

Turn right around and come back thru
> Gent 1 pulls line of six around toward center of set and prepares to go under arch the second time.
> Couple 4 turns around, walks back to position as line of six passes under arch to center of set.

Tie that knot like the cowboys do
> Gent 1 turns right and pulls the line through arch formed by last couple in line.

Now circle up six and keep it straight
Pick up two and make it eight
> Gent 1 breaks circle with left hand and picks up couple 4 on left side.

Circle eight and here we go.
> (Use any appropriate break.)

Repeat calls for couples 2, 3, and 4.

FORWARD UP AND BACK

Couples 1 and 3 go forward and back
Forward again and right and left thru
Right and left back in the same old track
Circle up four in the middle of the floor
> Break for circle of four.

Couples 2 and 4 go forward and back
Forward again and right and left thru
Right and left back on the same old track
Circle up four in the middle of the floor
> Break for circle of four.

Head ladies chain and chain right back
Side ladies chain and chain right back
Now all four ladies chain
Grand chain your ladies.
> Break for eight.

Variation

1 and 3 right and left thru
2 and 4 right and left thru
1 and 3 right and left back
2 and 4 right and left back
Head ladies chain
Side ladies chain
Head ladies chain and chain 'em back
Side ladies chain and chain 'em back
All four ladies chain
Grand chain the ladies.

FORWARD UP SIX

First and third balance and swing
Now whirl your girl to the right of the ring
> Gent 1 twirls lady 1 to gent 2. Lady 1 stands to the left of gent 2 to form a line of three, facing center.
> Gent 3 whirls lady 3 to gent 4. Lady 3 stands to the left of gent 4 to form a line of three, facing center.
> Gents 1 and 3 remain in home positions.
> Join hands in each line.

Forward up six and back you go
> Lines of three go forward and back.

Two gents loop with a do-sa-do.
> Gents 1 and 3 execute a do-sa-do.

Now right hand up and left hand under
> Gent 2 twirls the left-hand lady under the arch formed with right-hand lady to gent 3. Right-hand lady is twirled outside and over left-hand lady to gent 1. Gent 4 twirls the ladies in the same manner with his left-hand lady going to gent 1 and his right-hand lady going to gent 3.

Twirl those girls and go like thunder
Form new threes and don't you blunder
> Gent 3 now has lady 4 on the right and lady 1 on the left. Gent 1 has lady 2 on the right and lady 3 on the left. Two new lines of three are formed.

Repeat call three times beginning with "Forward up six and back you go," to return ladies to the right side of original partner. Then use any appropriate trim.

> **Note:** Vary the call "Two gents loop with a do-sa-do" by calling "Two gents loop with a right elbow" or "Two gents loop with a left elbow."

MILAGRO SQUARE

First four lead to the right
    Couples 1 and 3.
Go around that couple and take a little swing
    Couple 1 separates, lady goes right, gent goes left,
    and swings *three times* around behind couple 2.
    Couple 3 does the same around couple 4.
Center couples form a ring and circle once around
    While couples 1 and 3 swing, couples 2 and 4 circle
    once around in center of set.
Pass right through, just you two
    Couples 2 and 4. Do not turn back.
And around that couple and take a little swing
    Couple 2 moves forward, separates and swings
    behind couple 3. Couple 4 moves forward, sepa-
    rates, and swings behind couple 1.
Center couples form a ring and circle once around
    While couples 2 and 4 swing, couples 1 and 3 circle
    once around in center of set.
Pass right through, just you two
    Couples 1 and 3. Do not turn back.
And around that couple and take a little swing
    Couple 1 moves forward, separates, and swings
    behind couple 2. Couple 3 moves forward, sepa-
    rates, and swings behind couple 4.
Center couples form a ring and circle once around
    While couples 1 and 3 swing, couples 2 and 4 circle
    once around in center of set.
Pass right through just you two
    Couples 2 and 4. Do not turn back.
And around that couple and take a swing
    Couple 2 moves forward, separates, and swings
    behind couple 3. Couple 4 moves forward, sepa-
    rates, and swings behind couple 1.
Center couples form a ring and circle once around
    While couples 2 and 4 swing, couples 1 and 3 circle
    once around center of set.
Pass right through, just you two
    Couples 1 and 3. Do not turn back.
Circle with the next and around you go
Break right into a do paso
Take her home and everybody swing.

Repeat calls for couples 2 and 4 or side four.

SALLY GOOD'IN

First gent out and swing Sally Good'in
    Gent 1 swings right–hand lady Sally Good'in with
    right arm around.
Now your Taw
    Gent 1 swings own partner left arm around.
Swing that girl from Arkansas
    Gent 1 swings opposite lady (Arkansas) with right
    arm around.
Then swing Sally Good'in
    Gent 1 swings Sally Good'in with left arm around.

And now your Taw
    Gent 1 swings own partner right arm around.
Now don't forget your old Grandma
    Gent 1 swings corner lady (Grandma) with left arm
    around.
Home you go and everybody swing
    Swing with waist swings.

Repeat call with gents 1 and 2 leading out and doing
the figure simultaneously.
Repeat again with gents 1, 2, and 3 leading out and
dancing the figure simultaneously.
Repeat, fourth time, "All Four Gents" leading out and
dancing the figure simultaneously.

SIDES DIVIDE

First four forward and back
    Couples 1 and 3.
Forward again on the same old track
Swing in the center and swing on the side
    Gent 1 swings lady 3, gent 3 swings lady 1.
    Simultaneously couples 2 and 4 swing.
Now swing your own and sides divide.
    Couples 1 and 3 swing own partners in center.
    Side couples separate, ladies go left, gents right.
    Move one quarter around set, meet opposite and
    swing.
Circle four in the middle of the floor
    Couples 1 and 3.
Sides divide and swing some more.
    Sides separate. Move one quarter around set, meet
    partner and swing.
Do paso and don't get sore.
    Couples 1 and 3 in center.
Sides divide and swing some more.
    Sides separate. Move one quarter around set, meet
    opposite and swing.
Up the river and around the bend
Sides divide and swing again
    Sides separate, meet partners in original home
    position and swing.
And promenade your corners all
    Gents have new partners.
Hold that gal don't let her fall
Promenade around the hall.
    Promenade new partner home.

Repeat call for couples 2 and 4.
Repeat from beginning until ladies are back in home
positions.

TEA CUP CHAIN

The patter figure Tea Cup Chain was choreographed
by Mrs. Pat Morrison Lewkowicz of Chicago, formerly
from Austin, Texas. She worked out the figure of the
coffee table using tea cups from her collection as
ladies and gents, thus the name "Tea Cup Chain."

Later she worked it out with members of the Lone Star Square Dance Club of Austin, Texas.

General Directions: Tea Cup Chain is a symmetrical figure in which all couples begin moving simultaneously. The head and foot gents always send their ladies to the center and receive a new lady from the gent on the left. The side gents always send their ladies to the gent on their right and receive their lady from the center. Head and foot ladies start with the right hand and continue alternating right, left, right, etc. The side ladies start with the left hand to partner and continue alternating left, right, left, etc. Gents alternate similarly, taking whichever hand is extended to them. The ladies progress counterclockwise, moving to the right-hand gent each time. When the gent receives a lady, he turns her in place as in a regular ladies chain, always backing up in place. When he receives a lady's left hand, he turns her counterclockwise. If he receives her right hand, he turns her clockwise and sends her to the center or side as the case may be.

Specific Figure Directions: All couples begin moving simultaneously.

Head and Foot Ladies: The ladies move to the center, grasp right hands and turn three quarters around clockwise in the center; give left hand to side gent. Lady 1 goes to gent 2 and lady 3 goes to gent 4, who turns ladies counterclockwise.

Side Gents: Pass ladies on to the right-hand gent. Gent 2 sends lady 1 to gent 3 and gent 4 sends lady 3 to gent 1, who turns ladies around with the right hand clockwise.

Head and Foot Gents: Send ladies to the center. Ladies grasp left hands and turn counterclockwise one and a fourth in the center and give right hand to side gents. Lady 1 goes to gent 4 and lady 3 goes to gent 2.

Side Ladies: Side gents turn their ladies around counterclockwise and send them to the gent on the right. Lady 2 goes to gent 3 and lady 4 goes to gent 1.

Head and Foot Gents: Turn ladies around with the right hand clockwise and send them to the center. Ladies grasp left hands and turn counterclockwise one and one-fourth in the center and extend right hand to side gent. Lady 2 goes to gent 4 and lady 4 goes to gent 2.

Side Gents: Turn ladies clockwise and pass them on to the right-hand gent. Lady 2 goes to gent 1 and lady 4 goes to gent 3.

Head and Foot Gents: Turn ladies clockwise and send them to the center. They grasp right hands and turn three quarters clockwise and go on to original partner who turns them in place.

Notes: (a) Once the figure "Tea Cup Chain" is called, any patter may be used to fill in the execution time. (b) All couples work together so that while two are turning in the center, two ladies are being turned on the side and passed on to the right-hand gent. (c) The figure is usually repeated twice. (d) Select an opening and break to suit the figure.

SINGING CALLS

HURRY, HURRY, HURRY

Records: EZ 733; Grenn 12223; Windsor 4405B.

Cassette: "Smoke on the Water" Square Dance Classics by Bob Dalsemer, TC 123C (with calls), TC 124C (without calls).

Basics: Ladies chain.

Opener

Everybody swing your partner
Swing 'er high and low
Swing that next girl down the line [to the left]
Don't let 'er go
Cross the hall and swing your own
And swing and swing and swing
Promenade that pretty girl around the ring.

Figure

First couple lead to the right
Circle four around
Leave that girl, go on to the next
And circle three around
Take that couple on with you
And circle five hands round
Now leave those four
And join the line of three [on the corner beside part-ner]
Ladies chain across the hall
But don't return
Chain those ladies down the line
Watch 'em churn
Turn and chain across the hall
Don't you fall
Chain the line and swing your honey home.

Break

Allemande left with your left hand
'Round the ring we go
It's grand old right and left

(continued)

Walk on your heel and toe
When you meet your honey boys
Try a do–sa–do [or swing 'er high and low]
Promenade that pretty girl right on home
Hurry, hurry, hurry, hurry home.

Sequence: Opener, figure, and break for each couple.

ALABAMA JUBILEE

Records: EZ (LP) 506; Folkraft 1136; Windsor 4144, 4444.

Cassette: "Smoke on the Water" Square Dance Classics by Bob Delsemer, TC 123C (with calls), TC 124C (without calls).

Basics: Sashay, promenade, allemande left, grand right and left.

Four little ladies promenade inside of the ring
    Ladies move in single file, counterclockwise, around inside of set.
Back to your partner and give him a swing
Sashay 'round your corner girl
    Either sashay or do–sa–do.
Bow to your partner boys, give her a whirl
Now four little gents promenade inside of the ring
    Gents move single file, counterclockwise, inside of set.
Sashay 'round your partner, give your corner a swing
    Either sashay or do–sa–do.
You promenade just you and me
    Gents promenade corner lady.
To the Alabama Jubilee, yeah man
To the Alabama Jubilee.

Break

Turn the left–hand lady with a left hand 'round
    Turn corner once around. All turns with forearm grasp.
A right to your partner go all the way 'round
    Turn partner once and a half.
The right–hand lady with a left hand 'round
    Turn right–hand lady twice around.
Now swing your little honey
    Waist swing.
'Till her feet leave the ground
It's an allemande left, a right and left grand
Meet your little honey, take her by the hand
You promenade, just you and me
To the Alabama Jubilee, yeah man
To the Alabama Jubilee.

Repeat figure and break three times until ladies are returned to original partners.

HELLO DOLLY

Caller: Marshall Flippo.

Music: The Texans.

Record: Blue Star #1729, flip side.

Basics: Allemande thar, box the gnat, half–square thru, star thru, wheel and deal.

Intro, break, ending

Four ladies chain across that ring, turn 'em all a left–hand swing
Then roll away and circle, don't take long
Do an allemande left and allemande thar, right and left the four gents star
You're going you're still going you're still going strong
Shoot that star full around like that, with the corner girl you box the gnat
Pull her by and turn your own and then [promenade]
Promenade fellas, have a little faith in me fellas
Dolly's never going 'way again.

Figure

The head two couples half–square thru, then do–sa–do the outside two
Face the same little girl, star thru [and then]
Pass on thru and wheel and deal, star thru the center two
Half–square thru, then do–sa–do that outside two again
Star thru and pass thru, and wheel and deal go two by two
Centers pass on thru and then swing [promenade]
Promenade fellas, have a little faith in me fellas
Dolly's never going 'way again.

MAÑANA

Record: Windsor 4887.

Basics: Forearm turns, with all ladies.

Opener

Now you honor your chiquita
Give your corner girl a weenk
Allemande left your corner
Grand old right and left I theenk
Now when you meet your enchilada
Do–sa–do her neat
Swing your chili pepper and
Promenade the street.

Figure

Vaqueros star across the set
A left–hand turn that girl
Star back home again real quick

Another left-hand whirl
A right arm 'round your corner
Give your own a left-arm swing
Now promenade that corner girl
And everybody sing
Mañana, Mañana,
Mañana is good enough for me.

Chiquitas star across the set
A left-hand turn that man
Star back home and turn your hombre
With the old left hand
A right arm 'round your corner
Give your own a left-arm swing
Now promenade your corner girl
And everybody sing
Mañana, mañana,
Mañana is good enough for me.

Break

Allemande left your corner
And pass right by your own
Allemande right your right-hand girl
And leave your own alone [pass by]
Now allemande left your corner
And give your own a swing
Promenade to Mexico
And everybody sing
Mañana, mañana,
Mañana is good enough for me.

> **Sequence:** Opener, figure, break, figure, break.

JUST BECAUSE

> **Caller:** Mike Michele.
>
> **Record:** Western Jubilee No. 500.
>
> **Cassette:** "Smoke on the Water" Square Dance Classics by Bob Dalsemer, TC123C (with calls), TC124C (without calls).
>
> **Basics:** Allemande left, allemande right, grand right and left, ladies chain, see-saw, star.

Opener

Honor to your partners and to your corners all
Swing that opposite lady, she's the one across the hall
Now run away back home, swing and whirl your own
Thank your stars the bird ain't flown
Allemande left with the ol' left hand

Partner right and a right and left grand
Hand over hand around that ring
Right and left with the pretty little thing
Now promenade your partners, boys, shout and sing
Because, just because.

Figure

Now the two head ladies chain across, chain right over that ring
Send 'em right on back, take your own and give her a swing
Side two ladies chain across, chain right over that ring
Send 'em right on back, take your own and give her a swing
Allemande left your corner, allemande right your partner
Swing your corner lady around and around
Now promenade that corner, boys, shout and sing
Because, just because.

Break

It's all around your corner, that the gal we call Grandma
See-saw round your partner, she's the prettiest in the hall
All four gents center and star with the ol' right hand
Circle to your corner with a two-time allemande
Turn 'em once, turn 'em twice, back right off and bow real nice
Then a grand ol' right and left around the ring

> **Note:** All four gents step to center, form a right-hand star, walk all around new corner. Gents take corners with left forearm hold breaking their star and walk two complete turns around with corners. At the end of the turns, gents should all be facing counterclockwise around the set, ladies clockwise. Slip hands down from forearm hold to a hand hold, step back arms length and bow, then take partners right hand for the grand right and left.

Now promenade that dear old thing,
Throw your heads right back and sing
Because, just because.
(On meeting partners across set, promenade home.)

Repeat figure and break three more times.

GENTLE ON MY MIND

Caller: Bob Ruff.

Music: Wagon Masters.

Records: Wagon Wheel WW911. EZ Album 5, LP506.

Basics: Weave the ring, ladies chain, pass thru, right and left thru, roll away.

Opener, break, closer

Allemande your corner
Do–sa–do your own
Four men make a left–hand star around
Turn your partner right
Your corner allemande
Partner do–sa–do
Weave the ring now
Meet partner, do–sa–do, promenade.

Figure

Four ladies chain
Turn your girl and then
1 and 3 go right and left thru
Turn your girl
Roll away–circle left
Four girls pass thru
Turn left, go single file
Men pass thru, swing
Promenade.

Sequence: Opener, figure twice for 1 and 3, break, figure twice for 2 and 4, closer.

MARIANNE

Record: Folkraft 1282, flip side.

Basics: Ladies chain, cross trail, box the gnat.

Opener and ending

Four little ladies chain across
You turn 'em with your left hand
You chain those ladies back again
You turn your Marianne
Do–sa–do your corner, do–sa–do your own
Bow to your corner, but swing your own (hurry up now).

Chorus

All day, all night, Marianne (promenade 'em)
Down by the seaside along the sand (sing it)
Even little children like Marianne (swing 'em)
Down by the seaside along the sand (square sets).

Figure

Head two couples pass thru
Around just one you know
Go down the middle and cross trail thru
Around just one you go
Box the gnat at home
Four gents a left–hand star around
Now go back home and do–sa–do
Your corner swing (don't rush me).

Chorus.

Sequence: Opener, figure twice for head couples, figure twice for side couples, ending.

The chorus is not repeated after the ending. Last line: But swing your Marianne.

OLD-FASHIONED GIRL

Caller: Bruce Johnson.

Records: Instrumental: Windsor 7504A. With call: Windsor 4405A; Lloyd Shaw E–31.

Basics: Ladies chain, right and left thru, single-file turn back.

Opener

Honor your old-fashioned girl
Hold her close and swing and whirl
Then promenade that ring
Promenade in single file
Lady in the lead, Indian style
Gents step out, ladies left–hand star
Do–sa–do your honey when she comes around to you
Swing 'er once or twice just like her daddy used to do
Promenade that gal–she's just like the gal
That married dear old dad.

Figure

Head gents swing your maids
Take those girls and promenade
Just halfway 'round that ring
Now right and left thru across the middle
Hurry boys keep time with the fiddle
Chain right, your right–hand ladies chain
All four ladies chain across the hall
Chain 'em right back and don't you let 'em fall
Promenade that pearl
She's just like the girl
That married dear old dad.

Break

Do-sa-do your corner girl
Go back home and swing and whirl
Swing like your daddy said
Allemande left with your left hand
Right to your partner, right and left grand
Hand over hand around the ring you go
Do-sa-do your honey
When she comes around to you
Swing her once or twice
Just like her daddy used to do
And promenade your old-fashioned girl
She's just like the girl
That married dear old dad.

> **Sequence:** Opener, figure twice for 1 and 3 (second time, left-hand ladies chain), break, figure twice for 2 and 4, break.

DON'T LET THE GOOD LIFE PASS YOU BY

> **Caller:** Bob Vinyard.
>
> **Records:** Red Boot 118, Dance Ranch 601; S.D.T. 4001.
>
> **Basics:** Weave the ring, square thru.

Opener, middle break, closer

Circle left
Did you ever lie and listen to the rain fall?
Did you ever own a homemade apple pie?
Left allemande then turn the partner right
Left allemande then weave the ring
Man was made for loving not for buying
Do-sa-do around then promenade
Look my friend there's happiness in living
Somewhere between broke and being free.

Figure

Heads [sides] square thru four hands around now
Face the sides make a right-hand star
Go once around heads [sides] star by the left
Pick up that corner arm around
Back out, circle round the ring now
Swing the nearest girl promenade
Look my friend there's happiness in living
Just don't let the good life pass you by.

Center break

Did you ever hold a woman while she's sleeping?
Did you ever sit right down and have a cry?

Closer break

Did you ever hold a hand to stop the trembling?
Did you ever watch the sun desert the sky?

Tag

Just don't let the good life pass you by.

> **Sequence:** Opener, figure twice for heads, middle break, figure twice for sides, closer, tag.

HAPPINESS IS

> **Caller:** Wait McNeal.
>
> **Music:** Rhythmaires.
>
> **Record:** Belco #B-109.
>
> **Basics:** Roll away to a half-sashay, square thru, swing thru.

Opener, break, and ending

Four ladies chain, go straight across that ring
Turn the girls, roll away, you circle left and then
You roll away again, your own a do-sa-do
Allemande the corner and promenade your own
Happiness is, happiness is, happiness is
Different things to different people
That's what happiness is.

Figure

Now heads [sides] square thru four hands around you go.
Do-sa-do with that corner one you know
You swing thru and then, boys trade again
Swing the corner lady and you promenade that ring
Happiness is, happiness is, happiness is
Different things to different people
That's what happiness is.

> **Sequence:** Opener, figure twice heads, break, figure twice sides, ending.

> **Note:** "Boys trade" means that the two men who just turned each other in the swing thru, turn again halfway around so that each man meets his corner lady on the outside for a swing.

CHIME BELLS

> **Record:** Grenn 25316.
>
> **Basics:** All around left-hand lady, right and left thru, star thru.

Intro, break, ending

Walk around that corner, then you seesaw your taw
Join hands circle round that hall
Allemande the corner, do-sa-do your own
Four men star by the left around you go

(continued)

Turn the partner by the right and go left allemande
Come back and promenade around the ring (all the way)
Chime bells are ringing on the mountain so high
Upon a summer's eve.

Figure

Four ladies chain, turn a little girl and then
Heads promenade halfway you go
Down the middle go right and left thru, turn the gal I say
Star thru, pass thru, circle up four halfway
Swing that corner girl and go left allemande
Come back do-sa-do and promenade
Chime bells are ringing, on the mountain so high
Upon a summer's eve.

Alternate ending

Sleep my little lady on a mountain so high
Upon a summer's eve.

GOODBYE MY LADY LOVE

> **Caller:** Chip Hendrickson.
>
> **Record:** Top 25306.
>
> **Basics:** All around left-hand lady, weave the ring, promenade three-quarters, right and left thru.

Intro, break, and closing

Circle to the left, eight hands around you go
Walk all around the corner girl, seesaw your partner
Men star by the right, you turn it once around the set
Allemande left the corner, and you weave the ring
[Singing] Goodbye my lady love, farewell my turtle dove
When you meet your darling, you do-sa-do
Promenade her back to me, and love her so tenderly
So goodbye my lady love, goodbye.

Figure (twice for heads, twice for sides)

Heads promenade three-quarters, 'round the ring
Side couples right and left thru, turn your girl and pass thru
Circle four halfway, one-quarter more
Right and left thru, turn your girl and cross trail
Go to the corner, allemande left, well go forward two and then
Right and a left, full turn 'round and promenade
[Singing] Goodbye my lady love, so long my turtle dove
Promenade her home, well by and by.

> **Tag at end:** Goodbye my lady love, goodbye!

A FOOLER A FAKER

> **Caller:** Bob Fisk.
>
> **Music:** The Blue Star Rhythmaires.
>
> **Record:** Blue Star #1962, flip side.
>
> **Basics:** All around your left-hand lady, weave the ring, dive thru, pass thru, square thru.

Intro, break, ending

Walk around that corner girl, seesaw your partner
Join hands and circle 'round that ring
Men star right now go once around that ring, pal
Left allemande, now weave the ring
Weave in and out around that ring and when you meet your maid
Do-sa-do around, hey promenade
You're a fooler, a faker, a little heartbreaker
You're the sliest gal I've ever known.

Figure

1 and 3 you promenade, go halfway around now
Down the middle and square thru you do
Four hands around go hey do a do-sa-do
Once around and then go right and left thru
Dive thru, pass thru and then
Hey swing the corner girl and then promenade her, Joe
You're a fooler, a faker, a little heartbreaker
You're the sliest gal I've ever known.

TIE ME KANGAROO DOWN

> **Caller:** Andy Andrus.
>
> **Music:** Blue Star Band
>
> **Records:** Blue Star #2011, flip side; EZ 5012.
>
> **Basics:** Four ladies chain, right-hand star, do-sa-do, allemande left.

Opener, middle break, and closer

Four ladies chain across, Jane
Turn 'em left around,
Chain back across, Jane
Promenade her around (all together now)
Tie me kangaroo down sport,
Tie me kangaroo down,
Tie me kangaroo down sport, Tie me kangaroo down.

Figure

Heads go up and back, Jack,
Do-sa-do around,
Make a right-hand star and turn it once,
Once around that old town,
Allemande the corner girl, Earl
Do-sa-do your own,

Swing that corner gal, Al
Promenade her back home (all together now)
Tie me kangaroo down sport,
Tie me kangaroo down,
Tie me kangaroo down sport,
Tie me kangaroo down.

Promenade patter (second change for heads)

Loose me tie when I die, Si
Loose me tie when I die,
Don't you go and cry, Si
Loose me tie when I die.

Promenade patter (second change for sides)

Tan me hide when I'm dead, Fred
Tan me hide when I'm dead,
So they tanned his hide when he died, Clyde
And that's it hanging on the shed.

> **Sequence:** Opener, figure twice for 1 and 3, middle break, figure twice for 2 and 4, closer.

HOUSTON

> **Caller:** Bob Ruff.
>
> **Record:** Wagon Wheel 924.
>
> **Basics:** Allemande left, weave the ring, pass thru, star right, swing, do paso.

Opener, middle break

Circle left and around you go
Circle left you do a do paso, your partner left
Turn your corner by the right
Partner courtesy turn, everybody circle left again
Circle left just a little bit more
Left allemande and weave the floor
In and out and when you meet her, you swing
Swing your lady and promenade the ring
Promenade to Houston, Houston, Houston.

Figure

1 and 3 (2 and 4) pass thru, separate go around 2
Home you go and do–sa–do your lady too
2 and 4 pass thru, separate around 2
Home you go and do–sa–do your lady too
All the men star right around the land
With your corner girl you go left allemande
Do–sa–do your partner, your corner swing
Keep this lady and promenade the ring
Promenade to Houston, Houston, Houston.
Twice for head couples, twice for side couples.

IF THEY COULD SEE ME NOW

> **Caller:** Bob Ruff.
>
> **Record:** Wagon Wheel 915.
>
> **Basics:** Swing, allemande, grand right and left, do–sa–do, promenade, forearm turn, courtesy turn.

Opener, middle break, ending

All four ladies promenade inside, once around that ring
Come on back and swing, your partner you swing
Join hands and circle, go walking hand in hand
Allemande that corner, do the right and left grand
Grand old right and left you go until you meet your own
Do–sa–do your lady, promenade her home
Promenade your lady, go struttin' high and low
If my friends could see me now.

Figure

Ladies center back to back; men promenade outside
Once around you go, turn your partner by the left (forearm)
(Turn) your corner right (forearm)
Your partner courtesy turn (to face center of set)
Men center back to back, ladies promenade outside
Pass this guy, promenade the next, say "Hi"
Promenade this partner, go struttin' high and low
If my friends could see me now.

> **Sequence:** Opener, figure twice, middle break, figure twice, ending.

SMOKE ON THE WATER

> **Caller:** M. R. "Pancho" Baird.
>
> **Records:** Western Jubilee No. 598; EZ 526.
>
> **Cassette:** "Smoke on the Water" Square Dance Classics by Bob Dalsemer, TC 123C (with calls), TC 124C (without calls).
>
> **Basics:** Allemande left, star, grand right and left, turn back, sashay, pass thru.

I. Opener

Now you allemande left your corner
Then you walk right by your own
Right hand swing ol' Sally Goodin
  (Right–hand lady)
Swing left hand there at home
Those four little ladies to the center
Make a star with your right hand
Then allemande left your corner
Partner right go right and left grand.

Break

There'll be "Smoke on the Water on the land on the sea"
Right hand to your partner, turn around and go back three
Let's do a left, a right, a left–hand swing
Go all the way around, right hand to your partner
Twirl her home and settle down
  (Don't promenade, should be at home position)

(continued)

II.

Four gents center make a circle
  (Circle left)
You turn it once around, go back home sashay your
partner (Pass right shoulders go back to back)
Gents star right when you come down
Turn that star out in the center
'Til your corner comes around
Then you allemande left your corner
Grand right eight go round the town

Repeat break: "There'll be Smoke on the water, etc."

Figure

Head gents bow down to your partner
Swing that lady round and round
Pass right through right down the center

Separate go round the town
(Lady goes right gents go left to home position)
Then you walk right by your corner
Sashay round your partners all
(All sashay partners passing right shoulders then
back to back)
Then you allemande left your corner
Grand right eight go round the hall

Repeat break: "There'll be Smoke on the Water, etc."
Repeat II call: "Four gents center, etc."
Repeat figure for "Side gents."
Repeat break: "There'll be Smoke on the Water, etc."
Repeat opener: "Now you allemande left, etc."
Repeat break: "There'll be Smoke on the Water, etc."

6
Contra Dance

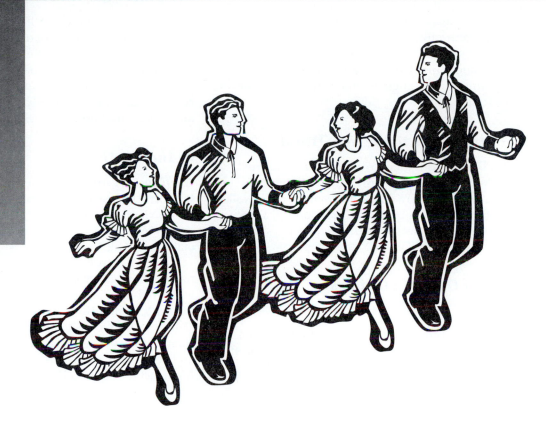

HISTORY

Country dances were the rage of the people of Eng–land during the 17th century. These consisted of Rounds and Longways. The English country dances, called *contre-danse*, traveled to France and Holland about 1680. The dances were polished and embell-ished for the courts; the royal families enjoyed them, too. The Longways and Quadrilles spread through Europe in many directions–and returned to England, now called "contra dances."

■ *Playford Collection*

John Playford, a talented musician and bookseller, collected and wrote dance descriptions and tunes from 1650 to 1728. These were a series of books, known as the *English Dancing Master—Plaine and Easy Rules for the Dancing of Country Dances*, with the *Tunes for Each Dance*. There were 17 printings; the last included 900 dances.

This collection reflected the dances of the villages and London society. Rounds, squares, and contras were all represented. Those coming to the New World between 1660 and 1800 brought their country dance and Playford's books.

■ *English, Scottish, and Irish Influence*

The English loved to dance and were known as the "dancing English." The peasantry and bourgeoisie developed all kinds of complexity of crossovers, interweaving, and partner changes. Most dances were quite simple and danced whenever an opportunity presented itself.

The Scots followed their Country and Highland dancing with passion. The men came to the floor like a drill square. If music was not available, they'd provide their own tune and danced until too tired for more. It was not a social occasion nor opportunity for flirtation. The Reels and Longway dances were popular in Scotland and continue to be danced in smaller communities.

Both the English and Scots displayed exactness in steps and variety in their figures.

The Irish have a natural flair for music and dance. Dancing a jig took place at all meetings or at the crossroads. Each village had its own piper. If no musician was present, villagers would dance to their own music, which was called "lilting" a tune.

Many contra tunes were written for the Irish harp. Irish tunes such as "White Cockade," "Irish Washer-woman," and "Turkey in the Straw" came with the immigrants to New England and were popular contra dance tunes.

■ Contra Dance to the New World

Contra Dances with their great popularity traveled to the New World. The British brought them to the 13 colonies. They were enjoyed by people of all walks of life. They were danced in the ballrooms of Virginia, the public assemblies, the barns, the taverns, and the kitchens of New England.

■ Contra Dance in California before the Gold Rush

The Spaniards brought Contra Dance to the coastal ports of South America. La Contradanza was danced in Spain in the early part of the 18th century. Carl Vega gives a date of 1850 for its arrival in Buenos Aires; others give earlier dates spreading through South America and Mexico. Alfred Robinson describes La Contradanza at a baile in San Diego in 1829. The country dances–Lancers, Quadrilles, Contras, Varsouvienne, Waltz–came from the South traveling northward up the California coast as far as Sonoma.

When the Americans from the East came to California by the overland routes, La Contradanza was out of fashion.

La Contradanza is a longways dance, with minor sets of two couples. As many as 18 figures were danced with a waltz chorus between each figure.

Today sometimes La Contradanza is performed for special Fiestas in Santa Barbara or Monterey.*

■ French-Canadian Influence

As the fun-loving French-Canadians have migrated into New England, they have become a part of the contra scene. The French-Canadian musicians have joined ranks with the others, and their fiddle tunes are frequently used for contras. One of the major influences is the long swing, 8 to 16 counts.

■ Yankee Musicians

It is interesting to note that live music has always been a part of the contra dance scene. A fiddler or two in the community or itinerant fiddler played in the kitchen for listening or dancing. For larger groups, a town hall was used with several violins, clarinet, cornet, organ, and eventually a piano, double bass, and flute. A traditional orchestra was in place.

■ And Yet They Live

The pioneers carried their square dances to every new territory. The fashionable dances like the Polka, Waltz, Varsouvienne, Quadrilles, and Lancers came along and were promoted by the dancing masters and societal events. Still, the contras persisted in New England.

Northern New Englanders continued dancing contras despite the newer dance manuals (call books), which did not include the contras. The dancing masters such as Elias Howe, Edward Ferraro, William B. DeGarmo, C. H. Cleveland, Jr., and Thomas Hill, claimed they were unfashionable. Perhaps the Irish and Scots clung to the customs of their native lands. It is a fact that Contra Dance was kept alive in the

*Czarnowski, Lucille. *Dances of Early California Days*, Palo Alto, CA: Pacific Books, 1950, pp. 89–107. Lucille Czarnowski was a Professor of Dance at the University of California, Berkeley, and Chairman of the Research Committee of the Folk Dance Federation of California. In the 1930s and 1940s, she collected oral histories, recorded music and songs of two generations, and researched extensively the personal memoirs of travelers and pioneers and books of early California folklore at libraries and museums. Her book (pp. 17–25) gives an excellent description of the social setting on the great ranchos, mission pueblos, and presidio towns. The frequent social gatherings and Californians' passion for dancing are conveyed.

smaller gatherings called "junkets," "heel burners," or "kitchen dances."

■ National Square Dance Revival and Country Dance

Three books and efforts contributed to renewed interest in Square Dancing. Henry Ford commissioned Benjamin B. Lovett of Massachusetts in 1926 to write *Good Morning*, a collection of quadrilles, contras, and couple dances. Lloyd Shaw of Colorado published *Cowboy Dances* in 1939, a collection of Western square dances. In New England, Ralph Page and Beth Tolman produced *The Country Dance Book* in 1937, based on articles they had written for *Yankee* Magazine. These people each sparked renewed interest in country dancing with all levels of society.

■ The First Contra Dance Revival—Ralph Page

During the '30s, the Depression Era, Ralph Page started calling square dances in Keene, New Hampshire. The country folk came to dance–squares, circles, lines, fox trots, waltzes, contras. They called the occasion a "square dance."

In 1943, in the midst of World War II, Ralph began calling Square and Contra Dances weekly at the YWCA in Boston. Servicemen and women and many students in the greater Boston region discovered the fun and spirit of Contra Dance at the Boston Y. For 24 years, Ralph made the weekly trip to Boston from Keene. Ted Sannella, one of many future contra callers, started dancing with Ralph at the Boston YMCA and became a world class caller/teacher and author of two books.*

A lifelong occupation and love of dancing came to Ralph naturally. Irish minstrels and musicians, and even a dancing master, were all part of his Scotch-Irish heritage. An excellent musician, he composed many tunes for dancing. He was recognized as an outstanding Square Dance caller, but it was in the realm of Contra Dancing that he truly left his mark as a teacher, caller, and writer.

---

*Sannella, Ted. *Balance and Swing*. Boston: Country Dance and Song Society of America, 1982.

–––. *Swing the Next*. Boston: Country Dance and Song Society of America, 1996.

Ralph Page is fondly remembered as the dean of American Contra Dancing. Ralph was born January 28, 1903, in Munsonville, New Hampshire, and died February 21, 1985, in Keene, New Hampshire.

Like the dancing masters of yore, he urged decorum on the floor. He believed in smooth dancing, and he felt we should dance our American folk dances with pride and a "wee bit of elegance." He set the pace with a twinkle in his eye.

Ralph was a popular teacher at major dance camps and schools across the United States. Internationally, he had successful teaching tours in Canada, Japan, and England. With his longtime partner and wife, Ada, he founded the New Hampshire Folk Dance Camp. His leadership was ever present in New England and was especially evident with his founding of the New England Folk Festival Association (NEFFA) in 1944 with Mary Gillette and Philip Sharples.

Northern Junket, a magazine devoted to New England folk dance, particularly Contra, was begun by Ralph in April 1949, and he published and edited the periodical until his death.

With his dedication to dance and love of history, many hours were spent in research and working with local historical societies. As a result, he assembled a significant collection of dance music, old dance books, and manuscripts. The following books are to his credit: *The Country Dance Book*, *The Ralph Page Book of Contras*, *An Elegant Collection of Squares and Contras*, and *Heritage Dances of Early America*. Together, these significantly enrich our understanding of past and present New England dance.

■ The Country Dance and Song Society and Other Organizations

The Country Dance and Song Society (CDSS)† started in 1915 as a group solely concerned with English Dances. Soon square and contra were included. CDSS is the largest organization that offers many services to contra dancers and groups. It publishes a magazine, membership directories, books, videos, and records. CDSS also sponsors dance camps and research, offers tax exempt status and attractive insurance packages to groups, and maintains a research library. The New England Folk Festival Association (NEFFA) and the

---

†CDSS refer to Appendix B, Organizations and Resources p. 487.

Intercollegiate Outing Club Association (IOCA) also contributed to the revival.‡ Suddenly, even orchestras were sponsoring the country dances.

Many organizations around the United States promote Contra Dancing and offer services. Some focus nationally, others serve a particular area; some are long established, while others are relatively new. The following groups suggest a broad coverage: The John C. Campbell Folk School, Berea, Kentucky, The Lloyd Shaw Foundation, Bayou Bedlam Contra Dance, North Texas Traditional Dance Society, Bay Area Country Dance Society in California, Wannadance, Seattle, Spokane Folklore Society and Folklore Village, Wisconsin.

■ The Second Contra Dance Revival

During the 1960s, the club square dance program negatively influenced many of the New England country dances. By the late '60s and early '70s, another generation of enthusiastic students and young people became interested in contra dancing, which fell into the "back to nature" realm. Some of these new callers had also learned from Ralph Page, Tony Parker, and Dudley Laufman. Dudley, in particular, encouraged young musicians to play for dances, thus adding new zest to the scene.

After Ralph, Ted Sannella (1928–1995), in a natural steadfast manner, stepped up to the plate to lead the national Contra Dance scene. He traveled across the United States and abroad always promoting the highest quality of dance and giving enormous energy to the Ralph Page Library and Legacy Weekend and the future of contra dance.

Now, they called the dance "a Contra Dance."

By the mid '70s, Contra Dance had spread to the West Coast, Mid–Atlantic and Midwest. The current revival continues today in the four corners of the United States.

■ Contra Dance Research

The University of New Hampshire, Durham, houses both Ralph Page's personal collection of dance and music books and the Country Song and Dance Society Library, which is available for research. Many colleges have advanced degrees in folklore and encourage dissertations relating to dance.

■ Contra Dancing Moves into the 21st Century

Contra dancing has made a big leap forward in popularity, not only across the United States, but internationally as well. Several factors have contributed to the increased enthusiasm. The interest of musicians has kept pace with the expansion of Contra dancing. They enjoy dancing and providing live music for dancing, adding "zing" to the dance floor. The availability and talent of bands specializing in Contra music continues to grow. They bring fresh energy to old tunes, introduce appropriate music, and compose new melodies. They have joined rank with callers and teachers with a common cause. The continued mobility of leaders, dancers, and musicians from New England to the West Coast, North, and South have all added to the Contra dance scene.

Expressions change. People will say "they are going to a Contra dance." In actuality there may be a few squares and round dances during the evening. People are looking for a dance activity to which they can come independently, meet friends and new people, and not have the pace and rigidity of the Club Square Dance program. It is interesting to note that squares are still popular, but they are the golden oldies of the '50s–'60s that the contra dancers enjoy. More people are using the term "country dancing" again. Country dancing is the umbrella term for contra, square, couple, mixers, and even a few line dances. The contra groups enjoy perfecting their round dance skills like the waltz and add other dances to their repertoire like English country dancing, Swing, Cajun, Salsa, Clogging, and even the Hambo.

Camps, workshops, and visiting callers have multiplied, with a focus on Contra and then one or two added attractions like Cajun, Country Western, caller workshops, and special musicians' clinics. The organization of the weekly dances tends to be minimal. The free spirit of the contra dancer resists a "constitution" and "limited membership."

With all the enthusiasm, the group faces some of the dilemmas that the square and round dance people had with standardization, proliferation of new dances, and burnout. Family dance camps are coming back as a way to sustain those who are having their families later. Interesting research has been stimulated. Many fine books appear yearly. Talented musicians have the opportunity to play. But few callers and musicians can make a living on this alone. The annual Ralph Page Legacy Weekend, the Ralph Page Library collection, and the CDSS library all contribute to the scholarship of researching Contra Dance.

Once again the tradition of Contra Dancing is firmly established. People enjoy dancing contras for the same reasons as long ago. The sense of community and fellowship is strong. It's part of our heritage. It's "good fun." Yes, Contra Dancing moves into the 21st century with vigor!

---

‡Refer to details, pp. 5–11, Sannella, Ted, *Balance and Swing.*

CONTRA DANCE BASICS

By Penn Fix, Spokane, Washington

■ Starting the Contra Dance Set

A contra dance set consists of two lines of dancers facing about four feet across from one another. The caller and musicians are at one end of these lines, referred to as the **top** of the set. The **bottom** of the set is farthest away from the caller. In these two lines, partners are across from each other with the women in the line on the caller's left and men in the line on the caller's right.

Before teaching the dance, the caller announces, "Take hands four." The couple at the top of the set takes hands to make a circle of four with the next couple. Then the next two couples join hands in a circle followed by the next and the next. The couple nearest the caller in each of these circles is referred to as the **active couple.** The other couple in each circle is the **inactive couple.** Note that a couple can start at the bottom of the set without another couple.

The active couple dances with the inactive couple below through a sequence of dance figures. A progression figure within the sequence will result in the active and inactive couples changing places. When the sequence begins again, the active couple is dancing with a new inactive couple. Eventually the active couple will reach the bottom of the set with no inactive couple with which to dance. Inactives will reach the top with no actives to dance. As **neutral couples,** they both will rest out at the top and bottom for a sequence, or one time through the contra dance. They then return in reverse roles: inactives are now actives, progressing down the set, and actives are now inactives, progressing up the set.

■ Formations in the Contra Dance

Once the dancers have taken hands four, the caller then must align them in the correct formation. There are four major formations used in Contra Dancing.

THE IMPROPER/CROSS OVER FORMATION
(duple improper).

The partners in the active couple in each circle change places with each other before the dance begins. See Diagram 1. When couples have reached the top or bottom of the set and are waiting out as neutral couples, they must remember to change places with their partners before reentering the dance.

THE PROPER/NOT CROSS OVER FORMATION
(duple proper).

The active couple in each circle does not change places before the dance. See Diagram 2. While wait-ing out at the top or bottom, couples do not change places with their partners.

THE BECKET FORMATION.

Partners are alongside one another to start the dance. See Diagram 3. The couples in the line on the caller's left progress down while the couples in the line on the caller's right move up. There are no designated actives or inactives in this formation.

THE TRIPLE FORMATION.

The active couple joins with two inactive couples in a circle of three couples. The call is "Take hands six." Triple contras are usually proper. See Diagram 4. The inactive couple that has reached the top of the set must wait out *two sequences* of the dance. When ready to reenter as an active couple, there will then be two inactive couples below them. As an active couple nears the bottom of the set with only one inactive couple to dance, both couples continue the dance sequence with an imaginary third couple. After this sequence, the top couple is at the bottom and waits out just one sequence before reentering as an inactive couple.

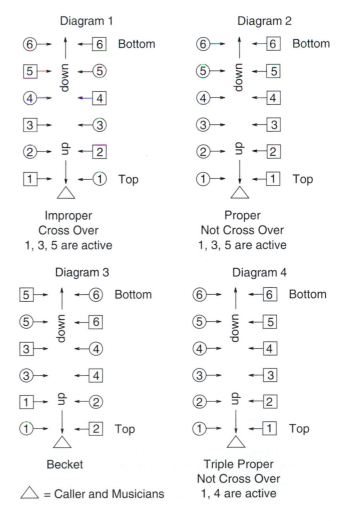

Diagram 1

Improper
Cross Over
1, 3, 5 are active

Diagram 2

Proper
Not Cross Over
1, 3, 5 are active

Diagram 3

Becket

△ = Caller and Musicians

Diagram 4

Triple Proper
Not Cross Over
1, 4 are active

■ Music and Timing

The Contra Dance and the music played for the dance are structurally married. The tunes played for Contra Dances have two parts, referred to as A and B. Each part has eight measures. For a contra dance, the tune is repeated twice in a sequence of AABB. The sequence of dance figures known as a Contra Dance is as long as a tune played AABB. When the tune repeats the AABB format, so too does the Contra Dance.

For dancers and caller alike these tunes played in AABB sequence translate to 64 counts. Thus a sequence of figures is 64 counts long. Most of the Contra Dance figures have assigned counts of 16, 8, or 4 in length. These counts are the beats of the music. Dancers must execute each step on the beat of the music and use the proper number of counts for each dance figure. If done in this manner, the dancer remains in time with both the dance and the tune and thus is not late or early for the next figure.

■ The Role of the Caller

The caller is actually a prompter. The calls are cues that give direction to dancers with a minimal amount of rhyming patter. The caller's responsibility is to choose a dance appropriate for the group and sequence in the program and then teach it to the dancers. This teaching occurs during the walk–through before the music begins. During this time, the caller has an opportunity to teach specific figures if the dancers are unfamiliar with them and to make the dancers aware of the specific sequence of figures of this dance.

After the walk–through, the caller returns the dancers to their original spots before starting the dance.

Once the Contra is underway, the caller must rely on abbreviated cues. For example, a ladies chain may have to be taught during the walk–through but during the actual dance, the caller prompts by simply saying, "Ladies chain."

The call itself must precede the actual movement so timing of the call is critical. It is essential for the caller to know how long figures take and how the figures fit the music. During the sequence of figures the caller must prompt two counts before the actual figure begins.

The calls are usually directed to the active couples in the set. In Becket formation dances where there are no actives or inactives, the call is directed to partners and neighbors.

The beginning of the dance can be the most difficult for a caller since the initial prompt must be done before the music starts. When working with musicians, the caller can request a short musical introduc-

tion, often referred to as "four potatoes." This two or four beat introduction allows the caller to prompt the first figure before the figure begins. When using recorded music, the caller must know the records so he or she can cue properly because some recorded music does not have introductions.

The dance can be repeated 10 or even 20 times. If the dancers are new to contras, then shorter is better, maybe 10 times through the dance. If the dance is symmetrical with actives and inactives dancing the same figures at the same time, then a shorter number of times through the dance is warranted. If the dance is assymmetrical in which the active couple is doing all the swinging and the inactives have little action, then the dance should be repeated 15 or 20 times.

After the dancers become familiar with the sequence of a dance, the caller can reduce or even stop prompting during that particular dance. Remember, dancers are cued not only by the caller but also by the music.

The ending of a dance can be a good deal easier if before the evening begins, the caller and musicians agree to ending signals. As the Contra Dance is nearing the end, the caller signals to a previously designated member of the band, "Two more times." This signal means that the musicians will play the tune two more times through. This signal is usually made in the B2 part of the dance. The caller then calls the dance two more complete times. In the final B2, he can reinforce communication by turning to all the musicians and saying, "We are going out." The dance ends immediately after the B2. The caller invites the dancers to thank their partners and the band and find another partner for the next dance.

■ Dance Sources

The caller draws from a number of sources for Contra Dances. True to its traditional nature, word–of–mouth and direct participation are two major sources for dances. Also, new dances are being composed almost daily. In the folk tradition these new compositions are offered freely to the Contra Dance community. While there are no restrictions in terms of user fees, the acknowledgement of the composer when known is expected after the walk–through.

The Appendix offers a wide variety of resources in its Bibliography Music (records and cassettes), videos, national organizations with services, and magazines.

■ Card File

Callers record dances in many ways, but the most popular remains a card file system. Note that the card records the date and location that the caller–teacher learned the dance; the name of the person that taught the dance (in our example the teacher and originator of the dance are the same person, but both pieces of information are handy); proper, improper, triple, or becket; and key cues, which are capitalized. On the back, any helpful information for teaching purposes and interesting facts are listed. It is wise to record the dance as taught because, in referring to it later, there is less error. The card may be carried to the dance and used for a quick refresher.

PIERCE'S HALL STROLL		Lady of Lake '85
		By Fred Breunig
		Duple, improper
A1:1	LADIES DO-SI-DO	
2	GENTS DO-SI-DO left shoulder 1½ & go to PARTNER	
A2:3	Everyone SWING your OWN on sides of set	
4	(long swing) end (1s face down, 2s face up) escort position	
B1:5	"STROLL" promenade along lines, turn as couple	
6	And RETURN look for opposite couple	
B2:7	RIGHT HANDS ACROSS turn 1½ round	
8	GENTS DROP OUT to original side	
	Ladies continue to turn right to LADIES CHAIN HALFWAY	

Community hall, East Putney, Vt., where Fred B. calls dances. Composed for the Sesquientennial, 1982.

Note:

#2 Gents LEFT shoulder do-si-do
1½ to face partner on her side

#6 Must recognize opposite couple at end of promenade
Star position—shake hands

#7 Emphasize turning STAR 1½, until Gents get back to their original (improper) sides! Must turn star with *DETERMINATION* or Not on Time

#8 At end of Ladies ½ Chain, gents can direct (lead) ladies into their do-si-do of next lady

■ Music Sources

Today's Contra Dance revival is built squarely on the shoulders of musicians. Live music has powered the continued interest in contras.

Irish, Scottish, English, French–Canadian, and even some Southern and Western hoedown tunes have found their way into the repertoires of Contra Dance musicians. Most of these tunes are Jigs, Reels, Horn-pipes, and even Marches written in 6/8, 2/4, and 4/4 meter. While the New England Chestnuts have tunes long associated with the dances, contemporary dances do not. Any tune can be played so long as it stays within the structure of 32 bars or 64 beats.

More important than the choice of tunes is the manner in which they are played. Musicians must play at a tempo that matches the walking step used by dancers. In addition they should phrase their music to help dancers associate the beginning and ending of the figures, which parallel the ending and beginning of the parts of the tune. Some tunes are chosen to match the character of the dance. Jigs are bouncy; Reels energetic and flowing. The music should reflect the spirit and buildup of the dance. Musicians can make the music match the excitement as the dance builds up to a high point.

Callers may use recorded music. However, because the majority rely on live music sources, a limited number of recorded sources are available.

See the Bibliography, Tune Books p. 501 and Appendix D, Contra p. 491.

■ Contra Dance Figures

THE BASIC STEP

A light rhythmic **walking step** to the beat of the music is used throughout the dance. Starting on the right foot is recommended. The arms hang freely at the side unless they are used to execute a dance figure.

THE SWING

Contra dancers live to **swing!** Almost all sequences have a swing and many crescendo into a swing. The hand holds vary in different parts of the country, but the swing position (right parallel) is the most common. Both dancers step into the swing on the right foot. A walk around or buzz step may be used. Knees are slightly bent. Counter balance is important, with feet close together, upper bodies bowed. The length of the swing is often 12 or 16 counts and not less than 8.

THE BALANCE

The **balance** (4 counts) often comes before a swing. It was originally intended as an introduction or greet-ing. Preceding a swing, two dancers take hands (either both hands or right hands) and step forward toward each other, back from each other, and then directly into the swing. This figure has developed over the years to a step on the right foot moving for-ward and slightly to the right of the partner lifting the free left foot in a kicking or swinging motion, fol-lowed by rising on the ball of the right foot. Weight is then transferred by stepping on the left foot, backing up slightly, and moving left of the partner. The right foot swings in front and then followed by rising on the ball of the left foot. Often the stepping on the right and left feet is accompanied by heavy stomps, which once inspired Ralph Page to note the dancers sounded like "a herd of lovesick water buffalo."

A balance may also occur when dancers are joined by hand in a line of four or along contra lines.

OTHER CONTRA DANCE FIGURES

Common figures found in both traditional square and contra dancing include **ladies chain** (a full chain over and back, 16 counts), **half chain,** (over and courtesy turn but no return, 8 counts), **do–si–do** (8 counts), **promenade** (8 counts), **forward and back** (8 counts), **allemande** turns (4 counts), **right and left thru** (a full right and left over and back, 16 counts), and **half right and left** (over and courtesy turn but no return, 8 counts). See the Glossary for details on these figures.

■ *Teaching Suggestions*

STARTING BECKET DANCES

An easy way to get dancers into the becket formation is to start from a proper Contra Dance formation. Announce, "Take hands four and top couples in each circle cross over." Once couples are in the Improper formation, then "Take hands four again and circle left one–quarter round." Now partners are along side each other and are facing another couple across the set. See Diagram 3, p. 181.

THE ROLE OF THE ACTIVE

In proper and improper contras, the caller prompts to the active couple. For example, "Swing the one below" directs the active man to swing the inactive woman and the active woman to swing the inactive man in their circle of four.

Becket contras have no active or inactive couples. The caller prompts to partners, men, and women. In a circle of four, **your neighbor** is the person of the opposite gender who is not your partner.

Because of the popularity of symmetrical dances in which every couple is dancing the same figure at the same time, the roles of active and inactive are less defined. In some instances, *your neighbor* has replaced *your inactive* in the call. For example, "Swing the one below," can be replaced with "Swing your neighbor."

THE ROLE OF THE INACTIVE

In assymetrical contras, the actives will dance figures while the inactives either are watching or assisting. Since the calls are directed to the actives, the inactives must know what to do without being prompted. The inactives also play an important role in the management of the formation. For example, when the actives go down the center of the set, and before they can come back to cast off, the inactives can straighten the lines out by making sure they are not too far away from their partners across the set nor too far away from the next inactive up and down the set. In addition some contras creep away from the top of the set. Inactives can help by taking one step up toward the caller each time the actives go down the center. The other role the inactives play is as assistants to the actives. They accept them in cast–offs and allemande turns in contra corners.

SCILIAN CIRCLE

The movement up and down the Contra Dance set can be confusing at first. Many newcomers become disoriented while waiting out at the top or bottom of the set. Perhaps an easier way to teach the progression and transition from one contra sequence to the next is through the scilian circle formation. Couples face couples clock– and counterclockwise in a big circle. Men have their partner on their right side facing the other couple. Essentially this formation is similar to an improper/cross over contra but without a top or a bottom. No one waits out a turn. See page 63.

CONTRA CORNERS

To start **contra corners** (16 counts), the active couple is below their original inactives in a Proper/Not Cross Over formation. Contra corners are across the set for each active person. The first contra corner is diagonally right from the active person; the second contra corner is diagonally left. For the call "turn contra corners," active partners meet in the center of the set and take right hands, turn halfway, and drop hands. They turn their first corner (the one diagonally right) with left hands all the way around and again drop hands. Active partners turn three–quarters around in the middle of the set with their right hands. They then turn the second corners (the one diagonally left) by the left hand all the way around and wait for the next call. In contra corners, the actives use their right and left hands, alternately; the corners always use their left hand to turn an active person. Each turn is 4 counts. See diagram 5.

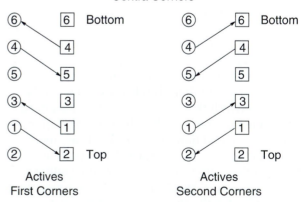

Diagram 5
Contra Corners

THE GYPSY

The **gypsy** (8 counts) can best be described as a do-si-do except that the two dancers always face each other, maintain eye contact, and never turn their backs to one another. In a right shoulder gypsy, the two move clockwise around each other; in a left shoulder gypsy, they travel counterclockwise.

HEY FOR FOUR

In a **hey for four** (16 counts), four dancers are in a line going across the set; the center two are facing one another and the other two are on the outside facing the center of the set. They weave without touching hands, moving in a figure eight pattern with an additional loop in the middle. In the most common formation, the center two are women and the outer two are men. To begin, two women face each other and pass right shoulders. Traveling toward the opposite side, the women pass left shoulders with approaching man. The women continue making a loop to left to face center, pass next man left; women pass right in center, pass man left, loop to the left to face center, pass next man left and are back in original position. The men follow the path of the woman in front of them by passing left shoulders with the woman, right shoulders with the man in center, left with the other woman, and loop left to face center. Men return passing the woman left, men pass right in center, then woman left, loop left and are home.

■ Dance Levels

The contra dances selected in the following section are divided by ability levels: Beginning, Intermediate, and Advanced. Since most students using this book are newcomers to contras, Beginning dances are divided further into three categories. *Beginning (1)* dances introduce the basic figures. *Beginning (2)* dances build on the content learned and applied in a different manner. *Beginning (3)* dances include those with the hey figure. *Intermediate* dances introduce the becket formation to students. And the *Advanced* dances can challenge both teacher and students!

BEGINNING 1	BEGINNING 2	BEGINNING 3
Aw Shucks!	Chili Pepper #4	Delphiniums and Daisies
Broken Sixpence	Contra for Margie	Roll in the Hey
Easy Does It	Jed's Reel	Symmetrical Force
Lady of the Lake	Small Potatoes	
The Nova Scotian	Salmonchanted Evening	
The Tourist		

INTERMEDIATE	ADVANCED
Becket Reel	Brimmer & May Reel
Chorus Jig	British Sorrow
Dance Gypsy	CDS Reel
Pierce's Hall Stroll	Dancing Sailors
Roadblock Reel	Hull's Victory
Shadrack's Delight	The Other Mary Kay
Silver Lake Waltz	Petronella
Weave the Line	Rory O'More
With Thanks to the Dean	

■ Contra Dance Tunes Composed by Ralph Page*

McQuillen's Squeezebox

Ralph Page

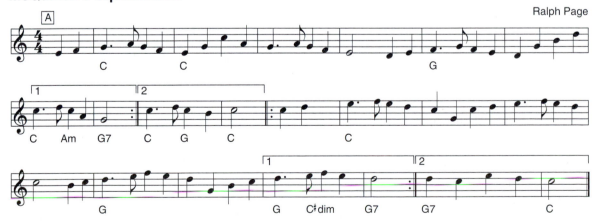

*Gone a Rovin', Patriot's Jig and McQuillen's Squeezebox—all original tunes composed by the late Ralph Page—are included by permission of the Estate of Ralph Page.

Gone A-Rovin'

Ralph Page

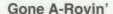

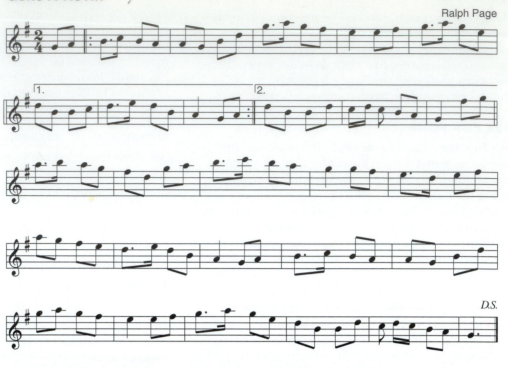

Patriot's Jig

Ralph Page

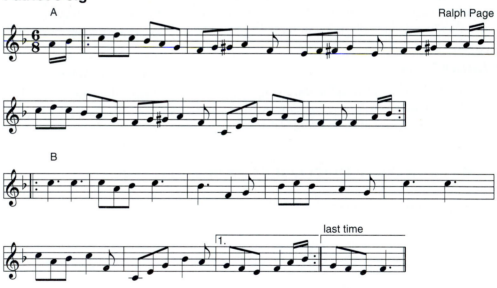

Aw Shucks!*

AW SHUCKS! IS A CONTEMPORARY contra composed by Carol Kopp. The inspiration for *Aw Shucks!* arose from the square *Northern Lights* along with the need for an easy and interesting dance. The title was inspired by the spirit of the southern Appalachian mountains.

Record: Teaching Record–Lloyd Shaw 343 (Carol Kopp calls on one side) "Combination Rag" by Strings & Things.

Music: Jig or Reel.

Contra Formation: Duple, Improper/Cross Over.

Level: Beginning 1.

DIRECTIONS FOR THE DANCE

A1 **Active couples sashay down the center** (8 counts). Actives take two hands and slide eight counts down the center. Inactives, in the mean time, move up the line to take the place left by the active next to them.

Active couples sashay back to your neighbors (8 counts). Actives stop between the original inactives below. Actives stay in the center facing their part–ner. Don't change sides. Stay crossed over.

A2 **Actives clap** (4 counts). Actives clap own hands, then partner's right hand, then own hands, and partner's left hand.

Actives turn to face neighbors and clap (4 counts). Turn away from partner to face the inactive behind you on the outside. With the inactive, clap own hands, then inactives' right hands, then own hands, and inactives' left.

Actives swing neighbors (8 counts). After clapping, swing the same. Men fin–ish the swing with the women on the right facing down the set. Join hands with couples across the set.

B1 **Down the center four in line** (6 counts).

Turn as couples (2 counts). With the one you swung, turn as a couple to face up the set. Join hands four in line again.

Come back up and bend the line (8 counts). Return to place and bend the line.

B2 **Ladies chain over and back** (16 counts). After the chain, actives step into the center to sashay. Remember the next inactive to dance with is now below the actives.

Aw Shucks! (continued)

---

*Aw Shucks! is included by permission of Carol Kopp, Streetsboro, OH.

Becket Reel

ECKET REEL IS AN ORIGINAL DANCE by the late Herbie Gaudreau of Holbrock, Massachusetts. He named it "Becket Reel" in honor of Camp Becket in the Berkshire mountains of western Massachusetts, where he called this dance while attending Charlie Baldwin's square dance camp. In some parts of New Hampshire it is known as Bucksaw Contra or Reel. It is similar to *Slaunch to Donegal*.

This was the first dance using this formation. The name of the dance became synonymous with the name of this formation, the Becket formation.

Record: Grenn 12239.

Cassette: "Woodchopper's Reel," Kitchen Junket ALC 200 A/BC.

Music: Any preferred traditional type reel, "Reilly's Own," Cole, M. M., *One Thousand Fiddle Tunes*; "Reel a Pitou," Page, Ralph, *An Elegant Collection of Squares*, p. 91.

Contra Formation: Becket formation. Refer to p. 181, Diagram 3.

Level: Intermediate.

DIRECTIONS FOR THE DANCE

A1   **Allemande left your corner once around** (4 counts). Corner is person alongside you who is not your partner. At the top and bottom, the corner is across the set. The corner remains the same person throughout the dance.

A2   **Opposite ladies chain over and back** (16 counts).

B1   **On the left diagonal right and left thru** (8 counts). Each couple does a right and left through with couple in opposite line on left diagonal. Courtesy turn partner to face middle of set. If there is no one to right and left thru, do not cross the set, but wait.

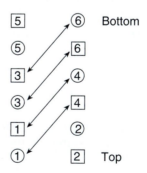

Straight across, do a right and left thru (8 counts). From lines, each couple does a right and left thru with couple directly opposite. Courtesy turn partner to face middle of set.

```
        5  ◄    ► ③   Bottom
        ⑤  ◄    ► 3
        6  ◄    ► ①
        ⑥  ◄    ► 1
        4  ◄    ► ②
        ④  ◄    ► 2   Top
```

B2   **Same two couples star by the left. Back by the right** (16 counts). As you come out of right–hand star, movement flows into left allemande at the beginning.

Brimmer & May Reel*

B RIMMER & MAY REEL IS A contemporary contra, composed by Dan Pearl in 1979. He had been dancing for about six months when he came up with this sequence, which owes a lot to Ted Sannella's "Patriot Jig." The Brimmer & May School was the site at that time of a large contra dance in the Boston area. This is the description of the dance as modified, for the better, by the folk process.

Music: Reel.
Contra Formation: Duple, Improper/Cross Over.
Level: Advanced.

DIRECTIONS FOR THE DANCE

A1   **Swing the one below** (16 counts). Actives swing the inactives.

A2   **Right and left thru** (8 counts). Do not right and left back.

Actives swing in the center (8 counts). Finish the swing facing down the set with women on the right of their partners.

B1   **Down the center four in line** (4 counts). Join hands across the set. Actives are in the middle with two women next to each other and two men next to each other in line. Go down the set and then stop but continue facing down.

Actives California twirl to their neighbor (4 counts). Actives drop hands with their neighbors, California twirl (see Glossary), and make an arch with their

Brimmer & May Reel (continued)

─────────────
*Brimmer & May Reel is included by permission of Dan Pearl, Southborough, MA.

partners. Then they face one another and pass right shoulders to face the one they swung in A1. Actives drop their joined hands.

With the handy hand, actives turn their neighbor twice around (8 counts). Active man turns inactive woman with left hands; active woman turns inactive man with right hands. After the actives have finished the turns, they face up the set as a couple; the inactive couple falls in behind them.

B2   **Up the center as couples, actives leading** (4 counts). Taking large steps, return two by two; actives are proper, not cross over and inactives are improper, cross over.

Actives cast out below the original neighbors (4 counts). Actives turn out one place to end below the original inactives; inactives have in the meantime moved up to take the position where the actives were before the cast-off. Inactives turn to face the original actives now below them. All join hands in a circle.

Circle left halfway round (4 counts). Couples are now back in their original cross over position

Pass thru up and down (4 counts). Actives pass right shoulders with inactives onto the next couple to swing.

British Sorrow

B*RITISH SORROW IS A* traditional Contra, "New England Chestnut".

Record: Lloyd Shaw 169 (flip) (4/4) or preferred march.

Music: Suggested tunes, "Jack's Life" or "The Tower of London Quickstep," Page, Ralph, *The Ralph Page Book of Contras*, p. 7.

Contra Formation: Triple, Proper/Not Cross Over

Level: Advanced.

DIRECTIONS FOR THE DANCE

A1   **Active couples cast down the outside below two** (8 counts). Active couples turn out (man left, woman right) and walk down outside of set past two couples. Counts 7–8, cut into center of set. Facing up the set, partners join inside hands.

Up the center and cast off (8 counts). Walk up the center, separate, and cast off with inactive couple (couple 2); active's arm around inactive's waist. Active couples have progressed one position down.

A2   **Right–hand star with the couple below** (8 counts). Active couple and the couple below (couple 3) form a right–hand star.

Left–hand star with the couple above (8 counts). Active couples move naturally into left–hand star with the couple above (couple 2).

B1   **Circle six to the right** (16 counts). All three couples join hands and circle right once around, falling back into lines at end of sequence. Actives are between #2 and #3 dancers.

B2   **Right and left thru with the couple above** (8 counts). Active couple and couple above (the couple with whom they cast off) right and left thru.

Right and left back (8 counts).

■ Notes

1. During the walk–thru, it is important to identify the triple set of couples dancing together. The active couples move down one position each time the dance is repeated. The active couples remain the lead couple in the triple set until they reach the foot. The relative position of the inactives changes too. At the top of the set, inactives wait two times to become active. (See 4th sequence.) Toward the bottom the *active continues to dance* with an imaginary 3rd couple (ghost) until they are at the bottom. Otherwise, the last couple will never move up.

	1st	2nd	3rd	4th	5th
bottom		ghost			ghost
	9	9	7	7	7
	8	7	9	9	4
	7	8	8	4	9
	6	6	4	8	8
	5	4	6	6	1
	4	5	5	1	6
	3	3	1	5	5
	2	1	3	3	2
top	1	2	2	2	3

2. The same dance with actives cross over (improper) is known as Ottawa Special.

Broken Sixpence*

BROKEN SIXPENCE IS AN original dance by Don Armstrong.

Record: Lloyd Shaw 155/156 (flip) or lively Contra music.
Contra Formation: Duple, Improper/Cross Over.
Level: Beginning I.

DIRECTIONS FOR THE DANCE

A1   **Do–si–do the one below** (8 counts). Actives face down the set, inactives face up. Actives do–si–do the one facing.

         Men do–si–do (8 counts). Men do–si–do in center of set.

Broken Sixpence (continued)

---

*Broken Sixpence included by permission of Don Armstrong, Macks Creek, MO.

A2   **Women do–si–do** (8 counts). Women do–si–do in center of set.

Actives swing in the center (8 counts). Swing in center of set, ending with woman on man's right, facing down the set. Active couple is between the inactive couple (couple below) in a line of four.

B1   **Down the center four in line** (6 counts). Join hands in line of four. Walk down the set.

Turn alone (2 counts). All four release hands, turn individually to face up the set.

Come back home (8 counts). Join hands. Walk up the set four in line. At home bend the line to form a circle.

B2   **Circle left once around** (8 counts).

Star by the left (8 counts). From left-hand star, turn away from the couple dancing with and move naturally into beginning of dance to "do–si–do the one below."

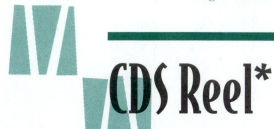

CDS Reel*

CDS REEL IS A CONTEMPORARY CONTRA. It is an original dance by the late Ted Sannella, composed in September 1984. The Country Dance Society (CDS) is the publisher of Sannella's books, *Balance and Swing* and *Swing the Next*.

Record: "Golden Wedding Reel," Hold the Mustard HTM IL.
Music: "Swinging on a Gate," Sannella, Ted, *Balance and Swing*, p. 69.
Contra Formation: Duple, Improper/Cross Over.
Level: Advanced.

DIRECTIONS FOR THE DANCE

A1   **Swing your neighbor** (8 counts). Finish the swing with woman on the man's right facing across the set.

All go forward and back (8 counts). Join hands in line, move four steps forward, four steps back.

A2   **Big circle, all go left** (8 counts). Top couple joins hands and bottom couple joins hands to complete the **oval,** which moves left.

Big circle, go right back to place (8 counts). **Oval** moves right. **Note:** each man locates his partner to form left-hand star, on call.

B1   **Left–hand star three–quarters with the opposite two** (8 counts). Active couple with original inactive couple above forms left-hand star, turn three-fourths around.

All swing your partner (8 counts). Men turn right to swing woman behind. Woman ends on man's right side.

B2   **Men allemande left, go once and a half** (8 counts). Two men allemande left, once and a half.

Swing your neighbor (8 counts). Men will swing the same person as the beginning; women ends on man's right side. Active couples have progressed on position.

*CDS Reel is included by permission of the late Ted Sannella.

Chili Pepper #4*

CHILI PEPPER #4 IS A contemporary Contra composed by Steve Schnur. In keeping with the "folk process," Schnur wrote a series of Chili Peppers (4 in total) back in 1981–82. During the summer of '81, he attended Pinewoods Dance Camp in Plymouth, Massachusetts. Bob Howell presented a dance, Green River, written by Glen Nickerson of Kent, Washington, which contained a "veer left" figure in A2. Chili Pepper was based on that figure.

Music: Jig or Reel.

Contra Formation: Duple, Improper/Cross Over.

Level: Beginning 2.

DIRECTIONS FOR THE DANCE

A1   **Do–si–do the one below** (8 counts). Actives do–si–do the inactive below.

Circle left once around (8 counts). The same two couples circle and then both couples drop hands with neighbors but retain the nearest hand of partner. It is helpful for the women to take note of each other so they can look for each other during the promenade back.

A2   **With your partner, veer left and promenade as couples along the line** (6 counts). These couples pass each other by the women's right shoulders and in the direction they are facing. Promenade along the nearest line. Active couples go down the active men's line while the inactive couples go up the inactive men's line. Take smaller steps for the promenade. As couples reach the top or bottom, turn right and continue up or down the other side of the set.

Promenade back (6 counts). Take bigger steps back.

Women allemande left half way to your neighbor (2 counts). When the couples who circled together in A1 meet, the two women take left hands and turn to face their neighbor: for active women, it's the inactive men; for inactive women, it's the active men.

B1   **Balance and swing your neighbor** (16 counts). Active men swing inactive women; active women swing inactive men. Finish the swing with the women on the right facing into the center. Join hands along the lines.

B2   **In long lines, go forward and back** (8 counts).

Actives swing your partner in the center (8 counts). Actives step into the center to swing. Finish the swing facing down the set with women on the right. Do–si–do with the inactive below to start again.

---

*Chili Pepper #4 is included by permission of Steve Schnur, Trenton, NJ.

Chorus Jig

CHORUS JIG IS A TRADITIONAL CONTRA, a "New England Chesnut." The tune, "Chorus Jig," is a Reel (2/4), not a Jig (6/8).

Record: "Chorus Jig," Canterbury Country Dance Orchestra F & W 3L.

Cassette: "Chorus Jig," New England Chestnuts, Vol. 1 & 2 ALC 203/4C.

Music: "Chorus Jig," Page, Ralph, *An Elegant Collection of Contras and Squares*, p. 39; *Fiddler's Fakebook*, p. 68; *New England Fiddler's Repertoire*, No. 96.

Contra Formation: Duple, Proper/Not Cross Over.

Level: Intermediate.

DIRECTIONS FOR THE DANCE

A1   **Actives down the outside and back** (16 counts). Each active walks down the outside of the set, turning on counts 7–8, and return to place.

A2   **Actives down the center and back, cast off** (16 counts). Active couples, holding inside hands, walk down the center, counts 7–8, turn alone. Return to original position. Cast off, counts 5–8, arm around the inactive person, progressing one position down.

B1   **Turn contra corners** (16 counts).

B2   **Actives balance and swing** (16 counts). End swing facing up the set, moving to go down the outside below the person you cast off.

Note: Turn contra corners–inactive person receives two consecutive turns, both left–hand turn, by two different people.

Contra for Margie*

CONTRA FOR MARGIE IS A CONTEMPORARY contra composed on Oct. 19, 1992, by the late Ted Sannella. Paul McCullough, a dear friend, had asked Sanella to write a contra for his girlfriend, Margie. Ted dedicated the dance to Margie Davis of Portland, Oregon.

Music: Jig or Reel.

Contra Formation: Duple, Improper/Cross Over–Double Progression.

Level: Beginning 2.

Contra for Margie is included by permission of the estate of the late Ted Sannella and publisher, Country Dance and Song Society. Contra for Margie appears on p. 82, Sannella, Ted. *Swing the Next*. Haydenville, MA: Country Dance and Song Society, 1996.

DIRECTIONS FOR THE DANCE

A1   **In long lines, go forward and back** (8 counts),

    Actives swing in the center (8 counts). Finish the swing with women on the right of partner facing down the set. Actives join hands with the inactives who are on the outside.

A2   **Down the hall four in line, inside couple arch** (8 counts). Actives are in the center. Actives raise their joined hands to make an arch.

    Ends duck under, actives face up, come back up, two by two (8 counts). Inactives duck under this arch to finish facing up the set as couples and return up the set. The actives retain joined hands, turn inward toward partner to face up and follow the inactives. The first progression occurs here.

B1   **Circle left once around with new neighbors** (8 counts). The actives turn to face the new couple below them and circle left.

    Do-si-do the same (8 counts). Actives do-si-do the same inactives whom they circled in B1.

B2   **Balance and swing the same neighbors** (16 counts). Finish the swing with the women on the right facing across the set. The second progression occurs here. The actives will next dance with the inactives below. Join hands along the line.

Dance Gypsy*

Dance Gypsy is a contemporary contra composed by Gene Hubert.

Music: Jig.

Contra Formation: Becket.

Level: Intermediate.

DIRECTIONS FOR THE DANCE

A1   **Down the center four in line** (6 counts). To start, as couples turn to face down the set, with the women on right of partner, join hands in line with couple across the set.

    Turn as couples (2 counts).

    And return. Bend the line (8 counts). Join hands.

A2   **Circle left three-quarters round** (8 counts).

    Swing your neighbor (8 counts). Men are swinging the left-hand women. The swing occurs on the men's original side. Finish the swing facing a couple on the right diagonal across the set.

B1   **Ladies chain on right diagonal** (8 counts). If there is no couple on right diagonal, do not chain.

    Left-hand star straight across (8 counts). Star with the couple straight across the set.

Dance Gypsy (continued)

*Dance Gypsy is included by permission of Gene Hubert, Graham, NC.

B2 **All balance and swing your partner** (16 counts). Partner is in the next left hand star up or down the set in B1. Couples swing on their original side. Finish the swing with women on right of their partners, facing down the set. Join in a line of four with couple across to start the dance again.

Note: Neutral couple resting out remains as a couple in the line on the caller's right if at the top of the set and in the line on caller's left, if at the bottom. After the ladies chain, these couples with the new women from the chain should line up as if waiting to enter as an Improper/Cross Over dance.

Dancing Sailors

DANCING SAILORS IS A contemporary contra composed by the late Ed Shaw. Al Olson served as a consultant. Shaw and Olson had known each other as sailors, thus Ted Sannella suggested the name.

Music: Reel.

Contra Formation: Duple, Proper/Not Cross Over.

Level: Advanced.

DIRECTIONS FOR THE DANCE

A1 **Actives down the outside below two** (8 counts). Actives go down the outside of their own lines past the next two inactive couples.

Meet in the center and return up the set (6 counts). Actives come into the center to meet, face up as a couple, and go back up the center.

Cast off (2 counts). Actives cast off with their inactives (both turn). Finish in long lines facing across from partner. Actives are now below their inactives.

A2 **Turn contra corners** (16 counts). Actives finish the contra corners by turning with their second corners. Actives are now facing their partners in the center of the set.

B1 **Hey for four on left diagonal with second corners** (16 counts). This hey is done on a diagonal with the active couples and their second corners. Actives begin the hey passing right shoulders with partner. Note that the inactives are not dancing the hey with their partners. See diagram.

Bottom	⑥	6		Bottom		6
	③	3			③4	
	④	4			3①	
	①	1			④1	
Top	②	2		Top	②	2

At start of contra corners   At start of hey with second corner

B2 **Swing your partner in the center of the set** (16 counts). Actives meet after the hey in the center to swing. Timing is important! The actives flow out of the hey into the swing. If late on the swing, a balance preceding the swing helps beginners to get the timing. After swinging, the actives must finish the swing facing up the set so that they are in the proper/not crossover formation. They then cast out to start the dance again. Remember, the inactives to cast off with are the new ones below.

Delphiniums and Daisies*

*D*ELPHINIUMS AND *D*AISIES IS A contemporary contra, composed by Tanya Rotenberg in 1985 for her parents on their 20th wedding anniversary. These flowers were used in her mother's wedding bouquet.

Music: Jig.

Contra Formation: Duple, Improper/Cross Over.

Level: Beginning 3.

DIRECTIONS FOR THE DANCE

A1 **Allemande left the one below once and half** (8 counts). Actives turn the inactives below. Women finish facing the center of the set.

Ladies chain (8 counts). Women chain to partner. Do not return.

A2 **Hey for four** (16 counts). Women begin by passing right shoulders in the center of the set.

B1 **All swing your partner** (16 counts). Couples swing on the side they first started the hey. Finish the swing with the woman on the right of her partner, both facing the couple across the set.

B2 **Circle left three–quarters round** (8 counts). Join hands with the couple across the set. It's the same couple you just completed the hey with. Circle left three–quarters ending in original position.

Allemande right the same one below once and half (8 counts). Actives turn the same inactives as in A1, and everyone progresses to the next to start the dance again.

Delphiniums and Daisies is included by permission of Tanya Rotenberg, Philadelphia, PA.

Easy Does It*

EASY DOES IT IS A contemporary contra, composed by the late Ralph Page.

Music: Jig or Reel.

Contra Formation: Duple, Improper/Cross Over.

Level: Beginner I.

DIRECTIONS FOR THE DANCE

A1 **Do–si–do the one below** (8 counts).

Swing the same (8 counts). Men finish the swing with the women on their right facing into the center of the set.

A2 **Ladies chain over and back** (16 counts).

B1 **Promenade across the set** (8 counts). In promenade position with one you swung in A1, pass left shoulders with the couple across, turn as a couple, and face into the center of the set.

Right and left thru (8 counts). Do not right and left back.

B2 **Left–hand star** (8 counts). With the same couple star once around.

Right–hand star (8 counts). Change hands and star in the opposite direction back to place. Then turn away to face the new couple to start the dance again.

Hull's Victory

HULL'S VICTORY IS A traditional Contra, A "New England Chestnut". This dance honors the battle between the U.S. ship *Constitution*, commanded by Captain Isaac Hull, and the English ship, *Guerriere*, commanded by Captain D'Acres.

Record: Traditionally danced to tune of the same name.

Cassette: "Hull's Victory," New England Chestnuts, Vol. 1 & 2 ALC 203/4C.

Music: "Hull's Victory," Cole, M. M., *One Thousand Fiddle Tunes*, p. 103; Page, Ralph, *An Elegant Collection of Contras and Squares*, p. 57.

Contra Formation: Duple, Proper/Not Cross Over.

Level: Advanced.

---

*Easy Does It is included by permission of the estate of the late Ralph Page and publisher, The Lloyd Shaw Foundation. Easy Does It appears on p. 16, Page, Ralph. An Elegant Collection of Contras and Squares. Denver, CO: The Lloyd Shaw Foundation, 1984.

DIRECTIONS FOR THE DANCE

A1   **Actives right hand to your partner, left hand across to the inactive** (4 counts). Active couples walk to center, join right hands, turn halfway and, still holding hands, join left hands with neighbor (inactive) across set. The inactive man has to make an adjustment stepping up the line and turning face down to accept the left hand of the active woman. Men face down the set, women up.

            Balance four in line (8 counts). Balance four in line, step forward, touch; step back, touch.

            Allemande left your inactive twice around (8 counts). Actives drop partner's hand, and allemande left neighbor twice around.

A2   **Allemande right your partner once around** (4 counts). Actives allemande right once around and form a line of four again.

            Balance four in line (4 counts).

            Actives swing in center (8 counts). End swing with woman on man's right facing down set. Join inside hands.

B1   **Down the center** (6 counts). Active couple walks down the set.

            Actives turn as a couple (2 counts).

            Come back, cast off (8 counts). Couples walk up the set and cast off with original neighbor. Two men turn, arm around waist, as a couple; two women do same, to face center. Active couples have progressed one position.

B2   **Right and left thru over and back** (16 counts). Same two couples right and left over and back.

            Note: Use pigeon–wing position for balance and allemandes.

Jed's Reel*

JED'S REEL IS A contemporary contra, composed in 1983 by Penn Fix for his nephew.

        Music: Reel

        Contra Formation: Duple, Improper/Cross Over

        Level: Beginning – 2

DIRECTIONS FOR THE DANCE

A1   **Do–si–do the one below** (8 counts).

            Ladies do–si–do (8 counts).

A2   **Men balance to each other** (4 counts). Men take right hands with one another and balance.

Jed's Reel (continued)

Men do–si–do (6 counts).

Men allemande right once and a half (6 counts). Finish this turn facing partners.

B1 **All balance and swing your partner** (16). End the swing with the women on the right of their partners facing across the set.

B2 **Promenade across the set** (8 counts). Active couple passes left shoulder with inactives to change places. Turn as couples to face the center of the set. And join hands.

Circle left three–quarters round (6 counts).

Pass thru up and down (2 counts). Pass right shoulders with the original inactive onto the next.

Lady of the Lake

LADY OF THE LAKE IS A traditional Contra, a "New England Chestnut."

Cassette: "Lady of the Lake," New England Chestnuts, Vol. 1 & 2 ALC 203/4C.
Music: "Miller's Reel," Cole, M. M., *One Thousand Fiddle Tunes.*
Contra Formation: Duple, Improper/Cross Over.
Level: Beginning 1.

DIRECTIONS FOR THE DANCE

A1 **Balance and swing the one below** (16 counts). Actives balance and swing the inactive below.

A2 **Actives balance and swing in the center** (16 counts). Actives swing their partner. Finish the swing facing down with active woman on the right.

B1 **Actives down the center** (6 counts). Active couples, inside hands joined walk down the center.

Turn alone (2 counts). Turn alone to face up the set.

B2 **And come back, cast off** (8 counts). Join hands, return to original position, cast off, walk around inactive person, progressing one position down. Inactive does not turn.

Ladies chain over and back (16 counts). Ladies chain with original inactives.

The Nova Scotian

THE NOVA SCOTIAN IS AN original dance by Maurice Henneger of Halifax, Nova Scotia, and was arranged by the late Ralph Page in 1954.

Records: "Glise a Sherbrooke," Folk Dancer MH 45 10073; "Portland Fancy," Fretless FR 203.

Music: "Speed the Plough," Cole, M. M., *One Thousand Fiddle Tunes.*

Contra Formation: Duple, Improper/Cross Over.

Level: Beginning I.

DIRECTIONS FOR THE DANCE

A1   **Allemande left with the one below** (4 counts). Active couples allemande left the inactives.

       Come back to the middle and swing your own (12 counts). Active couples swing in center set. Finish the swing facing down with the active woman on the right.

A2   **Go down the center three in line** (6 counts). Active couple and inactive woman (active man has a woman on either side of him, partner on his right, inactive woman on his left) take six walking steps toward bottom of set.

       Right hand high, left hand under, return to place (10 counts). Active man makes an arch with his right hand and his partner's left; left–hand woman walks under this arch as man's partner walks to other side, taking left–hand woman's place in line. Man now turns under his own right arm (4 counts). All are now facing up the set. Line of three returns to place with walking steps.

B1   **Ladies chain** (8 counts). Women chain to opposite side, courtesy turn. **Do not return.**

       Circle left once around (8 counts). Same two couples join hands and circle left.

B2   **Right and left, over and back** (16 counts). Same two couples right and left through across the set and back. They then turn away from each other to face the next in line to start the dance again.

The Other Mary Kay*

T HE *OTHER MARY KAY* is a contemporary contra composed by Tom Hinds.

Music: Jig or Reel.
Contra Formation: Becket.
Level: Advanced.

DIRECTIONS FOR THE DANCE

A1   **Circle left three–quarters round** (6 counts). Join hands with couple across the set and circle so that couples are facing up and down the set.

    Pass through up and down (2 counts). Pass right shoulders with the original neighbor (#1) and face the next neighbor (#2).

    With the next, do–si–do (8 counts). With the new neighbor (#2) do–si–do. Afterwards, turn to face the original neighbor (#1).

A2   **Star left with original neighbors** (8 counts). With couple that you circle with in A1, star once around back to the new neighbor (#2).

    Swing the new neighbor (8 counts). Swing the neighbor you do–si–do with in A1. Finish the swing facing across the set. The rest of the dance is done with this second couple.

B1   **Men allemande left once and a half around** (8 counts). Two men in the couples facing across from one another, turn by the left to face partners.

    Half a hey for four (8 counts). Men start by passing right shoulders with partners on the outside of the set. Women next go to the center and pass left shoulders; then pass the opposite partner on the other side of the set.

B2   **All balance and swing your partner** (16 counts). All couples are swinging on the original side of the set. Finish the swing facing across the set. The couple you heyed with in B1 is the same couple you start the dance with again.

    Note: Neutral wait out as if it is an improper/cross over dance even though it is in Becket formation.

---

*The Other Mary Kay is included by permission of Tom Hinds, Faber, VA.

Petronella

PETRONELLA IS A traditional Contra, a "New England Chestnut." It is an original dance introduced by Nathaniel Gow of Edinburgh, Scotland, in 1820. Gow's version danced a poussette; the American version is a right and left thru.

Record: Traditionally danced to tune by same name. Folkraft 1139, F & W 3L.

Cassette: "Petronella," New England Chestnuts, Alcazar ALC 203/4.

Music: "Pat'nella," Page, Ralph, *An Elegant Collection of Contras and Squares*, p. 73.

Contra Formation: Proper/Not Cross Over.

Level: Advanced.

DIRECTIONS FOR THE DANCE

A1 **Active man drops between two, join hands** (4 counts) **and balance** (4 counts). To start, the active man turns into the center, between and just below the inactives. He is facing up the set. At the same time, his partner turns into the center, facing down. Then all four join hands to balance to the right and then to the left.

Diagram A. First balance

        [1]

   ②   [2]

     ①

Turn to the right a quarter round (4 counts) **and balance** (4 counts). All drop hands, turn individually clockwise 360° and moving a quarter around. All face in and join hands and balance right and left.

Diagram B. Second Balance

       [2]

  [1]   ①

    ②

A2 **Turn to the right a quarter 'round** (4 counts) **and balance** (4 counts).

Diagram C. Third Balance

     ①

 [2]   ②

   [1]

Turn to the right a quarter 'round (4 counts) **and balance** (4 counts).

Diagram D. Fourth Balance

    ②

 ①   [1]

  [2]

Starting with A1, actives turning into the center, the turn and balance is repeated a total of four times.

Petronella (continued)

B1 **Down the center, turn alone** (8 counts). The inactive couple quickly moves into their original position so that the active couple may walk down the center. Each person turns alone, counts 7–8.

Back to place and cast off (8 counts). Active couple returns to original position, separate and walk around the one below and progresses down the set one position.

B2 **Right and left thru** (8 counts). Active couple and couple above right and left thru, two men passing right shoulders with opposite two women. No hands used in right and left thru. Two men and two women turn as a unit.

And right and left back (8 counts).

Pierce's Hall Stroll*

PIERCE'S HALL STROLL IS A comtemporary Contra. It is an original dance by Fred Breunig, composed for the Sesquicentennial (1982) of the community hall in East Putney, Vermont, where Fred calls a monthly dance.

Music: A march like "Scotland the Brave."

Contra Formation: Duple, Improper/Cross Over.

Level: Intermediate.

DIRECTIONS FOR THE DANCE

A1 **Ladies do–si–do** (8 counts).

Gents do–si–do left shoulder once and a half (8 counts). Men will end on same side as partner.

A2 **All swing partners** (16 counts). After swinging, take escort position. Active couple on men's side face down the set, inactives on women's side face up the set.

B1 **"Stroll"** (8 counts). All couples promenade in the direction facing. Those approaching end of the set turn to follow behind other line. Dancers are promenading in a continuous ellipse, counterclockwise. Counts 5–8, couples wheel around to face opposite direction.

And return (8 counts). All couples promenade in the reverse line of direction (clockwise) to original position.

B2 **Right hands across, turn once and a half** (8 counts). Each minor set forms a star with right hands joined as in shaking hands (not a "box star" position).

Gents drop out to original side. Men will have progressed one position.

———————

Pierce's Hall Stroll is included by permission of Fred Breunig, Putney, VT.

Ladies continue to turn by the right into ladies chain halfway (8 counts). Ladies chain away from partner to opposite. Courtesy turn. Women will be on original side and have progressed one position.

Note All couples are equally active in this dance. This dance illustrates the notion that the term *inactive* is a misnomer.

Roadblock Reel*

ROADBLOCK REEL IS A contemporary contra, composed by Bob Dalsemer.

Music: Jig or Reel.
Contra Formation: Duple, Improper/Cross Over.
Level: Intermediate.

DIRECTIONS FOR THE DANCE

A1 **In long lines, go forward and back** (8 counts).

Pass thru across (4 counts). Everyone changes places with their partners by passing right shoulders across the set. The actives turn to face the inactives below.

Allemande right the one below (4 counts). Once across the set, actives turn inactive below about three–quarters round. Finish this turn with women in the center. They join left hands and continue to hold right hands with their neighbors.

A2 **Across the set balance in line** (4 counts). In an ocean wave, balance to the right and left.

Women allemande left halfway (4 counts). Turn to face partners.

All swing your partner (8 counts). Finish the swing facing down the set with women on right of partner. Join hands with the couple across the set.

B1 **Down the center four in line** (6 counts). Actives are on the left side, inactives on the right.

Turn alone (2 counts). All drop hands, turn to face up and join hands again.

Come back four in line (6 counts). Bend the line (2 counts).

B2 **Circle left three–quarters round** (6 counts). After the circle, couples are back to where they started the dance in A1.

Swing the original one below (10 counts). Men finish the swing with women on their right facing across the set. This progression move occurs at the very end of the dance. Begin again by going forward and back and actives then dance with the next below.

*Roadblock Reel is included by permission of Bob Dalsemer, Brasstown, NC.

Roll in the Hey*

ROLL IN THE HEY IS A contemporary Contra, composed by Roger Diggle. This dance was composed in January 1985 with the idea of testing the transition, "hey for four passing right shoulders in the center, then circle left with someone new." The test has been successful. This contra is similar to the dance "The Bluemont Reel" by Warren Hofstra.

Music: Jig.

Contra Formation: Duple, Improper/Cross Over.

Level: Beginning 3.

DIRECTIONS FOR THE DANCE

A1   **Circle left once around** (8 counts). Actives circle with inactive couple below.

       Swing the one below (8 counts). Actives swing the inactives, finishing the swing with women on the right facing across the set.

A2   **Circle left three–quarters round** (6 counts). The same couples circle round. Finish the circle with partners on the men's original side.

       All swing your partner (10 counts). Everyone swing your partner on the men's original sides. Finish the swing with the woman on the right of her part-ner facing across the set and join hands along the lines.

B1   **In long lines, go forward and back** (8 counts).

       Ladies chain (8 counts). Do not return but finish with the women ready to return to the center of the set.

B2   **Hey for four** (16 counts). Women start the hey passing right shoulders in the center of the set. This hey ends after the men pass by the right shoulders in the center for the second time. Couples then progress to the next couple. Actives move down and inactives up to join in a circle with the new couples.

_____

*Roll in the Hey is included by permission of Roger Diggle, Madison, WI.

Rory O'More

RORY O'MORE IS A traditional Contra, a "New England Chestnut." Samuel Lover, the grandfather of Victor Herbert, wrote the words and music of "Rory O'More."

Records: Traditionally danced to tune by same name.

Cassette: "Rory O'More," *New England Chestnuts*, ALC 203/4C.

Music: Cole, M. M., *One Thousand Fiddle Tunes*, p. 62.

Contra Formation: Couples 1, 3, 5, and so on, active, *do not* cross over (duple, proper.)

Level: Advanced.

DIRECTIONS FOR THE DANCE

A1   **Actives cross over and down the outside. Down below one** (8 counts). Actives pull by with right hands joined, crossing to opposite side; walk down the outside of line, go around one person, and cut into middle of set to meet partner.

     Up the center, cross over. Cast off and actives join hands in the center (8 counts). Walk up the center, release hands, cross to own side, woman crossing in front of partner; cast off, walk around the couple originally below the active couple, to face center. Active couples have now progressed one position down. Active couples move to center of the set, partners join right hands, and join left hands with adjacent active couple. Three lines will exist, two on the outside (inactive dancers) and one in the middle (active couples).

A2   **Balance right and left and slide right** (8 counts). Actives balance right and left. Release hands, take three slides and a step to right, past partner. Join left hands with partner and right hands with neighbor.

     Balance left and right and slide left (8 counts). Actives balance left and right. Release hands, take three slides and a step to left, past partner.

B1   **Turn contra corners** (16 counts). Actives turn contra corners.

B2   **Actives balance and swing in center of set** (16 counts). At end of swing, dancers back into their own line, below the original inactives and ready to dance with the next inactive below.

Salmonchanted Evening*

SALMONCHANTED EVENING IS A contemporary Contra, composed by Steve Zakon in March 1987. Steve wrote the dance in honor of the band Fresh Fish, just before going on a three–week tour with them. Originally the dance was called "Not Tonight, I've Got a Haddock." Within a week it was renamed "Salmonchanted Evening"–a nonsense word, a delightful play on the words "some enchanted evening."

Music: Smooth tunes, well–phrased, such as Jigs.

Contra Formation: Duple, Improper/Cross Over.

Level: Beginning 2.

DIRECTIONS FOR THE DANCE

A1 **Allemande right below once and a half** (8 counts). Actives allemande with inactives once and a half. End with both men in center.

Men allemande left once and a half (8 counts). Men end on opposite sides facing partner on the other side.

A2 **All Gypsy partner on the side** (8 counts). Gypsy with partner by the right shoulder.

All swing your partner (8 counts).

B1 **Chain the ladies over and back** (16 counts).

B2 **Right and left thru** (8 counts). Right and left thru, courtesy turn. *Do not return*.

Circle left three–quarters (6 counts). Join hands and circle left three–quarters. Active couples will face down the set; inactive couples will face up the set.

Pass through (2 counts). Actives pass right shoulders with the inactives below and progress to the next inactive couple.

Salmonchanted Evening is included by permission of Steve Zakon, East Sullivan, NH.

Shadrack's Delight*

SHADRACK'S DELIGHT IS A contemporary Contra. It is an original dance by Tony Parkes. The dance was named for Betty and "Shadrack" McDermid.

Records: Well-phrased Jig. "Lamb Skinnet," Folkraft 1501; Lloyd Shaw 193/194 (flip).
Music: Scottish Jig suggested.
Contra Formation: Duple, Improper/Cross Over.
Level: Intermediate.

DIRECTIONS FOR THE DANCE

A1   **Do-si-do the one below, go one and a quarter** (8 counts). End in a line of four across the set, actives face down the set, inactives face up the set.

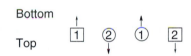

Balance four in line (4 counts). Begin balance to the right and then left. Look at the person in the direction of the balance.

Turn half by the right (4 counts). Turn neighbor by the right halfway, continue to hold hands with neighbor. Men meet in the center, take left hands. Actives end facing up the set, inactives facing down the set. Join hands in line of four.

A2   **Balance four in line** (4 counts).

Men turn half by the left (4 counts).

All swing your partners (8 counts). End with woman on right side of man, line of four, facing down the set, hands joined.

B1   **Down the center four in a line** (6 counts).

Turn as a couple (2 counts). Both men turn their partner so that the women remain on the right side of men and face up.

Return to place, cast off (8 counts). Cast off counts 5–8; each couple, arm around waist, take four steps, turning out to face center.

B2   **Right and left thru a cross** (8 counts). Counter turn. Do not return. Active men will have progressed one position down.

Same two ladies chain (8 counts). Courtesy turn. Do not return. Women progress one position down, progression complete.

Note: Sometimes danced without the cast-off for a smoother transition in the women's line.

Shadrack's Delight is included by permission of Tony Parkes, Arlington, MA.

Silver Lake Waltz*

S ILVER LAKE WALTZ IS A contemporary Contra, composed by Erna–Lynne Bogue, who wrote the dance while living by the shores of Silver Lake near Dexter, Michigan. She writes, "The dance had some of the peaceful symmetry and gentle romance of the lake." There are many "Silver Lakes" in the country and people always think it's about "their" Silver Lake.

Record: "Midwinter Blossom" (track 12) on *A Band Named Bob*, CD.

Music: 32 bar Waltz.

Contra Formation: Duple, Proper/Not Cross Over.

Level: Intermediate.

DIRECTIONS FOR THE DANCE

A1   **Actives half figure 8 through the couple below** (8 counts). Finish the half figure 8 above the inactives but now crossed over. Actives take right hand with partner.

Actives balance forward and back (4 counts).

Actives change places (4 counts). Active woman turns under joined hands.

A2   **Inactives half figure 8 through the couple above** (8 counts).

Inactives balance forward and back (4 counts).

Inactives change places (4 counts). Inactive woman turns under joined hands.

B1   **Actives join both hands and sashay two steps down the center** (4 counts).

Actives sashay back two steps (4 counts).

Actives cast unassisted around the inactives to progressed places (4 counts).

B2   **All waltz partner once around the current neighbors** (8 waltz steps). Couples take closed position. Taking 8 waltz steps, turning clockwise, same actives and inactives waltz around one another counterclockwise back to progressed place and remain proper/not cross over position.

Silver Lake Waltz is included by permission of Erna–Lynne Bogue, St. Scholastica Monastery, Duluth, MN.

Small Potatoes*

$\mathcal{S}$ MALL POTATOES IS A contemporary Contra, composed by Jim Kitch.

Music: Jig or Reel.
Contra Formation: Duple, Improper/Cross Over.
Level: Beginning 2.

DIRECTIONS FOR THE DANCE

A1   **Balance and swing the one below** (16 counts). Actives swing with the inactive below, finishing the swing with woman on the right facing across the set.

A2   **Circle left once around** (8 counts). The circle starts and ends in this progressed position with actives below the original inactives.

Ladies chain (8 counts). Women chain to their partners but do not return.

B1   **Women do–si–do** (8 counts). Finish by turning to face partner.

All swing your partner (8 counts). Finish the swing with women on the right of the men facing across the set.

B2   **Circle left three–quarters round** (6 counts). Join hands with the couple across and circle back to original positions in A1.

Pass through up and down (2 counts). Drop hands and pass right shoulders with original inactives onto the next couple.

Actives do–si–do with your new neighbor (8 counts). Begin the dance again with this same inactive couple by balance and swinging.

---

*Small Potatoes is included by permission of Jim Kitch, Phoenixville, PA.

Symmetrical Force*

S YMMETRICAL FORCE IS A contemporary Contra, composed by Fred Feild in 1979. The founder of the Chicago Barn Dance Company, Feild incorporated southern Appalachian figures in this dance to interest contra dancers in squares and big circle dances.

Music: Reel.

Contra Formation: Duple, Improper/Cross Over.

Level: Beginning 3.

DIRECTIONS FOR THE DANCE

A1   **Do–si–do inside first, then outside with the ones below** (8 counts). Also known as a mirror do–si–do, the actives start the do–si–do by both going down the center of the set, splitting the inactives and going around the outside of them back to place. The active man starts by passing left shoulders and active lady, right shoulders.

            Allemande the ones below *twice* **around with the handy hand** (8 counts). Active man turns inactive lady with left hand while active woman turns inactive man with right hand. Finish with the actives in the center of the set.

A2   **Actives swing your partner** (16 counts). Actives end the swing facing down the set with woman on right of partner. Join hands with original neighbors on the outside of the line.

B1   **Down the center four in line** (6 counts). Actives are in the middle of the line of four.

            Actives back under own joined hands, while inactives turn in to face up (2 counts). Without dropping any hands, the actives bring their joined hands over their heads, turn away from their partners, and bring their arms down in front of them. The arms end up crossed in front forming two leaves of a clover.

            Come back up (8 counts) in a line of four.

B2   **Inactives join hands on top and circle left** (8 counts). After returning four in line, the inactives join their free hands on top to complete the four–leaf clover. The circle of four then moves to the left.

            Inactives arch, actives go through, unwinding (4 counts.) Inactives raise their joined hands and pull actives under their arch. All continue to hold joined hands in a circle.

            Actives then go under again to the next (4 counts). Actives go through the arch of the inactives and thereby go down the center to the next inactive couple to start the dance again. Remember both active man and woman remain in the center of the set for the do–si–do.

Symmetrical Force is included by permission of Fred Fields, Tucson, AZ.

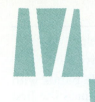

The Tourist*

THE TOURIST IS A contemporary Contra. It is an original dance by the late Ted Sannella, 1970. This version was arranged by Ralph Page.

Record: "Frenchie's Reel," Fourgone Conclusions, Front Hall FHR 029.
Music: "Lamplighter's Hornpipe," Cole, M. M., *One Thousand Fiddle Tunes.*
Contra Formation: Duple, Improper/Cross Over.
Level: Beginning I.

DIRECTIONS FOR THE DANCE

A1   **Down the outside of the set, turn** (8 counts). Active couples (1, 3, 5, and so on) turn out and walk down outside of set, behind their own respective lines, eight steps. Counts 7–8, each turns toward center of set.

Come right back (8 counts).

A2   **Into the center with a do–si–do** (8 counts). Active couples step to middle of set and do–si–do.

Circle four hands once around (8 counts). Actives join hands with the active couple below, circle left once around.

B1   **Balance and swing the one below** (16 counts). Active balance and swing the same inactive as in A2. Finish the swing facing across the set, ready to ladies chain.

B2   **Ladies chain over and back** (16 counts).

Weave the Line*

WEAVE THE LINE IS A contemporary Contra, composed by Kathy Anderson.

Music: Jig or Reel
Contra Formation: Duple, Improper/Cross Over – Double Progression
Level: Intermediate.

Weave the Line (continued)

---

*The Tourist is included by permission of the late Ted Sannella.
*Weave the Line is included by permission of Kathy Anderson, Indialantic, FL.

A1 **Actives star left below** (8 counts). Actives star with inactives below.

Circle left once around (8 counts). Actives with the same inactives circle.

A2 **Weave the line past two couples** (8 counts). Holding inside hands with partner, progress past two couples. Actives move to the left to pass the first inactive couple, women passing right shoulders. Then moving to the right, they pass the second inactive couple, men passing left shoulders. Actives are now facing a third inactive couple. At the ends, neutral couples immediately turn as couples to face into the set and reenter.

Actives as individuals do–si–do inactives #3 (8 counts). Drop hands with partners and do–si–do the inactive in the third group.

B1 **Actives balance and swing inactives #2** (16 counts). After the do–si–do with the inactive #3, everyone turn away to face the inactives #2 to balance and swing. Finish the swing, facing across the set and join hands along the lines.

B2 **In long lines, go forward and back** (8 counts).

Actives swing your partner in the center (8 counts). Actives finish the swing facing down the set to star left with the next couple who was originally inactive #3.

Note: In this double progression dance, the actives progress through two inactive couples during a single sequence and begin the dance sequence again with the third inactive couple.

With Thanks to the Dean*

Wᴵᵀʜ Tʜᴀɴᴋs ᴛᴏ ᴛʜᴇ Dᴇᴀɴ is a contemporary dance composed by Steve Zakon in 1985. This dance salutes the dean of Contra Dancing, Ralph Page. Steve wrote the dance in Ralph's memory to thank him for his efforts to keep Contra Dancing alive and vital for generations to follow.

Music: Smooth flowing tunes, usually Reels.

Contra Formation: Duple, Improper/Cross Over and Double Progression.

Level: Intermediate.

DIRECTIONS FOR THE DANCE

A1 **Allemande left below, go once and a half** (8 counts). Actives allemande left the one below, turn once and a half. End with women facing to the center.

Ladies chain (8 counts). Courtesy turn. Do not chain back.

A2 **Ladies allemande right** (4 counts). With right hand, women turn once round to face partner.

All swing your partner (12 counts). Everyone swings partner. Finish swing with women on right of partners, facing into the center of the set.

---

*With Thanks to the Dean is included by permission of Steve Zakon, East Sullivan, NH.

B1   **Circle left, once around** (8 counts). Join hands with the couple across the set and circle left once. All couples slide to the left (along the line), picking up the next couple (first progression). Men take responsibility to slide left with your partner.

Bottom   ③ ④
             ③ ④
             ① ②
Top   ① ②

Start and finish of circle left once around.

Couples move left along the line (2 counts).

Circle left with the next three–quarters round (6 counts). Finish the circle with the actives facing down and inactives facing up, ready to do–si–do with one another.

Bottom   ③ ⑥
            ③ ⑥
            ① ④   Bottom   ⑥ ⑥
            ① ④   ③ ③
            ②   ④ ④
Top   ②   Top   ① ①

Start of circle left three–quarters around.   **End of circle left three–quarters round.**

B2   **Do–si–do the second inactive** (8 counts). With the ones you circled three–quarters, do–si–do.

Allemande right the same once and a half (8 counts). The active couple progresses one position down at the end of the allemande (second progression). The left hand is free to start the dance over with "Allemande left" with a new couple.

Bottom   ⑤ ⑤
            ③ ③
            ⑥ ⑥
            ① ①
            ④ ④
Top   ② ②

7
International Folk Dance

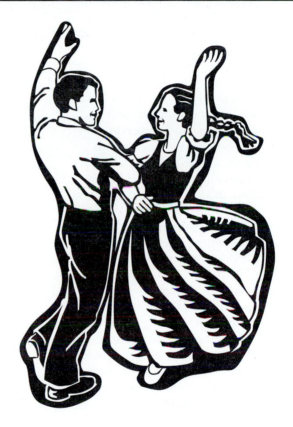

INTRODUCTION

Throughout human history nothing has approached the significance of dance. Indeed, it has been the basis for the survival of social systems in every decade. The story of people and their culture from ritual to art is the history of *Folk Dance.* In the transition from rite to art, the social and pleasurable qualities of Folk Dance have survived above all the rest. In each dance, however, we still can find a storehouse of traditions that were an intimate part of the culture of the people from whom the dance is derived. Although cultural traces become dim with time, there is more to a folk song than its tune and more to a dance than its movement. In these ongoing traditional expressions are recorded the early and ever-growing and –changing social lives of a people. These folk traditions are living history.

In the 1800s and 1900s Folk Dance persisted around the world in different forms. The tradition of institutions teaching dance in Asia (refer to pp. 16–19) has kept it alive. Africa and South America also have an infrastructure to foster their dance culture.

The impact of the modern industrial revolution in both Europe and America threatened to blot out the natural flow of folk expression. The threatened disappearance of folkways, songs, music, costumes, and dances spurred governments, private individuals, and organizations into concerted efforts to preserve these traditions. Organized efforts to revive interest in folk traditions began at different times in different countries, but in each the main thrust was to collect, note, and preserve in national repositories the finest possible examples of folk song, dance, music, costume, and art.

FOLK DANCE MOVEMENT

In Sweden, Arthur Hazelius created the Nordiskz Museet, or Northland Museum, to house rare folk dances and folk art. In 1893, the Friends of Swedish Folk Dance was formed. This and other organizations have worked to make this phase of Swedish culture known to every generation. The revival movement led to formation of the Danish Folk Dance Society in 1901. In 1911, Cecil Sharp, an English writer and musician, helped found the English Folk Dance Society. Branches of this society have been established throughout the British Commonwealth and America.

A series of events prior to the outbreak of World War II marked the revival of the Folk Dance movement in Europe. In 1928, the International Congress of Popular Arts was held in Prague. Thirty–one nations attended the Congress, convened by the Assembly of the League of Nations. The purpose was to study the geographical distribution of the different artistic forms of folk life and to compile records and devise methods for encouraging and preserving the popular arts still in existence. In 1935, the English Folk Dance Society and the British national Committee on Folk Arts sponsored an International Folk Dance Festival in London. In 1939, a second Congress was held in Stockholm, Sweden. Some 3,000 delegates and officials attended. The program provided opportunity for presentation of papers, discussions, and dance demonstrations by the various national groups in attendance.

After World War II many performing groups traveled to share their culture around the world. There is an eagerness to know and appreciate the different cultures. Sol Hurok brought the Russian Moiseyev Dance Ensemble to the United States. He brought folk lore to the theater and the theater to folk lore. One foreign group after another comes to delight Americans and descendants of each culture. American dance groups travel abroad to perform and be a part of international festivals. The Brigham Young Folk Dancers is one of many American groups that travels annually. The Folk Dance movement in the United States is spread like a patchwork quilt from coast to coast. Clubs, ethnic groups, and specialized performing groups are the backbone of the movement. Some regional organizations and a few state federations exist. In contrast to the highly organized and standardized American Square Dance movement, the International Folk Dance movement and the Contra/Country Dance groups are best described as diverse, autonomous, and fragmented. However unorganized it is at the regional and national level, the movement is bound together by the most universal adhesive known–the desire among participants to share their love of dancing dances from around the world.

The largest concentration of Folk Dance groups is found in major urban areas, such as New York, Seattle, Chicago, Detroit, San Francisco, and Los Angeles, where there is a greater mix of ethnic groups. Folk Dance groups were typically sponsored and housed by institutions whose aims included fostering of international understanding. College and university campuses, YMCAs, YWCAs, settlement houses, and churches were therefore popular locations for Folk Dance groups.

Physical Education classes at both public schools and college level have influenced International Folk Dance classes by offering classes and research, maintaining performing groups, and sponsoring foreign teachers on the circuit. With the advent of physical education classes as an elective at the college level, Folk Dance classes are few or have been dropped. But Folk Dance groups continue in the evening recreational program.

A major boost to International Folk Dance was felt in 1940 when the New York World's Fair and the San Francisco World's Fair introduced Folk Dance as an attraction for public participation. The enthusiastic response by the general public led to the formation of two major centers for the lay–folk dance movement: the Folk Dance House founded by Michael and Mary Ann Herman in New York City and Chang's International Dancers formed by Soon Chang in San Francisco. The California Folk Dance Federation, Country Song and Dance Society (CDSS), and New England Folk Festival Association (NEFFA) have promoted Folk Dance. These East–West urban strongholds of international dancing have produced thousands of folk dancers who have, in turn, spread the fun and enjoyment of Folk Dance throughout America.

■ Dance Sources

Educators and educational institutions have played a role in research, teaching, and fostering the use of Folk Dance in schools and recreation programs. In the early 1920s, physical educators, recognizing the value of dance in human neuromuscular development, drew from Folk Dance for the content of gymnastic dance routines. Movement from Irish Jigs, Italian Tarantellas, and American Virginia Reel were incorporated into these dance sequences. Paralleling the use of Folk Dance in gymnastics, Folk Dance was also developing as a separate subject in physical education classes and the early playground movement. Elizabeth Burchenal and C. Ward Crampton were two early researchers and collectors of traditional Folk Dances as they were being performed in European countries. By the beginning of the 20th century, Folk Dance was widely used in physical education in secondary schools and colleges.

Elizabeth Burchenal's research and collection of dance materials from original European sources brought a wealth of Folk Dance materials to schools and recreation programs in the early 1900s. As chairman of the Folk Dance committee of the Playground and Recreation Association of America, she was instrumental in introducing Folk Dance to a wide audience and training many teachers over several decades. Burchenal became the first president of the American Folk Dance Society, which was formed in 1916.

Mary Wood Hinman, a physical educator of exceptional vision, worked to provide an appropriate and meaningful way for ethnic groups to perform and share their cultural heritage with other Americans. Her work resulted in a series of Folk Dance courses being offered at the New School of Social Research in New York City in 1933. The courses were designed to provide an opportunity for various ethnic groups to teach their native songs and dances to people of all backgrounds. With the same philosophy in mind, Hinman was instrumental in establishing Folk Festival Councils in other American cities.

Another source of Folk Dance materials for the thirsty American folk dancer is the touring teachers. Guided tours to European dance festivals with authoritative leaders give the tour group an opportunity to see the real thing. Dance enthusiasts make full use of new innovations in sound technology for recording authentic music and filming dance as they travel from festival to festival. Participant interest in new dances increases as they tire quickly of old ones. This spurs the traveling researchers to comb the European countryside for more and more dances. The continued demand for new dances has been somewhat answered by more specialization in a single type of dance or a single nationality. These dance groups along with international groups give the added dimension of choice.

■ Camps

The *Folk Dance camp* concept became a popular vehicle for dancers and leaders alike to enjoy a total folk experience by learning about other cultures through dance, crafts, songs, games, costumes, and ethnic foods. They even have a chance to celebrate a Swedish Christmas in July! Jane Farwell established the first such camp at Oglebay Institute in West Virginia in the early 1940s. Jane Farwell is easily the "Johnny Appleseed" of Folk Dance camps since she organized and conducted successful camps from Florida to Maine. The idea spread, and in the late 1940s and early 1950s camps influenced by her idea or led by her enthusiasm were in operation across America.

Today the Folk Dance camp is the prime vacation choice for thousands of folk–dancing Americans. Camps attract the top teaching professionals who represent specific ethnic groups. Camp programs include complete syllabi of material taught, adventures in gourmet foods from many nationalities, special classes in folk singing, expert guidance in making costumes, and more often than not all of this *and* college credits! Folk Dance camps have come a long way since Jane Farwell and her campers "washed their faces in the May morning dew midst the fairy rings on a West Virginia hillside."

■ Performing Groups

International Folk Dance performing groups are predominantly associated with, sponsored by, or brought into existence on an American college or university campus. Then ethnic groups developed performing groups, and folk companies like Aman surfaced. Performance demands made it necessary for many groups to develop full–time professional staff to take care of their rehearsal and performance needs. Several of the more outstanding groups have made the step to a full professional dance troupe. These highly skilled and brilliantly costumed groups give concerts and conduct classes and workshops in the communities in which they perform. Performing groups acquire extensive costume collections, acquire musical instruments unique to the nationalities they represent, and develop musicians for orchestral accompaniment. Members of the group actively participate in the research into the background of the dances and nationalities they represent. Groups travel extensively at home and abroad and are often invited to perform at important national festivals. Groups may perform in 100 or more concerts each year.

These attractive and polished young college students often tour as ambassadors and official representatives of the United States State Department. Many groups offer aspiring high school dancers a unique opportunity to combine education with travel through full college scholarships. And, not unlike professional athletics, some performing groups are in the process of developing a "farm system" to train future dance performers.

■ Research and Advanced Studies

Academia and institutions like the Smithsonian and Library of Congress are stimulating interest and research in folklore here and abroad. Tracing, preserving, and reexamining the early records of dance in the United States have opened up new areas of interest, careful research, and desire to preserve this information. Libraries are being established to house existing collections and correspondence. Advanced degrees are offered to folklorists with a focus on dance.

■ Trends

The social and recreational aspects of Folk Dancing are still paramount over teaching and learning within the strict framework of authenticity. The enthusiasm for International Folk Dance has tapered down. Yet some groups are as strong as ever. Dance groups show an avid interest in nonpartner circle and line dances. Balkan and Israeli dances have become widely popular. Groups who love Kolos are tagged as having "kolomania"! Women find the freedom of modern times in the nonpartner dances; no longer must they wait to be asked to dance.

The generalist teacher has given way to the specialist. Teachers specialize in line dances or dances of a single nationality. The number of male Folk Dance teachers has had an impact on the role of men in dance in general. Teachers, leaders, and participants are becoming more tolerant of the variations found in a dance. There is a greater tendency to see variations and differences in dances as a result of "natural processes" in the culture from which the dance comes and in its application and use by Folk Dance groups.

Perhaps as a result of the popularity of folksingers like Peter, Paul, and Mary, dancers dusted off guitars and violins and once again accompanied Folk Dance. Interest in playing ethnic instruments sparked. Accompaniment with live music and musicians "sitting in" with the band gave a burst of new enthusiasm. The singing of folk songs during intermission or before a meal has become popular.

Another trend is the resurgence of ethnic dance in the ethnic communities of the United States. For instance, the Greek, Scandinavian, Philippine, and Japanese promote their native dance through their young people who enjoy performing for the public at festivals. Young and old will dance at their weddings and social events. They want to keep these traditions alive.

■ Future

Interest in national cultural heritage has continued and accelerated as a new millennium dawns. Efforts to preserve the knowledge and practices of the past have provided a wealth of information and artifacts from which dancers and dance scholars alike can draw for greater appreciation and understanding of dance's role in the cultural life of nations.

Each of the dances included in this chapter contains bits and pieces of the culture from which it comes. The story behind the dance reflects the history, geography, climate, religion, lifestyle, and

dance characteristics of the national group from which it is derived. Knowing the background and influence of these components of a dance gives depth and added dimension to teaching and performing. Learning Folk Dance, therefore, carries with it a greater responsibility than merely teaching or performing a physical skill. It is an opportunity to develop appreciation for the customs and traditions of other cultures, to discover that the language of Folk Dancing can be a common bond between people of all nations, and to learn that differences can become exciting adventures in discovering real similarities.

UNDERSTANDING FOLKWAYS ENHANCES DANCE

■ Eastern and Western Culture

Cultural influences in the form of borrowing and exchanging occur wherever two or more cultures meet along political or geographical boundaries. The Balkans are a historic example of an area that has for centuries been the meeting place for both Eastern and Western culture. Of the many ethnic groups passing in and out, the major cultural influences came from the Slavs, who dominated from about the sixth century A.D. to the Middle Ages; the Romans, both pagan and Christian; and the Ottoman Turks, whose influence lasted into the 19th century.

The Balkans are an ethnic mixture made up of four cultural groups: Greeks, Slavs, Daco–Romans, and Albanians. Linguistically they are represented by seven groups: Romans, Slovenians, Serbo–Croatians, Macedonians, Greeks, Albanians, and Bulgarians.

The long period of domination meant isolation from cultural movements going on in western Europe, and it caused the Balkan people to turn to their native folklore for identity and inspiration. Isolation worked to enrich their cultural heritage and served to make the Balkans an extensive storehouse of folk materials.

■ Geography and Climate

Worldwide, people have found homes in the desert, steppes, plains, river valleys, and mountains. Each of these settings influence lifestyle in its own unique manner. People who live in mountain terrains tend to be more isolated and less mobile, and they learn to make use of small spaces. It is under these conditions that traditions, folkways, and material cultures are most likely to be found intact and better preserved. The people of the southern Appalachian mountains in the southeastern United States are an example. In contrast, people living in fertile plains, river valleys, or broad plains are more accessible and mobile. These groups, by virtue of their environmental setting, are more exposed to cultural exchange. The dance of mountain people, therefore, should reflect an economical use of space and a uniformity in execution due to lack of cultural borrowing or exchanging. The dance of people living in more accessible settings should reflect a potpourri in style, steps, and lack of uniformity.

Climate is regarded as being a major influence on the quality of dance movement. Although it is a factor, it should not be regarded as an inflexible influence because climatic zones do not adhere to rigid lines of demarcation. Generally, dance movements of people living in a warm climate are fluid, flowing, and slow. They contain few strong, abrupt, or energetic motions. In extremely cold climates, dance movements are perceived to be strong, vigorous, and energetic, with sustained action. They often include acrobatic movements and contrary body actions. In temperate climates with a more gradual change in seasons and temperatures, dance movement is more balanced between vigorous and quiet sustained actions. The climate tends to prune out extraneous movements.

■ Religion

Dance in the form of pagan rituals was primitive people's means of supplicating the gods. These rituals were performed to communicate with the unseen forces that were perceived to sustain and regulate human survival. With the advent of Christianity, pagan rituals lost their magical content but remained in form and structure to become the earliest known forms of Folk Dance. The Morris, Sword, and Maypole dances are examples.

Historically, dance has been an integral part of Christianity and Christian ritual. The "Hymn of Jesus" described in the apocryphal Acts of John, A.D. 120, was a sacred dance in which the Apostles joined hands and circled slowly around Christ, singing a hymn. The mystical circle symbolized the protection of the Church from the outer world. In the early 12th century, Rabbi Hacin ben Salomo taught Christians to perform a choral dance around the altar in St. Bartholomew at Qauste in the Spanish province of Zaragoza. Ecclesiastical dancing survived in France as late as the 17th century.

The Protestant movement generally frowned on dance, albeit ambivalently. In New England during the Revolutionary years, everybody danced, including the minister, who found his niche in the community via the Ordination Ball. Although the fiddle was said to be the Devil's instrument, dance was credited with developing manners and discipline in the young.

■ Music

Rhythm is important in Folk Dance music. Rhythm is the musical beat that drives dance movement. It is organized and structured sounds. Rhythm is the musical sound that catches the essential style and quality of movement in a Folk Dance. Authentic music and rhythm are important in keeping the ethnic flavor and spirit of a Folk Dance from being lost.

There are cultural variations in rhythm structure. Western culture is accustomed to 2/4, 3/4, and 6/8 meter with groupings of four, eight, and sixteen bars or measures. In Eastern culture, the Western-type meters are rare, except for 2/4. Irregular rhythms dominate, with 5/16, 7/8, and 11/16 being common. Musical phrases and dance phrases do not always coincide with groupings of three, five, and so forth, bars or measures.

The first musical instrument was the human voice; therefore no culture has been without music or some type of musical instrument. Musical instruments played a major role in the spiritual life and rituals of primitive societies.

The drum—a dried animal skin stretched over a hollow log and beaten to produce sounds—is often believed to be the oldest instrument. Some believe wind instruments, with a simple reed blown on to produce a tone, to be first. Still others point to the hunter's bow, which produced a "twanging" sound when the arrow was released. In Africa, the drum was used for dance ritual and communication and was so important that it was referred to as "the pulse of life." The oldest music in America is that of American Indians. Their musical instruments—drums, rattles, bells, and rasps—are nearly as old as human society.

Much of what is known about music in ancient times has been passed along by story and legend. Hard evidence depicting musical instruments, however, has come from surviving pottery, sculpture, tomb paintings, and cave carvings. The Egyptians had great orchestras of flutes and string instruments. Thousands of years ago, the Chinese had royal orchestras of drums, bells, and gongs. In the Old Testament, Jericho was blown down by the sound of seven shofars.

European instruments have counterparts in simple form in Africa and in more elaborate form in Eastern countries. Instruments used for folk music and dance are largely those native to or invented by a particular national or ethnic group. The accordion, for example, was invented in Berlin in the 1820s by Friedrick Buschmann and has been a staple of German folk music and dance. In Sweden, the fiddle is the favorite instrument, although old-time dances are done largely to accordion music. Philippine dance instruments reflect a diverse cultural background. Native rhythm instruments, sticks, bamboo poles, and coconut shells are used along with castanets and Spanish guitars. The study of musical instruments is fascinating, and it is significant in keeping the total background and spirit of folk dancing in perspective.

■ Costumes

Costumes have an interesting and unique effect on the characteristic dance movements of the dancer. The style and range of movement is freed or restricted by the material and cut of the skirt, coat, or trousers. Headdress and footwear also have an interesting effect on qualities of movement. The effect costumes have on dance movement is an important element in studying the style and background of the dance.

Historically, costumes or clothing have served to protect from the elements, accommodate an occupational use, distinguish or give status, and represent a national or ethnological group. The Folk Dance costume is worn by national or ethnic groups and by members of International Folk Dance groups all over the United States. Costumes add an exciting and dramatic dimension to Folk Dancing.

■ Holidays, Festivals, and Special Occasions

Dancing is a social event and, as such, is an integral part of the calendar of events in all cultures. Sundays and holidays are common times when work ceases and families and friends can get together for fun and fellowship, with music and dancing as a special way to express the joy of the occasion. Weddings are times for the traditions and customs of a group to be shared, when all are made merrier by music and dance befitting the occasion.

Friends, neighbors, relatives, and often whole communities gather for cooperative work in the form of barn raisings, corn shuckings, or quilting bees. These occasions feature tables laden with potluck food and all the trimmings topped off with music and dancing until the wee hours of the morning.

Religious holidays are times of food, fiesta, and dancing. Celebrations may be in honor of a favorite saint and, as such, include mass, a festive parade, and music and dancing in the streets. In nonreligious groups, tribal or group tradition and custom may call for celebration by sacrificial offering to ancestral spirits and performance of ritual dancing.

Seasons are worldwide times of celebration. Christmas, harvest time, and midsummer are major times to roll out costumes, customs, decorations, food, and dance. Christmas is a time for elegant balls, caroling, and dancing around the Christmas tree. Harvest time, where older traditions still hold, is a community and family time to share work and play together. These are times when special traditions and customs are renewed.

AFRICA

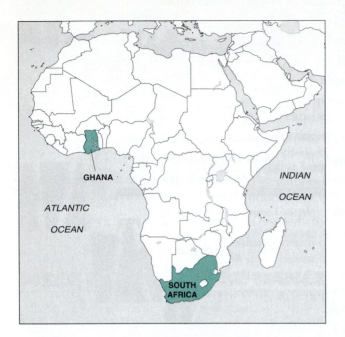

GHANA

ATLANTIC
OCEAN

INDIAN
OCEAN

SOUTH
AFRICA

Africa is divided into two parts by the Sahara Desert. The Arab culture influences the north. The southern part is poor and least developed. The landing of the Portuguese at Cape Good Hope in the last part of the 15th century opened the door for other European countries to join in the general exploitation of natural resources and, more tragically, human resources in the form of slaves. However, wherever slaves went, they carried with them the rich mythology, graphic, piastic art and music with a highly developed rhythmic structure.

The African tradition of oral rather than written communication was the basic reason for Westerners' general lack of understanding of African arts and traditional dance. Percussion and improvisation are the chief characteristics of traditional dance. Drums are the heartbeat of Africa and they control and follow dance movement. Improvisation is taught and learned through traditional gestures, which are the words of the dancers. Dance is an intricate part of the daily life in every village. Children are cradled by the rhythm of walking, working, and dancing. Dance is the main avenue of communication and is an expression of life and all its emotions. Refer to History of Africa pp. 4–6.

Borborbor
Ghanaian

BORBORBOR IS PRONOUNCED *BOW-BOW-BOW* and means "bend down." Borborbor is danced mostly in the central part of the Volta Region of Ghana. Dance was originally a medium of recreation, relaxation, and courtship. After a hard day's work and a big evening meal, young adults would gather in the open under the moonlight to dance away the day's toils. This gathering is also a place where single males look for future wives. Borborbor has evolved into a popular social dance. It is danced at funerals, outdoor events, weddings, church services, and parties. Beatric Feddy, Phd, Ghana, presented this dance during the Hoolyeh Folk Dance Festival in 1998.

Music: Cassette* "Saa Ml," by Ardey Allotey.

Formation: Solo: facing line of direction, circle formation.

Props: One handkerchief for each hand; Kleenex may be used as a substitute.

Step: Walk.

DIRECTIONS FOR THE DANCE

Meter 4/4

Mea. Counts

Part I: The Wave

1	1–2	Feet: With weight on the left foot, place the right foot diagonal right forward, bending down on the left knee at the same time. Shake hips on the down beat.
		Arms: Raise right arm up as if waving (arm goes up, as the foot goes out).

Borborbor (continued)

Cassette available from Ardey Allotey, PO Box 19006, Portland, OR 97219.

	3–4	Feet: Bring right foot back to left, slightly straighten the legs.
		Arms: Lower right arm as foot is brought back.
2	1–4	Repeat measure I
3	1	Step right forward
	2	Step left forward
	3	Step right forward
	4	Jump on both feet in place
4–6		Repeat dance on left side
		Repeat measures 1–6 until the music changes.

Part II "Look at Him, Look at Her, Shaking His/Her Hips"

Each dancer may choose which direction to travel (small steps & touches). There are three choices: Travel to another dancer and dance around them. Turn in place. Move in line of direction.

1	1	Step right in place.
	2	Touch left to left side, accent left hip to left side.
	3	Step left in place.
	4	Touch right foot to right side, accent right hip to right side. During this footwork hands are waist level, spinning clockwise around each other.
2	1–4	Repeat measure 1.
		Repeat measures 1–6 until the music changes.
		Repeat the dance from the beginning.

Style: Knees slightly bent, constantly moving the hips. Lean slightly forward from the waist.

Gahu

Ghanaian

GAHU IS PRONOUNCED *GA-NEW.* Some sources support that *Gahu* literally means "money dance" (ga = money, hu = dance/drum). It is believed that *Gahu* originated from the Republic of Benin, spread to parts of Nigeria where Ghanaian fishermen adapted it from their Nigerian hosts. Today Gahu is a very popular communal entertainment danced by communities especially during celebrations. Beatric Feddy, Phd, Ghana, presented this dance during the Hoolyeh Folk Dance Festival in 1998.

Music: Cassette* "Saa Ml," by Ardey Allotey.

Formation: *Solo:* facing line of direction, single circle. *Partner:* Double circle, hands not joined, facing line of direction.

Props: One handkerchief for each hand; Kleenex may be used as a substitute.

Step: Walk.

Cassette available from Ardey Allotey, P.O. Box 19006, Portland, OR 97219.

DIRECTIONS FOR THE DANCE

Meter 2/4 • Directions are the same for man and woman.

Mea. Counts

Part I

1	1	Touch right foot diagonally right forward, leaning diagonally right forward, gesturing your right forearm diagonally forward, parallel with your right foot. Steps are small in length.
	2	Step with your right foot where you touched, gesturing elbow again.
2	1–2	Repeat Measure 1 on the left side

Repeat measures 1–2 until the music changes.

Break: Raise arms above your head, shake handkerchiefs, and say "Hoooo."

Repeat Part I until the music changes.

Part II:

Partners face each other. While dancing Part II, arms are at your side with yours elbows bent.

Move elbows back and forth, mimicking a wing movement of a bird.

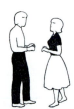

1	1	Step side right with right foot
	2	Step right with left foot crossing in front of right
2	1	Step side right with right foot
	2	Lean a little right and slightly lift left foot
3–4	1–2, 1–2	Repeat to the left

Repeat measures 1–4 until the music changes. It will vary from song to song.

Break: Raise arms above your head, shake handkerchiefs, and enthusiastically call out "Hooooo."

Part III: Show your money   VOCALS

1	1	Facing slightly towards center and bending over a little at the waist, touch your right foot forward in line of direction. Pat your right hip with your right hand where a back pocket would be.	Mo
	2	Step with right foot where you touched your right foot and pat your right hip again.	ney!
2	1	Facing slighty to your right, standing tall (knees still bent a little), touch your left foot forward in line of direction. Extend your right hand forward at waist level, palm facing up (to show the people sitting down the money you have taken from your pocket).	I have
	2	Step with left foot where you touched your left foot.	it!

Break: Raise arms above your head, shake handkerchiefs, and say "Hooooo."

Repeat the dance from the beginning

Style: Knees slightly bent, constantly moving the hips side to side. Lean slightly forward from the waist.

Pata Pata

South African

P*ATA* P*ATA*, PRONOUNCED *PAH-TA PAH-TA*, is a composed dance of African-type movements.

Record: Miriam Makeba, Reprise 0732, High/Scope LC 84–743–350.

Formation: Scattered, all facing music. The last phrase includes a quarter turn clockwise; therefore, each repeat faces a different wall.

Style: Many variations. Body, hand, and arm movements are very improvisational.

Steps: Touch–step, walk, heel–toe swivel.

DIRECTIONS FOR THE DANCE

Meter 4/4

Introduction: no action.

Beats

1	Beginning right, touch toe diagonally forward and snap fingers.
2	Step right beside left and clap.
3–4	Repeat beats 1 and 2 using left foot.
5	With feet close together, weight on balls of feet, turn heels out and together, elbows bent waist high, turn elbows out and in.
6	Weight on heels, turn toes out and in, hands out and in.
7–8	Repeat action of beats 5 and 6.
9	Weight on left foot, lift right knee across in front of left leg, rotating right leg in.
10	Touch right toe to right side.
11–12	Repeat action of beats 9–10.
13	Step on right foot, pivoting one–quarter turn clockwise and kick left leg forward and clap.
14–16	Facing a new wall, back up three walking steps (left, right, left.)

Tant' Hessie

South African

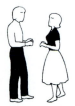

TANT' HESSIE IS A SOUTH AFRICAN dance meaning "Aunt Esther's white horse." Huig Hofman introduced this dance at the University of the Pacific Folk Dance Camp in 1962.

Record: Folkraft 337–006B, High/Scope LC 84–743–041.

Formation: Double circle, partners facing, man on the inside.

Steps: Walk, buzz step swing.

DIRECTIONS FOR THE DANCE

Meter 2/4 • Directions are the same for both man and woman.

■ *Measures*

1–4   Introduction: no action.

Part I

1–2   Beginning left, walk four steps toward partner, right shoulders adjacent to form a single circle and nod.

3–4   Take four walking steps back to place.

5–8   Repeat action of measures 1–4 with left shoulders adjacent.

Part II

9–12   Do–si–do partner passing right shoulders with eight walking steps. Eye contact and flirt.

13–25   Do–si–do partners passing left shoulders with seven walking steps. Snap fingers and engage in eye contact as passing partner.

26   Step on left foot toward partner, extend arms at shoulder height reaching upward, and yell "HEY."

Part III

27–34   Take shoulder–waist position, stepping into the swing with the right foot, lean away from partner and swing slowly with a buzz step turning clockwise. Bend knee on the step, body rises on the push step. End swing with man's back to the center of circle.

Repeat dance with a new partner on left, man moving forward to meet next woman; woman walks back to meet him on first four walking steps.

■ NOTE

1. The music suggests a slight swagger, jaunty attitude, snapping of the fingers, and flirtation. The swing is a comfortable speed to learn the buzz step. Let the body sink and rise.

2. *Tant' Hessie* is an excellent mixer and dance to use early in the program.

ALPINE REGION— SWITZERLAND, AUSTRIA, AND GERMANY

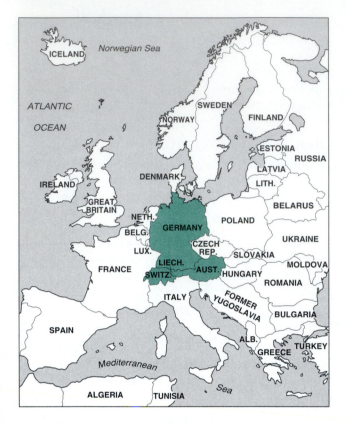

Dance Characteristics

Despite the differences in language, religion, politics, and geography, Switzerland, Austria, and Germany share many similarities in dance, particularly in the Alpine region. The most popular couple dances are the Waltz, Polka, and Schottische. The Ländler is a common dance with many variations. It is basically a courting dance in character: the man leads the woman through many figures in 3/4 or 4/4 time, and eventually the couple ends in closed position, revolving together around the dance floor. In 3/4 time, a flat–footed, even Waltz (smooth) rhythm is maintained, and it is thought to be the forerunner of the Viennese Waltz. The *Schuplatter* is also well known in the Alpine region as a part of the Ländler or as a solo dance for men. Characteristically, the men stamp their feet and slap their knees, thighs, boots, or lederhosen to the rhythm of the music. The dance originated with the woodcutters in their free time, as a possible imitation of a grouselike wild bird during mating season.

The ritual dances are danced on special occasions, particularly at carnival time. Sword dances and dance–dramas like the English ones are a part of carnival. Dance formations tend to follow the usual European patterns of Longway Sets, Quadrilles, squares, or circles.

Folk Dancing in Switzerland

By Karin Gottier, Tolland, Connecticut.

The dances of eastern Switzerland are very similar to those of alpine Germany and Austria, while the dances of the western Swiss cantons are related to those of France and in the south, to those of Italy. Most Swiss dances are couple or group dances using the steps of the popular ballroom dances of the 19th century: Mazurka, Waltz, Polka, Schottische, and Gallop. Perhaps because of the austerity of the Calvinist period, few traditional dances survived, and many of the contemporary Swiss folk dances are reconstructions based on traditional dance figures that were collected and set either to traditional tunes or to melodies especially composed for these dances. Very few ritual dances have remained, and those are usually danced at "driving out winter" ceremonies, carnival, spring and harvest celebrations, and at the time of the ascent and descent of the cattle from the high pastures. There is literary evidence that Switzerland still knew "dances of death" until the middle of the last century. One such source is Gottfried Keller. In his novel *Der grüne Heinrich*[*] he describes a funeral dance:

> We immediately hurried outside to where, on the corridor and stairs, the crowd began to pair off and form a procession, for without a partner no one was allowed to go up. I took Anna by the hand and fell into line which began to move, led by the musicians. They struck up a lugubrious mourning march, to the rhythm of which we marched three times around the attic, which had been converted into a ballroom, and formed a large circle. Hereupon seven couples stepped into the center and executed a lumbering old dance with seven figures and difficult jumps, kneefalls and intertwinings, accompanied by resounding clapping. After the spectacle had gone on for some time, the host appeared and went through the rows thanking the guests for their sympathy; here and there whispering into the ear of a young man–in such a way that all could hear–that he should not take the mourning too much to heart and to leave him (the host) now alone with his grief. Moreover, the host recommended that the youth should rejoice again in life. Whereupon he walked away and climbed down the stairs with lowered head as if they led directly to Tartarus.

---

*Gottfried Keller, *Der grüne Heinrich*, München: Wilhelm Goldmann Verlag.

The musicians suddenly switched to a gay "Hopser," the older people withdrew and the young swept shouting and stamping across the groaning floor.

In character Swiss dances are more sedate and earthbound than their German counterparts. Among folk dance groups, great emphasis is placed on precision of detail in the placement of hands and arms and in the holds between partners.

The Swiss Folk Dance movement has from its inception been a branch of the Swiss Costume Association (Schweizerische Trachtenvereinigung), which fosters and encourages the practice of all aspects of folk art. One of the pioneers in the field of Swiss Folk Dance was Luise Witzig. After having come into contact with the German and English folk dance movement, she recognized the importance of folk dance research and its significance to the work of the Costume Association. She began to conduct dance workshops in which she transmitted the results of her research work. This encouraged others to collect and notate existing material in their immediate areas. The Swiss Costume Association then made it its task to systematically collect old tunes and dance figures that were still to be found, especially in the Alpine areas. Because early researchers were able to find only fragments, many Swiss dances are reconstructions or new creations. By 1935 it was possible to publish the first collection of dance notations. Since then, this organization has released records, books, and pamphlets on the dances of all cantons. It also conducts annual folk dance leader training courses and folk dance workshops, always insisting on high standards of accuracy and precision.

Alongside the Folk Dance movement of the Swiss Costume Association, there exists the Association of Folk Dance Groups (Arbeitsgemeinschaft Schweizer Volkstanzkreise), which is a collective member in the Swiss Costume Association. This organization was formed in 1956 and consists of independent dance groups that practice all forms of European folk dancing and sponsor specialized workshops in the dances of a given country, conducted by an expert in that particular field. The objectives and practices of the Folk Dance Association are very similar to the recreational folk dance movement in the United States.

D'Hammerschmiedsg'selln German

D'HAMMERSCHMIEDSG'SELLN IS pronounced *duh-HAM-mair-shmeets-guh-sehln* and means "the journeyman blacksmith." This Bavarian dance was originally performed by men only. The intrigue of the clapping pattern has made it a popular dance. It was introduced by Huig Hofman from Belgium at Stockton, California, and Moorehead, Kentucky.

Dance A While CD: #16. "D'Hammerschmeidsg'selin."

Records: Folkraft 1458; High/Scope RM 7 and CD; LS E 19.

Cassette: High/Scope RM 7.

Formation: Set of four dancers, two couples, woman on partner's right (a) or four men, partners facing each other (b).

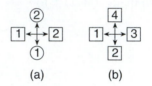

(a)   (b)

Steps: Step–Hop, Waltz.

Clap Pattern:

Counts	Two measures = 6 counts
1	Both hands slap own thighs as knees flex slightly.
2	Clap own chest, body turning slightly left.
3	Clap own hands together.
4	Opposites clap right hands.
5	Opposites clap left hands.
6	Opposites clap both hands.

DIRECTIONS FOR THE DANCE

Meter 3/4 • Directions are same for both man and woman, except when specially noted.

■ Measures

Introduction: no action.

Clap Pattern

1–16   If two couples, the men start clap pattern (count 1) and continue through measure 16. The two women start clap pattern on count 1 of measure 2 and continue through measure 16. Couple one will be on count 4, clapping opposite dancer's right hand when couple two begins. Or, if four men, man 1 and man 3 start; man 2 and man 4 start on measure 2.

Figure I. Circle

17–24	All four join hands. Beginning left, take eight step–hops, circle moving clockwise.
25–32	Reverse direction, taking eight step–hops, circle moving counterclockwise.

Clap Pattern

1–16	Repeat action of measures 1–16.

Figure II. Star

17–24	Form right-hand star. Beginning left, take eight step–hops, star revolving clockwise.
25–32	Form left-hand star. Take eight step–hops, star revolving counterclockwise.

Chorus, Clap Pattern

1–16	Repeat action of measures 1–16.

Figure III. Large Circle

17–24	Circles of four open out to form one large circle. Beginning left, take eight step–hops, circle moving clockwise.
25–32	Reverse direction, taking eight step–hops, circle moving counterclockwise.

■ VARIATION (MIXER)

1–16	Clap pattern.
17–24	Figure I or II repeat circle left or right–hand star.
25–32	Take corner for new partner. Closed position. Man beginning left, woman right, take eight Waltz steps, turning clockwise, dancing anywhere. Form a new set with a new couple to start clap pattern.

■ NOTES

1. During circle figure, arms should be firm and dancers should lean slightly back, using centrifugal force, which adds zest to the dance.
2. The inner action of partners and couples in the precision of performing the clap pattern adds to the fun–loving spirit of the dance.

Dr Gsatzlig*

Swiss

Dr Gsatzlig means "exactly" and is from Appenzell, Switzerland. Jane Farwell learned this dance there and introduced it across the United States in 1954. Later, Farwell corrected one of the figures slightly, which accounts for two different versions. Although the music is written in 2/4 meter, it has the quality of a Schottische.

Record: Folk Dancer MH 1114.

Music: L. Witzig and A. Stern Pub. Hug and Co., Zurich 12 *Schweitzer Tanze.*

Position: Closed, man's back to center of circle, man's left, woman's right arms extended toward line of direction.

Steps: Side Step, Schottische, Two–Step.

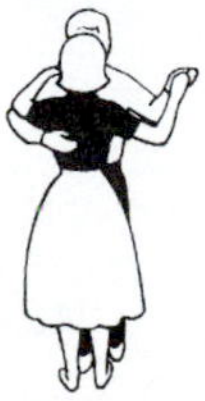

Dr Gsatzlig (continued)

*Dr. Gsatzlig included by permission of Jane Farwell, Folklore Village Farm, Dodgeville, Wisconsin.

DIRECTIONS FOR THE DANCE

Meter 2/4 • Directions are for man; woman's part reverse.

■ *Measures*

	1–4	Introduction.
	I.	**Dr Gsatzlig (Side Step)**
A	1–2	Beginning left, take four side steps forward, moving in line of direction.
	3	Take two side steps in reverse line of direction, swinging joined hands sharply down, elbow bending, upper arm shoulder high.
	4	Take two side steps in line of direction, arms extended toward line of direction. Joined hands always point in the direction traveling.
	5–8	Beginning right, repeat action of measures 1–4, traveling in reverse line of direction.
A	1–8	Repeat action of measures 1–8.
	II.	Heel and Toe Schottische
B	9	Open position. Beginning left, take one heel and toe.
	10	Take one step–close–step–close in line of direction. Weight remains on left.
	11–12	Swinging joined hands sharply down, elbow bending, upper arm shoulder high, face reverse line of direction. Beginning right, repeat action of measures 9–10, moving in reverse line of direction.
	13–16	Closed or shoulder–waist position (latter preferred). Beginning left, take four slow Two–Steps (Swiss Schottische steps) turning clockwise, progressing in line of direction.
B	9–16	Repeat action of measures 9–16.
	III.	Dr Gsatzlig (Side Step)
A	1–8	Repeat action of Figure I, measures 1–8.
	IV.	Schottische
C	17–18	Man faces line of direction, crossed arms held on chest; woman faces man, back to line of direction, hands on hips, knuckles toward body. Beginning left, take two Schottische steps (step close step–hop) (Swiss Polka) in line of direction. Both move diagonally toward center, then away from center, always progressing forward.
	19–20	Take four slow step–hops in line of direction, man stamping left on first step, woman turning clockwise twice.
	21–24	Repeat action of measures 17–20.
C	17–24	Repeat action of measures 17–24, with right hands joined, free hand on hip. The woman turns clockwise under man's raised arm.
	V.	Dr Gsatzlig
A	1–8	Repeat action of measures 1–8.

■ **ROUTINE**

AABBACCAABBACCA. The record, Folk Dancer MH 1114, allows for this sequence.

The Swiss dance movements are small and precise. Keep the steps simple without much extension of the knee or foot. The side steps are little steps; do not scrape the foot, but lift each foot. Turn head and focus eyes on the direction of travel during the side steps. The abrupt change of direction and focus of a large group is very effective. Keep free hands on hips. Keep step–hops low and subdued. Jane Farwell refers to it as a *leisurely dance*.

■ **NOTES**

1. It is fun to sing "la–la–la" during the specific tune for Dr Gsatzlig.
2. Add a few shouts "ya'hoo'hoo'hooy" any time.
3. In Switzerland, they call a Polka a Schottische and a Schottische a Polka. Since this book is used primarily by Americans, the terms *Schottische* and *Polka* as defined by Americans are used.

Kanonwalzer

German

ACCORDING TO NOTES FROM Michael Herman, *Kanonwalzer* was made from a field tape collected by Hugh Thurston. This dance is very effective for outdoor festivals and large groups and is a good closing for special parties.

Record: Folk Dancer MH 001.

Formation: Couples in several concentric circles, minimum *three* circles, hands joined. Could be adapted for no partners.

Steps: Waltz step throughout dance.

DIRECTIONS FOR THE DANCE

Meter 3/4 Directions are the same for man and woman.

■ *Measures*

No introduction

Figure I. Circle Left

1–8   Inner circle, beginning left, travel left, eight Waltz steps. Outer circles watch.

As the inner circle starts a new figure, the next circle dances the first figure. When the second circle starts the next figure, the third circle begins, dancing what the circle in front of it just finished doing, and so on.

The result is that each circle will be doing something different, always picking up the next figure from what the circle in front just did.

There is no set order of figures. Here are some suggestions.

Figure II. Circle Right

Figure III. To the Center and Back

Figure IV. Man Kneels, Woman Dances Around Man

Kanonwalzer (continued)

Figure V. Woman Kneels, Man Dances Around Woman

Figure VI. Back Grasp Hold, turn clockwise 4 or 8 Waltz steps and counter clockwise 4 or 8 Waltz steps. On right and left elbow, turn.

Figure VII. Join Right Hands, woman twirls under raised arms as man travels around the outside.

Figure VIII. Standing in Place, patty–cake clapping with partner.

Figure IX. All Dancers Travel to the Center and Out.

Note: It is a good idea to circle left and right between figures to make it easier for the outer rings to follow.

Krüz König*

German

"KRÜZ KÖNIG" IS A GERMAN dialect expression for *Kreuz König*, which means "king of clubs." Heinrich Dieckelmann, a German folkdancer and pianist, composed the tune and made a present of it to his friend Ludwig Burkhardt in 1924. Burkhardt immediately contacted Folk Dance groups in Hamburg and Berlin for ideas. Four couples in a square was very common in northern Germany. There was a desire for dances with more vivacity and more difficult figures. One day the dance was born, with no claim to steps or figures of ancient origin. Krüz König was a new Folk Dance. Ludwig Burkhardt was well known for his leadership in teaching German Folk Dance to young people and teachers and for his early publications of German Folk Dance. He described his dance in *Kneveler, das Tanzbuch mit "Krüz-König,"* Bärenreiter Verlag Kassel, 1927.

> **Record:** "Folk Dancer" MH 1022 or "Tanz" SP 23 030.
>
> **Music:** Herman, Michael, *Folk Dances for All,* p. 89.
>
> **Formation:** Set of two couples facing, woman to right of partner, hands joined in a circle of four.
>
> **Steps:** Running steps, step–hop steps, Mazurka steps, Achtervör steps: step left foot to left, step right foot close behind left, step left foot to left and right across left. **Note:** This is like a grapevine step, but is *not leaped.* It is danced very close to the ground.

Key to symbols:

Man facing forward □

Woman facing forward ○

DIRECTIONS FOR THE DANCE

Meter 3/8

■ *Measures*

1–4   Introduction: no action.

---

*Krüz König directions translated by Karin Gottier, Tolland, CT.

Figure I. Circle of Four

1–4	Beginning left, circle left with one Achtervör step and eight running steps.
5–8	Repeat measures 1–4.

Figure II. Wings

1–8 repeat	Partners take conversation position. Men hook left elbows to form a line of four. Formation turns counterclockwise with 24 running steps. At the end of this figure, men release hold and women take a small step to the right to face center.

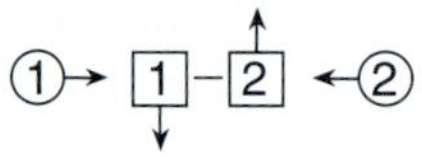

$$①→ \boxed{1}-\overset{\uparrow}{\underset{\downarrow}{\boxed{2}}} ←②$$

Figure III. Straight Chain

9–10	With two step–hops men change places by giving left hands. Women dance two step–hops in place. Each man is now facing the opposite woman.

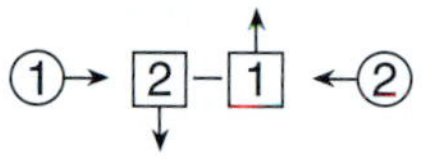

$$①→ \boxed{2}-\overset{\uparrow}{\underset{\downarrow}{\boxed{1}}} ←②$$

11–12	With two step–hops men change places with women by giving right hands. The women are now on the inside of the set.

$$\boxed{2}→ ①-\overset{\uparrow}{\underset{\downarrow}{②}} ←\boxed{1}$$

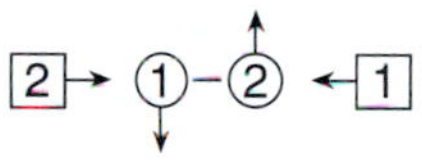

13–14	With two step–hops women change places by giving left hands to each other while men dance two step–hops in place. Women are now facing their original partners.

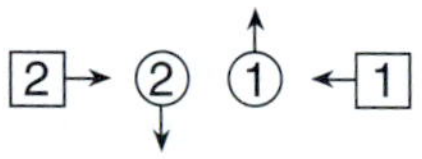

$$\boxed{2}→ ②\ \overset{\uparrow}{\underset{\downarrow}{①}} ←\boxed{1}$$

15–16	Original partners give right hands and change places with two–step hops. Men are now on the inside of the set.

$$②→ \boxed{2}-\overset{\uparrow}{\underset{\downarrow}{\boxed{1}}} ←①$$

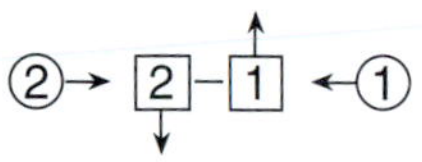

9–14 repeat	Repeat measures 9–14 returning to original place. Women are still on the inside.

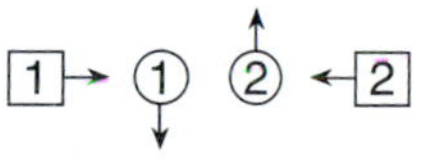

$$\boxed{1}→ ①\ \overset{\uparrow}{\underset{\downarrow}{②}} ←\boxed{2}$$

Krüz König (continued)

| 15–16 repeat | With extended right–hand grasp, man pulls partner with momentum and half–turn counterclockwise to his right side to place. At the same time, men release women's right hand and take their left. All join hands to form a circle of four. |
| | **Note:** This figure should be executed with well–stretched arms and a large floor pattern. |

Figure IV. Circle of Four, Circle of Two with Mazurka

17–20	Beginning left, all dance four Mazurka steps clockwise. Release hold with corner.
21–22	Take two–hand hold with partner. Continue to turn clockwise with two Mazurka steps.
23–24	Without changing hold or direction, couples turn twice clockwise with six running steps.
17–22 repeat	Repeat four Mazurka steps in circle of four and two Mazurka steps turning with partner.
23–24 repeat	Repeat the six running steps turning partner; however, turn only once with three running steps and change to a right–hand hold. Men lead their partners to the center with right arms well extended, so that women stand in the center *right shoulder to right shoulder*, facing in opposite directions. Men take corner woman's left hand in their own left.

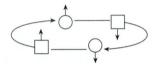

Figure V. "King of Clubs"

25–28	**Women on inside:** The two men run 12 steps clockwise, turning the two women, who form the center axis, with them.
29–32	**Men on inside:** Left hand is released. With six running steps, man leads woman by the right hand outward to his place, taking her place in the center, standing right shoulder to right shoulder with the opposite man. Each woman takes the left hand of corner man into her own.
	They run clockwise with six steps, turning the men, who form the axis of the formation, with them.

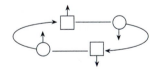

| 25–28 repeat | **Women on inside:** With six running steps women release left–hand hold and lead their partners by the right hand outward, taking men's place in the center. Both men take left hand of corner woman in own left and continue to turn the set clockwise with six running steps. |

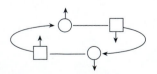

| 29–32 repeat | **Men on inside:** Repeat measures 29–32 with women dancing on the outside and men on the inside. During the last measure, men make half a jump-turn clockwise and join hands in a circle of four. Men will have their original partner on their left and the corner woman, who is now their new partner, on their right. The dance is repeated one more time with the new partner. |

Styling note: The last figure should be danced with well-stretched arms. Dancers on the outside of the formation need to pull away from center of the set with their left arms. All stand very tall. In circle figures, the momentum is established by pulling away from the center of the set, or from partner. The character of the entire dance is one of restrained energy and controlled strength.

Man in the Hay

German

MAN IN THE HAY IS danced to the tune of an old German folk song "A Farmer had a Pretty Wife." The song is well known in Scandinavia.

Dance A While CD: #3. "Man in the Hay."

Records: Folk Dancer MH 1051; High/Scope RM 3 LP and compact disc.

Cassette: High/Scope RM 3, Folk Dancer MH 1051, Folkraft 1051.

Music: Burchenal, E., *Folk Dances of Germany*, p. 28.

Formation: Set of four couples in Square Dance formation.

Steps: Skip, slide.

DIRECTIONS FOR THE DANCE

Meter 6/8 • Directions are same for woman and man, except when specially noted.

■ Measures

	1–4	Introduction: All join hands and swing arms forward and back briskly, standing in place. The movement is small and staccato. Keep elbows straight and stand in close formation.
	I.	**Circle**
A	1–16	Beginning left, take 16 skips clockwise. Repeat counterclockwise.
		Chorus
B	9–10	Head couples take closed position. Man beginning left, woman right, take three slides to center and pause or stamp.
	11–12	Man beginning right, woman left, take three slides back to place and pause or stamp.
	13–16	Man beginning left, woman right, take six slides across set to opposite side, men passing back to back. Step left, bring right foot to left and hold. Do not turn.

Man in the Hay (continued)

| | 17–20 | | Repeat action of measures 13–16, returning to home position, woman passing back to back. Man leads with right foot, woman left. |
| | 9–20 | | Side couples repeat action of measures 9–20, B. |

		II.	**Women's Circle**
A	1–8		Four women join hands in circle. Beginning left, take 16 skips clockwise. Men clap.
			Chorus
B	9–20		Repeat action of measures 9–20, 9–20, B.
	9–20		

		III.	**Men Circle**
A	1–8		Four men join hands in circle. Beginning left, take 16 skips clockwise. Women clap.
			Chorus
B	9–20		Repeat action of measures 9–20, 9–20, B.
	9–20		

		IV.	**Basket**
A	1–8		Head couples form circle, men's arms around women's waists, women's arms around men's shoulders. Beginning left, take 16 skips or slides clockwise. A brisk buzz step may be used here with the right foot in front of the left and so vigorous the women are swept from their feet. Keep basket hold firm and lean back.
			Chorus
B	9–20		Repeat action of measures 9–20, 9–20, B.
	9–20		

		V.	**Basket**
A	1–8		Side couples repeat action of Figure IV, measures 1–8, A.
			Chorus
B	9–20		Repeat action of measures 9–20, 9–20, B.
	9–20		

| | | **VI.** | **Circle** |
| A | 1–8 | | Take 14 skips clockwise and end with a bow to the center of the circle with hands still joined. |

■ VARIATION

Arrange all the squares so that they are directly behind and beside another square, so that the couples may slide through several squares and return to original position during the chorus.

Measures 13–16, B, man beginning left, woman right, take eight slides across set and on through as many sets as they can go, men passing back to back. Measures 17–20, B, repeat action of measures 13–16, returning home, women passing back to back.

1. Eshatt ein Bauer ein schönes Weib,
   die blieb so gerne zu Haus,
   sie bat oft ihren lieben Mann,
   er sollte doch fahren ins Heu,
   er sollte doch fahren ins Heu,
   er sollte doch fahren ins
   ha ha ha, ha ha ha,
   Heu, juch hei, juch hei, juch hei,
   er sollte doch fahren ins Heu.

2. Der Bauer dachte in seinem Sinn:
   Die Reder, die sind mir gut!
   Ich will mich hinter das Haustor stelln,
   will sehr, was sie wohl tut.
   Will sagen, ich fahre ins Heu.
   etc.

3. Da kommt geschlichen ein Reiters–
   knecht, zum jungen Weibe hinein,
   und sie umfängt gar freundlich ihn,
   gab stracks ihren Willen darein.
   Mein Mann ist gefahren ins Heu.

4. Er faste sie um ihr Gürtelband,
   und schwang sie hin und her;
   der Mann, der hinter dem Haustor
   stand, ganz zornig trat er hervor:
   Ich bin nicht gefahren ins Heu!

5. Ach, trauter, herzallerliebster Mann,
   vergib mir diesen Fehl!
   Ich will ja herzen und lieben dich,
   will kochen dir Mus und Mehl.
   Ich dachte, du wärest ins Heu.

6. Und wenn ich gleich gefahren wär
   ins Heu und Haberstroh,
   so sollst du nun und nimmermehr
   einen andern lieben also.
   Da fahre der Teufel ins Heu!

1. A farmer had a pretty wife who was so happy to stay at home and who encouraged him to go out and work in the Hay.

2. One day he thought to himself "Aha! I will hide behind the door and see what she does. I will tell her I'm going to work in the Hay."

3. Then a stable boy came steathily in to the young wife, who greeted him most warmly, saying "My man is away in the Hay."

4. He grasped her around the waist and whirled her 'round and 'round; the husband standing behind the door entered in a rage, saying "I didn't go to the Hay!"

5. Ach, beloved husband forgive me this error! I will love and cherish you and will cook you porrage and jam. I thought you were in the hay.

6. (Husband:) And ever if I were away in the Hay, never shall you love another one. Then the devil would go into the Hay!

Sonderburg Doppelquadrille

German

SONDERBURG DOPPELQUADRILLE IS A German variant of the Danish dance based on the dance description (Dunsing and Dunsing 1946) by Paul and Gretel Dunsing.

Records: Folkraft 1163; World of Fun LP 4, Side B–1.

Music: Dunsing, Gretel and Paul, *Dance Lightly*, p. 16.

Formation: Two lines facing each other, four couples in each line. Head couples are two couples on each side of line nearest head of set. Foot couples are two couples on each side of line forming remainder of set.

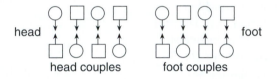

Steps: Walk, Polka.

DIRECTIONS FOR THE DANCE

Meter 2/4 • Directions are same for man and woman, except when specially noted.

■ Measures

I. Two Circles

1–16   Head couples and foot couples join hands and form two separate circles. Beginning left, take 16 walking steps to left, circle moving clockwise; then take 16 walking steps to right, circle moving counterclockwise, ending in original formation (two lines).

II. Heads Down Center

17–24   Head four join inside hands with opposite dancer and take eight walking steps moving down center of set (toward foot) and on eighth step turn individually to face reverse line of direction. Join inside hands and take eight walking steps forward to return to place.

25–32   Foot four repeat action of measures 17–24, moving toward head of set and back to place.

III. Four Circles

17–32   Opposite couples join hands. Take 16 walking steps, moving to left, and take 16 walking steps moving to right, ending in original position.

        IV.   Chain

33–40   Opposite couples execute grand right and left in small circles, four dancers each. Opposite dancers join right hands, pass, left hand to partner, and so forth, ending in place and bowing to partner.

41–48   Repeat action of measures 33–40.

        V.   Polka

33–48   Couples take closed position or shoulder–waist position. Man beginning left, woman right, take 16 Polka steps turning clockwise, progressing in line of direction around oval circle formed by two lines, back to place.

■ **VARIATION**

Measures 33–40, opposite couples may execute right and left through across the set, then back to place, instead of grand right and left.

Spinnradl zu Dritt*   Austrian

Various forms of this dance were collected in the Alpine regions of Bavaria, Austria, and the German settlement areas of Czechoslovakia. The most widely danced variant was collected by Hermann Derschmidt in 1924 in Klaffer, Upper Austria, and published by him and Erna Schützenberger in their five–part collection, *Spinnradl-unser Tanzbuch.*

Record: Tanz EP 58 129, "Osterreichische Tänze"; Tanz EP 58 118, "Volkstänze aus dem Sudetenland," series I; Folkraft 1474.

Formation: One man between two women. He holds their outside hands, while they join their inside hands behind his back. All face line of direction, left shoulder to the center. Arms are loosely stretched.

Steps: "Dreierschritt" (triple-walking step): a smooth, unaccented walk in 3/4 time. One triple-walking step requires three walking steps. Jump, light running steps.

DIRECTIONS FOR THE DANCE

Meter 3/4

■ *Measures*

1–4   Introduction

1–8   Beginning left, all move forward with eight triple–walking steps. These steps are danced close to the ground, smoothly and unaccented. Man looks alternately at the left and right woman.

9   On count 1, man pulls women forward. As their joined hands pass over his head, he bends his knees briefly and immediately stands up again. The

Spinnradl zu Dritt (continued)

*Spinnradl zu Dritt directions translated by Karin Gottier, Tolland, CT.

joined hands of the women are now in front of him. On counts 2 and 3 the right woman turns once counterclockwise with two steps. She now stands between the man and left woman. (All hands should be held closed together. *Do not* release hold.)

10   As man and left woman form arch by lifting their joined hands, right woman slips under the arch by bending her knees briefly on count one. She continues moving to the right side of man. On counts 2 and 3 the left woman begins to make a clockwise turn.

11   While left woman continues to turn under her own arm to the right on count 1, the man begins to turn left on counts 2 and 3. All are back to the beginning position.

12–14   Repeat measures 9–11. This time the left woman slips through the arch, which is formed by man and right woman. The right woman turns out counterclockwise and the man clockwise.

15   All move forward with three short, light running steps.

16   All execute a *silent*, soft jump on both feet. Repeat measures 9–16.

Note: *At no time do the dancers back up.* The action moves forward over the head of the turning person. The movements of measures 9–16 flow into each other. The dancers do not remain in place but continue to move slightly forward in the line of direction. The character of the dance is smooth and flowing. The steps are danced close to the ground with no accent. The jump is soft, elastic, and silent.

Hermann Derschmidt writes in the collection *Spinnradl-unser Tanzbuch* "the man must see that the 'ducking under' does not occur backwards, rather through the pulling of joined hands over head by the other two partners . . . the 'ducking under' must occur exactly on the first count, during the second and third count each partner in turn prepares to duck under" (Erna Schützenberger and Hermann Derschmidt, *Spinnradl-unser Tanzbuch*, p. 15, Musikverlag Josef Preissler, Munich, 1974).

BALKAN COUNTRIES

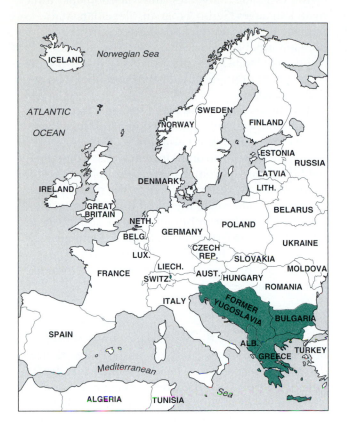

■ Introduction

The Balkan Peninsula includes the former Yugoslavia grouping of Croatia, Bosnia, and Serbia along with Bulgaria, Greece, and Albania. Originally occupied by Slavic tribes, the area has seen a steady flow of outside influences, including Greeks, Romans, Crusaders, and Turks. Different areas have come under the influence of pagan, Roman Catholic, Greek Orthodox, Bulgarian Orthodox, and Moslem religions. As different countries have emerged from Ottoman Turkish control, boundaries have been established and national unification developed.

The Balkan Peninsula is rich in folk art, music, dance, and tradition. The fact that these countries have remained more agrarian for a longer period of time than other western European countries has made it possible to visit villages in remote areas and find people still wearing their native dress daily and performing traditional dances.

The Folk Dance tradition is a living one. The Sunday hora, a social get-together including dance, is a common custom in small and large communities. Each village has one or several places set aside for a dance: the square, the threshing circle, a barn or a hall for inclement weather, the wide porch of a home, or a level clearing or meadow.

The *Chain Dance* (circle), open or closed, is the common dance among the Balkans, but it is referred to by different terms and with different spellings (*Kolo*, Serbia; *Hora*, Romania; *Horo*, Bulgaria; *Oro*, Macedonia; and *Xopos*, Greece [pronounced *hó-rohs*]). The same words are used for the social occasion and the dance. There are many old tunes and songs for the Hora, and newly composed tunes still use the complex rhythms that are associated with Balkan music. The rhythm of the songs relates to the length of syllables and goes back to Greek poetry and drama.

Some of the dances originated with the craft guilds; for example, the *Butcher's Dance*, the *Shepherd's Dance*, and the *Tailor's Dance*. Others were named for the place of their origin, and the ritual dances frequently were related to pagan ceremonies that were adapted to another religion. Originally, the chains were for men or women alone. The men's movement is more exuberant and dynamic, and the opportunity for the leader to show off is always present. Women have traditionally kept their movement more restrained, with feet closer to the floor and eyes downcast.

Such couple dances as the Waltz, Schottische, and Polka did not begin to appear until after 1876, when the Western style began to influence the peasant dances. Today, it is common to include Kolos (Horos) with the Ballroom Dances.

■ Greece

DANCE CHARACTERISTICS

Dance was a common theme on ancient vases and many frescoes in Byzantine monasteries. The Greek word *chorus* means dance. The chorus in the tragedies sang and danced. The continuity of dance tradition among the Greeks persists through their history, through ancient Greece, Byzantium, 400 years of slavery to the Turks, the uprisings, the establishment of Greece as a sovereign kingdom, the European influence, and the social and political reforms following World Wars I and II.

Greek dance has always been an integral part of the people's lives. It is characterized by the display of human emotions, expressing great joy, exuberance, sorrow, aspirations, and hopes. It is a living tradition that may be found at cafés, bars, and religious celebrations, wherever people meet.

Modern Folk Dancing in Greece can be classified in a variety of ways. One is according to rhythm. There are the *Syrtos* or *Kalamatianos*, 7/8 meter; the *Tsamiko*, 3/4 meter; and the *Hasápikos* (sometimes referred to as the Butcher's Dance), 2/4 meter. Some Folk Dances are remnants of ritual drama, such as the survival of the hobby horse during carnival. Sometimes they are classified according to formation: circular, pair, or solo.

Most of the dances follow the circle or the broken circle formation; although men and women used to dance alone, they now dance together without partners. In the broken circle, the leader (traditionally a man, unless it is a women's dance) is on the right-hand end, holding two handkerchiefs, one in his right hand, away from the body, to wave and signal variations in step, and the other joining the leader to the next person in the line. The leader improvises steps in time with the music, displaying his ingenuity and skill. As the leader, he encourages the group to become one as they keep the basic step going. In small villages, the leader may use this opportunity to display his personality to the opposite sex. The element of competition among leaders is always present, as one attempts to surpass another. A second dancer can join the leader in improvisation. Occasionally the leader moves to the opposite end and the next person in line becomes the leader.

The body is firm and upright. The women traditionally move in a simple and dignified manner, with footwork close to the ground and eyes downcast. The man is more exuberant in his dance style, leaping, twisting, and turning, but always in time to the basic rhythm. The different regions have definite styles and traditions.

MUSIC

Greek folk music is a monophonic mixture of ancient Greek scales and Byzantine church music. Only the music of the Ionian Islands reflects Western music. Usually the rhythms are 5/4 or 5/8, 7/8, or 9/8 (which are the rhythms of the tragedies). The dance steps are slow and quick, corresponding to the length of syllables of words, rather than to the beat. Musical meter was based on poetic meter.

The dances are performed with the accompaniment of the dancers' singing or folk instruments. The string instruments are the lyra, the violin, the lute, the santouri (dulcimer), the mandolin, and the bouzouki. The wind instruments are the pipiza, the comemusa, the clarinet, the pastoral flutes, the gaida (bagpipe), and the zurna. The percussion instruments include drums, bells, triangles, défi (small tambourines), krotala (wooden spoons), and finger cymbals.

The musicians, not more than four or five, usually stood in the middle of the dancers and responded to the mood of the occasion. Certain instruments and combinations were typical of specific regions.

■ Former Yugoslavia

DANCE CHARACTERISTICS

In 1945, the Federal Republic of Yugoslavia was established. It was comprised of six republics (Serbia, Croatia, Slovenia, Macedonia, Montenegro, and Bosnia–Hercegovina) and was surrounded by seven nations (Austria, Hungary, Romania, Bulgaria, Greece, Albania, and Italy); it included four nationalities (Serbs, Croatians, Slovenics, and Macedonians), three main languages (Serbo Croatian, Slovenian, Macedonian), three main religions (Eastern Orthodox, Roman Catholic, and Moslem), and two alphabets (Latin and Cyrillic). The great diversity that this represents speaks dramatically for the turmoil of this section of Europe.

The music, dance, and art of this area have much in common. The Kolo is danced in all parts of the former Yugoslavia, but variations exist because of past influences. In strong Moslem areas, women may not be visible; in Croatia, Slovenia, and North Serbia, as the result of Western influence, the men and women may alternate; the silent Kolos have resulted from the Turkish prohibition of native song; and where the Austro–Hungarian Empire dominated the northern section, the influence of the Catholic Church and the church calendar and Western music and dance are seen.

STYLE

The Kolos combine the Slavic dance traits of liveliness, gaiety, quickness, and gymnastic footwork. The dancers are relaxed from head to foot. The leader frequently carries a handkerchief, waving it to signal step changes or in rhythm to the music. The leader passes it to the next person to relinquish the position.

Serbia emerged as a nation at the end of the seventh century. The clans were fighting each other within; the Greek church and the Roman Catholic Church each were struggling for domination in the Balkans; and the Turks, Russians, and Austrians were pressing from the outside. The Serbian culture is rich with much influence from Turkey. Serbian dances usually move to the right. The steps are quite small, the upper body is "quiet," with most action below the knee. The soft leather, moccasin–type shoe, called *opanci*, allows for the rolling forward and backward action of the foot.

Macedonia is divided into three parts. Of the total population, 40 percent are Macedonian, 50 percent Greek–Macedonian, and 10 percent Bulgarian–Macedonian. Located in the high mountains, the people are separated by streams and rivers; yet they share common traditions. Rich in timber, wheat, and minerals, Macedonia controls the route from central Europe down the valleys to the Aegean Sea. Enemies have always desired Macedonia because of this pathway.

MUSIC

The tone of the music of this region reflects intense feelings from sadness to gaiety. Occasionally a dancer will shout, expressing momentary emotion. The basic instruments are the svrala or frula (shepherd's pipe), the gaida (bagpipe), the gusle (fiddle), and the drum.

■ Bulgaria

DANCE CHARACTERISTICS

Although the area was originally occupied by Slavic tribes, the Bulgars, a Finno–Ugrian nomadic tribe, became established. Eventually the Slavic princes were driven out, but the ancient Slavic culture persisted, including the language, as the Bulgars settled and intermarried. Bulgarian music and dance reflect the influence of Greece, the Roman Empire, and the Ottoman Empire. Yet, in the mountainous regions, dance and rituals exist that show little influence of the invaders and are almost identical to those of Yugoslavia and southeast Russia.

The social aspect of Bulgarian dance tradition is a part of the Sunday Horos, festivals, and country fairs. The customs (Joukowsky 1965) and dance are closely interrelated. The Chain Dances (Horos) are the most popular. The Bulgarians dance with "devotion and dignity" and in general appear solemn as they move through complex rhythms. The upper body is "quiet," with most of the action in the feet. The skillful dancer is very light on his or her feet, almost "not touching the ground." The footwork is very precise. One word in the name of a dance frequently describes the character of the dance, for example, Tropanko Horo (stamped). There is great variety in steps, and the opportunity for the dancer to improvise and add personality is inherent. Although most Horos move to the right, some move to the left; some move forward and backward with slight movement to the right or left. The tempos vary from slow to fast.

Through the names of Horos, it is suggested that the dance may be of Bulgarian, Romanian, or Turkish origin. Over the years, the Horos have changed to meet the dancing tastes of the people of specific places and times. The Chain Dances used to follow very definite forms (closed, broken, led from one or two ends, straight line dance, crooked, and so on).

There are also solo and couple dances, *Ruchenitsa* being the most common and the liveliest.

STYLE

Different styles are associated with different regions. In southwest Bulgaria, the dances are small stepped and lively; in the north, they are more free, with humor and gaiety. The Thracian dances are slower and more solemn and yet they are punctuated with stamps; the Drobrudza dances display more emotion, with the dancer's whole body moving at a moderate tempo and knees slightly bent.

Then there are the ritual dances. Some relate to nature, emphasizing the belief in the magic that certain dances are said to hold; others relate to religious holidays, marriage, and so forth. In Bulgaria, carnival dances and customs occur the week preceding Lent and at other feast days in the year.

It is only recently that modern Ballroom Dancing has reached the villages.

MUSIC

Singing, mostly by women, while dancing the Horo is very common. The words express a wide range of moods. In some areas, diaphonal songs are common, two or three singing and then two or thee others responding. Sometimes the folk instruments in various combinations are used as accompaniment. The instruments include three kinds, wind instruments like the gaida (bagpipe), various pipes, and the common whistle; string instruments like the gudulka, the gusla (a mandolin type), and the lute; and percussion instruments, including various sizes of drums and tympans. In place of folk instruments, orchestras of clarinets, violins, and drums are becoming popular, as is the use of military bands in small villages.

The most common meter is 2/4. But Bulgarian rhythms of unequal beats (5/16, 7/16, 9/16, and 11/16 meter) are characteristic of their music.

Hasápikos

Greek

ASÁPIKOS MEANS "BUTCHER'S DANCE." Whereas the Americans call this dance Hasápikos, the Greeks refer to it as *Serviko* and reserve the word *Hasápikos* for the slow Hasápiko. This dance, known by different names, is common throughout the Balkans, the character of the variations differing.

Records: Festival 3513; Folk Dancer MH 4052; Folkraft 1021 "The Paro," Folkraft LP 3 and 8; High/Scope RM 4, LP and compact disc; Worldtone 10025.

Cassette: High/Scope RM 4.

Formation: Broken circle, arms extended, resting on adjacent dancer's shoulder (right in back of adjacent dancer's left), *T* position.

Steps: Walk, slide, step swing.

DIRECTIONS FOR THE DANCE

Meter 2/4

■ *Measures*

| | I. | **Basic Step** |

1   Line always progresses to right. Beginning right, step to right, step left behind right.

2–3   Take two step swings, stepping right, then left, in place.

Variation

1   Cross in front and step–hop swing: Beginning right, step right, step left, crossing in front of right.

2–3   Take two step–hop swings in place.

II. **Turn**

1   Release arms, raise overhead, and, beginning right, take two walking steps, making one complete turn clockwise. Resume *T* position.

2–3   Repeat action of basic step, measures 2–3.

III. **Progressive Turn**

1   Leader makes one turn while others in line dance basic step.

2–3   Repeat action of basic step, measures 2–3.

1–3   Leader and second dancer make one turn and then two step swings, while others dance basic step. Each time the next dancer joins the dancers turning until the whole line is turning on measure 1. Or the leader may call "oli" ("all turn") after two or three dancers are turning with the leader.

IV. **Slide**

1–3   Beginning right, take six slides (two per measure) in line of direction. Toward end of musical phrase, take smaller steps to change pace back to basic step.

	V.	**Slide–Step Swing**
1		Beginning right, take two slides, moving in line of direction.
2–3		Take two step swings in place.
	VI.	**Leap Pas de Basque**
1		Beginning right, leap to right, leap left behind right.
2–3		Take two pas de basque steps in place.
	VII.	**Twisting Step**
1		Moving to right, feet together, weight on heels, pivot toes to right side (count 1) weight on toes, pivot heels to right (count 2). Knees slightly bent, body twists with each pivot.
		Repeat action as long as desired.
	VIII.	**Skip Pas de Basque**
1		Face slightly right. Beginning right, take two skipping steps in line of direction.
2–3		Face center. Hop left slightly and take two pas de basque steps in place.

- **NOTES**
    1. The Greeks in the cafés cross in front and the Folk Dancers cross behind.
    2. The leader indicates the order of figures.
    3. The leader holds a kerchief in his or her right hand, arm raised, elbow bent, hand about the level of head, and signals change by twirling the kerchief.

- **STYLE**

The dancer's movement responds to the music. The step swing is more of a step lift, the knee bending slightly and straightening (body rises slightly) on the step. If the leader is a man, he shows his virtuosity by performing fancy acrobatic steps in time with the music, still leading the line. They are not as vigorous as Tsamiko.

Lesnoto

Macedonian

LESNOTO, OR *LESNO*, IS A COMMON dance type in the regions of Macedonia and former Yugoslavia. Prior to World War II, the Macedonians traditionally danced it in separate lines; one for men and one for women. Currently, men and women dance together, particularly in the city, and when only the basic steps are performed.

Records: FEZ 701; Folk Dancer MH 3037; Folkraft 1552; Folkraft LP–25, Side A, Band 5.

Formation: Broken circle, hands joined, held at shoulder height, *W* position.

Steps: Walk, step swing.

Lesnoto (continued)

DIRECTIONS FOR THE DANCE

Meter 7/8 • Directions are same for man and woman.

■ *Measures*

I. Basic Pattern

1   Face slightly right. Line travels right. Beginning right, step right (slow), lifting left knee across right (quick); step left diagonally to right (crossing in front of right foot) (quick).

2   Facing center, step right sideward to right, bending knee slightly, body rises as leg straightens (slow); men lift left knee in front so that thigh is parallel to ground (quick, quick); women lift left foot just off the ground and touch toe lightly in front of right foot.

3   Step left sideward to left, bending knee slightly, and body rises as leg straightens (slow); men lift right knee in front so that thigh is parallel to ground (quick, quick); women lift right foot just off the ground and touch toe lightly in front of left foot.

■ *Variations*

II. Turn

1   Release hand hold. Turning once clockwise, step right to side, pivoting to face out of circle (slow) step left, pivoting to face the center of the circle (quick, quick). Line continues to travel right. Men crouch slightly while turning. Rejoin hands.

2–3   Repeat action of measures 2–3 of the basic pattern.

III. Squat (Men Only)

1   Repeat action of measure 1 of the basic pattern.

2   Facing center, men squat with weight on balls of both feet, almost sitting on heels; knees face forward (slow), body rises, weight on right, lifting left knee as in basic pattern, measure 2 (quick, quick).

3   Squat with weight on balls of both feet (slow), body rises, weight on left, lifting right knee as in basic pattern, measure 3 (quick, quick).

IV. Combination

1–3   Variations II and III may be combined with both men and women turning on measure 1; and on measures 2–3, men dance squats and women dance the basic pattern.

V. Step–Hop

If the tempo is fast, add a step–hop on measures 2–3 with the knee lift.

■ NOTES

1. No introduction. Start dancing at the beginning of a phrase.
2. The variations may be introduced in any order at the discretion of the leader.

■ STYLE

When men and women dance in same line and join hands shoulder level, with right elbow bent downward and right palm facing upward, holding next dancer's left hand, left arm is held diagonally out to left side, with left palm facing downward and held by next dancer's right hand. Men (only) form separate line, using a shoulder hold; women use hold described above. Leader on right end holds handkerchief in right hand above head for signaling changes. The step is very simple; the subtlety of body movement reflects the Macedonian interpretation of the music and mood. The following suggestions will enable dancers to "catch the flavor" of the dance:

1. Hold the hands in the *W* position, slightly in front.

2. The footwork in Macedonia is light, close to the ground; not really bouncy or on "tippy toe."

3. In measures 2–3, during step lift of knee, there is a subtle double bounce following the step. The knee flexes slightly twice after the step. Cue: Slow quick quick, slow quick quick. Step flex flex, step flex flex.

4. Leader signals the variations by waving a handkerchief in a circle above head, anticipating a variation. To signal the turn, the right hand moves in front of the chest on the step left, swing right. This cues the line that a Two–Step turn follows.

Misirlou

Greek-American

THE ORIGIN OF *MISIRLOU* IS most interesting inasmuch as it originated at Duquesne University in Pittsburgh (Holden and Vouras 1965). In 1945, Professor Brunhilde Dorsch, hoping to find a Greek dance for a program, contacted a Greek–American student, Mercine Nesotas, who taught several Greek dances to the dance group. The group enjoyed the dance *Syrtos Haniotikos* the most; Miss Nesotas called it the Kritikos. Because the appropriate music was not available, someone suggested that the steps be adapted to a slower piece of music, Misirlou. This dance was taught by Monty Mayo of Pittsburgh at Oglebay Folk Dance Camp, Wheeling, West Virginia, in 1948. It is danced all over the world now–even by Greeks.

Record: Folkraft 1060; High/Scope RM 8 LP and compact disc; Festival 4804, 3505 (Vocal).

Cassettes: Dancecraft 162006; High/Scope RM 8.

Music: "Misirlou," by M. Roubanis, Colonial Music Publishing Company, 168 West 23rd Street, New York, NY.

Formation: One large broken circle, hands joined, lead dancers at right end of line.

Steps: Two–Step, grapevine.

DIRECTIONS FOR THE DANCE

Meter 4/4

■ *Measures*

1   Beginning right, step in place (count 1). Hold (count 2). Pointing left toe in front of right, describe an arc to left toward right heel (counts 3–4). Circle moves counterclockwise.

2   Step left behind right (count 1). Step right to side (count 2). Step left across in front of right (count 3), and pivot counterclockwise a half–turn on left to face reverse line of direction (count 4).

Misirlou (continued)

3   Beginning right and moving clockwise, take one Two–Step.

4   Step back on left (count 1). Step right to side, body facing center (count 2). Step left across in front of right (count 3). Hold (count 4).

▪ **NOTE**

The dancer at the right end of the broken circle leads the line in serpentine fashion, coiling it counterclockwise, then reversing and uncoiling it clockwise, while executing the dance pattern.

▪ **VARIATION**

Measure 4: Beginning left, take one Two–Step backward, moving counterclockwise, and on last step pivot right on ball of left foot to face center.

Pljeskavac Kolo*

Serbian

P*LJESKAVAC KOLO,* PRONOUNCED *PLYE-skah-vahts KO-lo,* means "clapping Kolo." It is a Serbian Folk Dance, a quick, easy, and charming introduction to the Kolo.

Dance A While CD: #12. "Pljeskavac Kolo."

Records: Canadian MH 1009; Carousel Cr–701 (45 EP); Folk Dancer MH 1009; Folkraft 1548, Festival 4817.

Cassette: Dancecraft DC 387.

Formation: Broken circle, joined hands held down.

Steps: Walk, stamp.

DIRECTIONS FOR THE DANCE

Meter 2/4

▪ *Measures*

I.   Walk, Step in Place

1   Beginning right, take two walking steps (slow, slow) diagonally forward. Circle moves counterclockwise.

2   Beginning right, take three steps (quick, quick, slow) pivoting one–half turn to left (slow).

3   Beginning left, take two walking steps backward (slow, slow). Circle continues to move counterclockwise.

4   Beginning left, take three steps (quick, quick, slow) pivoting one–half turn to right (slow) to face line of direction.

1–4   Repeat action of measures 1–4.

*Dance arranged from the dance description by Michael Herman and reproduced here by permission of Folk Dance House, New York.

II.   Stamps and Claps

5–6   Face center. Beginning right, take two walking steps (slow, slow) toward center. Stamp three times right, left, right (quick, quick, quick).

7–8   Beginning left, take two walking steps (slow, slow) backward, away from center. Clap hands three times (quick, quick, quick).

5–8   Beginning right, repeat action of measures 5–8.

▪ NOTES

1. Each walking step is done with a bounce and tremble of the entire body.
2. The leader may use a skip step instead of a walking step. Dancers follow the leader and use skip step too.
3. Spontaneous Kolo shouts ("Veselo" . . . "hoopat svp–hup, hup, hup, tss, tss, tss," . . . or "ceceya") add to the interest of this dance.

Rumunjsko Kolo   Serbian-American

Records: Folk Dancer MH 1010; Folkraft 1402; Festival 4811.

Formation: Broken circle, joined hands held down.

Steps: Schottische, rock, stamp, step–hop.

DIRECTIONS FOR THE DANCE

Meter 4/4

▪ *Measures*

Introduction. Dancers stand in place and feel the basic rhythm for the first four measures and start with part II or they may begin on the first beat with part I.

I.   Step–Hop, Schottische

1–4   Face line of direction. Beginning right, take two step–hops and one Schottische step, turning on hop to face reverse line of direction. Moving backward in line of direction and beginning left, take two step–hops and one Schottische step, turning on hop to face center. On each hop, free foot swings forward. Circle moves counterclockwise.

II.   Rock Stamp

5   Face center. Beginning right, cross right over left (count 1), rock back onto left (count 2), rock forward onto right (count 3), hop right and swing left forward into position to repeat (count 4).

6   Beginning left, cross left over right (count 1), rock back onto right (count 2), rock forward onto left (count 3), hop left and swing right forward into position to repeat (count 4).

Rumunjsko Kolo (continued)

| 7–8 | Beginning right, cross right over left (count 1), rock back onto left (count 2), rock forward onto right (count 3), hop right and place left beside right (weight remains on right) (count 4). Stamp left three times (counts 1–3), hold (count 4). |
| 9–12 | Beginning left, repeat action of measures 5–8. Finish with stamp on right. |

▪ STYLE

The dancers are close together, standing straight, hands joined below waist level. The basic body movement comes from below the hips, knees relaxed. The footwork is close to the floor. The body does not sway on the rock, but the rock comes from the knees. Leader at right end leads line in a serpentine fashion, coiling and uncoiling while traveling.

Sarajevka Kolo*

Bosnian

SARAJEVKA KOLO IS PRONOUNCED *SAH-rah-yev-kah KO-lo*. The dance was introduced in this country by Michael Herman.

Records: Folk Dancer MH 1002; Folkraft 1496.

Formation: Broken circle, joined hands held down. Dancer at each end of circle places free arm behind back, fist clenched.

Steps: Step–hop, grapevine, pas de basque, walk, step-touch.

DIRECTIONS FOR THE DANCE

Meter 2/4

▪ *Measures*

		I.	**Fast Music**
A	1–2		Face slightly right. Beginning right, take two step–hops, line moving right.
	3		Facing center, step right to right side, step left behind right (grapevine).
	4–6		Beginning right take three small pas de basque steps (right, left, right).
	7		Face slightly left. Beginning left, take two walking steps to left.
	8		Step–hop left, turning on hop to face slightly right. The hop is a lift, ball of foot does not quite leave the floor.
			Repeat action of part I, measures 1–8 three times.

Sarajevka Kolo included by permission of Michael Herman, director of Folk Dance House, New York.

Meter 4/4

II.   Slow Music

B   1   Beginning right, take two slow walking steps, line moving right.

2   Facing center, step right to right side, step left behind right, step right, touch left near right.

3   In place, step left, touching right near left; step right, touching left near right.

4   Beginning left, take three walking steps, line moving left. Pivot on left (count 4) to face right.

1–4   Repeat action of part II, measures 1–4.

■ NOTES

1. Since there is no introductory music, dancers may wait through the fast music and begin dancing with part II, slow music.

2. The sequence of the music is AABBAAAABBAAAA, and so forth.

Savila Se Bela Loza*

Serbian

SAVILA SE BELA LOZA IS PRONOUNCED *SAH-vee-lah say BAY-lah LOH-zah*, and means "a (grape) vine entwined in itself." The dance comes from Sumadija, Serbia. Dick Crum and Dennis Boxell introduced this dance in this country.

Dance A While CD: #20. "Savila Se Bela Loza."

Records: Carousel CR–701 (45 EP); Festival 109; Folkraft 1496; High/Scope RM 6, LP and compact disc; LS E 43.

Cassette: High/Scope RM 6.

Formation: Broken circle, joined hands held down.

Steps: Run, Schottische.

DIRECTIONS FOR THE DANCE

Meter 2/4

■ *Measures*

Part I

1–9   Face slightly right. Beginning right, take 18 small running steps. Line moves right (counterclockwise).

10   Step–hop right in place, to change direction.

11–20   Face slightly left. Beginning left, repeat action of measures 1–10. Line moves left (clockwise).

Savila Se Bela Loza (continued)

---

*Savila Se Bela Loza included by permission of Richard George Crum.

Part II

21–22   Beginning right, take one Schottische step, moving right. Or, facing center, step right, step left behind right, step–hop right.

23–24   Beginning left, take one Schottische step, moving left. Or, facing center, step left, step right behind left, step–hop left.

25–32   Repeat action of measures 21–24 two times.

▪ VARIATIONS

1. Measures 21–22: Face center, step right slightly forward, step left in place, step right beside left; hop right.

   Measures 23–24: Beginning left, repeat footwork.

   Measures 25–32: Beginning right, repeat action of measures 21–24 of variation 1.

2. Part II, a hop, step, step, step–hop may be substituted for the Schottische step, traveling right and left or facing center and moving in place.

▪ NOTES

1. No introduction. Music for part I usually serves as an introduction, and dancers begin with part II.

2. During part I, measures 1–10, the leader on the right end may lead line anywhere, winding or coiling the line in a **counterclockwise** direction, even through an arch made by two of the dancers in the line. Measures 11–20, the dancer on the left end may lead line anywhere in a **clockwise** direction. The dancer on the left end never initiates the coiling; he coils only if the leader has coiled on measures 1–10. Neither the leader nor the end dancer should ever lead the line so that dancers will have their backs to one another.

▪ LYRICS

Singing these words while dancing adds a natural zest.

Verse I

A. Savila se bela loza vinova   A pretty grapevine entwined itself
     Uz tarabu vinova (repeat two times)   Along a fence, a grape (vine)
       (Repeat A)

B. Todor Todi podvalio   Todor tricked Toda
     Triput curu poljubio   Kissed the girl three times
       (Repeat B twice)

Verse II

A. To ne beše bela loza vinova   It was not a pretty grapevine
     Uz tarabu vinova (repeat two times)   Along a fence a grape (vine)
       (Repeat A)

B. Todor Todi podvalio   Todor tricked Toda
     Triput curu poljubio   Kissed the girl three times
       (Repeat B twice)

Verse III

A. Vec to beše dvoje mili i dragi   It was, rather, two lovers,
     Dvoje mili i dragi (repeat two times)   Two lovers
       (Repeat A)

B. Todor Todi podvalio   Todor tricked Toda
     Triput curu poljubio   Kissed the girl three times
       (Repeat B twice)

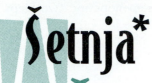

Šetnja*

Serbian

SETNJA IS PRONOUNCED *SHAYT-NYAH* and is from Sumadija, Serbia. This dance is frequently done at Serbian festive occasions. A young man pays a Gypsy musician to play and he gathers his friends to join his line as they dance around the area. Dick Crum introduced this dance to this country in 1955.

Records: Festival 4816; Folk Dancer MH 3029; Folkraft 1490.

Formation: Broken circle, left forearm held at waist level; right hand hooks and rests on left forearm of neighbor during slow music; joined hands held down during fast music. Leader at right end of broken circle.

Steps: Walk, step–hop.

DIRECTIONS FOR THE DANCE

Meter 2/4

■ *Measures*

| | I. | **Walk, Slow Music** |

1	Face right. Beginning right, take two walking steps (slow, slow) in line of direction.
2	Take three more walking steps (quick, quick, quick) moving in line of direction and face center (quick).
3	Moving away from center, step left behind right (slow), step right behind left (slow).
4	Step backward left (quick), step right next to left (quick), and step left across in front of right (slow).
5–8	Repeat action of measures 1–4 for slow music.

| | II. | **Step–Hop, Fast Music** |

Joined hands, held down.

1	Face right. Beginning right, take two step–hops in line of direction.
2	Moving in line of direction, take two steps (quick, quick); step–hop right, turning to face center on hop.
3	Moving away from center, step–hop left behind right, step–hop right behind left.
4	Step backward left (quick), step right next to left (quick), and step–hop left across in front of right.

Repeat action of part II, measures 1–4 until end of music.

Šetnja (continued)

---

*Šetnja included by permission of Richard George Crum.

1. No introduction. Start action with the beginning of a phrase.
2. During part I, the manner is quite casual, with flexing knees. Part II is more exuberant as the dancer runs, taking the step–hops and Two–Steps.

■ **LYRICS**

These words may be sung while dancing.

I. Dodji, Mile, u naš kraj, pa da vidiš, šta je raj. (repeat)

Hej, haj, u naš kraj, pa da vidiš šta je raj. (repeat)

II. Prodje, Mile propeva, i volove protera. (repeat)

Hej, haj, propeva, i volove protera. (repeat)

Syrtós

Greek

SYRTÓS IS THE MOST TRADITIONAL Folk Dance in Greece. Basic footwork is always the same but varies in styling. The music may be 2/4, 4/4, or 7/8 meter. *Kalamatianos*, a Syrtós from Kalamata, is 7/8 rhythm. Whatever the meter, it is counted slow, quick, quick. Syrtós means "to pull or lead," which is characteristic of the dance movement.

Record: Most Greek albums include a good Syrtós.

Formation: Broken circle, hands joined, shoulder high, elbows bent, *W* position. Dancer at either end of broken circle may place free hand on hip, fingers pointing backward, or arm extended, snapping fingers.

DIRECTIONS FOR THE DANCE

Meter 2/4

■ *Measures*

1   Face center. Beginning right, step to right (slow), step left behind right (quick), step right to right (quick).

2   Step left crossing in front of right (slow), step right to right (quick), and step left crossing in front of right (quick).

3   Step right, facing slightly left (slow), touch ball of left foot slightly forward toward center (slow).

4   Step left backward (slow), touch ball of right foot slightly behind left (slow). Repeat pattern throughout the dance.

■ **STYLE**

The leader may be a man or a woman. A kerchief is usually held between the first and second dancers in line. This allows the leader greater freedom to execute variations. The second dancer gives the needed support to the leader to perform acrobatic moves. The dancers continue the basic step.

■ **VARIATIONS FOR LEADER**

1. Measure 4: Leader makes one solo turn counterclockwise, spins on left, touches right.
2. Measures 1–2: Leader steps right (slow), makes two solo turns clockwise (quick, quick, slow, quick), and steps left (quick).
3. Measures 1–2: Leader makes three solo turns clockwise (slow, quick, quick, slow, quick, quick) and joins the group on measure 3, step point.

Tropanka

Bulgarian

THIS "LIVELY" STAMPING DANCE IS ideal for beginning an evening of fun with folk dancing for novice groups.

Dance A While CD: #6. "Tropanka."

Record: MH 1020.

Formation: Single circle, nonpartner dance. Joined hands, shoulder height, *W* position.

Steps: Walking, step–hop, stamp.

DIRECTIONS FOR THE DANCE

Meter 2/4

■ *Measures*

Walk and Stamp (Music A)

1–2   Beginning right, move with five quick walking steps (shuffle–like) counterclockwise, stamp left foot twice and pause.

3–4   Repeat beginning left, moving clockwise, stamp right foot twice.

5–8   Repeat measures 1–4 (Music A).

Step Hop and Stamp (Music B)

1–2   Face center, step hop on right, swing left slightly across right. Step hop on left, swing right slightly across left. Step on right in place and stamp left foot twice and pause.

3–4   Repeat measures 1–2 beginning left and end stamping right twice and pause.

5–8   Repeat measures 1–4 (Music B).

To Center and Back (Music C)

1–2   Beginning right, step hop twice toward center, step on right and stamp left twice.

3–4   Repeat measures 1–2. Moving backward, begin left.

5–8   Repeat measures 1–4 (Music C).

Note: During the move to center, joined hands are raised as dancers move in and lowered as they move out.

BRITISH ISLES

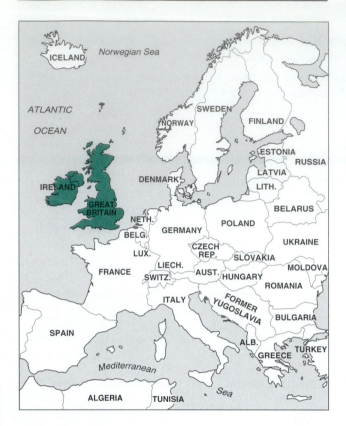

■ Introduction

The British Isles were settled by the Celts, who came across from the Continent, by the Milesians, a nomadic Celtic tribe who came to Ireland from northern Italy (Lombardy), and then by invaders from the Basque country (Gallicia). Scotland was settled by the Picts (of uncertain origin) and the Scots, who came from Ireland. Subsequent invading tribes (Romans, Angles, Saxons, Normans, Danes) influenced the culture of the British Isles. The Celts practiced Druid rites, which included dancing, and some of the pagan rites were retained during their conversion to Christianity. A constant exchange of culture existed among the English, the Irish, and the Scottish as the result of natural migration, war, and travel by sailors from one country to another. Hugh Thurston (1964; p. 5) has commented that the figures and the steps of the country dances during the period of 1720–1800 were so similar, with national characteristics lacking, that a particular dance could not be identified as English, Scottish, or even American.

■ England

DANCE CHARACTERISTICS

England's Morris and Sword dances are two ritual dance forms, performed for renewal and continuance of life, that have survived over the centuries. The third form is the country dance, a term that covers a variety of social dances. According to Douglas Kennedy, "These English country dances came directly from the folk in the form of rounds and squares and longways and contras. Having established themselves as fashionable ballroom forms, they continued through the times of the Stuarts, Commonwealth, the Restoration, Queen Anne and the Hanoverian line right into our own century."*

MORRIS DANCE

Morris Dance for centuries has been part of the spring Whitsuntide festival. Whit–Monday was the day for the Morris men to perform, a custom that was little known outside rustic villages in the English countryside until the 19th century. In 1899 Cecil Sharp observed an out–of–season Morris Dance performed by six men dressed in white shirts, adorned with ribbons and padded leg bells, as they pranced and "footed" it in the snow of winter on the outskirts of Oxford. From that experience, Sharp was inspired to delve into the music, dance steps, and history of the Morris. The result was *The Morris Book*, a five–part publication that has been an invaluable source of information concerning this ancient ritual.

The origin of the name Morris is shrouded in the mist of history and is speculative at best. The Whitsuntide custom goes back to before the Norman conquest. Whether the dance had a name then is not known. In addition, the Morris has been estimated to have been in existence since the 12th century. Scholars can only theorize about the name; however, the Moorish or Spanish origin of the name has generally been discounted.

In its early form the Morris included character actors such as the Squire, clown, and fool, any one of whom would act as the leader depending on the region and/or Morris tradition from which they came. Other characters taking part in this ancient dance–drama were the Hobby–horse, animal–men, and Maid Marion or "Betsy." During these early times the men dancers played a subsidiary role to the actors. In more recent times, the actors have become secondary to the dancers, who entertain with their spectacular athletic feats.

During its long history the Morris was plagued by ecclesiastical restrictions issued from Rome and Canterbury. In addition, the Puritans waged a vigorous campaign against this traditional rustic pastime. They succeeded in destroying so many of the countryside customs that not even Charles II could restore all the Morris customs and all the Maypoles! This attitude came with the Puritans across the ocean to the

---

*Kennedy, Douglas. *English Folk Dancing Today and Yesterday*. London: G. Bell and Sons, 1964, p. 112.

colonies where, as occurred in some American southern communities, the word "dance" had to be replaced with the word "game."

The last 50 years has seen a revival of the Morris in America. Contemporary times even find the Morris danced by women. Today there are three organizations: the Morris Ring for men only, the Women's Morris for women only, and the Open Morris for men and women. At present no Federation of Morris teams are based in the United States or Canada. Communication between groups and about group events is facilitated by the *American Morris Newsletter* published in Silver Spring, Maryland.

SWORD DANCE

The English Sword Dance is a technically intricate, exciting, and dramatic dance form handed down by example and oral tradition from the remote past. The dance, coupled with the play or dramatic action, has a half–magic and half–religious aura.

The Sword Dance Play consists of two aspects, dancers who blacken their faces or wear masks, and a retinue of characters consisting of (depending on region and tradition) the Hobby–horse, clown, the woman Beson Betty or Dirty Bet, and often a King, Queen, Lord, Lady, and a quack Doctor with his Jack. Although performed at other times of the year the Sword Dance's season traditionally was midwinter on Plough–Monday. It was through the absorbing and diligent work of Cecil Sharp that the details of this fast–dying dance tradition and the content and materials of the drama associated with it have been preserved. Sharp's three–part publication of *The Sword Dances of Northern England* remains today the invaluable source for information concerning this ancient custom.

The Sword Dance is distinguished by the type of instrument used. The Yorkshire tradition consisted of a long rigid sword made of wood or iron. The Northumberland and Durham version, which was shorter and more flexible, was called a Rapper. The dance is commonly referred to as the "Long Sword" or "Rapper" Dance.

The Rapper was fitted with handles at each end and a swivel at the hilt so that the blade could twist and turn within the hand. This turning feature coupled with the shorter blade allowed the dancers to twist and turn as individuals or for the whole group to literally turn inside out. *Stepping*, a highly skilled dance movement, was used to change patterns, alternating with the weaving of the swords in a figure. The Rapper style was acrobatic and breathtakingly exciting.

The very nature of the long sword with its more rigid blade eliminated the acrobatic elements found in the Rapper performance. The Long Sword Dance thus is more elaborate and ceremonial in nature yet still dramatic and fascinating. Common to both performances, however, were the "dramatis personae" of the ancient Plough Play, the "Lock," Knott, or Rose, and the "calling on" stage by accompanying actors or characters.

The Long Sword Dance always finished with a "Lock." In some traditions the "Lock" is tied around the neck of one of the accompanying characters, who then dies dramatically. In other traditions the beheaded actor simply gets up, brushes himself off, and leaves, thus signaling the end of the play. In still other traditions the beheading begins the dramatic part of the play. A mock–Doctor appears accompanied by his Jack to undertake a cure of the dead and restore him to life. The symbolism is that of fashioning new life from the ashes of the old, a repeated theme in Sword dance–dramas thought to be associated with the Mummers' plays.

The Rapper Dance tradition seems to be found mostly in the coal mining districts of northern England. Versions of the Rapper dance vary little, which is thought to be a consequence of its existence in closely knit coal mining societies. The design of the sword, its length, and versatility are thought to be a product of the iron workers of antiquity.

COUNTRY DANCES

By Kate Van Winkle Keller, Darnestown, Maryland, and George A. Fogg, Boston

English country dances came to notice in the late 1500s as group dances performed at court and in sophisticated private gatherings. The first publication was in 1651 when John Playford gathered up more than 100 country dances then currently popular in London society. They were in a number of forms: rounds, squares, two– and three–couple, and Longways sets; some were very simple ("Rufty Tufty"), others, more complex ("Chelsea Reach"). By 1690 when an eighth edition of his hugely popular book called *The Dancing Master* appeared, most of the old dances had been dropped in favor of a Longways progressive formation in which couples stand in parallel lines, men in one line facing their partners in the other. This formation persists today in traditional and Contra dances.

Longways country dances are performed in small groups within a larger set, the first couple in each "minor" set leading the figures. The dance has six or eight figures, such as back–to–back, hand–turn, circle, or lead through, that are arranged to fit the music and move the leading couple down one place. Each time the dance is repeated, the leading couple performs the figures again with a new subgroup in the set. The popularity of country dancing hinges on the repetitious nature of the figures and its flexibility. In the 17th and 18th centuries, steps were optional and were chosen by the leading couple to suit the company. The specific dance was also chosen for the occasion–those with more complex figures for elite dancers in public assemblies, simpler ones for dancers in barns and taverns.

Country dances served as an important cultural vehicle in British, European, and New World social settings between 1660 and 1800. Over this period, old court–oriented societies were replaced by materialistic middle–class people who displayed gentility and manners on the dance floor as badges of achievement. Country dances faded from view in the early 19th century as behavior and appearance ceased to be a defining social standard.

ENGLISH COUNTRY DANCING TODAY

English country dances flourish again today as a living tradition. In the 19th century, once it was acceptable to hold your partner in your arms in polite company, the Waltz and the Polka took over the ballrooms. Dancing was no longer something just to look at and admire, but something to enjoy physically, regardless of who was watching. But country dances persisted among country folk and were taught by rural dancing masters long enough to be remembered by the older generations when Cecil J. Sharp learned about them in the early 1900s. He collected and published a number and then sought their history in libraries. He interpreted old dance terms that had long gone out of use and took the lead in bringing English country dances back into vogue.

Since that time, modern dancing masters have created many new dances within the country dance form to fit the social mores of their day. Today on both sides of the Atlantic Ocean, many follow Sharp's lead seeking out and interpreting interesting old dances published by Playford, Bray, Walsh, Neal and, the Thompson family. Some are creating new material in the old forms, and others, such as Pat Shaw, have composed dances that synthesize traditional English, Scottish and American idioms.

The earliest country dances were danced with Renaissance steps such as single, double, and perhaps some steps from the showy galliard. In the 18th century, elite dancers adopted French steps such as *pas de bourrée*, minuet, *contretemps*, rigadoon, and *balancé*. Today most country dances are performed with a smooth dance–walk, bouncy sets, and occasional slipping steps or skipping.

MUSIC

Country dances are composed to popular tunes of all kinds: old ballad tunes, marches and arias by Purcell and Handel, elegant dances from the theater, and joyful fiddle tunes from countryside. English country dances are tied to their tunes and the same tune is played throughout the dance. Tunes usually comprise two or three repeated eight–bar phrases in duple or triple meter. Present tastes in the United States lean toward triple meter tunes, and many new and old dances in triple time are found on ball and class programs.

Although it is impossible to define a typical country dance tune, some qualities can be observed. Smooth melodic motion, distinct cadences, and harmonic and rhythmic drive are present in the most satisfying tunes. Because each phrase is usually repeated, full modulations are seldom present although tunes in AABA form often do modulate in the B strain, setting up a dramatic return to A ("La Belle Catherine").

Instruments to accompany early country dancing varied from a pipe and tabor (played by one person) to a full orchestra plus pipe organ as found at assemblies in 18th century Bath. Over the years, the fiddle was probably the most commonly used instrument. Today dances are usually accompanied by combinations of three or four instruments such as concertina, fiddle, flute, piano, accordion, harp, cello, and many others.

■ *Ireland*

DANCE CHARACTERISTIC

Despite a common background with the other British Isle countries, Ireland's dance and culture tend to be very different from Scotland's and England's. There are three types of Irish folk dances: Jigs, Reels, and Hornpipes. Jigs and Hornpipes are characterized by clog and tap steps, and Reels by shuffle or gliding steps. The dances follow traditional formations of solos, couples, and groups or sets. The specially trained solo dancers perform step dances based on clog or shuffle steps. The popular dances are Jigs and Reels (simple steps) in round, square, and Longway formations.

The tradition of Feis (a celebration of competitions among the poets, singers, musicians, storytellers, and dancers held after harvest in November) dates back to 1300 B.C. It has been suggested that it was originally a form of Thanksgiving. Different Celtic countries had a similar tradition but referred to it by other names. In the Feis contests, women were allowed to compete, and the minstrel in that period had more status than the warrior. The strong tradition of Feis is credited with keeping Irish folk music and dance alive. Despite difficult times when the Irish came to the United States, immigrant minstrels perpetuated their heritage, which has become a part of American folk music.

When the famous dancing schools–such as those at Limerick, Kerry, and Cork–were established, a polished style evolved and natural expressions were eliminated with emphasis placed on the footwork. Some of the spontaneity of expression was lost. But the dance schools and competitions are to be credited for keeping the Irish dance tradition vibrant.

STYLE

Characteristics of the Irish people, such as their keen sense of humor, happiness, wit, imagination, and superstition, prevail in their dances and music. The dancer is erect, hands at the sides, and face rather impassive. The range of movement is minimal. The distinguishing characteristic is the intricate and exact footwork. In the most difficult dances, there are about 75 taps per quarter minute. The control of the various sounds produced by the taps of heels and soles on the floor and against each other is of utmost importance in competitive dancing. Although the dances are based on five simple steps, improvisation and elaboration of steps are delightful characteristics of Irish dance.

MUSIC

Originally, the fife and harp were used for dance accompaniment. Today, fiddles, flutes, violins, and accordions are popular. Irish music is very lilting. The secondary rhythm of the tapping feet combines with the melody to create an interesting effect.

■ Scotland

DANCE CHARACTERISTICS

The unbroken history of Scottish dance has long been preserved as part of Scotland's strong national pride. The practice of regimental troops dancing to relieve tension before battle or to celebrate victories is one aspect of the Scottish heritage. After the 1745 rebellion when the English tried to end the clan system and suppress the Highland culture, the Scottish ways of dress, dance, and music became even stronger when they were forced underground. When the ban was lifted in 1782, Scotland's fierce national pride was stronger than ever. The Highland battalions, moving abroad and eventually around the world, wore their kilts and continued their ceremonies and dance traditions.

Another tradition, the Highland games, continues to stimulate interest through dance, bagpipe, and athletic contests. The Scottish Country Dance Society is to be credited with standardizing steps and techniques, setting up a system of exams and certificates, and publishing many Scottish dances.

Almost all Scots can dance several of their traditional dances. Today, during an evening of social dancing, a *Waltz Country Dance*, a *Petronella*, a *Skip the Willow*, or a *Highland Schottische* are usually included.

STYLE

The Scots are very enthusiastic about dance and have always entered into it with a great deal of zest. Highland solo dancing or competitive dancing, such as the *Highland Fling* and *Sword Dance*, are intricate and athletic. The carriage of the body is very erect and the supporting leg is kept straight. The toes are pointed at all times. Arms are used for balance. The hand and arms positions are exact; either the fists are at the hips, the arms curved over the head, with thumb and third finger touching, or one arm is held above the head and the other is held at the hip. The body movement is upward, with hopping or jumping off one or two feet on the first beat. This is referred to as *snap*. The feet beat in the air soundlessly. The body is propelled back upward into the air when the heel touches the floor. Elaborations of steps occur while the body is in the air.

MUSIC

Scottish Highland Dances have been performed traditionally to the music of the bagpipes, which have a nine-note scale. The lilting rises and falls of the tunes influence the dance style. The snap occurs when a sixteenth note is followed by a dotted eighth. Although the first note, the first beat, is light and gives impetus to the next note, which is stressed and louder, the intake of breath when playing the bagpipe has become the snap or sixteenth note. Only the bagpipe can express the peculiar quality and rhythm of Highland Dance music. The violin and piano are now played in many parts of Scotland for Reels and Jigs.

Bonny Prince Charlie Crossing the Frew*

Scottish

BONNY PRINCE CHARLIE CROSSING THE *Frew* depicts the crossing of Prince Charles at the Frew (1745), the only place to ford the river Forth from the north. The river winds back on itself, and the setting and the turnings depict the leaping from stone to stone. The dancers at the bottom of the set watch, as Charles himself did, until all have crossed. The final figure is the flight under fire and farewell to the south as the King's soldiers in King's Park fired only a few shots. Stirling Castle was held, and Prince Charles marched south, then back to Culloden and final defeat.

Record: Dance with Jim Johnson and his Band, FLPS 1853, or any 40–measure Jig in 6/8 time. (Fiesta Record Co., Inc., 1619 Broadway, New York, NY.)

Formation: Longway Reeltime dance. A four–couple set, three couples active, one couple inactive. Top of set indicated by first man's left shoulder.

Position: Feet in first position, hands at sides.

Steps: Skip change step, pas de basque, setting.

DIRECTIONS FOR THE DANCE

Meter 6/8 • Directions are same for man and woman.

■ *Measures*

1–16   Dance begins with honors, men bow, women curtsey. First and second couples set (2 measures), join right hands across, and wheel halfway around (2 measures) with two skip change steps.

Second and third couples set (2 measures), join left hands across, and wheel halfway around (2 measures) with two skip change steps.

First and fourth couples set (2 measures), join right hands across, and wheel halfway around (2 measures) with two skip change steps.

First couple dance half–figure–eight up and around fourth couple. First woman will pass in front of partner up and around fourth man to opposite side. First man dances up and around fourth woman to finish at bottom on original side with four skip change steps.

Fourth couple will step up on measures 15 and 16.

Man = □
Woman = ○   Top ← □ □ □ ○
                     ○ ○ ○ □

---

*This dance was choreographed by Mary McLaren Lindsay of Mesa, Arizona. Mrs. Lindsay is a certified teacher of the Royal Scottish Country Dance Society of Edinburgh, Scotland; she was born in Bannockburn and educated in the Stirling area. The dance is used by permission.

17–24   Second, third, and fourth couples advance and retire two skip change steps forward and backward. Join both hands, turn own partner halfway around with two pas de basque steps. Drop hands and fall back to sides on last two pas de basque steps. First couple stand at bottom for these last 8 measures. All dancers are now on original sides.

Man = ☐
Woman = ◯   Top ← ◯ ◯ ◯ ◯
                    ☐ ☐ ☐ ☐

25–32   Bottom couple casts up on their own outside of the set to top. (Dance slightly in on first measure toward each other as they cast). Meet each other and dance under bridges (arches) formed by second, third, and fourth couples with eight skip change steps.

33–40   Second with third, fourth with first, couples dance right and left. **Note:** Dancers retain original number through 1–40 measures.

Repeat dance from beginning with new first couple.

■ SCOTTISH STEPS AND FORMATIONS

Wheeling: A four-hand star or mill figure in which dancers turn with either the right or left hand. In this dance, it is used to change lines or turn half around.

Set or Setting: Two pas de basques in place, facing as directed.

Pas de Basque: Push off left foot and leap sideways onto right, weight on ball of foot. Close left foot into third position front and change weight onto ball of left foot. Step back (shift weight) onto right foot, keeping weight on ball of foot as left foot is extended forward in third position. Cues: Leap (count 1), step across (count 2), step in place (count 3). Step, beat, beat.

Skip Change Step: Begin in first position. Skip (hop) on left foot while extending right foot forward, knee straight and toe pointed. Step on right foot, keeping leg straight and firm. Close left to right in third rear position (remain on toes). Step forward onto right foot. Cues: Skip (hop), step, close, step.

Right and Left: Each dancer extends right hand to partner and changes places across the line; each dancer faces up or down the lines, gives left hand to other man or woman dancer, and changes places in line; each dancer gives right hand to partner and changes place across the line; each dancer gives left hand to other man or woman and finishes in original place. Cues: Across the line, up or down the line, across the line, and up or down the line.

Note: The symbols used to represent the man and woman are the reverse of those used by the Royal Scottish Country Dance Society.

The Bridge of Athlone

Irish

THE *BRIDGE OF ATHLONE* IS AN Irish dance that contains a figure representing the Bridge.

Record: *Rakes of Mallow,* High/Scope LC 84–743–041.

Music: *The Rakes of Mallow;* any good reel.

Formation: Longways set, even number of couples, facing each other, women on left side from the top.

Steps: Walk, side step (seven and two threes).

DIRECTIONS FOR THE DANCE

Meter 2/4 • Directions are the same for man and woman.

■ *Measures*

1–8	Introduction: no action.

Part I. Advance and Retire

1–4	Hands joined in a row. Beginning right, two lines walk toward each other and back up.
5–8	Repeat action.

Part II. Side Step

1–4	Hands still joined, side step to own right. (See side step analysis at end of dance.)
5–8	Repeat side step to left, now in original position.

Part III. Down the Center and Back

9–10	Couple 1, join both hands crossed, face to face, dance "seven" down the center.
11–12	Turning clockwise a half turn, dance "two threes."
13–16	Returning to top of set, dance "seven" and repeat half turn clockwise, dancing "two threes."

Part IV. Cast Off

9–16	Couple 1 casts off around the outside, walking sprightly, man left, woman right, to the bottom of the set. Other dancers follow the leaders.

Part V. The Bridge

1–8	Couple 1 joins two hands to form an arch at the bottom of the set. The other couples join two hands, go under the arch, and return to the top of the set.
	Couple 2 will now be at the top of the set; couple 1, at the bottom. When they reach this position, all face their partner and raise two hands to form bridges the length of the set.

1–8	Couple 1 releases hands. Woman walks up the set under the bridges, the man walks up the outside (men's line).
9–16	At the top, the man walks to the bottom under the bridges, the woman goes down the outside (women's line). When they reach the bottom, they face each other and become the bottom couple.

The dance is repeated (without the introduction) until all have had an opportunity to be couple 1.

■ SIDE STEP

Meter 2/4   Made up of two parts: "seven" and "two threes."

"Seven"

1–2	Moving sideward to the right, with a little jump (both feet off the ground), land on the toes, right heel over left toe (count 1). Step right a short step to the right (count 2). Step left toe to right heel (count 3). Step right a short step to the right (count 4). Step left toe to right heel (count 5). Step right a short step to the right (count 6). Step left toe to right heel, right foot lifted slightly (count 7). Hold (count 8). Repeat to the left, reversing the movements.

"Two Threes"   Each measure is counted: "one, two, **three.**"

1. Beginning right, step on toe behind the left heel, lifting the left foot slightly (count 1). Step left in place and lift right foot slightly (count 2). Step right behind left and lift left foot slightly (count **3** – actually 2 counts).

2. Repeat action of measure 1, beginning left.

The step may begin right or left. The step may be done in place or sidewards.

Butterfly Hornpipe* English (Warwickshire)

PRESENTED BY GEORGE A. Fogg at the Third Annual English Country Dance workshop at Lost Pines Dance Hall, Bastrop, Texas, fall 1992.

Source: *Community Dance Manual 1; Country Dances of Today 1* and Sharp, Cecil, *Country Dance Book 1.*

Original: Collected by Cecil J. Sharp.

Record: *Orange and Blue* ED 105.

Music: Any good hornpipe such as *Manchester* or *Rickett's,* also found in *Community Dance Manual 1* and *Country Dances of Today 1.*

Formation: Duple Minor Longways.

Step: Jaunty walking or 1, 2, 3 Hop; a low easy Schottische.

Butterfly Hornpipe (continued)

---

*Directions and permission to publish courtesy George A. Fogg, 40 Gray Street, Boston, MA 02116–6210.

Meter 4/4

■ *Measures*

Part A1

1–8   Right–hand star and left–hand back.

Part A2

1–8   Arching (over and under). (Ones over twos; then twos over ones and repeat.)

Part B

1–8   Couples swing and change places. In closed position, dance (Two–step or Schottische) one and one–half times around each other to change places.

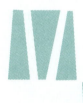

Dover Pier*

English

Source: Keller, K. and G. Shimer, *The Playford Ball*; Simons, A., *Kentish "Hops" 1.*

Original from: Preston's *Twenty Four Country Dances for the Year 1791.*

Record: *Five Country Dances from Printed Collections,* PR–EP 315.

Music: Barnes, P., *English Country Dance Tunes*; Keller, K. and Shimer, G., *The Playford Ball*; Simons, A., *Kentish "Hops" 1.*

Formation: Duple Minor Longways.

Step: Walking.

DIRECTIONS FOR THE DANCE

Meter 2/4

■ *Measures*

Part A1

1–8   All set twice and right hands across (right–hand star) halfway and fall back.

Part A2

1–8   Repeat A1 with the left hand star.

Part B1

1–8   First couple cross over and go below (second couple move up) and first couple two–hand turn one and one–half to end proper.

Part B2

1–8   Right and left with hands (4 changes).

Note from *The Playford Ball:* "The wharfs of Dover are the chief points of departure for the continent, being but twenty–one miles across the English channel to Calais in France."

---

*Directions and permission to publish courtesy George A. Fogg, 40 Gray Street, Boston, MA 02116–6210.

The First of April* English

Source: Porter, W. S., and A. and M. Heffer, *The Apted Book of Country Dances.*
Record: *Apted Country Dances*, Lib 1.
Cassette: *Barn Dancin' and Country Dancin'* BEE006
Music: Barnes, Peter, *English Country Dance Tunes I & II*; and Porter, W. S., and A. and M. Heffer, *The Apted Book of Country Dances.*
Formation: Duple Minor Longways.
Step: Walking and slipping.

DIRECTIONS FOR THE DANCE

Meter 6/8

■ *Measures*

Part A1
1–4 First and second couples right hands across (right–hand star) once around.

Part A2
1–4 The same couples left hands across, back again.

Part B1
1–8 First couple lead down the middle, lead back up, and cast down one place.

Part B2
1–8 Hands four (circle) left and back right (slipping).

---

*Directions and permission to publish courtesy George A. Fogg, 40 Gray Street, Boston, MA 02116–6210.

flowers of Edinburgh*   Scottish Reel

DANCES WITH JACOBITE NAMES, like *Flowers of Edinburgh*, may have been composed by the many fiddlers in Scotland. After the 1745 Rebellion, the pipes were banned. The Chiefs had their own fiddlers and the dances usually depict a famous battle, event, or, in many instances, a place name.

Records: Folkraft 1333; Scottish Dance Time Album Volume I, SMT 7028; or any eight–time, 32–measure Reel in 4/4 meter.

Formation: Longway Reeltime dance. A four–couple set involving three couples in each 32–bar repetition. Top of set is indicated by left shoulder of first man.

Steps: Skip change step, pas de basque, poussette.

DIRECTIONS FOR THE DANCE

Meter 2/4 • Directions are same for man and woman, except where noted.

■ *Measures*

1–6	Dance begins with honors, men bow, women curtsey.
	First woman turns round by the right, and casts off two places (i.e., dances down behind second and third woman, then crosses over and dances up behind second and third man to her partner's original position, Fig. 1). At the same time, first man follows his partner, crossing over and dancing behind second and third women, then up the middle to his partner's original position, Fig. 2. (Six skip change steps.)
7–8	First couples set to one another. Two pas de basques.
9–14	Repeat bars 1–6, but first man leads as in Fig. 1, and first woman follows, as in Fig. 2. First couples finish in original position. (Six skip change steps.)

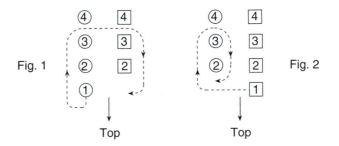

15–16	First couple set to one another. (Two pas de basques.)
17–24	First couple lead down the middle and up again. (Eight skip change steps.)

---

*This dance is used by the permission of the Royal Scottish Country Dance Society, 12 Coates Crescent, Edinburgh, Scotland, EH3 7AF. Patron–Her Majesty The Queen; President–The Earl of Mansfield; Secretary–Miss M. M. Gibson. Permission granted April 16, 1986.

25–32	First and second couples poussette. (This is the progression sequence).

Note: Men begin with left foot.

Repeat, having passed a couple.

Man = □
Woman = ○

Top ← ① ②

② ③ ④

① ③ ④

■ SCOTTISH STEPS AND FORMATIONS

Skip Change Step: Begin in first position. Skip (hop), on left foot while extending right foot forward, knee straight and toe pointed. Step on right foot, keeping leg straight and firm. Close left to right in third rear position (remain on toes). Step forward onto right foot. Cues: Skip (hop), step, close, step.

Pas de Basque: Push off left foot and leap sideways onto right, weight on ball of foot. Close left foot into third position front and change weight onto ball of left foot. Step back (shift weight onto right foot, keeping weight on ball of foot as left foot is extended forward in fourth intermediate position, toes down. Cues: Leap (count 1), step across (count 2), step in place (count 3). Step, beat, beat.

Poussette: Both hands joined at shoulder level, elbows at side, hands held firmly. Men begin with left foot. Couples dance eight pas de basque steps. The two couples change places by dancing along the sides of a square, couple 1 down the man's side, couple 2 up on woman's side. Couples dance one step away from center (measure 1); both quarter–turn on corner of square, pull with right hand–men now have backs to top of set. They are on sideline of set (measure 2); both travel up or down the set (measure 3); both quarter–turn, pull with right hand–men have backs to woman's side of set (measure 4); both dance to center of set (measure 5); both turn around to own sides (measure 6); all dancers fall back to sidelines. Dancers have now changed places (measures 7 and 8). **Note:** Pas de basque is used as a traveling step, moving forward and back. Cues: Away from center quarter–turn, up or down quarter–turn, dance into center turn half around, and fall back, fall back.

Set or Setting: Two pas de basques in place as directed.

Note: The symbols used to represent the man and woman are the reverse of those used by the Royal Scottish Country Dance Society.

Gie Gordons

Scottish

Records: Express 282; Folkraft 1162.

Cassette: Dancecraft DC 989; Dancecraft DC 162006.

Music: *Folk Dancer,* Volume 7, No. 4, p. 11.

Position: Varsouvienne.

Steps: Walk, Two–Step, pas de basque.

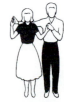

Gie Gordons (continued)

Meter 2/4 • Directions are same for both man and woman, except when specially noted.

■ *Measures*

I. Walk

1–2 Beginning left, walk four steps forward in line of direction. On fourth step, pivot clockwise to face reverse line of direction. Woman is now on man's left.

3–4 Continue walking backward four steps in line of direction.

5–8 Repeat action of measures 1–4 in reverse line of direction.

II. Two–Step

9–12 Man beginning left, takes four Two–Steps in line of direction, as woman, beginning right, turns clockwise under man's right arm four Two–Steps. Or man, beginning left, woman right, pas de basque out and in and man takes four walking steps in line of direction as woman turns twice clockwise under man's right arm.

13–16 Closed position. Man beginning left, woman right, takes four Two–Steps turning clockwise, progressing in line of direction. Or takes two Two–Steps turning clockwise, then man walks four steps forward progressing in line of direction as woman twirls under raised right arm. Assume Varsouvienne position.

Note: This dance may be done with inside hands joined instead of Varsouvienne position.

The Northdown Waltz* English

NOTE FROM *THE PLAYFORD BALL:* "The North Downs are a long ridge of hills running southwest from Rochester to Dover in Kent."

Source: Keller, K., and G. Shimer, *The Playford Ball;* Simon, A., *Kentish Hops (Third Pickings).*

Original from: Goulding & Cos., *Collection of New & Favorite Country Dances 1820.*

Record: Kentish Hops 2, KH 2.; *Kentish Hops* by Ring O'Bells BEE 007.

Music: Barnes, P., *English Country Dance Tunes: 1 & 11;* Keller, K., and G. Shimer, *The Playford Ball;* Simon, A., *Kentish Hops (Third Pickings).*

Formation: Duple Minor Longways.

Step: Walking waltz–three steps to the bar.

---

*Directions and permission to publish courtesy George A. Fogg, 40 Gray Street, Boston, MA 02116–6210.

DIRECTIONS FOR THE DANCE

Meter 3/4

■ *Measures*

Part A1

1–4 First woman and second man right–hand balance forward and back, then change places.

5–8 First man and second woman do the same.

Part A2

1–8 Repeat A1 back to original places.

Part B1

1–8 First couple leads down the middle and leads back to second couple's place (second couple moves up).

Part C

1–8 Take ballroom position and waltz completely around each other counterclockwise and end progressed.

Oslo Waltz

Scottish-English

THE *OSLO WALTZ* IS A LIVELY FAMILY–TYPE Waltz mixer. It is of Scottish–English heritage, set to a Norwegian folk song.

Records: Canadian MH 3016; Folk Dancer MH 3016.
Formation: Single circle, couples facing center, woman to the right of partner, all hands joined.
Steps: Waltz, Waltz balance, three–step turn.

DIRECTIONS FOR THE DANCE

Meter 3/4 • Directions are for man; woman's part reversed.

■ *Measures*

I. Waltz Balance and Lady Turn

1–2 Man begins left; all take one Waltz balance forward. Man begins right; all take one Waltz balance back.

3–4 Man begins left, Waltz balance steps in place as he turns left–hand woman from his left to his right side. Woman makes two clockwise turns in two Waltz steps.

5–16 Repeat measures 1–4 three times.

Oslo Waltz (continued)

II. Step–Swing, Three–Step Turn

Single circle, partners face in butterfly position. Man's new partner is woman on his right.

1–4   Man begins left, steps left to side, swings right across left. Steps right to side, swings left across right. Dropping hands, couples three–step turn individually toward center.

5–8   Man begins right; couples repeat step–swings and three–step turn to place.

III. Draw, Waltz

1–4   Butterfly position: Man begins left; couples take two step–draws toward center. Repeat two step–draws away from center.

5–8   Closed position: Man begins left; couples take four Waltz steps, turning clockwise, progressing counterclockwise around the circle.

Repeat dance from the beginning.

The Ragg*

English

Source: Jackson, R., and G. Fogg, *A Choice Collection of Country Dances.*

Original from: *A Choice Collection of Country Dances with their Proper Tunes, whereof many never before Published, and in an easier Method to be understood than ever yet Printed, Gathered, Composed and Corrected by Many of the Best Masters of this Kingdom.* Dublin Printed & sold by John & William Neal in Christ Church Yard (ca. 1726).

Cassette: Bare Necessities *Take a Dance*, FF90564, will fit. Use the tune "Take a Dance."

Music: Jackson, R., and G. Fogg, *A Choice Collection of Country Dances.*; Barnes, Peter, *English Country Dance Tunes 1 & 11.*

Formation: Duple Minor Longways.

Step: Walking.

DIRECTIONS FOR THE DANCE

Meter 6/8

■ *Measures*

Part A1

1–4   First couple cross over and go below to second place.

5–8   First couple two–hand turn once and a half.

Part A2

1–8   Second couple repeat A1.

---

*Directions and permission to publish courtesy George A. Fogg, 40 Gray Street, Boston, MA 02116–6210.

Part B1

1–8   Right– and left–hand star (hands across).

Part B2

1–4   Set twice.

5–8   Right, left, and right with hands (3 changes).

Original instructions:

1st cu: cross over and turn in 2d cu: place:
2d cu: ye same in their own places:
All 4 right hands across half round, and left hands back again:
All Shuffle, then right and left:

Road to the Isles Scottish

ROAD TO THE ISLES IS A FAVORITE marching song of the pipe bands. The tune called "Bens of Jura" was composed by Pipe Major MacLellan about 1890 with words by Dr. Kenneth McLeod. The original words are very similar to the song "Border Trail." The dance is relatively new in composition and is similar to the Scottish Polais Glide and the Douglass Schottische.

Records: Folk Dancer MH 3003; Folkraft 1095, 1416; World of Fun LP 3, Side B–5; High/Scope RM–5 Compact Disc.

Cassette: Dancecraft DC 989; High/Scope RM–5.

Music: Rohrbough, Lynn, Cooperative Recreation Service, *Sing it Again, Handy II*, p. 16.

Position: Varsouvienne.

Steps: Schottische.

DIRECTIONS FOR THE DANCE

Meter 2/4

■ *Measures*

    I.   Point, Grapevine

1   Point left toe forward to left.

2–3   Step left behind right (count 1), right to right side (count 2), left in front of right (count 1), and hold (count 2).

4   Point right toe forward to right.

5–6   Step right behind left (count 1), left to left side (count 2), right in front of left (count 1), and hold (count 2).

7–8   Point left toe forward (body leans backward), point left toe back (body leans forward).

Road to the Isles (continued)

9–12   Beginning left, take two Schottische steps in line of direction. Without releasing hands, turn clockwise on hop (count 2, measure 12) to face reverse line of direction. Woman is now on man's left.

13–14   Beginning left, take one Schottische step in reverse line of direction. Without releasing hands, turn counterclockwise on hop to face line of direction. Woman is now back in original position on man's right.

15–16   Stamp in place right, left, right.

▪ STYLE

The Scottish flavor may be added by precise and petite foot movement. Kicking the heel up on the hop of the Schottische step so as to flick the kilt is characteristic.

Siamsa Beirte

Irish

SIAMSA BEIRTE IS PRONOUNCED *SHI-um-suh BEHR-ti* and means "a frolic for two." Siamsa Beirte is a 2/4 Hornpipe time, *not* a Reel. Una and Sian O'Farrell introduced Siamsa Beirte at the Stockton Folk Dance Camp in 1956.

Dance A While CD: #21. "Siamsa Beirte."

Records: Folkraft 1422, "Bluebell Polka"; Robin Hood 8001; World of Fun LP–5, Side B–4; or any evenly phrased Irish Hornpipe.

Music: "Bluebell Polka," *Country Dancer*, May 1951, p. 16.

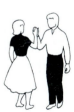

Formation: Double circle, partners facing, man's back to center, right hands joined at shoulder height and left hand hanging relaxed by side.

Steps: Threes, rock, Schottische.

DIRECTIONS FOR THE DANCE

Meter 2/4 • Directions are for man; woman's part reverse.

▪ *Measures*

1–8   Introduction: no action.

        "Threes" and Rock

1   Beginning right, hop in place, step to left on left, step right almost behind left, step left (counts *and* 1 *and* 2). Do not dip on second step.

2   Beginning left, repeat action in other direction (counts *and* 1 *and* 2).

3–4   Beginning right, hop in place; bringing left behind right, step on left, hop left; bringing right behind left, step on right, hop right; bringing left behind right, step on left; rock to side on right, rock to side on left (count *and* 1 *and* 2 *and* 1 *and* 2). The rock is side to side with feet close together, the right foot crossed in front of the left. Raise weight onto ball of foot and rock. The woman begins on the left foot but steps one foot behind the other as does the man.

5–8   Beginning with **left hop,** repeat action of measures 1–4 in reverse line of direction.

"Threes" and Change Over

9   Repeat action of measure 1.

10   Beginning with **left hop,** take one Schottische step to change places. Man moves around woman as she turns counterclockwise under joined right hands.

11–12   Repeat action of measures 9–10 and return to original position.

Irish Turn

13–16   Take both hands, crossed so that man's right joins woman's right on top and man's left joins woman's left underneath. Hold at shoulder height, elbows bent. Man pulls right hand toward him and down and under the left, rolling up so that the woman's forearms are resting on him. Beginning with right hop, take four Polka steps, turning clockwise, progressing in the line of direction. Irish Folk Dance teachers refer to this Polka (hop 1–3) as "turning threes." Both pull away slightly, remaining in a true facing position for this turn.

■ **STYLE**

The body is held erect but not stiff, with the head high; the steps are small, lively, and clean cut, with the toes pointing down.

■ **NOTE**

The rhythm hop step step step is taken in even rhythm (*and* 1 *and* 2) even though it is referred to as a Polka.

Three Meet*   English

T HREE MEET IS A DANCE OF greeting from northern England and Northumberland.

Records: Folkraft 1112, 1262.

Music: Gadd, May, *Country Dances of Today, Book 2,* p. 15; Kennedy, Peter. *Fiddler's Tune* Book 1. Tune: "When Daylight Shines," p 42.

Formation: Sets of three, two women and a man, or vice versa, arms linked, facing another set of three. All sets form large circle; alternately one faces line of direction, the other reverse line of direction.

Steps: Running step, buzz step.

Three Meet (continued)

---

*Dance arranged from the dance description by May Gadd, *Country Dances of Today, Book 2,* Country Dance Society of America, May 1951.

Meter 4/4

■ *Measures*

I. Forward, Back, and Change Sides

1–4   Take four steps, moving forward, four steps moving backward. Take eight steps on a diagonal to right, passing opposite set and turning counterclockwise a half–turn to face same set on opposite sides.

5–8   In new place, repeat action of measures 1–4 to return to original place.

II. Elbow Swing

9–10   Taking eight steps, the middle dancer turns right–hand partner with right elbow swing twice around in place.

11–12   Middle dancer takes eight walking steps, turning left–hand partner with left elbow swing twice around. On last two steps, the three in set cuddle up (arms reach around each other, middle dancer's arms underneath) to form a basket of three.

III. Basket in Line of Three

13–16   In cuddle position, sets progress diagonally to right passing each other, while turning clockwise with a buzz step (right foot crossed in front of left), and meet new set coming in opposite direction.

Repeat dance, each set dancing with new set.

■ **NOTE**

The English Country Dancers are particular about attacking each new phrase of music on time.

■ **STYLE**

The English running step is a light, bouncy, dignified half–walk and half–run step. The body is in a dignified easy posture. The free hand of each outside dancer in the set hangs free to the side. The middle dancer holds the arms of the two partners in closely to his or her sides so that the threes can move easily as a unit. As a dance of greeting, the spirit is as light–hearted as the music. The dancers enjoy visiting around the circle to each new set of three.

The White Cockade*

Scottish Reel

DANCES WITH JACOBITE NAMES, like *The White Cockade*, are believed to have been composed by the many fiddlers in Scotland. After the 1745 rebellion, the pipes were banned. The Chiefs had their own fiddlers and the dances usually depict a famous battle, an event, or a place name.

Records: Scottish Dance Time Album Volume 4; or any eight–time 32–measure Reel in 4/4 meter.

Formation: Longway Reeltime dance. A four–couple set involving three couples in each 32–measure repetition. Top of set is indicated by left shoulder of first man.

Position: Feet in first position, hands by side.

Steps: Skip change step, pas de basque, slip step, setting.

DIRECTIONS FOR THE DANCE

Meter 4/4 • Directions are same for man and woman.

■ Measures

1–8	Dance begins with honors to partner, men bow, women curtsey. First, second, and third couples set and cross over with two skip change steps giving right hands, then set and cross back with two skip change sets to original places, again giving right hands.
9–16	First couple leads down the middle and up again to top place in the middle of the dance. (Eight skip change steps.)
17–20	First couple casts off to second place on own side. Second couple steps up on measures 19–20. (Four skip change steps.)

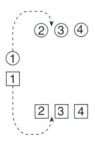

The White Cockade (continued)

*This dance is used by the permission of the Royal Scottish Country Dance Society, 12 Coates Crescent, Edinburgh, Scotland, EH3 7AF. Patron–Her Majesty The Queen; President–The Earl of Mansfield; Secretary–Miss M. M. Gibson. Permission granted April 16, 1986. [From Preston, *24 New Country Dances for the Year 1797*.]

| 21–24 | First and third couples dance four hands round to left. (Eight slip steps.) |
| 25–32 | Second and first couples dance rights and lefts with eight skip change steps. |

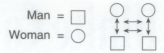

Repeat, having passed a couple.

- **NOTE**

Dance is repeated from second position, now involving third and fourth couples. Couple at the top stands and waits. At the end of the second sequence (32 measures), original first couple slips below the fourth couple, who now moves up. A new top couple starts the next 32 measures, or the third sequence. Once at the bottom of the set, the top couple becomes the new first couple.

- **SCOTTISH STEPS AND FORMATIONS**

Set or Setting: Two pas de basques in place facing as directed.

Skip Change Step: Begin in first position. Skip (hop) on left while extending right foot forward, knee straight and toe pointed. Step on right foot, keeping leg straight and firm. Close left to right in third rear position (remain on toes). Step forward onto right foot. Cues: Skip (hop), step, close, step.

Right and Left: Each dancer extends right hand to partner and changes places across the line; each dancer faces up or down the lines, gives left hand to other man or woman dancer, and changes places in line; each dancer gives left hand to other man or woman and finishes in original place. Cues: Across the line, up or down the line, across the line, up and down the line.

Slipping Step: This is used in all circles danced in Reel or Jig time, and in dances where the dancers join both hands to slip down, up or across the dance. The step is started from first position (i.e. heels together, feet turned out at right angles, with heels raised; take a step sideways with left foot (second position), bring right foot to left foot with heels touching (first position). Cue: step, together; step, together. Movements normally done in circles to the left and right.

- **NOTE**

The symbols used to represent the man and woman are reverse of those used by the Royal Scottish Country Dance Society.

Willow Tree

English

WILLOW TREE WAS COMPOSED BY Hugh Rippon, formerly with the English Folk Dance and Song Society, in 1968. It is based on the Dutch Folk Dance Gort Med Stroop.

Record: Folklore Village FLV 7802 (6/8 and 2/4); No Reels by The Old Swan Band FRR 0ll; Sold Out by Flowers and Frolics BR6.

Music: Medley of "Willow Tree," (6/8) "Wabash Cannonball" (2/4), "Golden Slippers" (2/4); Werner, Robert, *The Folklore Village Saturday Night Book*, p. 37; *English Dance & Song* Autumn 1963 Vol xxx, No. 3; *English Folk Dance & Song Society, Everyday Dances*, p. 14.

Formation: Longway set, eight couples. Head and foot couples are active; *do not cross over*.

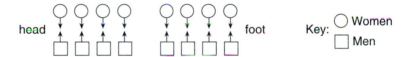

Note: No call. Could prompt.

DIRECTIONS FOR THE DANCE

Introduction: no action (4 counts).

A1, A2   **Partner change** (32 counts). Head couple, two hands joined, takes eight slides to foot of set (8 counts). Others clap hands. Head man leaves his partner at the foot, joins two hands with foot woman, and they take eight slides to head of set (8 counts). Foot man and woman #1 join two hands and take eight slides to head of set (8 counts). Foot man leaves woman #1 at the head of set and takes his original partner, two hands joined, and takes eight slides to return to original position (8 counts).

B1, B2   **Elbow Reel** (32 counts). Active couples, head and foot couples Reel, hooking right elbows with partner in middle of set, and turn clockwise once and a half, separate. Active men turn counterclockwise next woman in line, with left elbows hooked, once around as active women turn next man in line with left elbows hooked once around. Head couples move down, foot couple up the set turning alternately next person in line with left elbow and then partner with right elbow until active couples meet in middle of set (between couples 4 and 5). Each dancer is on original side. Head and foot couples join hands to form a ring of four, raise hands to form four arches.

Willow Tree (continued)

C1 **Cast out and Promenade** (16 counts).

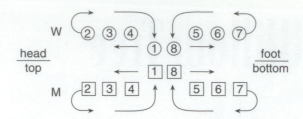

The remaining three head couples (2, 3, 4) face up the set; the remaining three foot couples (5, 6, 7) face down the set. Couples 2 and 7 individually cast out, walk down the outside of the set to the middle of set, move through arch made by head and foot couple; meet partner in center of ring of four, join inside hands. Couple 2 faces up, couple 7 faces down, move through the other arch, returning to head or foot of set. (*See diagram.*) Single–file, couples 3, 4, 5, and 6 move to head or foot of set, cast out, move through arches and promenade up or down set to next position.

C2 **Swing** (16 counts). All couples swing. Couples 2, 3, and 4 have moved up one position and couples 5, 6, and 7 have moved down one position. Couples 1 and 8 are now in the middle of the set.

■ **NOTES**

1. Repeat dance until all couples have been active once or twice.

2. Forearm grasp may be used for reel.

3. Eight couples work best, but adjustments for six to ten couples are possible. Divide set in half; e.g., three couples and four couples. The Reel can move faster or slower to complete.

4. The first figure must be danced to the proper music. The swing may be shortened or eliminated to accommodate those that are behind.

CANADA

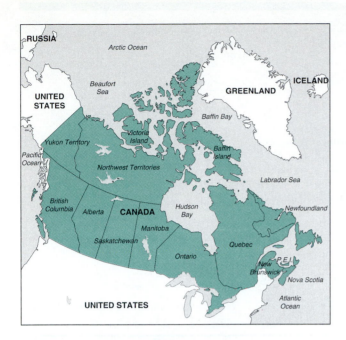

■ Discovery and Settlement

The Norse voyager, Lief Ericson, is purported to have sighted the east coast of Canada about A.D. 1000. Nearly 500 years later, in 1497, the Italian navigator, John Cabot, sailing under the sponsorship of King Henry VII of England, landed on the northeast coast of North America. A second voyage in 1498 took him as far south as Cape Cod.

French exploration of the Bay of Fundy, Nova Scotia, and the Gulf of St. Lawrence began in the early 1500s. Jacques Cartier ascended the St. Lawrence as far as present day Montreal and established a colony at Quebec. Settlers from Normandy and Picardy, along the English Channel, established Acadia in Nova Scotia in 1604.

In the ensuing 250 years, the French and English colonized the eastern seaboard of North America (Canada and the United States) and brought with them their culture, including music and dance.

The last half of the 18th century (1750–1800) saw the French lose their foothold in Canada, and their governance in North America was removed to Louisiana. The English held on to northeastern Canada, but lost out to the revolutionaries of the Thirteen Colonies.

The early part of the 19th century (1800–1840) saw a great influx of Scots to eastern Canada, settling in Prince Edward Island, Cape Breton, and Nova Scotia.

■ Population

Ninety percent of the Canadian population has settled mainly along the border of the United States. The cultural and ethnic origins of the population are represented primarily by British (English, Scottish, Irish, and Welsh), French and German groups, followed next by people of Ukraine, Italian, Dutch, Scandinavian, Polish, Jewish, and Russian backgrounds. Other groups include Native Americans, Eskimos, Asians, East Indians, other Europeans, and Africans.

■ Culture

The three main cultural influences of English, French, and Scottish people have shaped the present day traditions. The settlers who came to the New World brought with them their love of dancing 17th and 18th century dances. Scottish Highland dancing, Scottish Country dancing, Cape Breton step dancing, and French Canadian dance are very dominant. There is also a wide variety of European, Square and Contra dance similar to that in the United States.

■ Cape Breton

Cape Breton was originally inhabited by the Mi'kmaq Indians and in the 18th century was sparsely settled by the French. The present culture was influenced by the arrival of 30,000 Scots from the Highlands and Western Isles of Scotland, forced to leave between 1800 and 1850. This was a result of the Highland Clearances. Cape Breton became a stronghold of Gaelic culture. Its musical heritage, particularly a unique style and tradition of Scottish fiddling, thrives.[1]

The interrelationship of Cape Breton step dancing and rhythmic fiddle music is important in the preservation of each. An unbroken tradition of step dancing, solo form and social dancing, traces back to the earliest settlers from Scotland. The Strathspeys and Reels from Scotland were the original social dances. The introduction of the Lancer and Quadrille sets replaced the Scottish dances. It is an interesting course of Scottish country dancing both in Scotland and Cape Breton, coming, going, disappearing. The traditional Cape Breton fiddle music suited the new dances (Lancer and Quadrille), which thus survived. Today, step dancing has received great interest beyond Cape Breton. The tradition is kept alive by the explosion and interchange of recordings, publications, new compositions, traveling teachers, and musicians.

---

[1]Dunlay, Kate, and David Greenberg. *Traditional Celtic Violin Music of Cape Briton*, Mississauga, Ontario, Canada: DunGreen Music, 1996

La Bastringe

L A BASTRINGE IS A French Canadian mixer.

Dance A While CD: #2. "La Bastringe."

Record: Leg 120.

Formation: Couples in a single circle, woman on man's right.

Hand hold: W position.

Steps: Walk, Two–Step and buzz swing.

DIRECTIONS FOR THE DANCE

Meter 2/4 • Men and women use the same footwork.

Introduction: 20 counts

Mea.Counts

		Part I Walks
1–2	1–4	Beginning right take three steps to the center, counts 1–3. On count 4 tap left foot next to right.
3–4	5–8	Beginning left, take three steps back, counts 1–3. On count 4 tap right foot next to left.
5–8	1–4	Repeat action of measures 1–4
		Part II Two–Step *Keep arms in W position.*
1–4	1–8	Beginning right, take four Two–Steps in reverse line of direction
5–8	1–8	Four Two–Steps in line of direction.
		Part III Swing
1–2	1–4	Man lifts his left arm up and woman turns under clockwise.
3–8	5–16	Right parallel position, buzz step clockwise for 12 counts.
		Part IV Two–Step with partner
1–7		Open to shoulder waist position, facing line of direction, beginning right, take seven Two–Steps forward, progressing in line of direction.
8		Turning one–quarter counterclockwise (man backing up, woman moving forward) take one Two–Step left to face center. Join hands in W position around the circle and repeat the dance from the beginning.

The Saint John River

THE *SAINT JOHN RIVER* WAS COMPOSED BY Prudence Edwards, 1966. This Scottish country dance won first place in a contest to commemorate Canada's Centennial in 1967. Pru Edwards was a member of the Fredericton Scottish Country Dance Group, New Brunswick, and now lives in Galiano, British Columbia.

Music: 32 Bar Strathspey. *Brave of Balquidder*, Singing Birds; *The Bonnie Lass o' Bon Accord*; Mary Hamilton.

Record: *The Saint John River*, Stan Hamilton and his Flying Scotsmen, Volume 5, SMT 70–2.

Formation: Four couples in a four couple set. All face center of set.

Step: Strathspey.

1	①	Top
2	②	
3	③	
4	④	

DIRECTIONS FOR THE DANCE

Meter 4/4

■ Measures

Chord — Arms relaxed at sides, men bow from the waist. Women lift skirt slightly, right foot behind left and curtsy.

Arms are relaxed at sides unless specifically noted. The Strathspey step is used throughout the dance, man and woman always begin with right foot.

I. The Stream

1–8 — First woman casts behind the second woman, crosses the set and casts behind the third man, crosses the set, casts behind the fourth woman, crosses the set and finishes below the fourth couple on the opposite side. The woman glances coquettishly back at her partner occasionally to be sure he is following. First man follows his partner to finish below the fourth woman on the opposite side.

II. The Bridges and The Salmon Pools

9–16 — First couple, inside hands joined, dances up under the two–hand arch formed by the fourth couple (Measures 9–10); join two hands (arms graceful above waist–not stiff–man aiding the woman) and dances four Strathspey steps turning once and a half clockwise; inside hands joined dance up under arch formed by the second couple (Measures 15–16), finishing in original position.

III. The Reversing Falls

17–24 — First couple, man's right hand joins woman's right hand, dances down the middle and up, followed by the second, third, and fourth couples. At the bottom, the first man and woman turn toward each other and dance

The Saint John River (continued)

up the set. The second couple individually dance one step up, turn toward each other, man takes partner's right hand with his right hand and dances two steps down the middle. They separate and turn out two steps up, turn toward the middle, and join right hands and one step home. The third couple follows the second couple, two steps up, turns, join right hands in the middle, goes down two steps, separates and turns out, two steps up, turns and goes down two steps home. The fourth couple individually dances four steps on the outside to the top, touches hands *briefly* (almost a push away), turns out and dances four steps back to place.

The first and fourth couples must be alert to complete their path.

25–28   In straight lines, facing center, all four couples pass partner's right shoulders, dance back to back (do–si–do).

     IV.   **The River Meets the Sea**

24–32   First couple dances a right hand hey on own side to the bottom of the set; changing places with the second couple with right hands, third couple with left hands, and fourth couple with right hands to finish in fourth place facing center. First man and fourth woman make polite turns on last step (an extra quarter turn).

Repeat dance with new top couple.

Bow to partner at the end of the dance.

▪ NOTE

1. The Saint John River forms a portion of the border between New Brunswick and Maine and flows into the Bay of Fundy. On occasion, high tides flow upstream.

2. The figures reflect the various portions of the Saint John River as it moves through New Brunswick.

   The Stream (measures 1–8) describes the meandering course of the river as the man chases the woman.

   In *The Bridges and The Salmon Pools* (measures 9–16) couple one dances under an arch (bridge) and circles (as if in a pool).

   The Reversing Falls (measures 17–24) describes the action of the ebb tide as the river runs downstream over a shallow waterfall; the flow reverses with the incoming high tide.

   The River Meets the Sea (measures 25–32) has a wave–like back–to–back movement, and the head couple wends down the set as the Saint John River disappears into the sea.

CZECH AND SLOVAKIA

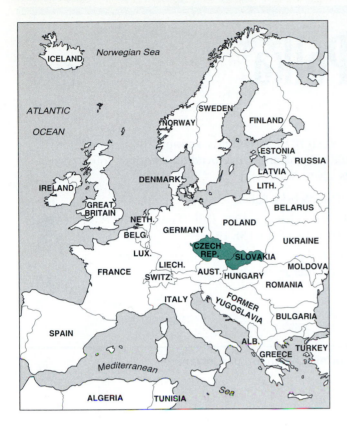

■ Dance Characteristics

As 1992 dissolved into 1993 so the former country known as Czechoslovakia dissolved its unity and by virtue of a "velvet divorce" peacefully became two separate political units, the Czech Republic and Slovakia. Despite the separation many common threads remain. The Czechs are of Slavic origin and speak a common Slavic language. Children's dances and games reflect some of the oldest elements found in Slavic culture and are similar to games and dances found in Poland, Russia, and the general Balkan region.

In the past, the two countries' rich mineral and agricultural resources attracted both Western and Eastern invaders, and migrating tribes and warriors have long used the rivers that flow from east to west.

During the 17th century, Bohemia, Moravia, and Slovakia were a part of the Austro–Hungarian Empire. English Country Dances and Western Court Dances were introduced. About that time, the Italians were invited to the courts. Consequently, the dance tradition of Czech and Slovakia has been influenced by both Western and Eastern culture. In the western regions, the folk songs are in the major key; in the east, in the minor key. In the west, where industrialization is more developed, the folk customs are preserved by societies and through holidays, but in the east, where it is more agriculturally oriented, many of the folk customs, including wearing traditional dress, are very much a part of daily life.

MUSIC

The oldest native instruments are the kobza (like a lyre), the viol, the lucec (hurdy–gurdy), the bagpipe, and the drum. A typical Slovakian folk band also includes a dulcimer and a violin. In southern Bohemia, the bagpipe is played alone or with a violin, and, in eastern Bohemia, the bands are composed of clarinets, violins, double basses, horns, and trumpets.

Doudlebska Polka*

Czech

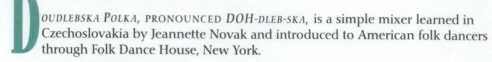

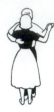

DOUDLEBSKA POLKA, PRONOUNCED *DOH-DLEB-SKA*, is a simple mixer learned in Czechoslovakia by Jeannette Novak and introduced to American folk dancers through Folk Dance House, New York.

Dance A While CD: #9. "Doudlebska Polka."

Records: Canadian MH 3016; Festival 114007; Folk Dancer 3016; Folklore Village 45; Folkraft 1413, LP–13; LSE 19.

Formation: Couples in closed position form one large circle or several smaller circles. Directions are for one large circle.

Steps: Polka, walk.

DIRECTIONS FOR THE DANCE

Meter 2/4 • The directions are for man, woman's part reverse.

■ *Measures*

1–4	Introduction: no action.

I. Polka

1–16	Beginning left, take 16 Polka steps turning clockwise, traveling in line of direction.

II. Walk and Circle

17–32	Open position, woman's free hand on hip. Man stretches left arm out to place hand on left shoulder of man in front as couples take 32 walking steps moving in line of direction. This action moves dancers toward center to form a ring of couples. As ring revolves counterclockwise, everyone sings "tra–la–la," and so forth.

III. Men Clap, Ladies Circle

33–48	Men face center of circle and clap hands throughout figure as follows: clap own hands (count 1), clap own hands (count *and*), clap hands of man on both sides, shoulder high (count 2). Women with hands on hips, take one half-turn clockwise to face reverse line of direction and take 16 Polka steps, progressing forward in reverse line of direction around men's circle.
	On last measure, each woman steps behind a man, and men turn around and begin dance again with new partner.

■ VARIATION

1. Measures 1–16, for beginners a heavy Two–Step and the Varsouvienne position or inside hands joined may be substituted.

2. Measures 33–48, the men may slap a thigh occasionally, duck down, or cross their own hands over when they clap neighbors' hands.

---

*Dance arranged from the dance description by Michael Herman and reproduced by permission of Folk Dance House, New York.

3. Measures 17–32, if group is large, form several small circles.
4. Measures 33–48, if more than one circle is formed, ladies may "cheat" by moving from one circle to another.

■ NOTES

1. Those without partners go to the center (the "lost and found" department) and meet the other one without a partner.
2. If there are extra people, extra men without a partner may join dance during star figure, and extra women may join ring as women Polka around outside.
3. Encourage group singing during the march, especially loud. It makes the dance fun!

Tancuj

Czech

CZECH FOLK DANCE PRONOUNCED *TON-TSOOY*.

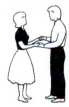

Record: Folk Dancer MH 1017.

Formation: Double circle, couples facing, hands joined. Men's backs to center of circle, women face center.

Steps: Two–Step, runs, hops.

DIRECTIONS FOR THE DANCE

Meter: 2/4

■ *Measures*

Part I. Step Together Step, Swing

1–2   Moving to men's left, women's right. Men step sidewards left, close right to left, step left and swing right across left. Women: step sidewards right, close left to right, step right and swing left across right.

3–4   Repeat moving in opposite direction. (Note: Swing joined hands vigorously.)

5–16   Repeat measures 1–4 three times.

Part II. Run

1–8   Partners take a right hip position. Place right hand on partner's left hip, hold own hand on own hip. Run clockwise 16 steps.

9–16   Change to left hip–to–hip position and run 16 steps counterclockwise.

Part III. Step Together, Step Swing

1–16   Repeat Part I, Step together, step swing.

Part IV. Heel and Toe

1–8   Partners move away from each other, men to center, women away from center. Hop on left, place right heel down, hop on left, place right toe down. Repeat hopping on right. Dance eight "heel-toe" movements away from partner.

Part V. Run

1–16   Repeat Part II, clockwise and counterclockwise run.

        Repeat dance from the beginning.

FRANCE

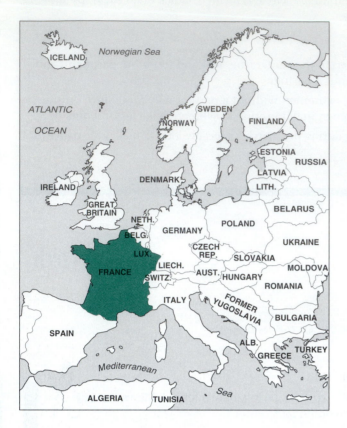

■ Dance Characteristics

Although originally settled by Celts, France, situated between the sea and the northern plains, with wide river valleys, was easily invaded by one group of settlers and warriors after another. Thus, the ancient dance rituals are quite varied. Although there are characteristics unique to different provinces, French dances tend to have many common features. The dances are simple in form, the behavior of dancers is very polite, and the movement is restrained. Many of the dances are based on one or two steps.

MUSIC

In Brittany, the tunes are sung or played on a biniou (bagpipe) and a bombarde (rustic oboe). For La Farandole, the dancers are preceded by musicians, who play the tambourin (small drumhead with a long body) with the left hand and the galoubet (an oboe-like instrument) with the right.

For La Bourrée, the native instruments are the cabrette (a simple form of bagpipe) and the vielle (an oval-shaped mandolin with a very short fingerboard and a resined wheel at the other end that is turned by a handle that strikes the strings as in a hurdy-gurdy). The cabrettaire (player of the bagpipe) often wears a band of small round bells on one ankle and taps the heel on the first beat of each measure to accentuate the rhythm.

Branle d'Ossau*

THIS IS AN OPEN CIRCLE DANCE FROM Gascogne Pyrénées: Vallée d'Ossau in Béarn. Marilyn M. Smith learned this dance from Pierre Corbefin in the summer of 1989.

Cassette: Marc Castanet et Michel Le Meur: *Raccord Duo Swing*, Side B, Band 1.

Formation: Open circle, traveling left (clockwise), hands joined, arms down, men and women alternate positions along the line.

Steps: Rocking step and as analyzed in dance description.

DIRECTIONS FOR THE DANCE

Meter 2/4 • Directions are the same for man and woman.

■ *Measures*

Introduction: Dancers may begin at the beginning of any musical phrase.

1 Traveling to the left, dancers face center: Step left (count 1), hop slightly on left bringing right leg over in front of left (count 2), step across on right in front of left (count *and*).

2 Backing up slightly in line of direction, step left, right, left (counts 1, 2, *and*).

3 Dancing in place, step on the right slightly behind the left (count 1), hop slightly on right while bringing left leg behind right (count 2), step on left slightly behind right, end facing the center (count *and*).

4 Facing center, step on right in front of left (count 1), step back on left in place (left foot is behind right) (count 2), step on right in place (in front of left) (count *and*). The movement resembles a "rocking step" in place.

Repeat dance from beginning.

---

*Dance description and permission to use *Branle d'Ossau* courtesy of Marilyn M. Smith. Cassette available from Marilyn M. Smith, 1560 Yardley Street, Santa Rosa, CA 95403

La Montagnarde*

L *A MONTAGNARDE* (*LAH MOHN-TAHN-YARD*) IS A bourrée from the Auvergne region of central France. It is done in "cortège" formation, which can accommodate any number of couples. Marilyn M. Smith learned the dance in France in 1986, and presented it at the University of Pacific Folk Dance Camp in 1987.

Cassette: "On Y Va," Side A/3, or "Lo Drac," Side A, Band 7.

Formation: Couples, one behind the other in a long column facing "up the set" (cortège). Woman to the left of man, right hands joined behind man's back, and left hands joined behind woman's back. Couples are spaced three to four feet apart and should maintain this distance.

Steps: Pas de bourrée, man's stamping pattern, man's right lateral pas de bourrée, woman's right lateral pas de bourrée, man's left lateral pas de bourrée, woman's left lateral pas de bourrée. Arms: During all right and left pas de bourrée steps both men and women have arms up, slightly forward, elbows bent, palms forward, and hands at or just above head level.

DIRECTIONS FOR THE DANCE

Meter 3/8

■ *Measures*

Introduction: An improvisation of the bagpipe (cabrette) plus three measures–no action.

I. Avance (Advance)

1–8   Couples in cortège formation move forward "up the set" with pas de bourrée steps. Eight measures is suggested but is not a fixed number when danced in the village or at a bal folk, but at the beginning of an 8-measure phrase and every 8 measures thereafter the "head couple" will begin Figure II.

II. Tour sur Place (Turn in Place)

1–4   Beginning left, the "head couple" turns once and a half clockwise in place with four pas de bourrée steps, and ends facing "down the set."

5–6   Same couple releases hands and separate, bringing arms up. Woman passes in front of man, moves diagonally forward to the right with two pas de bourrée steps, while man moves diagonally forward to left with two pas de bourrée steps. Man ends to left of and just beyond the man of couple 2. Woman ends to right of and just beyond the woman of couple 2.

7–8   Man dances man's stamping pattern. Woman turns once half counterclockwise to end facing "up the set."

---

*Dance contributed by Marilyn M. Smith and arranged from dance descriptions by Jack Peirce for the Folk Dance Federation of California, Inc. January 1988. Cassette available from Marilyn M. Smith, 1560 Yardley Street, Santa Rosa, CA 95403.

III. Croisement (Crossing)

1–4   Couple 1 dances right lateral pas de bourrée in the slot between couple 2 and couple 3, passing face to face.

5–8   Couple 1 dances left lateral pas de bourrée in the slot between couple 3 and couple 4, again passing face to face. In this figure man always faces "down the set" and active woman "up the set." Continue with this figure proceeding down the set until the couples meet at the bottom of the set, where they join hands in position for Figure I. Couples may do a clockwise turn.

Every eight measures the new "head couple" will begin Figure II, then continue "down the set" with Figure III. The cortège continues to dance the pas de bourrée moving "up the set," keeping three to four feet spacing between couples to accommodate those doing Figure III. **Note:** The dance can continue indefinitely!

■ STEPS

Pas de bourrée: Step forward on the left (count 1), step on the right beside or slightly forward of the left (count 2), step on the left slightly forward (count 3). The step alternates. It also may be done turning in place or marking time in place.

Man's stamping pattern (2 measures): *Measure 1:* Stamp left in place with weight (count 1), hold (count 2), hop on left (count 3). *Measure 2:* Stamp right kicking left forward from knee (count 1), hold (counts 2 and 3).

Man's right lateral pas de bourrée (4 measures): *Measure 1:* Facing "down the set" and traveling right, step on the left crossing in front of right (count 1), step on right to right (count 2), step on left beside or slightly forward of right (count 3). *Measure 2:* Step on right to right (count 1), step on left beside or slightly forward of right (count 2), step on right slightly to right (count 3). *Measures 3–4:* Man's stamping pattern.

Man's left lateral pas de bourrée (4 measures): *Measure 1:* Facing "down the set" and moving left, step on left to left (count 1), step on right beside left (count 2), step slightly left on left (count 3). *Measure 2:* Step on right crossing in front of left (count 1), step on left to left (count 2), step on right beside or slightly forward of left (count 3). *Measures 3–4:* Man's stamping pattern.

Woman's right lateral pas de bourrée (4 measures): *Measures 1–2:* Facing "up the set" and moving right dance measures 1–2 or man's left lateral pas de bourrée. *Measures 3–4:* Make one full turn clockwise with two pas de bourrée steps, beginning with the right. End facing "up the set."

Woman's left lateral pas de bourrée (4 measures): *Measures 1–2:* Facing "up the set" and moving left dance measures 1–2 or man's left lateral pas de bourrée. *Measures 3–4:* Make one full turn counterclockwise with two pas de bourrée steps, beginning with the left. End facing "up the set."

■ STYLE

Arms: During all right and left lateral pas de bourrée steps both man and woman have arms up, slightly forward, elbows somewhat bent, palms forward, and hands at or just above head level.

Generally the styling is very flat and smooth; the knees are slightly bent throughout. The dance may be done an indefinite number of times with any number of couples, but it is less effective with too few couples since the feeling of a long cortège or column of dancers would be lost.

La Tournijaire*

THERE ARE MANY VARIANTS OF THIS dance found in the Massif–Central. This particular variant from Auvergne is an arrangement of figures learned in France from Yvon Guilcher in summer 1984. Three other variants of this dance were observed in the Rouergue. Pronunciation: *lah-toor-nih-JIGH-ruh*.

Cassette: *Bal Folk en Californie* by Le Soleil, Side A/3.

Formation: Couples in a circle, woman on man's left. Hands joined, arms up in a *W* position.

Steps: Pas de bourrée, man's stamping pattern, Waltz.

DIRECTIONS FOR THE DANCE

Meter 3/8

■ *Measures*

Introduction (3 measures plus 1 count).

I. Ronde

1	Eight measures traveling to left: Facing center and traveling to the left, step on left to left (count 1), close right to left (count 2), step slightly sideward to left on left (count 3). Count 1 is a much bigger step to left than count 3. Styling is smooth, flat, gliding. Knees are slightly bent throughout.
2	Still facing center and traveling to left, cross right in front of left (count 1), step to left, cross right in front of left (count 1), step to left on left (count 2), close right to left (count 3).
3–4	Repeat measures 1–2.
5–8	Repeat measures 1–4, except on measure 8 dance pas de bourrée in place ready to change direction.
1	Eight measures traveling to right: Facing center and traveling right, step on left slightly behind right (count 1), step on right beside left (count 2), step on left beside right (count 3). **Note:** This step travels only slightly to the right. It is used as a transition step to change direction.
2	Step on right to right (count 1), step on left beside right (count 2), step on right slightly to right (count 3).
3	Step on left crossing in front of right (count 1), step on right to right (count 2), step on left beside right (count 3).
4	Repeat measure 2.
5–8	Repeat measures 3–4 two more times. On measure 8 dance pas de bourrée in place or travel only slightly to get ready for refrain, which follows.

---

*Dance description and permission to use *La Tournijaire* courtesy of Marilyn M. Smith. Cassette available from Marilyn M. Smith, 1560 Yardley Street, Santa Rosa, CA 95403.

Refrain

1–8   **Women:** Form a circle in the center, hands joined and arms up in *W* position. Women repeat Ronde figure traveling eight measures to the left as in Figure I.

       Men: Beginning left, dance individual clockwise turns while moving counterclockwise with a small flatfooted waltz step turning smoothly and continuously. End on measure 7 facing center. *Measure 8:* Step right in place (count 1), small step sideward left on left (count 2), close right to left (count 3). Men hold arms up and slightly forward palms forward.

9–16   **Women:** Reverse direction of Ronde and travel eight pas de bourrée steps to right as in Figure I.

       Men: Facing center, travel to left (clockwise) with basic pas de bourrée step as in Figure I of Ronde. Arms still up and slightly forward.

    II.   **Right and Left Hand Around**

1–8   Facing partner (woman is on man's left), join right hands (arms bent) and dance eight pas de bourrée steps traveling clockwise in a circle with partner beginning with left foot.

9–16   Facing "corner" (the woman on man's right), join left hands and dance eight pas de bourrée traveling counterclockwise in a circle with "corner." Man helps right–hand woman get into formation for the Refrain.

    Refrain

1–16   Repeat measures 1–16 of the Refrain.

   III.   **Panier (Basket Hold)**

1–8   Men form front basket hold by joining hands in front of women. (Women are already in a circle with hands joined from the Refrain. Women lower arms in this figure so men can form basket hold over their arms.) Circle travels to the left eight measures beginning with the left foot.

9–16   On count 1 of measure 9, change to regular hand hold (arms up in *W* position). Circle continues to travel eight measures to the left with basic pas de bourrée (Ronde formation) beginning with the left foot. Circle widens and picks up speed.

    Refrain

1–16   Repeat measures 1–16 of Refrain.

   IV.   **Chaîne**

1–2   Facing partner (woman on man's left), join right hands (arms bent) and begin right and left chain, men traveling diagonally left out of the circle, women traveling diagonally toward center of circle with two basic pas de bourrée steps, beginning with the left.

3–4   Give left hand to next partner, men traveling diagonally toward center of circle and women traveling diagonally right out of circle with two basic pas de bourrée steps beginning left.

       Note: Men travel clockwise, women travel counterclockwise around circle.

5–8   Repeat measures 1–4, traveling around the circle and chaining with partner's number 3 and partner's number 4.

9–10   With partner number 4, do two basic pas de bourrée steps turning one half turn counterclockwise around each other to face in opposite direction (the direction from which you came).

11–16   Repeat measures 1–6: Men now travel counterclockwise, women travel clockwise alternating right hand (measures 11–12) and left hand (measures 13–14), and end facing original partner. Dancers use measures 15–16 to get into closed social dance position with original partner. Man should end with back to center.

La Tournijaire (continued)

V. **Valse**

1–16 **Note:** (There is no Refrain after Figure IV Chaîne.) In closed dance position waltz 16 measures with partner. Man begins left, woman begins right, turning clockwise and traveling counterclockwise around the circle.

Ending: Musicians play an "ending" motif during which man may turn partner clockwise under their joined hands to finish dance.

■ **NOTE**

Man's stamping pattern may be used in Ronde measures 7–8; in Refrain measures 15–16; or in Panier measures 15–16. Refer to p. 291 for man's stamping pattern.

Mon Père Avait un Petit Bois

MON PÈRE AVAIT UN PETIT BOIS IS pronounced *mohn pair ah-veh tanh puh-tee bwah* and means "my father had a little woods." This dance is a Branle, a 16th–century court dance. Branle comes from *branler*, to shake, and is also known as "brawls."

This Branle was introduced at Mendocino Folk Lore Camp in 1963, by Madelynne Greene as taught to her in Normandie, France, in 1962 by Madame Jeanne Messager, leader of Ethnic Dance Group in Caen.

Record: "Branle Normand," Folkraft 337–002.

Formation: Single circle, hands joined and held down. No partners.

Steps: Walk, step–hop, branle.

DIRECTIONS FOR THE DANCE

Meter 4/4 • Directions are the same for all.

■ *Measures*

1–2 Introduction: no action.

1–2 Beginning right, take four walking steps (slow, slow, slow, slow). Circle moves counterclockwise.

3 Facing center of circle, step forward on right (count 1); hop on right, swinging left leg with knee bent backward (count 2); step left (count 3); hop on left, swinging right leg straight forward (count 4). Arms swing backward and body bends forward (counts 1–2), arms swing forward and body leans backward (counts 3–4).

4 Repeat action of measure 3.

| 5–8 | Repeat action of measures 1–4. |
| 9–12 | Beginning right, take eight branle steps. Branle step: Step right in place, left foot comes behind and just below right calf, softly touching (count 1), hop on right (count 2). Hands remaining joined, thrust right hand out to right, left elbow bending (count 1), maintaining arm position (count 2). Reverse footwork and arms for branle step, beginning left (counts 3–4). |

▪ LYRICS

This dance is frequently done to the singing of the song, unaccompanied.

1. Mon per'avait un petit bois
   d'ou venez–vous bell'promener avec moi
   Il y crossait bien cinq cents noix
   d'ou venez–vous belle D'ou venez–vous donc.
   d'ou venez–vous promener–vous promener la belle
   d'ou venez–vous bell'promener avec moi.

1. My father had a little woods
   Where do you come from, pretty (girl), stroll with me.
   There grew at least 500 nuts
   Where do you come from pretty girl, where do you come from.
   Where do you come strolling from pretty girl
   Where do you come from, pretty girl, stroll with me.

2. Il y crossait bien cinq cents noix
   d'ou venez–vous bell'
   Sur les cinq cents j'en mangais trois
   d'ou venez–vous bell'.

2. There grew at least 500 nuts
   Where do you come from pretty girl
   Out of the 500, I ate three
   Where do you come from pretty girl.

3. Sur les cinq cents j'en mangais trois
   d'ou venez–vous bell'
   J'en fus malade au lit des mois
   d'ou venez–vous bell'.

3. Out of the 500, I ate three
   Where do you come from pretty girl
   I was sick in bed for months
   Where do you come from pretty girl.

4. J'en fus malade au lit des mois
   d'ou venez–vous bell'
   Tous mes parents m'y venaient voir
   d'ou venez–vous bell'.

4. I was sick in bed for months
   Where do you come from pretty girl
   All my relatives came to see me
   Where do you come from pretty girl.

5. Tous mes parents m'y venaient voir
   d'ou venez–vous bell'
   mais non et n'y venais pas
   d'ou venez–vous bell'.

5. All my relatives came to see me
   Where do you come from pretty girl
   But no, and don't come
   Where do you come from pretty girl.

Rondeau de Garein*

A LINE DANCE FROM GASCOGNE AS learned by Marilyn M. Smith in Toulouse in the summer of 1986.

Cassette: "Suite des Rondeaux," *Bal Folk en Californie* by Le Soleil.

Formation: Line leading to the left (clockwise), hands joined right over left, arms bent at the elbows or hands joined down at the side. Alternate position for men and women along the line is preferable.

Step: As analyzed in dance description.

DIRECTIONS FOR THE DANCE

Meter 2/4

■ *Measures*

Introduction (4 measures)

1   Facing center, lift slightly on right (preparatory left count *ah*), step to left on left (count 1), step on right beside left (count *and*), step slightly to left on left (count 2).

2   Facing center, step on right crossing over in front of left (count 1), step to left on left (count *and*), step on right crossing over in front of left (count 2).

3   Step in place on left (count 1), bounce twice in place on left, kicking right forward slightly from the knee, (knee is bent) and retract right foot slightly (counts 2 *and*).

4   Step back slightly on right (count 1), with slight preparatory lift on right (count *and*), close left to right with left heel next to right toes turned slightly out to the left (count 2).

Repeat dance from beginning.

---

*Dance description and permission to use *Rondeau de Garein* courtesy of Marilyn M. Smith. Cassette available from Marilyn M. Smith, 1560 Yardley Street, Santa Rosa, CA 95403.

HUNGARY

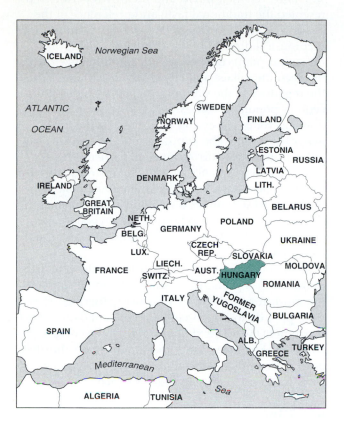

■ Introduction

By Andor Czompo, Professor Emeritus, Williamsburg, Virginia

Hungarian folk dances can be grouped into five major categories: Herdsmen's dances (Pásztor táncok), Leaping dances (Ugrós táncok), Maidens' round (Leány karikázó), Recruiting dances (Verbunk), and the Csárdás. To establish these categories certain principles of classification were applied, based on the analysis of the spatial, technical, musical–rhythmical, and functional characteristics of the dances. Each of these dance types also represents different historical periods reflecting certain socio–cultural conditions. Although these dances comprise the living dance repertory of the Hungarian peasantry, their existence and popularity vary greatly within Hungary, and show not just functional differences but varied geographical distributions as well.

The old layer of the Hungarian folk dances includes the Herdsmen's dances, the Leaping dances, and the Maidens' rounds. They date back to the Middle Ages and show similarities with other European folk dances of the same period. In addition to the Maidens' rounds, which are always danced in a closed circle with varied handholds and accompanied by singing, the boundaries of the other older dances are not always clear. Their formations in particular show great variety from male solo to group and mixed couple variations. The dance tunes that accompany these dances also belong to the old layer of Hungarian dance music as defined by Béla Bartók. Other ancient and common characteristics are the lack of physical contact (or maybe just a handshake hold) between the partners in couple dances and the unstructured, improvised mode of performance. In the dance repertory of the village folk in the 20th century, these dances reached the last stage of their natural existence. They are performed on rare occasions at weddings, family gatherings, or other festivities.

The recent, newer style of Hungarian folk dances, the *Verbunk* and the *Csárdás*, evolved and developed during the 18th and 19th centuries. Assuming a national character, they became the representative Hungarian dances both in Hungary and abroad.

The Verbunk (from the German word *werben:* recruiting) is the result of the 18th–century military recruiting practice, when musical entertainment and jollification were used to attract the attention of the young men and induce them to join the military service. The early Verbunk hardly differed from the male solo Leaping and Swineherd's dances; the technique, formation, and musical accompaniment adjusted later. In western Hungary a semicircle and circle form developed with a regulated structure, and often a dance leader was in charge. In eastern Hungary the dance maintained a solo form with a rich, highly improvised movement repertory of heel clicks, leg swings, and rhythmical boot–slapping. The earlier "Old Style" dance music, notated in 2/4 meter, changed to a more stately 4/4 beat with regular accents. This new style of music became very popular both in folk and national art music and continued in the popular Csárdás music well into the 20th century. Although it lost its military significance, the Verbunk is still danced on special occasions. During regularly organized dance events, the Verbunk is the first dance of the dance order, followed by a general couple Csárdás.

The Csárdás (from the word *csárda:* roadside inn) is the most recent, the most popular, and the most widely known Hungarian dance. It developed during the 19th century from earlier couple dances by adopting some Western European couple dance components, such as shoulder–waist and waltz positions for closer physical contact, and some turning elements. Improvised and unstructured, the Csárdás is usually danced in two parts. It begins with a Lassú (slow) section, where a Two–Step–like motif is dominant, performed mainly sideways. This is followed by a shorter Friss (fast) part, where turns and vertical movements dominate. The partners occasionally separate, providing an opportunity for the male to dance a solo, using motifs and patterns from the Verbunk.

After the Second World War the traditional lifestyle of the Hungarian peasantry changed drastically. The survival of the folk dances shifted to an institutionalized movement, emphasizing stage performance. During the 1970s and 1980s a new trend emerged, the so-called Tánchaz (dance house) movement. This is mainly an urban phenomenon. Devotees gather in clubs and youth centers to dance traditional folk dances to live music provided by village-style orchestras. The emphasis is on enjoyment, reestablishing the original purpose and function of folk dancing. There are still many well-known village folk ensembles, guarding traditional forms and principles with a conscious effort.

■ Dance Characteristics

STYLE

Hungarian folk dances comprise many stylistic traits depending upon their established types and are influenced by functional, emotional, spatial, and other specifics.

The *Maidens' rounds* are usually serene and lyrical with an increased dynamic range during the faster running part of the dance. The *Leaping* dances are light and playful due to their more individualistic and improvised nature. The *Herdsmen's* dances express control and skill, especially in the handling of implements. The *Recruiting* dances in circle form show a more regimented and disciplined style, while the soloistic, improvised form preserved the earlier, light *Leaping dance* character. In the *Csárdás*, which is basically a couple dance, the partners use technical synchronization and varied handholds with close physical contact to express the courting nature of the dance. Occasional separation and rejoining of the partners during the dance further enhance the teasing-flirting (csalogató) character of the *Csárdás*.

MUSIC

In the traditional village setting Hungarians preferred a small band of musicians to provide accompaniment for general dancing. Often these musicians were gypsies; however, their music and melody repertory represented the traditional taste and preference of the peasant population whom they served. L. Gulyas, former musical director of the Hungarian State Folk Ensemble, points out the significant difference between the village and city gypsy musicians: "While the repertory of the urban musicians includes 19th century popular music as well as international drawing-room pieces and dance music, the rural gypsy musician is the depository of the specific peasant culture which surrounds him, particularly in instrumental folk dance music." The instruments used by the small village bands are the violin, viola, double bass and sometimes a small dulcimer (cimbalom). The larger city gypsy orchestras use several violins and violas, cello, double bass, a large cimbalom, and a clarinet.

Traditional Hungarian folk instruments were used in the villages primarily as solo instruments providing music for small family or other gatherings. They were popular to accompany old types of dances. Such instruments were the duda (bagpipe), the citera (zither), the furulya (flute), and the nyenyere (hurdy-gurdy). These old instruments are enjoying a new revival and popularity in today's Tánchaz.

RESOURCE

A new VHS videotape, "Hungarian Recreational Folk Dances" by Andor Czompo, features demonstrations by the dancers of the Timar's Hungarian Folk Dance Ensemble in Budapest. The video demonstrates 17 dances and includes the three dances described in this book (*Csárdás Palócosan, Kiskandsztánc, Urgrós*) along with the dances *Körcsárdás* and *Ecseri Csárdás*, which were published in the fifth and sixth editions of *Dance A While*. "Hungarian Recreational Folk Dances" (45 minutes) is available from Andor Czompo, 100 Gleneagles, Williamsburg, VA 23188.

Hungarian Motifs*

TECHNICAL EXERCISES USING BASIC Hungarian folk dance motifs and their combinations are very useful in increasing the skill level and agility needed to perform Hungarian dances. The exercises may be done in a "follow the leader" style. First try each motif several times in the order listed, making changes at the half point or end of melodies. Later, leaders may arrange their preferred patterns and create new and interesting combinations.

Formation: Circle with a simple side–low hand hold or let individual dancers hold hands on hips and face the center of the room.

Music: Any good medium tempo (quarter note = 140–160 beats per minute) Verbunk, Csárdás, or Kanász–ugrós music in duple meter. Example; Hungaroton LPX 13031–32; Szatmári Verbunk or Dunántúli Ugrós or AC Special #3; Lassú Csárdás.

■ MOTIFS

1. **Knee Bends**
   Bend both knees slightly (counts 1–2), straighten both knees (counts 3–4).
   Note: The knee bends can be done in first position (feet together parallel) or second position (feet apart sideways parallel). Repeat the same way.

2. **Knee Bounces**
   Before count 1 bend both knees slightly. Straighten both knees with a slight accent (count 1), bend both knees slightly (count 2). Repeat the same way.
   Note: The preliminary knee bend is necessary only at the beginning. The knee straightenings coincide with the primary accent of the music.

3. **Side Close Step** (Single Csárdás step)
   Step on the right foot to the right side (counts 1–2), close the left foot to the right (no weight) (counts 3–4). Repeat with opposite footwork and direction.

4. **Double Csárdás Step**
   Step on the right to the right side (count 1), step on the left in place (beside right) (count 2), step on the right to the right side (count 3), close the left to the right (no weight) (count 4). Repeat with opposite footwork and direction.

5. **Step Hop**
   Step on the right in place (count 1), hop on the right in place (count 2). Repeat with opposite footwork.

6. **Cifra**
   Leap on to the right side (count 1), step on the left in place (count *and*), step on the right in place (count 2). Repeat with opposite footwork and direction.
   Variation: Cifra (Pas de Basque)
   Leap onto the right foot to the right side (count 1), step on the left in front of the right (count *and*), step on the right behind the left (count 2). Repeat beginning leap to left.

Hungarian Motifs (continued)

---

*Motifs arranged and permission to use courtesy of Andor Czompo. Music available from 100 Gleneagles, Williamsburg, VA 23188.

Variation: Back Cross Cifra

Leap onto the right foot to the right side (count 1), step on the left behind and across the right (count *and*), step on the right in front of and across the left (count 2). Repeat beginning leap to left.

7. **Leap Hop Kick**

Leap onto the right in place with a slight knee bend. At the same time lift the left in the back so the left lower leg is close to parallel with the floor (count 1); hop on the right in place. At the same time kick the left to forward–low position (count 2). Repeat beginning to the left.

8. **Run and Click**

Take two running steps, right and left in place (counts 1–2), close the right to the left with accent (slight heel–click) (count 3), pause (count 4). Repeat the same way.

9. **Heel Click**

Bend both knees slightly. At the same time open both heels (pigeon–toed) (counts 1–2), straighten both knees. At the same time close the heels together with a slight accent (counts 3–4).

Note: May be performed with these counts or twice as fast. Repeat the same way.

10. **Cross Jump Heel Click**

Jump into a "crossed position" (right foot in front of left) (count 1), jump into second position (feet apart and pigeon–toed) (count 2), jump into first position (feet together parallel, knees straight) (count 3), pause (count 4). Repeat the same way.

Csárdás Palócosan*

CSÁRDÁS IN PALÓC STYLE IS FROM north–central Hungary. This version is arranged by Andor Czompo.

Record and CD: Rounder 5005, side A, band 2, "Play the Bagpipe, Uncle John."

Formation: Independent couples. Partners face and join in a shoulder–shoulder position.

Motifs: Double Csárdás, Turning Csárdás, Two–Step.

■ **MOTIFS**

1. **Double Csárdás** (♩♩♩♩)

Step on the right, to the right side (count 1), step on the left beside the right in place (count 2), step on the right to the right side (count 3), close the left to the right with partial weight (count 4). Repeat beginning left.

2. **Turning Csárdás** (♩♩♩♩)

Step on the right in place turning one–quarter to the right (count 1), step on the left in place (count 2), step on the right in place turning one–quarter to the right (count 3), close the left to the right with partial weight (count 4).

3. **Two–Step** (♪♪♩)

Step on the left forward (count 1), step on the right in place (count *and*), step on the left forward (count 2). Repeat beginning right.

*Description and permission to use *Cárdás Palócosan* courtesy of Andor Czompo. Music available from 100 Gleneagles, Williamsburg, VA 23188.

Meter 4/4

■ Measures

Introduction: One note.

1–2   Double Csárdás twice starting to the man's right. Woman follows with opposite footwork.

3   Man executes the Turning Csárdás. Woman, following the man's lead, walks with three steps clockwise about halfway around the man (left, right, left) closing the right to the left with partial weight on the fourth count.

4   Double Csárdás to the man's left.

5–8   Repeat measures 1–4.

9   Double Csárdás to the man's right.

10–12   Two–Step three times. During Two–Step partners release hands and separate. Man makes a small circle to his left; woman with opposite footwork circles to her right. At the end they rejoin in Csárdás position.

Repeat the dance from the beginning four times.

Kiskanásztánc*

KIS MEANS SMALL, SHORT. KANÁSZTÁNC IS A swineherder's dance. This dance is a short version of a type of dance known as Kanásztánc. Although the majority of these dances are done with an implement (stick, shaft, small ax with a long handle), this version utilizes motifs that can be done without those implements. There are many sources for this dance. This arrangement is by Andor Czompo.

Records: Rounder 5005 "Jew's Harp Music," Side 1, Band 3, or any good moderate tempo Kanásztánc or Ugrós: AC #3, LPX 18007, LPX 18031–32; and CD.

Formation: Solo, i.e., single dancer, hands on hips.

Motifs: Steps and Hop, Back Cross Cifra, Close and Step.

■ MOTIFS

1. **Steps and Hop** (♩♩♩♩)

Step on right toward a right forward diagonal into a small knee bend (count 1), step back on the left (count 2), step on the right forward into a small knee bend (count 3), hop on the right, turning about 1/4 to the left, at the same time swing the left lower leg forward (count 4). Repeat beginning left.

2. **Back Cross Cifra** (♫♩)

Small leap onto the right to the right side (count 1), step on the left behind the right (count *and*), step on the right in front of the left (count 2). Repeat beginning left.

Kiskanásztánc (continued)

---

*Description and permission to use *Kiskanásztác* courtesy of Andor Czompo. Music available from 100 Gleneagles, Williamsburg, VA 23188

3. **Close and Step** (♪♪)

Starting position: Weight is on the left in a small knee bend. The right foot is right–side–low with a slightly bent knee. Close the right to the left with accent (heel click). At the same time straighten both knees (count 1). Small step on the right forward into a small knee bend. At the same time lift the left to the left–side–low position with a slightly bent knee. Repeat beginning right.

Individual dancers have hands or fists on hips. Start the dance at any time with the music.

DIRECTIONS FOR THE DANCE

Meter 2/4

■ *Measures*

1–4   Dance the Steps and Hop motif twice.

5–6   Dance the Back Cross Cifra motif twice.

7–8   Dance the Close and Step motif twice.

Repeat this sequence several times until the end of the music.

Note: For those who like to improvise, each motif may be done any number of times or in a different order.

Ugrós*

A CONTEMPORARY RECREATIONAL folk dance in Hungarian Ugrós style arranged by Andor Czompo.

Record and CD: Rounder 5005, side 2, band 6, "For a Birthday."

Formation: Solo, i.e., a single dancer, hands on hips.

Motifs: Touch and Step, Back Cross Cifra, Lift and Step with Claps, heel click.

■ MOTIFS

1. **Touch and Step** (♪♪)

Touch the right heel forward on the floor (leg straight) (count 1), step on the right in place (count 2). Repeat beginning left.

2. **Back Cross Cifra** (♫♪)

Small leap onto the right to the right side (count 1), step on the left behind the right (count *and*), step on the right in front of the left (count 2). Repeat beginning left in opposite direction.

---

*Description and permission to use *Ugrós* courtesy of Andor Czompo. Music available from 100 Gleneagles, Williamsburg, VA 23188.

3. **Lift and Step with Claps** (♪♪)

Lift the right knee forward and hit the right thigh with the right hand (count 1), step on the right in place. At the same time clap the hands together in the front (count 2). Repeat beginning left foot and hand. **Note:** Man can lift the leg forward with bent and turned out knee and hit the inside of the lower leg (boot top). **Variations on the clap:** Replace the single clap with a double

(♫) or triple clap. (♫♪)

4. **Heel Click** (♪♪♪)

Starting position: Weight on left. The right foot is right–side–low with a slightly bent knee. Close the right to the left with slight accent (knees are straight) (count 1), bend the knees and at the same time turn out (open) both heels (pigeon–toed) (count 2), close the heels together with accent and straighten knees (count 3), pause (count 4).

DIRECTIONS FOR THE DANCE

Meter 2/4

■ *Measures*

Individual dancers face the music or the center of the dance floor. Hands are on hips. During the dance individual dancers can turn and change facing direction at will.

	Introduction: the first full melody.
1–2	Dance the Touch and Step motif #1 twice (right and left).
3–4	Dance the Back Cross Cifra motif #2 twice (right and left).
5–8	Repeat measures 1–4.
9–10	Dance the Lift and Step motif #3 twice (right and left) with single claps.
11	Dance the Lift and Step motif #3 with double or triple claps.
12	Dance the Lift and Step motif #3 with left foot and hand.
13–14	Dance the Back Cross Cifra motif #2 twice (right and left).
15–16	Dance the Heel Click motif #4 one time.
	Repeat the dance from the beginning.

ISRAEL

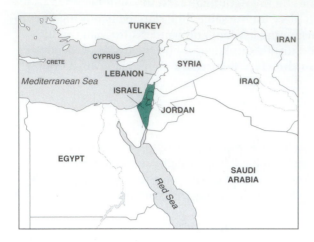

■ Clarification of Ethnic Names and Nationalities

The advent of the nation of Israel in the late 1940s has led to some confusion as to the origin of dances from that country and region. "Dances named 'Palestinian' are pre–Israel–Jewish. During that (pre–Israel) era the Palestinians were the Jews; the Arabs were Arabs. Now the Arabs are the Palestinians and the Jews are Israeli." *

■ Dance Characteristics

Since Biblical times Jewish dance[†] has been spiritual in nature and very much a part of the religious experience. As the Jews wandered about the world, they assimilated the culture of each new home into their own tradition. Dance has always been a part of the Jewish child's education and family life. During the Middle Ages, the popular "tanzhaus" (dancing hall) was established in the ghettos of France, Poland, and Germany, and Jewish dance leaders developed.

About 1736 Israel Baal Shem Tov, a young mystic who came from the Carpathian Mountains, inspired a new Jewish religious movement known as Chassidism (also spelled Hassidism). The movement flourished in the ghettos of Poland and eastern Europe. Baal Shem encouraged dance movement and singing with prayer to realize the nearness of God. A new ritual of dancing and humming in worship took place. Improvisation of dance "arose as a conscious attempt to create human joyousness out of misery."[‡]

With a long tradition of dance, the Jews immigrated to the new state of Israel (formed in 1948), bringing with them many diverse cultures and tradi-

tions. The Israeli Folk Dances danced today are dances they have brought from other cultures, like east European ones. But a large number of the currently popular Folk Dances have been created by such folk choreographers as Gurit Kadman, Sara Levi, Yoav Ashriel, Rivka Sturman, Dvora Lapson, and Dani Dassa. Using German interpretive dance techniques and old and newly composed tunes, they have blended dance movements from the Yemenites, the Arabs, the Druzi, the Kurds, and the Hassidim (the largest impact being played by the Yemenites).

The Yemenites, Jews originally from the southwest corner of Arabia, started immigrating to Palestine about 1910, and, in 1949 they were transported by airplane to the new state of Israel. Although the Yemenites had many things in common with the Arabs, their religion was different, and they could read and write. The Yemenites were a link with the Biblical Hebrews. They had maintained old religious and cultural patterns, songs in the language of the Bible, and dances of Oriental rhythm. Their dances were slow and gentle, gradually accelerating as danced to drumming, hand clapping, and singing. Their basic dance forms inspired a new trend in Israeli dances and the Yemenite step in many variations became a basic step. A group of well-known dances (*Dodi Li and Ma Na'avu*) came from the Song of Songs.

The dance of the Bukhara Jews[§] emphasizes hand movements. Their melodies are mostly in 3/4 and 6/8 meter and sound like a Iändler; therefore, people frequently mistake them for Bavarian dances.

The newly created Folk Dances involve a variety of themes: Biblical (*Shibbolet Bassedeh*, a harvest festival), the great need for water (*Mayim Mayim*); experiences that have occurred in modern times (*Sisu Yerusalyim*, choreographed after the Six–Day War, celebrates the joy of being in Jerusalem again), and discotheque dance (*Shir Hashalom*), referred to as "The Madison Avenue Dance" by Israelis. The movement in the dance rarely pantomimes its theme.

Line, circle, and couple dance formations are used. It is interesting to note that the Jewish Square Dance differs from European Quadrilles in that the women of the side couples stand on the left side of their partners so that two women or two men are at each corner. The woman was not to touch a "strange man."

Characteristically the total body is involved in movement, frequently with a fluid, undulating movement; the knees and ankles are flexible; hand movements may be reaching upward, clapping hands symbolic of clapping cymbals in ecstasy, or reaching behind the back in a mood of restraint.

The music, also a blend of many cultures, may be tunes from other lands or newly composed ones. The music on Israeli recordings could be identified as German, illustrating the many cultures that Israeli dance represents. The melodies have a strong rhythmic pulse.

---

*Following the publication of the 7th edition of *Dance A While*, Vyts Beliajus wrote the authors the above statement of clarification in a letter dated January 22, 1994.

[†]See "The Story of Jewish Dance," *Viltis*, October–November 1968.

[‡]Berk, Fred. *Ha-Rikud, The Jewish Dance*. American–Zionist Youth Foundation, Union of American Hebrew Congregations, U.S.A. 1972, 1975.

[§]See "Jews from Bukhara," by Vyts Beliajus in *Viltis*, May 1962.

Cherkessiya

TSCHERKESSIA OR *CHERKESSIYA IS A* dance for men from Circassia. They were followers of the Mohammedan faith, who sought religious freedom in the czarist days of Russia. They left southeastern Russia and migrated to Palestine and Syria. The Circassians were noted for their horsemanship. The rhythmic movement of the dance portrays either horses or riders.

Records: RCA EPA 4140; Dancecraft DC 74627; High/Scope RM 2, LP and compact disc; Merit AV LP; Worldtone 10040 (vocal), 10043 (instrumental); RCA LPM 1623.

Cassettes: Dancecraft DC 162303; High/Scope RM 2.

Music: Beliajus, V. F., *Dance and Be Merry*, Vol. I, p. 12; Chochem, Corinne, and Roth, Muriel, *Palestine Dances*, p. 31; Lapson, Dvora, *Dances of the Jewish People*, p. 34.

Formation: Groups of four or five dancers in a line, arms linked about one another's waist, or any number of dancers in a single circle.

DIRECTIONS FOR THE DANCE

Meter 2/4

■ *Measures*

Part I

A   1–2   Keeping the left foot in place, step right across left, step left in place, step back right, step left in place. As cross step is taken, body leans forward, left knee bends to give flexibility to movement. As backward steps are taken, body should lean back as far as possible.

       3–8   Repeat action of measures 1–2 three times.

Part II

B   9   Line or circle moves to the right. Beginning right, step to the side, step left behind right.

      10–16   Repeat action of measure 9 seven times.

■ VARIATIONS FOR PART II

1. 16 scissor kicks (cut steps) in front.
2. 16 scissor kicks (cut steps) in back.
3. Combination of scissor kicks in front and back.
4. Eight slow skips to the right (one per measure).
5. Keep feet together, move both toes, then both heels to the right.
6. Semicrouch position, execute a shuffle step, moving to the right.

■ NOTE

The action described in part II may be used each time or a different action selected from the variations may be used for each repeat of the B music. The dance should be started in a slow tempo. Each repetition becomes faster until a climax of great excitement is reached. If done in a line, each group moves independently, allowing the action of part II to carry it anywhere on the floor.

Harmonica*

H

ARMONICA MEANS "ACCORDION." The dance movements are symbolic of the action of an accordion. The dance was choreographed by Rivka Sturman.

Records: Folk Dancer MH 1091; Folkraft 1108; Worldtone 10030.

Music: Lapson, Dvora, *Dances of the Jewish People*, p. 13.

Formation: Single circle, hands joined and held down.

Steps: Grapevine, run, hop.

DIRECTIONS FOR THE DANCE

Meter 4/4

■ *Measures*

	I.	**Grapevine**
1		Moving counterclockwise, cross left in front of right (count 1), step right to side (count 2), cross left behind right (count 3), leap right to side with slight accent (count 4).
2		Continue moving counterclockwise and step–hop left (counts 1–2), step–hop right (counts 3–4).
3–8		Repeat action of measures 1 and 2 three times.
	II.	**Cross Step, Hop**
9		Beginning left, cross left over right (count 1), step right in place (count 2), step left in place (count 3), and hop slightly on left (count 4), turning body to left side on hop.
10		Beginning right, cross right over left (count 1), step in place (count 2), step right in place (count 3), and hop slightly on right (count 4), turning body to right side on hop.
11		Beginning left, repeat action of measure 9.
12		Moving clockwise, step–hop right (counts 1–2), step–hop left (counts 3–4).
13–15		Beginning right, repeat action of measures 9–11.
16		Moving counterclockwise, step–hop left (counts 1–2), step–hop right (counts 3–4).
	III.	**Friendship Circle, Swaying**
17		Place hands on upper arms of adjacent dancers. Dancers sway to left (counts 1–2), sway to right (counts 3–4). Action of feet may be step left, touch right to left; then step right, touch left to right.
18		Beginning left, moving clockwise, take four running steps.
19–24		Repeat action of measures 17–18 three times.

---

*Dance arranged from the dance description by Dvora Lapson, *Dances of the Jewish People*, 1954 (p. 13).

Hava Nagila*

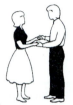

HAVA NAGILA MEANS "COME LET us be joyful." This couple dance is done to an old hora melody, "Hava Nagila."

Records: Folkraft 1110, 1116; High/Scope RM 4, LP and compact disc; Worldtone 10001; LS E 43.

Cassette: High/Scope RM 4.

Music: Lapson, Dvora, *Dances of the Jewish People*, 1954, p. 18.

Formation: Double circle, partners facing, man's back to center, two hands joined. Partners stand close together, elbows bent, and hands close in.

Steps: Walk, leap, hop, jump, running step.

DIRECTIONS FOR THE DANCE

Meter 4/4 • Directions are for both woman and man, except when specially noted.

■ *Measures*

		I.	**Pull Away and Circle**

A 1 Beginning right, take four steps backward, knees bend slowly taking body into crouch position by fourth step. Back remains fairly straight.

2 Beginning right, take four steps forward, moving immediately into left reverse open position (count 1). Stand straight with left elbow bent and close to body, right arm is straight across in front of partner. Turn clockwise in reverse open position (counts 2–4).

3–4 Repeat action of measures 1–2.

1–4 Repeat action of measures 1–4. On fourth measure, partners face line of direction and take back cross position.

II. Leap and Turn, Balance and Run

B 1–2 Beginning right, leap forward, body bending forward (count 1), step left beside right (count 2), step right back, body straightens (count 3), step left beside right (count 4). Repeat.

3 Drop left hands. Beginning right, take four steps, woman making three–quarters turn to face man who turns one–quarter clockwise to face her. Partners join left hands under right.

4 Beginning right, take four steps, woman in place, man turning a full turn clockwise under their joined upraised hands. Now in original starting position, with joined hands crossed.

Hava Nagila (continued)

---

*Dance arranged from the dance description by Dvora Lapson, *Dances of the Jewish People*, 1954 (p. 19).

	5–6	Man beginning left, woman right, take four balances to side. (Man–left, right, left, right; woman–right, left right, left.)
	7–8	Hook right elbows and extend left arm diagonally upward and outward. Take eight running steps around each other, turning clockwise once around to face original starting position. Drop hands and move apart about three feet.
	III.	**Clap, Hop, and Turn**
C	1	Bend over to right and clap hands to one's own right side about knee level (counts 1–2). Repeat bending to left (counts 3–4). Sing "Uru Uru Achim."
	2	Bend forward and clap in front (count 1), gradually raise hands to outstretched arm position, in three upward lifts (counts 2–4). Head follows hand positions. Sing "Uru Uru Achim."
	3	Hands on hips. Jump in place (count 1). Take three hops on right, extending left foot forward (counts 2–4).
	4	Repeat action of measure 3, hopping on left foot and extending right.
	5–6	Repeat action of measures 3–4.
	7	Repeat action of measure 3, letting left foot trail behind while turning clockwise around in place once on three hops.
	8	Repeat action of measure 4, letting right foot trail behind while turning counterclockwise around in place once on three hops.

■ LYRICS

A. Hava Nagila   Let's be joyful
  Hava Nagila   Let's be joyful
  Hava Nagila Venismecha   Let's be joyful
   Repeat A

B. Hava Neranena   Let's sing
  Hava Neranena   Let's sing
  Hava Neranena Venismecha Let's sing and be joyful
   Repeat B

C. Uru Uru Achim   Wake up, wake up, brothers

D. Uru Achim Belev Sameach   Wake up, brothers, with a happy heart
   Repeat D three times

E. Uru Achim   Wake up, brothers
  Uru Achim Belev Sameach   Wake up, brothers, with a happy heart

Hineh Ma Tov

THE WORDS *HINEH MA TOV* ARE taken from the Bible. Their meaning–"How good it is to dwell together as brethren"–admonishes people to live in the world as brothers, friends, and good neighbors.

Dance A While CD: #10. "Hineh Ma Tov."

Record: Folk Dancer MH 1091; Folkraft 1434, LP–2; Worldtone 10018.

Formation: Nonpartner circle or line dance. Lines may be composed of four to eight dancers moving freely in any direction.

Steps: Walk, twinkle, yemenite.

DIRECTIONS FOR THE DANCE

Meter 2/4

■ *Measures*

Part I

1–2 Beginning right, move counterclockwise four walking steps. Flex knees during slow walk, hold hands down and straight.

3–4 Beginning right, continue counterclockwise, run lightly eight steps. Run in a quick, prancing style.

Repeat measures 1–4.

Part II

5–6 Face center, raise joined hands to shoulder level. Leap softly onto right and bring joined hands down (counts 1–2). Twinkle: Step back on left (count 3), step right to left (count 4), step forward on left (counts 1–2). Stamp right softly beside left (counts 3–4). Weight remains on left. Hands remain down during twinkle.

7–8 Yemenite: Step right to side (count 1), shift weight back to left (count 2), step right across left (count 3). Repeat to left: Step left to left side (count 1), shift weight to right (count 2), step left across right (count 3), stamp right softly. Weight remains on left.

Repeat dance from the beginning.

■ WORDS

Hineh ma tov, uma naim (*hee-nay-ma-tov, ooma nayim*). She–vet a chim gam ya chad (*sheh-vet-akim-gahm-ya-khad*).

Hora

THE JEWISH PEOPLE, DISPERSED OVER THE earth for many years, have kept their religion alive, but many of the folk traditions have become broken or lost. When the people returned to Israel, they brought dances from their former homelands. The Sephardic Jews, who left Spain during the Inquisition, settled in the Balkan area. They danced the Balkan *Hora*, adopting it and incorporating it into their festivities.

The word *hora*, a Croatian–Serbian word, means "tempo" or "movement." Although the earlier Hora dances were probably a part of primitive agricultural rites (the leaps and high jumps in the dance suggest and were supposed to induce high growth of corn); the Hora became more subdued and restrained as the people danced it indoors in small spaces. As danced in Israel today, it has absorbed the flavor of the people living there and is once again danced outdoors.

> **Records:** Folk Dancer MH 1052, 1053; Folkraft 1110, 1118, 1431, 1476, LP-12; LS E 43.
>
> **Cassette:** Dancecraft DC 162303.
>
> **Music:** Chochem, Corinne, and Roth, Muriel, *Palestine Dances*, p. 15; Beliajus, V. F., *Dance and Be Merry*, Vol. I, p. 37.
>
> **Formation:** Single circle, hands on shoulders of person on either side, arms straight.

DIRECTIONS FOR THE DANCE

Meter 4/4

■ *Measures*

1–3   Moving counterclockwise, step right to side, place left behind right, and step right. Kick left in front of right while hopping on right. Step left to side, kick right across left while hopping on left.

This same pattern is repeated throughout the dance.

■ NOTE

Begin the Hora slowly to establish the rhythm, keep the tempo slow and the music soft, and then gradually accelerate the rhythm and increase the volume. If the group is large, it is interesting to have several concentric circles, some circles beginning with the right foot, moving clockwise, and others beginning with the left foot, moving counter-clockwise.

■ STYLE

If the movement of the dance begins mildly, with a tiny hop, it can build gradually to a larger hop as the tempo increases.

If dancers extend arms and lean back, keeping head up, the momentum is easier. Dancers should hold up their own arms, not press down on shoulders of the person to each side.

Ma Na'avu

M*A NA'AVU IS A LOVELY NONPARTNER CIRCLE* or line dance. The lyrics are from the Bible, Isaiah 52–57. The music was composed by Joseph Spivak, and the dance was choreographed by Rajah Spivak.

Records: High/Scope RM6, LP and compact disc: Tikva 45–102; Worldtone 10020; Festival FS 201 400, LS E 43.

Cassette: High/Scope RM 6; Festival FS 201.

Formation: Single open circle or single line, hands joined and held down.

Steps: Touch, twinkle, rocking, yemenite.

DIRECTIONS FOR THE DANCE

Meter 2/4

■ *Measures*

Introduction (4 measures).

1–2　Touch: Beginning right, touch right forward (count 1), touch right to side right (count 2). Twinkle: Step back onto right (count 3), step left next to right (count *and*), step forward onto right (count 4). Rock: Rock weight back onto left (count 1 *and*), rock weight forward onto right (count 2 *and*), rock weight back onto left (count 3), step right forward in place (count *and*), close left to right (count 4). Lift body upward as if taking a deep breath. Weight ends on right for repeat beginning left.

3–4　Repeat action of measures 1–2 beginning left.

5　Yemenite: Step right to side right (count 1), step left next to right (count *and*), step right forward and across left (count 2), turn to face counterclockwise by pivoting slightly on the right (count *and*). Move counterclockwise three steps left, right, left (counts 3 and 4). Bring joined hands to shoulder level during the three steps. End facing forward.

6–8　Repeat action of measure 5 three times.

Repeat dance from the beginning.

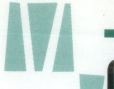

Mayim*

MAYIM IS A JEWISH FOLK TUNE. TRANSLATED, Mayim means "water." The dance movements express the joy of finding water in arid land and emulate the motion of waves as they break on the shore. The dance originated in a kibbutz on the shores of Galilee.

Dance A While CD: #18. "Mayim."

Records: Folkraft 1108, 1475 LP–12; High/Scope RM 5, LP and compact disc; Tikva LP 106; World of Fun LP 6, Side B–3; Worldtone 10040; LS E 19.

Cassette: High/Scope RM 5.

Music: Lapson, Dvora, *Dances of the Jewish People*, p. 8.

Formation: Single circle, hands joined and held down.

Steps: Grapevine (tscherkessia), running step.

DIRECTIONS FOR THE DANCE

Meter 4/4

■ **Measures**

1–2		Introduction: no action.
	I.	**Grapevine (Tscherkessia)**
1–4		Moving clockwise, cross right in front of left (count 1), step left to side (count 2), cross right behind left (count 3), step left to side with a light springy step, accenting step (count 4). Repeat three times.
	II.	**To Center and Back**
5		Beginning right, move to center with four running steps. Leap slightly, bending the knee on first step. Lift joined hands gradually above heads as dancers move to center. Sing "Mayim, Mayim, Mayim, Mayim" while moving to center.
6		Beginning right, repeat action of measure 5, moving away from center. Lower joined hands gradually down to sides.
7–8		Repeat action of measures 5–6.
	III.	**Run, Toe Touch, Clap**
1		Beginning right, move clockwise with four running steps; turn to face center.
2		Leap on right and touch left across front to right side (count 1); hop on right, touch left to side (count 2); hop on right, touch left in front to right side (count 3); hop on right, touch left to side (count 4).
3		Repeat action of measure 2, part III.
4		Leap on left, touch right in front to left side and clap hands directly in front at arm's length (count 1); hop on left, touch right to side and swing arms out to sides shoulder high (count 2); hop on left, touch right in front to left side and clap hands directly in front at arm's length (count 3); hop on left, touch right to side and swing arms out to sides shoulder high (count 4).
5		Repeat action of measure 4, part III.

---

*Dance arranged from the dance description by Dvora Lapson, *Dances of the Jewish People*, 1954, p. 8.

I.   1–4   V–Shav–tem Mayim Bi–Sa–Son, Mi–ma–Yi–Wey Ha–Y'Shu–ah

     3–4   V–Shav–tem Mayim Bi–Sa–Son, Mi–ma–Yi–Wey Ha–Y'Shu–ah

II. 5–6   Ma–Yim Ma–Yim Ma–Yim, Ma–Yim, V–Ma–Yim Bi–Sa–Son

     7–8   Ma–Yim Ma–Yim Ma–Yim, Ma–Yim, V–Ma–Yim Bi–Sa–Son

III. 1   Hey! Hey! Hey! Hey!

     2   Mayim Mayim Mayim Mayim

     3   Mayim Mayim Bi–Sa–Son

     4   Mayim Mayim Mayim Mayim

     5   Mayim Mayim Bi–Sa–Son

Ve' David

T HE FULL TITLE OF *VE' DAVID* IS *Ve' David Y'Fey Enayim*, meaning "And David of the Beautiful Eyes." It is a couple mixer choreographed by Rivkah Sturman.

Dance A While CD: #7. "Ve' David."

Records: Festival FS–201; Folk Dancer MH 1155; Folkraft 1432; High/Scope RM 3, LP and compact disc; Worldtone 10043.

Cassette: High/Scope RM 3; Festival FS–201

Formation: Double circle, couples facing counterclockwise. Woman to the right of partner, inside hands joined.

Steps: Walking steps.

DIRECTIONS FOR THE DANCE

Meter 2/4

■ *Measures*

Part I (Music A)

Introduction (6 measures)

1–2   Beginning right, walk forward four steps. Couples turn to face center, join hands in a single circle on fourth step. Walk away from center four steps.

3–4   Beginning right, walk four steps to center and four steps away from center.

Part II (Music B)

1–2   Men clap hands, women walk four steps to center, and four steps back to place.

3–4   Men clap hands and walk four steps to the center, turn to the right and walk four steps away from the center to new partner. New partner is the woman to the right of original partner.

5–6   Hungarian–turn position: Partner stand right side to right side, right hands on partner's left hip, left hands curved overhead. Turn clockwise eight "buzz–steps."

Repeat dance from the beginning.

ITALY

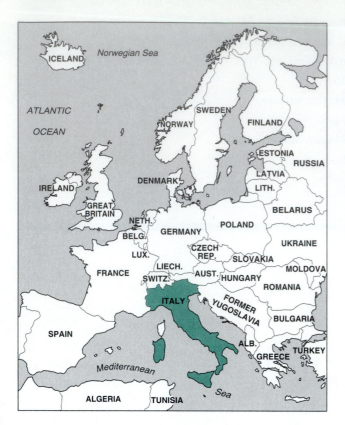

■ *Dance Characteristics*

Italian dance is not only an expression of the native Mediterranean people, but also reflects the influence of the invaders from Asia, northern Europe, and Africa. The dances are simple in form and pattern. The dances may be classified in the following groups: Processional and Religious Dances, Sword Dances, Chain Dances in closed or open circles, and Couple Dances. The *Tarantella*, which originated in the southern part of Italy, is one of the best-known dances.

STYLE

The dancers are free and easy. The body is held loosely, often swaying from side to side with arms held high in the air and the head erect. In the mountainous areas of Italy and in the Sword Dances, the steps are precise. Pantomime and flirtation are parts of the dance, especially in courting dances. The dances sometimes are accompanied by castanets or tambourines used by the dancers themselves.

Il Codiglione

I*L CODIGLIONE* MEANS "THE COTILLON" AND IS pronounced *eel koh-deel-YOH-neh.* Vyts Beliajus first saw this dance performed at Chicago's Hull House about 1928 by an Italian group of dancers, and he introduced it at Idyllwild in 1954.

Record: Folkraft 1426.

Formation: Double circle of couples, Varsouvienne position, facing line of direction.

Steps: Walk, pas de basque.

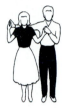

DIRECTIONS FOR THE DANCE

Meter 6/8

■ *Measures*

1–4	Introduction: no action.

I. Walk

1–16	Beginning left, take 32 walking steps forward in line of direction.
17–24	All join hands to form a single circle and take 16 walking steps to right. Circle moves counterclockwise.
25–32	Take 16 walking steps to left. Circle moves clockwise.

II. Two Circles

1–8	Women form circle and take 16 walking steps to left, circle moving clockwise. Men form circle around women and take 16 walking steps to right, circle moving counterclockwise.
9–16	Each circle moves in the opposite direction, women counterclockwise, men clockwise.

III. Basket

1–8	Men join hands and raise over and in front of women to form basket as women join hands. Woman remains to right of partner. Take 16 walking steps to right. Circle moves counterclockwise.
9–16	Women's hands remain joined. Men raise joined hands over women's heads, release hands, and reach under women's arms to rejoin hands in front of women and form basket again. Take 16 walking steps to left. Circle moves clockwise.

IV. Walk

1–16	Repeat action of measures 1–16, part I.
17–24	Men turn and walk clockwise single–file in reverse line of direction while women continue to walk counterclockwise in line of direction.
25–32	Reverse. All turn half around and men walk counterclockwise while women walk clockwise. Women turn on the last measure to Varsouvienne position, facing line of direction.

Il Codiglione (continued)

V. Walk, Pas de Basque, Do–Sa–Do

1–3	Varsouvienne position. Take six walking steps forward in line of direction.
4	Release hands. Partners turn to face and back away from each other two steps. End facing partner, man's back to center.
5–8	Snap fingers with arms outstretched above head and beginning right, take four pas de basque steps in place.
9–12	Lower arms to side and partners do–sa–do, passing right shoulders first, taking eight steps.
13–16	Partners do–sa–do, passing left shoulders first, taking eight steps and progress to new partner on left by moving diagonally left on last four steps.
1–16	Repeat action of measures 1–16.

VI. Ending

1–2	With feet slightly apart, take weight on right foot and clap hands (counts 1–3); pause (counts 4–6), step left and clap hands (counts 1–3); pause (counts 4–6).
3–4	Repeat action of measures 1–2.
5–8	Hook right elbow with partner and turn clockwise seven steps, then stop. Turn back on partner and clap hands overhead on last beat.

▪ NOTE

Directions above are given for the Folkraft record.

▪ STYLE

There should be smooth transitions when changing directions. The walking steps are on the ball of the foot; a flat walk is heavy and ugly. The hands are joined shoulder high, elbows down, without an extended arm. The body is carried high. The success of this dance depends on the style of execution. The body is high and light.

Sicilian Tarantella

THE *SICILIAN TARANTELLA* IS A flirtatious dance for four based on a number of typical Sicilian steps. Real tambourines add an exciting flavor to the dance. Snapping fingers and sharp hand claps may be substituted for shaking and hitting of tambourines.

Dance A While CD: #22. "Sicilian Tarantella."

Records: Folkraft 1173; High/Scope RM 6, LP and compact disc; Worldtone 10033.

Cassettes: Dancecraft DC 162105; High/Scope RM 6.

Music: Herman, Michael, *Folk Dances for All*, p. 45.

Formation: Sets of two, partners facing. Men are side by side and women are side by side. Couple 1 is nearest the music. Couple 1 may be designated the "head couple," couple 2 the "foot couple."

Steps: Step-hop, running steps.

DIRECTIONS FOR THE DANCE

Meter 6/8 • Directions are same for man and woman.

■ *Measures*

I.   Step Clap, Hop Swing

1   All dancers step left, clap hands (count 1). Hop on left, swing right across (count 2). Striking tambourine or claps should be made in front of dancer, not overhead.

2   Repeat measure 1, beginning right, and swing left across.

3–4   Beginning left, four running steps in place. Men snap fingers, women shake tambourines or snap fingers.

5–8   Repeat measures 1–4.

1–8   Repeat Part I.

II.   Runs Forward and Back

9–10   Beginning left, four runs forward toward partner. Dancers begin bending low. Men snap fingers, women shake tambourines or snap fingers.

11–12   Beginning left, four runs backward away from partner. Dancers slowly straighten up and raise arms upward. Men snap fingers, women shake tambourines or snap fingers.

13–16   Repeat measures 9–12.

9–16   Repeat Part II.

III.   Run and Turn

17–20   Man 1 (head) and woman diagonally opposite (foot) run toward each other, hook right arms, turn once around and return to place.

21–24   Man 2 (foot) and woman 1 (head) repeat action of measures 17–20.

17–24   Repeat measures 17–24, turning with left arms.

IV.   Do–Si–Do

1–4   Man 1 (head) and woman diagonally opposite (foot) run toward each other; pass right shoulders, back to back; pass left shoulders, and dance backward to place. Do not fold arms across chest. Snap fingers as dancers pass each other.

5–8   Man 2 (foot) and woman 1 (head) repeat action of measures 1–4.

1–8   Repeat action, except pass left shoulders when moving forward and right shoulders when running backward to place.

9–12   Dancers face a quarter–turn to the right; hands on hips, left shoulders to center of circle, move counterclockwise with eight skipping steps.

13–16   Repeat measures 9–12, right shoulders to center of circle.

V.   Stars

17–20   Dancers form a left–hand star and move counterclockwise with eight skipping steps.

21–24   Repeat measures 17–20, forming a right–hand star and moving clockwise.

■ **NOTE**

This arrangement is based on a piano score of 24 measures. Recordings may only have eight measures of Music A and eight measures of Music B. The dance may be done with only four parts to best fit the recording.

LITHUANIA

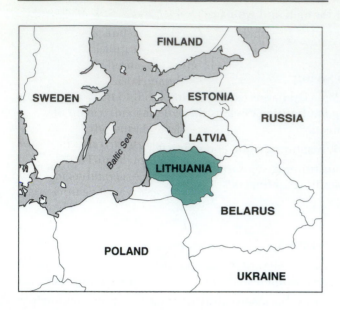

■ Dance Characteristics

Folk Dancing in Lithuania was related to the way of life and reflected the chores and the various aspects of farm life. Although the older dances were slow and restrained, in later years they became livelier. Eventually, the polka arrived on the scene from Poland and became an integral part of Lithuanian Folk Dance. According to Vyts Beliajus, the Polka was flat footed with more body bounce than foot hop because the farmers wore wooden shoes and, if their feet came too far off the ground, the shoes would fall off.

The Lithuanians and Poles hop on the fourth count. The first Three steps are low, short, and bouncy.

Kalvelis

THE NAME MEANS "THE YOUNG BLACKSMITH." The clapping action imitates the beating of the hammer on the anvil. The dance was introduced to the United States by Vytautas Finadar Beliajus, noted Lithuanian dance teacher.

Record: Folk Dancer MH 1016.

Formation: Couples in a single circle facing center. Woman on man's right.

Steps: Polka, stamping, skips.

DIRECTIONS FOR THE DANCE

Meter 2/4

■ *Measures*

Music A	**Part I. Circle Polka**
1–8	Circle counterclockwise with seven polka steps. End with three stamps on the eighth measure.
1–8	Repeat circling clockwise.
Music B	**Chorus. Claps and Skips**
9	Clap left hand onto right, right onto left.
10	Repeat left onto right and right onto left.
11–12	Hook right elbows with partner and turn once around with four skips.
13–16	Repeat claps, hook left elbow, and turn once around with four skips.
9–16	Repeat all of Music B.
Music A	**Part II. To Center and Back**
1–4	Women dance three polka steps to center, stamp three times.
5–8	Repeat back to place.
1–4	Men dance three polka steps to center, stamp three times.
5–8	Repeat back to place. (**Note:** Men's dance action should be vigorous.)
Music B	Repeat Chorus.
Music A	**Part III. Grand Right and Left**
1–8	Partners face, join right hands. Dance Grand Right and Left for 16 polka steps to meet new partner. (**Note:** Music A is repeated.)
Music B	Repeat Chorus with new partner.

Variations on Part III: Men stand in place as women weave to the right with 16 polka steps. Repeat Chorus with new partner. Women stand in place as men weave around circle with 16 polka steps, ending, if all goes well, with partner. Repeat Chorus with original partner. Instead of the Grand Right and Left, take ballroom position with partner and dance 16 polkas around the circle. Repeat Chorus.

Repeat dance from the beginning.

Klumpakojis

*K*LUMPAKOJIS MEANS "WOODEN FOOTED" OR "clumsy footed." It is frequently translated erroneously as "wooden shoes." It is a form of the Finger Polka–type Folk Dance found the world over. Notice its similarity to the Swedish Klappdans, the Dutch Hopp Mor Annika, and the Danish Siskind.

Records: Folkraft 1419; Worldtone FDLP 2.

Cassette: Dancecraft 162402.

Formation: Double circle, couples side by side, inside joined, free hands on hips, facing line of direction.

Steps: Walk, stamp, Polka.

DIRECTIONS FOR THE DANCE

Meter 2/4 • Directions are for man, woman's part reverse.

■ *Measures*

I. Walk

1–4 Beginning left, take eight brisk walking steps in line of direction, turning toward partner to face reverse line of direction on last step.

5–8 Join inside hands, free hands on hips. Take eight walking steps in reverse line of direction.

1–8 Face partner, joining right hands, right elbow bent, left hand on hip. Partners take eight steps, walking around each other clockwise. Join left hands and take eight steps, walking counterclockwise.

II. Stamps, Claps

1–4 No action (counts 1 *and*, 2 *and*). Then stamp three times. No action (counts 1 *and*, 2 *and*). Clap own hands three times.

5–8 Shake right finger, right elbow bent, at partner (counts 1–3), hold (count 4). Shake left finger, left elbow bent, at partner (counts 1–3), hold (count 4). Clap right hand of partner and turn solo counterclockwise in place once with two steps. Facing partner, stamp feet three times quickly.

1–8 Repeat action of measures 1–8, Part II.

III. Polka

1–8 Varsouvienne position. Beginning left, take 16 Polka steps forward in line of direction. On last two Polka steps, man moves forward to new partner.

■ NOTES

1. Zest is added to the dance if dancers shout "hey hey" or "ya–hoo" spontaneously during the Polka sequence.

2. This dance may be used to introduce either the Two–Step or the Polka step.

MEXICO

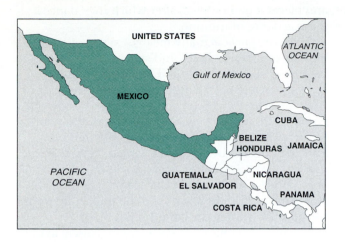

■ *The Dance in Mexico*

By Nelda G. Drury, Associate Professor, Emeritus, San Antonio College, San Antonio, Texas.

If you were to visit Mexico you would probably find a civil or religious celebration or parade in which dances are featured. Dance is an integral part of Mexican life. The costumes worn by the dancers add a high note of color to the occasion. Let's take a look at the history of the dance in Mexico. Three phases become immediately apparent: pre–Hispanic, the period of conquest, and the dances of modern Mexico.

PRE-HISPANIC

The first inhabitants of Mexico were the Nahuas, Toltecas, Zapotecas, Mixtecos, Totonacos, and Mayas. Each group made dance a part of their existence. They taught their children to dance even before they attended school, for they believed it an essential part of growing into adulthood. Unfortunately, little is known about these ancient dances. Our knowledge of them is derived from ancient codices that have been discovered and from the writings of some of the priests who entered Mexico with Hernán Cortez.

These sources indicate the importance of dance to native Mexicans. They performed dances in their religious celebrations that often lasted several days. The dances were performed in concentric circles with the eldest of the group in the center directing the change of steps. Participants of higher rank were bestowed a place in the inner circle closer to the center. These dances had many similarities to those of ancient Egypt. Dances were performed before going off to war or as tribute to the god of rain or other gods as the occasion required. They were also performed in adoration of the sun or the moon. Some of the gods were bloodthirsty so human sacrifices were part of the rituals.

The Deer Dance is one of the few pre–Hispanic dances that has survived in its pure form over the centuries. It is a dance of the Yaquis from the states of Sonora and Sinaloa. It enacts the killing of a deer and is considered a classic of this era.

Dance accompaniment was predominantly by percussion instruments and woodwinds, such as flutes usually made of bamboo canes. These instruments were elaborately decorated and very colorful. A few instruments that have survived the ravages of time may be seen in the Museum of Anthropology and History in Mexico City.

PERIOD OF CONQUEST

In the second phase of the dance in Mexico a new lifestyle evolved with the arrival of the Spaniards. This period is characterized by astounding changes. The people were confronted with new customs, new ideologies, a new religion, new beliefs, and even a new language! Along with the Spanish conquistadors came evangelists bringing Christianity to the New World. When the new religious leaders realized the importance of dance in the life of the Indians and found that it could not be suppressed, they adapted the dances to Christian rituals. If the native Indians held a festival to honor one of their idols or gods, the priests would substitute a Christian saint in its stead. The Spanish introduced new dance rhythms and new string instruments.

The blending of the two cultures produced the *danza Mestiza,* which rapidly spread to all the states of the republic. These dances were warlike reenactments of the conquest. One of the most famous dances of this type is *La Danza de la Pluma* (dance of the plumes). In the dance, from the state of Oaxaca, the performer dons a splendid headdress that is covered with feathers, beads, and mirrors in beautiful designs and breathtaking colors. The dance simulates the struggles between the Indians and the Spaniards. The choreography is simple, but the steps are quite difficult. The dance is performed by men only and is very popular even today.

Most of the dances of this era are of the same type. Examples are *Moros y Cristianos* (Moors vs. Christians) and the *Danza de los Diablitos* (devils). There are also dances of pre–Hispanic origin that have had their music and costumes embellished by the European influence. Examples of these are *La Danza de los Quetzales* (quetzal is a bird) from the state of Puebla and *La Danza de los Voladores* from Papantla, Veracruz. The latter is sometimes called the dance of the "Flying Indians."

Dances that depict the work ethic are demonstrated by such dances as *Los Sonarjeros,* a planting dance, and *La Tortuga del Arenal,* which reenacts the gathering of turtle eggs, an important part of the diet of the Juchitecas. Most of these dances were performed at fiestas and in the courtyard of the church, a custom that still exists. Every region has its own *danzas mestizas*, which correspond to its own way of life. Each embodies a reminder of what used to be and an acceptance of the new.

DANCES OF MODERN MEXICO

The third phase of the dance of Mexico evolved from the intermarriage of the Spanish with native Mexicans. As time went by, the children of this union, called *Mestizos*, began to acquire more and more of the Spanish customs and slowly discarded that which was purely indigenous. During the colonial period other nationalities also added their influence. The French who came with Maximilian brought the ballroom dances that were popular in the courts of Europe (*Bailes de Salon*) such as the Polka, Waltz, Schottische, Mazurka, and Varsouvienne. The Germans favored the northern part of Mexico and left their stamp on the music and dance of that region. Dance, however, took a new direction. Each region developed its own *zapateado* (footwork) and with it, its own jarabe.

El Jarabe Tapatío is considered the national dance of Mexico. From the state of Jalisco, it is the most popular of all the Jarabes. It is a dance of courtship and tells about the Charro (young cowboy) who has taken a fancy to a beautiful "China" (young señorita) and decides to visit her and declare his passion. She shares the same feelings but does not want to seem overanxious. So she shyly repulses his advances. Dejected over the rejection, he goes off to a cantina where he imbibes a little too much tequila and proceeds to get a little tipsy. On coming to his senses, he decides to try once more to show his serious intentions. He throws his most prized possession, his sombrero, at her feet and allows her to dance in the brim.

Upon observing the manifestation of his true love for her, as a gesture of acceptance, she picks up the hat and places it on her head, after which they dance a *Diana*, a dance of triumph.

The word *jarabe* actually means a syrup or sweet mixture of different herbs and sugars. In music it is a medley of different tunes and in dance it consists of steps characteristic of a particular region. These are truly Mexican dances, Indian in origin and influenced by the Spanish, giving them the true flavor of Mexico. The most popular, recognizable, and best known of the Jarabes are *Jarabe Tapatio, Jarabe de la Botella* (Jalisco), *Jarabe Michoacano, Jarabe Tlaxcalteco,* and *Jarabe Mixteco.* Yucatan has produced the Jaranas; the Huapango is from Huastica; and the polkas are from the northern part of the country.

Music is also unique to each region. Jalisco, in the central part of Mexico, has mariachis or groups of strolling, singing musicians using the violin, different sized guitars, and more recently the trumpet. The typical musicians of Veracruz use the harp and violins and sing in a high pitch. The music of the north includes the guitar and accordion, often a button accordion, and in the south the marimba and the jaranas. Music has had deep influence on dance and vice versa.

An added attraction is the colorful costumes worn in each of the different regions of Mexico. From the predominantly white costumes from the warm climates of Veracruz and Yucatan, to Jalisco's colorful and beribboned costumes, to the heavy woolen skirts of Michoacan, to the fringed leather garments of the vaquero (cowboy) of northern Mexico, there are more than 600 regional costumes. Dance in Mexico is the spontaneous manifestation of the feelings, the passions, and the pleasures of its people.

El Jarabe Tapatío*

EL JARABE TAPATÍO IS OFTEN REFERRED TO AS the Mexican Hat Dance. It is considered to be the national dance of Mexico. Refer to p. 322 for further background. The more proficient dancer will add steps and flourishes; others will simplify the dance.

Records: Folkraft R 4127; Imperial 1002; Peerless 1918; Victor 23–5901.

Formation: Any number of couples scattered informally around the dance area. Partners face each other or the front with inside hands joined, man's right holding woman's left.

Jarabe step: The basic step is like a very small two–step with accent on the first count. Example: step forward on right foot (count 1), step on left foot close to right instep (count 2), step forward on right foot. Repeat starting with left foot. This counts as two Jarabe steps, six counts, one measure. There are many styles of *Jarabe* step execution, such as: count 1 being done with just the heel, or the second count being done with the heel, rather than the whole foot. The steps should be very small since the music is very fast.

Steps: Jarabe step, heel toe, stamp, run, buzz step, chug.

DIRECTIONS FOR THE DANCE

Meter: 6/8 • Directions are the same for both woman and man.

Roll of music   **Introduction:** Length of roll of music varies. The woman turns to her left under partner's joined hand and both move away from each other about three short steps. Man's hands are held low behind his back, woman holds skirt out to side. Body should lean forward slightly.

■ *Measures*

Part I

8 measures   **A.** Beginning right, move toward partner using 14 basic Jarabe steps. Stamp right foot and hold. At this point couple should be in center of stage, right shoulder to right shoulder with partner.

8 measures   Continue in same direction to partner's place with 12 Jarabe steps, turning to right on 13th and 14th steps, and stamp on right. Now facing partner.

Cue words: Heel step, toe step.

8 measures   **B.** Step on right heel slightly in front of left foot, small step forward on left foot, step on right toe slightly back (but not behind) left foot, very small step forward on left foot. Use same floor pattern as **A** to partner (center) and stamp. Seven heel step, toe steps to the center and stamp. Continue across and turn to face partner and stamp.

El Jarabe Tapatío (continued)

---

*Directions by Nelda Drury, Associate Professor, Emeritus, San Antonio College, San Antonio, Texas.

8 measures	Pass right shoulders and continue to own original place, seven more heel–toe steps, turn to right to face partner, and stamp.
8 measures	**C.** Using 14 Jarabe steps, go all the way to partner's place, turn and stamp right.
Meter 3/4	

Part II

4 measures	Take 3 running steps toward partner (right, left, right), then cross left over right to do a full turn to right (in center, close to partner). Continue to opposite side, with three runs and cross left over right to a half–turn right to face partner. The running should be done lightly, like scissor kicks, straight legs lifting the free foot high from the hip. Pass by right shoulder.
4 measures	**Turns:** Beginning right, take three buzz steps, turning right, stamp left. Turning left, repeat stepping left, stamp right.
4 measures	Repeat turns to right and to left. The stamp should be done facing toward partner.
12 measures	Repeat first 12 measures, runs and turns.

Part III Borrachito (Drunken) Step

	This is like a waltz step. Fall forward onto right foot (count 1), step on left close to (and behind) right ankle (count 2), step on right foot (count 3). Repeat, starting with left foot. Dip right shoulder slightly forward when falling onto right foot. Dip left shoulder when falling onto left foot.
6 measures	Beginning right, take six borrachito steps, traveling to opposite side. Do not stop at center.
2 measures	Cross right foot over left and dance six little rocking steps while turning to the right (clockwise) in place. End facing partner.
8 measures	Repeat all, crossing back to original side.
Meter 2/4	

Part IV Hojas de Té

	Hojas de te are the rhythmic words for practicing this step. This step is similar to Part I B; just add a chug to it. Step on right heel, step left. Step on right toe, step left, chug.
8 measures	Beginning right, take seven of these steps to center and stamp. Right shoulder to right shoulder with partner. Continue to other side, step left, turning right, stamp right. Each should be in own original place, facing partner.

Part V

6 measures	Run lightly forward, right, left, right, and cross left over right do full turn (pivot) to right (clockwise) ending with right shoulder toward home. Beginning right, take four push steps back to place. Push step is similar to buzz step, without turning, but traveling in straight line. The number of push steps varies according to proficiency.
6 measures	Repeat runs toward center; right, left, right, and cross left over right, do full turn, remain in center. Man throws hat on the floor at woman's feet during these push steps. Take 6 push steps, facing partner, leading with left shoulder, traveling around hat clockwise.

Part VI

8 measures	Left shoulder leading, stepping on left foot, dancers move around the hat with 16 push steps.

8 measures	The man and woman travel around the hat in opposite directions: man clockwise, woman counterclockwise. End up at own side.
	Woman leaps lightly into brim of the hat, cross right over left and dance six rocking steps (weight onto right, lifting left heel, pointing left toe down, then transfers weight onto left, lifting right heel). During these rocking steps, maneuver to end up on woman's original side. Use last two measures to get out (step, jump, leap, whatever) of the hat, onto "her" side. Today the woman seldom leaps into the hat, because they want to save the hat.
	Man's step like a polka. (Lunge or fall forward on right, lifting left heel high in back, step on ball of left, step on right. Repeat starting with left.
3 measures	**Interlude:** Woman sinks down, picks up hat with both hands, places hat on her head. Man swings right leg over her head, crosses right over left, pivots to left. Man extends his right hand to her left hand to help woman up, and she rises. They stand side–by–side facing front, inside hands joined.
Meter 2/8	

Part VII

8 measures	Take 4 light running steps forward, four backing up to place. Repeat four forward, four back.
8 measures	Hop on left, at same time place right heel out to right (count 1), hop on left, at same time cross right in front of left and touch right toe to floor (count *and*), hop on left, at same time place right heel to right (count 2), bounce lightly on both feet (count *and*). Repeat starting left. Repeat all.
8 measures	Take four running steps forward, four backward. Skip in place. Raise joined inside hands, woman turns left under that arch. Man kneels on left knee, woman places left foot on man's right knee. Woman holds her skirt out to the side with right hand, man extends left arm out, and both lean away from each other and hold pose!

Jesucita En Chihuahua*

*J*ESUCITA EN CHIHUAHUA IS A vigorous and exciting polka from northern Mexico. This is a choreographed sequence, arranged by Señora Alura Flores de Angles.

> **Records:** Folkraft 1513; Peerless 3248; Polka 1489 (Pepe Villa); Victor 70–7609; National 4511.
>
> **Formation:** Couples in Varsouvienne position facing the line of direction.
>
> **Steps:** Two–Step, walk, heel toe, slide, step–close, stamp.

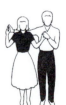

Jesucita En Chihuahua (continued)

---

*Directions by Nelda Drury, Associate Professor, Emeritus, San Antonio College, San Antonio, Texas.

DIRECTIONS FOR THE DANCE

Meter 4/4 • Directions are the same for both woman and man.

■ *Measures*

Part I

8 measures — Beginning right, take 16 Two–Steps in line–of–direction. Use last two measures, without releasing hands, to do a half–turn to right and face reverse line of direction. Woman remains on outside. Turn as in Road to the Isles (p. 273), measure 12.

Part II

8 measures — Beginning right, take 16 Two–Steps in reverse line of direction. Use last two measures to do a half–turn to left to face original line of direction. Woman remains on outside.

Part III

8 measures — Take 4 walking steps forward (right, left, right, left) (4 counts). Release left hand. Take four more small walks forward while woman turns right under held hands (4 counts). Rejoin left hands and repeat this combination three more times. Four times in all.

Part IV

8 measures — Repeat Part I. Take 16 Two–Steps forward. Do not turn around, do not reverse.

Part V

8 measures — Lower joined right hands to woman's waist. Both stamp forward with the right, close left foot up to right foot. Step back with right, draw left foot back toward right foot. Take eight of these steps, maneuvering to turn clockwise.

8 measures — Repeat same footwork, but turn counterclockwise.

Part VI

Cue words: Heel, toe, heel, toe, slide, slide, slide, bounce.

8 measures — Hop on left foot and at same time touch right heel to right side. Hop on left foot and at same time cross right in front of left and tap right toe to the left of left foot. Repeat heel toe. Take two slides to the right, step right to side (like a gallop) and bounce on both feet. Beginning left, repeat to the left. Repeat all.

Part VII

8 measures — Repeat Part V, forward, close, back, close, for eight measures, turning clockwise.

Part VIII

8 measures — Repeat Part I, 16 Two–Steps in line of direction.

Part IX

8 measures — Repeat Part III, walk and woman turns.

Part X

8 measures — Face partner, take closed position, man's back to center. Man beginning left, woman right, step to man's left side, close with right. This step is similar to the Merengue. Take 16 step–close steps in line of direction. End with a stamp.

La Cucaracha*

THE SONG THAT ACCOMPANIES THE dance was popularized during the Mexican Revolution. There are many versions of La Cucaracha. An original version and an adapted version for recreational groups are presented.

Records: DL P5; DC 162105 LP; EZ 5009; FD LP5; Folkraft 1458; R 4134; Merit AV Album 5.

Cassette: DC 162105 C.

Formation: Couples scattered informally around the dance area. Partners face each other, man's left shoulder, woman's right shoulder toward the front. Man places thumbs in belt, woman holds skirt out to the side.

Steps: Walk, stamp.

DIRECTIONS FOR THE DANCE

Meter 3/4 • Footwork is the same for man and woman, both beginning right.

■ *Measures*

Part I

1	Step on right foot diagonally across left, step back on left in place, step back right in place.
2	Step on left foot diagonally across right, step back on right in place and hold (count 3).
3–4	Spin to left with four steps (left, right, left, right). Hold (counts 2, 3).
5–8	Repeat measures 1–4, beginning with left foot, toward the right. Face front.
9–16	Repeat measures 1–8 facing front.

Part II

17–18	Beginning right, walk forward diagonally left three steps (right, left, right). Stamp left twice (no weight).
19–20	Walk back to place (left, right, left). Stamp right foot twice (no weight).
21–24	Repeat measures 17–20 diagonally right. Face partner for measures 25–32.
25–32	Repeat measures 17–24 to partner's right shoulder and back to place, then to partner's left shoulder and back to place.

■ VARIATION (LA CUCARACHA, ADAPTED)

Formation: Couples in a circle, facing center, both beginning right.

Part I

1–8	Action of measures 1–8 is original version, facing center of circle.
9–16	Repeat measures 1–8 facing partner.

La Cucaracha (continued)

---

*Directions by Nelda Drury, Associate Professor, Emeritus, San Antonio College, San Antonio, Texas.

Part II

17–24   Action of measures 17–24 is original version to partner's right shoulder and back, then to left shoulder and back.

25–26   Weave the ring **three places:** Walk three steps to partner's right shoulder (right, left, right), stamp, stamp.

27–28   Continue forward to next person's left shoulder with three walks and two stamps.

29–32   Continue forward to next person's right shoulder with three walks and two stamps. This is a new partner.

31–32   Join both hands, walk four steps, turning 3/4 around and face center, woman to right of man, drop hands.

La Raspa

FREQUENTLY, *LA RASPA* IS CALLED *Mexican Hat Dance* by the public. The true Mexican Hat Dance, *Jarabe Tapatio*, is an entirely different dance.

Records: Coast 7018; EZ–716; Folkraft 1457; High/Scope RM 3, LP and compact disc; Merit AV LP; World of Fun LP 6, Side B–5; Worldtone 10042.

Cassettes: Dancecraft DC 887; Dancecraft DC 162303.

Music: Sedillo, Mela, *Mexican and New Mexican Folk Dances*, p. 36.

Position: Partners face, man holds clasped hands behind back, woman holds skirt, or two hands joined.

Steps: Bleking step, running step.

DIRECTIONS FOR THE DANCE

Meter 2/4

■ *Measures*

Part I

A   1–4   Beginning right, take one bleking step.

5–8   Turn slightly counterclockwise away from partner (right shoulder to right shoulder) and, beginning left, take one bleking step.

9–12   Repeat action of measures 1–4, facing opposite direction (left shoulder to left shoulder).

13–16   Repeat action of measures 1–4, facing partner.

Part II

B   1–4   Hook right elbows, left hands held high. Take eight running steps, clapping on eighth step.

5–8   Reverse direction, hook left elbows. Take eight running steps, clapping on eighth step.

9–16   Repeat action of measures 1–8, B.

- **VARIATION**

Measures 1–8: Take 16 running steps, right elbows hooked. Measures 9–16: Reverse and take 16 running steps.

- **ICEBREAKER**

No partners, all stand in single circle. Turn slightly left and right for action of measures 1–16, A; run in line of direction and reverse line of direction for action of measures 1–16, B. Halfway through record, everyone may take a partner.

Las Chiapanecas*

LAS CHIAPANECAS IS A WOMAN'S DANCE from the state of Chiapas.

Records: EZ 716; Folkraft 1483; LS E 20.

Formation: There are many options. As a couple dance, both on same foot, moving in the same direction, or opposite feet, moving in opposite direction. As a solo dance, dancers scattered, or group dance with a lot of choreography.

DIRECTIONS FOR THE DANCE

Meter 3/4

- ### *Measures*

Part I

1	Beginning left, step left in place (count 1), hop on left (count 2), step on right diagonally forward left, across left (count 3).
2	Step on left in place (count 1), hop on left (count 2), step backward on right (count 3).
3–6	Repeat measures 1 and 2 two more times.
7–8	Do four stamps, left, right, left, right (no weight on last stamp).
9–16	Repeat measures 1–8 to the right, starting with right.
17–32	Repeat measures 1–16.

Part II

1–3	Beginning right, turn to right with three–step turn or take three waltz steps.
4	Lean slightly to right and clap hands twice about shoulder high.
5–8	Repeat measures 1–4 to the left, beginning left.
9–16	Repeat measures 1–8.

Las Chiapanecas (continued)

---

*Directions by Nelda Drury, Associate Professor, Emeritus, San Antonio College, San Antonio, Texas.

Part III A

1	Beginning right, step to right (count 1), tap left heel close to right (count 2), step on left close to right (count 3).
2–3	Repeat measure 1 two more times. Three times in all.
4	Two stamps, right, left (no weight on left).
5–8	Repeat measures 1–4 to left, starting with left.
9–14	Repeat measure 1 six times.
15–16	Do a pivot turn to right (step on right, cross left over right and turn).

Part III B

17	Beginning left, step to left on left (count 1), hop left and at same time lift right foot (keep it close to left ankle) (count 2), step on right close to left (count 3).
18–32	Repeat pattern of Part III A to the left, substituting the "lift" instead of tapping heel.

■ VARIATION

Part I and/or Part III: Individuals may waltz around, turning instead of suggested pattern.

Santa Rita*

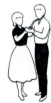

*S*ANTA *R*ITA IS A COUPLE DANCE from northern Mexico.

Records: CBS – E.P.C. 393; Folkraft 1513.

Formation: Couples in semi–open position, facing line of direction, in a circle.

Steps: Two–Step, slide, polka.

DIRECTIONS FOR THE DANCE

Meter 2/4 • Directions are for man; woman's part reverse.

■ *Measures*

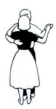

Part I

1–4	Beginning left, take four Two–Steps forward. In Mexico this is called a polka. There is no hop, but rather a scuff forward on the foot that starts the Two–Step.
5–6	Closed position, man's back to center of circle. Cross left over right, cross right over left. Stamp left foot three times, weight ends on left.
7–8	Step right to right side, close left to right, step right (like a Two–Step to side). Stamp left twice (no weight).
9–16	Repeat measures 1–8.

---

*Directions by Nelda Drury, Associate Professor, Emeritus, San Antonio College, San Antonio, Texas.

Part II

17	Closed position, man's back to center of circle. Moving to the left side, step left, close right, step left.
18	Cross right over left, cross left over right.
19–20	Repeat measures 17–18 in reverse line of direction, beginning right.
21–32	Repeat measures 17–20 three more times.

Part III Polka

33–48	Closed position. Take 16 Polka steps (traditional real polka, not a Two–Step). Turn clockwise while progressing in line of direction.

Part IV Wrap Up

49–50	Join two hands, man's back to center of circle. Beginning right, balance forward (right shoulder near right shoulder), balance away (backward).
51–52	Both hands remain joined, man lowers right hand, woman's left, as woman turns to her left (counterclockwise), taking two small Two–Steps, under her right hand, his left. Lower joined hands. Partners are side by side, woman to right of man.
53–54	In wrap position, balance forward, balance backward, using 2 small Two–Steps.
55–56	Unwind her back to place.
57–58	Balance forward (left shoulder to left shoulder), balance backward.
59–60	Wrap up woman to man's left side. Man's left, woman's right hand stays down. The woman turns to her right (clockwise) taking two small Two–Steps, under her left hand, man's right. Lower joined hands.
61–64	In wrap up position, facing line of direction, balance forward, balance backward, balance forward, balance backward. Do not unwrap.

Part V

65–68	In wrap up position, take four small Two–Steps in place (right, left, right, left).
69–72	Take seven push steps sidewards right (counts 1–7). Bounce on both feet on count 8.
73–80	Repeat measures 65–72 to the left, starting with left foot.

Interlude

81–82	Dancers are facing line of direction, woman on left side of man. Release man's right hand. Beginning left, woman takes a three–step turn to her left.
83–84	Release inside hands and both turn. Man does a four–step–turn to his left (left, right, left, right) in place. Woman does one and a half turn to right, with four steps (right, left, right, left). She ends up in front of man. Closed position, man facing line of direction.

Part VI Apache Step

May be done cheek-to-cheek, bend forward at the waist, "tush" protruding in back.

85–86	**Man's step:** rock forward onto left foot and push joined hands (man's left) forward (count 1). Step back onto right foot (back at home position) (count 2). Step far back with left foot, pull joined hands back, toward man's left hip (count 1). Step on right foot, it never left home (count 2).
87–88	Repeat measures 85–86.
89–92	Man walks forward eight steps: step forward left, at same time right heel turns up and out, right toe remains on floor.

Santa Rita (continued)

93–100	Repeat 85–92 starting with right. Bring joined hands to man's left hip.
85–88	Woman's step is the opposite. Beginning right, woman rocks back and forward, back and forward.
89–92	Then she walks backward eight steps. If possible, do "broken ankle" step. Step back on right, at same time turn left ankle to left so that left edge of foot is on the floor, do not put weight on turned ankle.
93–100	Repeat starting left.

Part VII

Closed position, man facing line of direction.

Cue words: Heel, toe, slide, close, step; cross, cross, close, bounce.

101	Hop on right and tap left heel to left side. Hop on right and cross left foot over right ankle, left toe taps floor.
102	Step left to side, close right to left, step side left, toward center.
103–104	Cross right over left, cross left over right. Close right foot to left foot. Bounce on both feet.
105–108	Repeat measures 101–104 to right, starting with right.
109–116	Repeat measures 101–108.

Part VIII

| 117–132 | Repeat Part I, measures 1–16. |

Part IX

| 133–148 | Repeat Part II, measures 17–32. |

Part X

| 149–161 | Repeat Part I, measures 1–16. |

POLAND

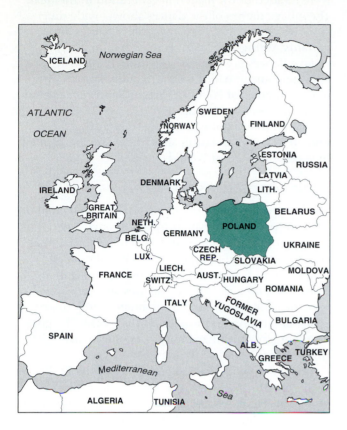

■ *Dances of Poland*

By Jacek Marek, Mansfield, Massachussetts

Poland, a country roughly the size of New Mexico, is truly unique in the diversity reflected in its cultural inheritance. It is unlikely you will find anywhere in the world a comparable heritage, which includes some 15,000 folk songs, more than 1,000 dances, hundreds of carols, more than 200 folk costumes, and a distinctive range of ethnic customs and rites.

Folk culture and arts are vital components of Polish national heritage. They manifestly assert themselves in the unflagging popularity of folk song and dance groups and ensembles basing their work on folk motifs. Polish folk music determines its national musical style; Polish folk orchestration is among the richest in the world. One needs only to mention the names Chopin, Szymanowski, Moniuszko, Wieniawski, and to remember the world-wide successes of the prominent Polish contemporary composers Gorecki, Lutoslawski, and Bacewicz. All are indebted to inspiration drawn from the inexhaustible resources of Polish musical folklore.

DANCE FOLKLORE

Our knowledge of Folk Dance dates primarily back to the 19th century, although there are some brief dance references from the Middle Ages and the Renaissance.

Some dance music also survives containing elements of rural tunes; there are 17th and 18th century paintings showing peasant dancing. Generally, however, few resources focus on peasant culture. To follow the development of folk dance in Poland one has to understand the historical context.

About the time that Christopher Columbus was discovering America, the Jagiello dynasty ruled most of east-central Europe. This was called the "Golden Age" in Polish history. Soon, however, privileges granted to the middle class gentry (szlachta) gradually weakened the state. Class egoism and shaky political structures eventually emptied the treasury, debilitated the standing army and crippled the administration. As a result, Poland was partitioned between Russia, Prussia, and Austria and for a period of time (1795–1918) did not even exist on the political map of Europe.

Ironically, this contributed to the preservation of folk culture. The oppression of the partitioning powers–German and Russian especially–caused an unusual resistance in the Polish people, manifested in their attachment to native customs, family rites, music, dance, and costume. By wearing Polish folk dress, they kept alive the distinctive identity of their country even though it no longer existed on the political map. Strong occupants' reprisals provoked even more intense reactions. Poles struggled to preserve their cultural identity and to regain unity and political independence.

Toward the end of the 18th and at the beginning of the 19th century, a particular interest in peasant culture became evident. Individuals, societies and groups, began to turn to folk traditions as a repository of pure and untainted national values. They were also in hopes of gaining the support of the peasant masses for the independence movement and restoration of the Polish state. With the tendency of the mid-19th century Romantic period to glorify aspects of rural life, privileged society began to introduce certain "folk" dances at sleighing parties, masquerades, and other courtly occasions. Especially popular were *Krakowiak, Mazur,* and *Chodzony,* later called *Polonez.* These dances in modified form first swept into drawing rooms at home and abroad and later, in even more modified form, were brought to the stage under the direction of the ballet masters of the day. For the first time, collectors of folklore also included dance. The marked development of social and economic structures gave rise to political changes within Polish society. The general economic development, though uneven in the three different administrations (Poland was partitioned at that time), strengthened democratic tendencies in all of Poland. The position of the peasantry was getting stronger, which led to a blossoming of folk culture. A reform giving freedom to the peasants led to the rise of an individual economy. A wealthy village society was established, and colorful costumes appeared all around the country. The second half of the 19th century was the period of the most exuberant flowering of traditional folk culture, which became the symbol of Polish national culture. Today's folk culture–and especially Folk Dance–is derived from the standards of that period.

The outbreak of World War I created a situation Poles had hoped for through three generations: The three co–partitioning powers were fighting among themselves. Upheaval in Russia swept away the tsarist regime, and the entry of the United States into the war gave Poland independence in 1918. After an independent Polish state was restored, national themes, including so–called Folk Dances (actually free impression on folk dance themes by dancers and ballet masters) appeared on professional stages. The national repertoire began to grow. Organizations, societies, and institutes were created, aimed at the propagation and cultivation of traditional Polish folk culture. During the 1930s Folk Dance was introduced to the youth movement and to schools. Groups in folk costumes presenting folk dance, music and customs performed at various state and local festive occasions. Also, some professional work was initiated in collecting peasant dances. Unfortunately, most of those works were destroyed in World War II.

After the war, well–organized ethnographic work on dance began. Publications appeared containing professional documentation of the entire dance folklore of many regions. In addition, research methods were established and results published.

Simultaneously, the progress of industrialization and urbanization of the Polish countryside substantially altered the ethnographic picture. Large scale migration led to mixing of regional traditions. Traditional village dances, with some exceptions, have only become relics. Yet, there were (and are) communities where traditional folk culture survives, although transformed in form and content. In some places the old traditions are treated with respect, if not reverence, and used to demonstrate national pride and patriotism.

DANCE CHARACTERISTICS

Folk dance preserves the customs and rites of the family and community and is entertaining as well.

There is a visible transition of dance heritage; dances were handed down from one generation to the next. The village names of the dances show a wide diversity. The same dance may have many names and variants. Youngsters learn dancing by imitation.

Five dances are currently identified as Polish national dances, which were originally known only in certain areas of Poland: *Polonez (Polonaise)*, *Krakowiak*, *Mazur*, *Kujawiak* and *Oberek*.

In addition to these, there are numerous others known as regional dances since they were performed in specific regions of Poland.

CONTEMPORARY SITUATION

The historical wind of democracy, which in the fall of 1989 swept Communism away, simultaneously brought both new hopes and difficulties to the people in Eastern and Central Europe. For almost 50 years Poland had used folk groups as propaganda tools. Costumes, instructor's salaries, and free travel were provided for hundreds of amateur folk dance groups that traveled throughout the world. The government also subsidized hundreds of festivals throughout Poland.

Coincident with the disappearance of the Berlin Wall–that ghostly symbol of the so–called "Cold War"–government funding for folk groups, and for all cultural activities, ended. By the early 1990s, more than half of the previously viable folk groups had disappeared from the folkloristic map of Poland due to the lack of funds. Among the survivors one may find not necessarily the most ethnographically valuable but more likely those able to adapt to the challenges of a free market. All must be self–supporting and thus constantly seeking financial aid.

Can we predict the future of the Polish Folk Dance movement? The Polish economy in recent years is among the fastest growing in the developing countries. It is possible by the end of the next decade, that Poland may make up for a half century of Communist depravation. The Folk Dance movement (at least in its recreational form) will probably recover. With more money in their pockets, people will be able to better afford participation in cultural activities–hopefully, including Folk Dance.

Tramblanka–Polka Mazurka

TRAMBLANKA (*TRAM-BLANK-AH*) IS A couple dance from the region of Opoczno in the Mazowsze region in central Poland. Its most popular version was introduced for the first time by the State Ensemble "Mazowsze."

Music: "Dance of Poland."

Formation: Couples around the circle in escort position, facing line of direction. Woman to the right of partner puts her left arm under man's folded right arm. Outside hands free.

Steps and Styling

1. *Mazurka Step*–2 measure sequence:
   Measure 1–hop on right foot (count 1); slide on left foot to the left (count 2); step on right closed to left foot (count 3).
   Measure 2–three running steps in place, left, right, left foot.
   In measures 3–4 repeat action of measures 1–2 with opposite footwork and direction.

2. *Running Steps*–Steps are small, light, and bouncy. Do not kick feet up in back, but keep them close to the floor and don't prance. Body is held erect and proud. Occasionally man may typically move his head back and forth sideways rhythmically.

DIRECTIONS FOR THE DANCE

Meter 3/4

Introduction: Four measures, no action.

■ *Measures*

Part I Running on the Circle

1–3	Beginning with outside foot (man–left, woman–right) couple runs in line of direction, with three steps per measure, nine steps in all. At the same time outside fists move rhythmically forward/backward, with three movements per measure.
4	With three accented steps couple makes one–half CCW turn in place (man backward, woman forward)
5–7	Another nine running steps three per measure in line of direction.
8	With three accented steps couple makes one–quarter CW turn in place (man forward, woman backward) end facing center.
9	Three running steps forward (toward center).
10	Three accented steps in place, lean forward.
11–12	Three running steps backward ended with two accented steps facing partner, woman back to line of direction.

Tramblanka–Polka Mazurka (continued)

---

*Directions by Jacek Marek. Cassette available from Jacek Marek; 874 West Street, Mansfield, MA 02048, e–mail: jmarek@ziplink.net.

Part II Mazurka in Semi–open Position

1–3   Leaning into direction of movement do three sliding Mazurka steps (one per measure) toward center: man hops on right foot and slides on left, woman opposite.

4   Three accented steps in place (man: left–right–left; woman: right–left–right). Remain in closed position; joined man–left, woman–right hands curved overhead.

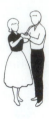

5–7   Repeat action of measures 1–3 symmetrically, toward outside of the circle.

8   With three accented steps do one–quarter CW couple turn in place (man ends back to center).

9–11   Repeat action of measures 1–3 in line of direction.

12   Two accented steps away from partner. End with right hand on hip, and left arm bent with thumb up.

Part III Running Do–Sa–Do.

1–3   With nine running steps (three/measure) move diagonally forward to your left, then make do–sa–do in CW direction around partner passing right shoulders first and backing up passing left shoulders. Move left arms as in Figure I.

4   Three accented steps in place.

5–8   Repeat action of measures 1–4 in CCW direction passing left shoulders first then backing up passing right shoulders.

9–12   Hook right elbow with partner and turn once CW in place with nine running steps, both moving left arms as in Figure I. On last measure dance two stamping steps to end in closed ballroom position, man back to center.

Part IV Mazurka with Half Turns

1–2   Leaning into line of direction couple makes one sliding Mazurka step, then makes half CW turn in place with three running steps (woman ends back to center).

3–4   Repeat action of measures 1–2 with opposite footwork.

5–8   Repeat action of measures 1–4. End up in open position facing center of the circle.

9–10   Three running steps toward center followed by three accented steps in place.

11–12   Three running steps backward toward outside of the circle, followed by two accented steps.

    Repeat whole dance from the beginning two more times.

Walczyk "Ges Woda"

WALCZYK "GES WODA" (VAL-CHIK GENSH VOH-DOM) IS A couple dance in 3/4 meter from the Lublin region in eastern Poland. The name derives from the first words of the accompanying song, sang by the "Mazowsze" State Folk Ensemble. The suggested variant is done as a mixer with changing partners. Arrangement is by Jacek Marek. "Walczyk" is a soft meaning of the word "walc" = waltz.

Music: "Dances of Poland."

Formation: All facing center join hands at shoulder's level. Woman to the right of partner.

DIRECTIONS FOR THE DANCE

Meter 3/4

■ *Measures*

1–4	Introduction: no action.
	Part I Joined Hands
1	Step to right on right foot, swing left foot in front of right (bent knee) in direction of movement.
2	Step on left foot in line of direction, bend right knee. Keep knees close.
3–4	Repeat action of measures 1–2 one more time, except in 4th measure make one–quarter CCW turn on left foot.
5–8	Repeat action of measures 1–4 with opposite footwork and in opposite direction (begin with right foot), end in facing position (Woman back to line of direction).
	Part II Couple Walk, Waltz
9–12	In closed position, beginning with man left foot forward, woman, right foot backward, do four Waltz–type steps in line of direction (step–step–close/no turns); man ends back to the center.
13–16	Beginning man left, woman right foot, do four Waltz steps in line of direction with right couple turns (half turn per measure, two full turns in all).

Interlude Circle with Partner, Change Places

Join both hands with partner (right/left, left/right) and with three Waltz–type steps do one and one–quarter couple turn in place (measure 1–3), then open to face center position, man to the right of partner.

Repeat dance from the beginning four more times; each time in measures 9–16 Waltz with a new partner.

---

*Directions by Jacek Marek. Cassette available from Jacek Marek; 874 West Street, Mansfield, MA 02048, e–mail: jmarek@ziplink.net.

ROMANIA

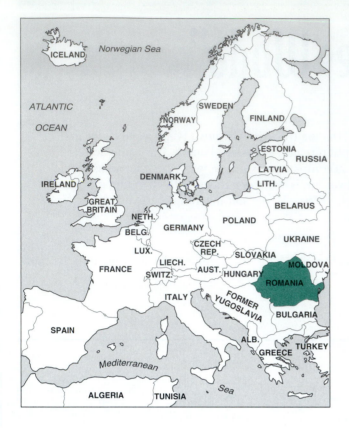

■ Background

The Roman Empire extended its influence in the northeast as far as Romania, and, despite a history of many ethnic influences (Slavic, Turkish, and Germanic), the language, based on Latin, has remained a unique feature of this Balkan country.

Romania is generally considered to be divided into six major folk regions: Oltania, Multania, Banat, Dobruja, Moldavia, and Transylvania. Each major region is, in turn, subdivided into several minor regions, all of which have their own unique folklore.

In general, the dances are quite fast, with intricate footwork, including heel clicks and stamping in complex, rhythmic patterns. Traditionally, the men's movements in the dance are stronger than the women's.

Major dances done in a circle or a line include:

- *Hora*
- *Bruil:* Loosely translated as the "belt," usually done holding on to the neighbor's belt. *Bruil* was originally intended for men.
- *Sirbia:* Serbian–like, usually incorporates a lifting and a flicking of the foot.

The principal couple's dance is the *Invirtitia* (turning dance). This dance form has many patterns, and in a traditional setting, the man leads his partner similar to American Swing dance.

A notable characteristic of Romanian dancing is the shouts or "crying out" of the dancers during the dance. These vocalizations are know as *strigaturi*. A saying in Romania goes: "Those who dance and do not shout, they deserve a crooked mouth." Strigaturi are always shouted out in rhythmic harmony with the music. Some are simple, as "Hey *una*" (Hey, one), or as complex as a poem.

Traditional dancing in Romania is connected to many aspects of village life. The most prominent example occurs most Sundays. The Sunday dance event is referred to as the *Hora*, or *Joc*. People gather together to socialize and dance. In some areas, this event takes place in the village square. In northern Transylvania, a special structure, called the *ciuperca** (or "mushroom"), houses the dance event. As the influence of modernization has spread to the village, attendance at the *Hora* has declined. For many, watching TV programs of Romanian football has replaced the traditional dance event.

Traditional dancing may still be performed in cities during wedding celebrations and other special events. Contemporary dances and traditional dances can be observed on the same dance floor to a mixture of popular and folk songs.

■ Music

Traditional music of Romania has unique qualities for each of the major folklore regions. In *Banat*, many wind instruments are played; the most common is the *taragot*. In *Muntenia* a portable *tambal*, similar to a hammered dulcimer, is popular. In *Dobrogea*, instruments display influences from Turkey and Bulgaria. The one common instrument to all regions is the violin. Several other stringed instruments are played in conjunction with the violin. The accordion, not a traditional instrument, is also played in most Romanian music today. The rhythms are frequently syncopated, in 2/4 meter.

---

*The shape of the roof resembles the top of a mushroom.

Alunelul

Romanian

Alunelul, pronounced *ah-loo-NAY-loo*, means "little hazelnut."

Dance A While CD: #8. "Alunelu."

Records: Canadian MH 1120; Folk Dancer MH 1120; Folkraft 1549; High/Scope RM 5, LP and compact disc; National 4573; Worldtone 10005.

Cassette: High/Scope RM 5.

Formation: Single circle, all facing center, hands on shoulders of person on either side, arms straight. Small circles of eight to ten dancers are best.

Steps: Step, stamp.

DIRECTIONS FOR THE DANCE

Meter 2/4

■ *Measures*

B	1–4		Introduction: no action.

I. Five Steps

A	1–2	Beginning right, take five steps sideward; step right to right side, step left behind right, step right to right side, step left behind right, step right to right side. Circle moves counterclockwise. Stamp left heel twice, close to right.
	3–4	Beginning left, repeat the action of A, measures 1–2. Circle moves clockwise.
	1–4	Repeat the action of A, measures 1–4.

II. Three Steps

B	5	Beginning right, take three steps sideward; step right to right side, step left behind right, step right to right side. Circle moves counterclockwise. Stamp left heel once.
	6	Beginning left, repeat the action of B, measure 5. Circle moves clockwise.
	7–8	Repeat action of B, measures 5–6.

III. One Step

	5–6	In place, step right, stamp left heel close to right once; step left, stamp right heel close to left once; step right, stamp left heel close to right **twice.**
	7–8	Beginning left, repeat action of part III, measures 5–6, reversing foot pattern.

■ NOTES

1. Dancers need to be light on their feet; use small, precise steps; and support weight of their own arms. Do not let arms sag, and hold heads erect.

2. The tempo of the music of some recordings accelerates at the end. The dancers enjoy the competitiveness of testing their agility of footwork with the musicians. A leader can adjust the speed of control if using a variable record player.

Hora De Mina*

HORA DE MINA IS PRONOUNCED *Hoar-ah deh MU-nuh*. This dance was learned by Mihai David while a member of the Romanian State Folk Ensemble, 1965–68.

Record: Gypsy Camp Vol. 3.

Formation: Circle, hands joined, held at shoulder height, *W* position.

Steps: Walk, Two–Step.

DIRECTIONS FOR THE DANCE

Meter 2/4

Mea.	Counts	
1–16		Introduction: no action.
		Part I Walks and Touch In and out of center
1–2	1–4	Beginning right take three steps to the center, counts 1–3. On count 4 tap left foot next to right.
3–4	5–8	Beginning left, take three steps back, counts 1–3. On count 4 tap right foot next to left.
5–16		Repeat action of measures 1–4 three more times.
		Part II Walk, Two–Step Travel in line of direction
1–2	1–4	Facing reverse line of direction, beginning right, take four steps moving back in line of direction.
3–4	5–8	Pivot on left foot, face line of direction, beginning with right, take two Two–Steps in line of direction.
		Repeat action of measure 1–4 three more times; on last Two–Step, bring arms down.
		Part III Walk, Lift, Walk, Stamp In and out of center
1–2	1–4	Beginning right take four steps to the center, rising arms to *W* position by count 4.
3	5–6	Step side right with right, count 5, lift left leg (knee bent), count 6,
4	7–8	Step side left with left, count 7, lift right leg (knee bent), count 8.
5–6	1–4	Beginning right take four steps back, lower arms down by count 4.
7	5–6	Step side right with right, count 5, stamp left heel (no weight) next to right, count 6, lift arms to *W* on count 5.
8	7–8	Step side left with left, count 7, stamp right heel (no weight) next to left, count 8.
		With count 7, lower arms down.
1–8		Repeat action of measure 1–8, leaving arms in *W* on last count.
		Repeat the dance from the beginning

---

*Permission to use *Hora De Mina* courtesy of Mihai David, Los Angeles. Records available from Mihai David, 2940 West Lincoln Blvd., Suite D, Anaheim, CA 92801.

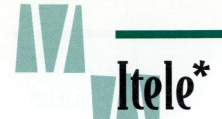

Itele*

Romanian

ITELE IS PRONOUNCED IT-EL-LAY This dance was learned by Mihai David while a member of the Romanian State Folk Ensemble, 1965–68.

Record: Gypsy Camp Vol. 2.
Formation: Short lines, belt hold, or hands joined in front basket hold.
Steps: Grapevine.

DIRECTIONS FOR THE DANCE

Meter 2/4

Mea. Counts

		No Introduction
		Part I Grapevine
1	1–2	Beginning right, step right in front of left on count 1, step left to side on count (1 *and*), step right behind left on count 2, and step left to side on count (2 *and*).
2–7		Repeat action of measures 1 six more times.
8	1–2	Step right foot in place on count 1, step left foot in place on count (1 *and*), step right foot in place on count 2.
9–16		Repeat action of measures 1–8, with opposite footwork.
		Part II Stamps in Place
1	1–2	Beginning right, stamp the right foot forward, taking weight, leaving the left foot in place, on count 1, step in place with left on count (1 *and*), step in place right on count 2, step in place left on count (2 *and*).
2–3		Repeat action of measure 1 two more times.
4		Step right foot in place on count 1, step left foot in place on count (1 *and*), step right foot in place on count 2.
5–8		Repeat actions of measures 1–4, with opposite footwork.
9–16		Repeat actions of measures 1–8
		Repeat dance from the beginning

Notes: Dancers need to be light on their feet, using small, precise steps.

---

*Permission to use *Itele* courtesy of Mihai David, Los Angeles. Records available from Mihai David, 2940 West Lincoln Blvd., Suite D, Anaheim, CA 92801.

Sibra Din Cimpoi*

Romanian

SIRBA DIN CIMPOIE IS PRONOUNCED *SIR-BUH DIN CIM-POI* This dance was learned by Mihai David while a member of the Romanian State Folk Ensemble, 1965–68.

Record: Gypsy Camp Vol. 1.

Formation: Medium length lines facing center with hands on shoulders of person on either side, arms straight.

Steps: Steps, stamp, leap.

DIRECTIONS FOR THE DANCE

Meter 2/4

Mea.	Counts	
		No Introduction
		Part I Step lift (*Sirba* step), side behind
1	1	Beginning right, step in place on count 1, hop on right foot while lifting left leg (knee bent) on count (1 *and*).
	2	Repeat actions of count 1, with opposite footwork.
2	1	Beginning right, step side right on count 1, step left behind right on count (1 *and*).
	2	Repeat actions of count 1.
3–16		Repeat action of measures 1–2 seven more times.
		Part II Sirba, Stamp, Leap in Place
1	1	Beginning right, step in place on count 1, hop on right foot while lifting left leg (knee bent) on count (1 *and*).
	2	Repeat actions of count one, with opposite footwork.
2	1	Repeat action of measure 1, count 1.
	2	Step left in place on count 2, stamp right foot next to left on count (2 *and*).
3	1	Step forward with right foot on count 1, bring left foot to right heel on count (1 *and*). Left knee pointing slightly side left.
	2	Step back with left foot on count 2, stamp right foot next to left on count (2 *and*).
4	1	Step right in place on count 1, swing left leg in front on count (1 *and*).
		Leap on to left foot in place on count 2 (knee slightly bent), step right in front with a straight leg on count (2 *and*).
5–8		Repeat actions of measures 1–4.
		Repeat dance from the beginning.

Note: The *Sirba step* is usually considered a step lift in place. Sometimes there is a quick flicking action of the foot during the lifting.

*Permission to use *Sirba Din Cimpoi* courtesy of Mihai David, Los Angeles. Records available from Mihai David, 2940 West Lincoln Blvd., Suite D, Anaheim, CA 92801.

RUSSIA

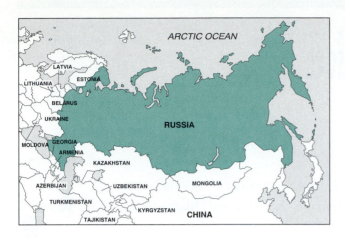

■ Dance Characteristics

The former Union of Soviet Socialist Republics (USSR), a political unit, was made up of 16 republics and many cultures (Slavs, Turks, Ugrian tribes, Mongolians, and Tartars). Movement of people and inter–marriage have existed for a long time. Consequently, a great variety of dance is found in Russia, reflecting these many cultures.

The term *Russian dance* refers to a geographical location in central Russia. These are typical north Slavic dances: fast and slow, musical phrases of six or eight measures, including many prysiadka (knee bend) variations for the men.

Many of the dances favored by American folk dancers come from the Ukraine, where the Cossacks lived. Cossack dancing is reflective of the spirit of fearless soldiers and superb horsemen. It is exuber–ant, exciting, and characterized by fast running, leap–ing, and pas de basque steps and by the difficult knee bend or *prysiadka* steps, used by the men. Also charac–teristic are turning, spinning, stamping, and heel clicking. The Ukrainian dancers are unsurpassed for their vitality, competitive spirit, and endurance.

Georgia is located at the eastern end of the Black Sea. The language of Georgia (belonging to the Turki–Tartar group) relates to that of the Basques. The tall, stately men dance on the tip of their toes, moving at varying tempos but always maintaining an illusion of floating constantly through space.

The Western influence on Russian dance is limited to the Court Dances and contact with Poland.

STYLE

The Russian dances are characterized by emotional expressiveness. The movements are fluid in the warm countries and very vigorous in the cold countries. The Russian dances are not always set. On the inspi–ration and the mood of the dancer, the steps are changed.

MUSIC

The song–dances are sung by choirs with musical accompaniment. There are also ceremonial dances performed today with only vocal accompaniment. When Peter the Great tried to Westernize the musical tastes of his people, native instruments were banned. The people then sang for the dancers. But, in the courts, imported classical instruments and Western Court Dances became very popular.

Russian music uses the pentatonic scale (five notes in an octave). The stretching or leaping that is fol–lowed by a sustained position in dance coincides with the characteristics of the pentatonic scale.

During the latter part of the 17th century and the early part of the 18th century, peasant dances and folk songs became popular with all classes. The Russ–ian minstrels are credited with making the balalaika popular. Eventually, even the aristocrats became interested in learning to play it.

Alexandrovska

A*LEXANDROVSKA* IS A RUSSIAN BALLROOM DANCE, probably named in honor of Czar Alexander.

Records: Folk Dancer MH 1057; Folkraft 1107; Worldtone 10031.

Music: Fox, Grace, *Folk Dancing in High School and Colleges,* p. 10; Beliajus, V. F., *Dance and Be Merry,* Vol. 1, p. 22.

Position: Partners face, two hands joined.

Steps: Waltz, draw step.

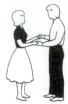

DIRECTIONS FOR THE DANCE

Meter 3/4 • Directions are for man; woman's part reverse.

■ *Measures*

	I.	**Face to Face, Back to Back**

1 — Beginning left, take one draw step to left.

2 — Step left to side (count 1), release man's left hand, woman's right, pivot on left back to back, swinging joined hands and right foot forward (counts 2–3). Join other hands shoulder high. Release right hand.

3 — Beginning right, take one draw step in line of direction.

4 — Step right to side, touch left to right, weight remaining on right.

5–8 — Beginning left, repeat action of measures 1–4 in reverse line of direction. In measure 6, joined hands are swung down and back as partners pivot, bringing them face to face.

9–16 — Repeat action of measures 1–8.

II. Woman's Turn

1 — Partners face, inside hands joined, outside hands on hip. Beginning left, take one draw step in line of direction (counts 1–3).

2 — Man repeats draw step to left as woman turns clockwise once with two steps (right, left) under man's right arm (counts 1–3).

3–4 — Repeat action of measures 1–2, part II. On last draw, man touches right to left, woman takes three steps in the turn (right, left, right).

5–8 — Man beginning right, woman left, repeat action of measures 1–4, part II, in reverse line of direction.

9–16 — Repeat action of measures 1–8.

III. Skating

1 — Promenade position. Beginning left, take one Waltz step forward in line of direction.

2 — Take one Waltz step, turning toward partner to face reverse line of direction. Movement continues in line of direction.

3–4 — Take two Waltz steps backward, moving in line of direction.

5–8	Repeat action of measures 1–4, part III, in reverse line of direction.
9–16	Repeat action of measures 1–8, part III.

IV. Waltz

1–2	Closed position. Beginning left, take one draw step to side, step left to side, touch right to left, weight remaining on left.
3–4	Beginning right, repeat action of measures 1–2, part IV, to right side.
5–8	Take four Waltz steps, turning clockwise, progressing in line of direction.
9–16	Repeat action of measures 1–8, part IV.

Korobushka

*K*OROBUSHKA, ALSO SPELLED *K*OROBOTCHKA, MEANS "little basket" or "peddlar's pack." According to Michael Herman (1941), this dance was originated on American soil by a group of Russian immigrants, following the close of World War I, to the Russian folk song, "Korobushka."

Dance A While CD: #11. "Korobushka."

Records: Canadian MH 1059; EZ 6009; Folk Dancer MH 1059; Folkraft 1170; World of Fun LP 3, Side B–4; Worldtone 1005; High/Scope RM 8 LP and compact disc.

Cassette: High/Scope RM 8.

Music: Beliajus, V. F., *Dance and Be Merry*, Vol. I, p. 20.

Formation: Double circle, partners facing, man's back to center. Two hands joined or man crosses arms on chest, woman places hands on hips.

Steps: Hungarian break step, Schottische, balance, three–step turn.

DIRECTIONS FOR THE DANCE

Meter 2/4 • Directions are for man; woman's part reverse.

■ *Measures*

I. Schottische Step

1–2	Beginning left, take one Schottische step away from center of circle. Extend right foot on hop.
3–4	Beginning right, take one Schottische step toward center of circle.
5–6	Repeat action of measures 1–2.
7–8	Hungarian break step (cross–apart–together).

II. Three–Step Turn

9–10	Drop hands. Man and woman beginning right, take one three–step turn or one Schottische step, moving away from each other.
11–12	Beginning left, repeat three–step turn or Schottische back to place.

Korobushka (continued)

13–14	Join right hands. Man and woman beginning right, balance together, balance back.
15–16	Man and woman beginning right, change places with four walking steps, woman turning counterclockwise under man's arm.
17–24	Repeat action of measures 9–16, returning to original starting position.

- **MIXER**

One may progress to a new partner on the last three–step turn, measures 19–20, by taking turn in place, balancing with a new partner, and changing sides. The man progresses to the woman in front of him at the completion of the three–step turn in place. Before dancers cross over, the man may identify his new partner as the next woman in the line of direction.

Troika

*T*ROIKA MEANS "THREE HORSES." THE dance symbolizes the three horses that traditionally drew sleighs for the Russian noble families.

Dance A While CD: #13. "Troika."

Records: Canadian MH 1059; EZ 5009; Festival 3617; Folk Dancer MH 1059; Folkraft 1170; World of Fun LP 3, Side B–3; High/Scope RM 2 LP and compact disc.

Cassette: High/Scope RM 2.

Music: Herman, Michael, *Folk Dances for All*, p. 7; Neilson, N. P., and Van Hagen, W., *Physical Education for Elementary Schools*, 1954, p. 373.

Formation: Set of three, man between two women, facing line of direction, inside hands joined, outside hands on hip.

Step: Running step.

DIRECTIONS FOR THE DANCE

Meter 4/8

- *Measures*

	I.	**Run Forward**
1–4		Beginning right, take 16 running steps in line of direction. The first four runs may be done diagonally right, second four, diagonally left, and last eight straight forward.
	II.	**Arch**
5–6		Right-hand woman moves under arch made by raised arms of man and left-hand woman with eight running steps. Man runs in place and follows right-hand woman turning under his left arm. Left-hand woman runs in place.

7–8	Left-hand woman moves under arch made by raised arms of man and right-hand woman with eight running steps. Man runs in place and follows left-hand woman turning under his right arm. Right-hand woman runs in place.
III.	**Circle**
9–11	Set of three join hands in circle and run 12 steps clockwise.
12	Stamp left, right, left, hold.
13–16	Repeat action of measures 9–12, moving counterclockwise.

■ STYLE

The knees should be lifted high and the body and head held high.

■ MIXER

The man may move forward to the next group of three as the stamps are taken in the last figure.

SCANDINAVIA

By Gordon E Tracie*

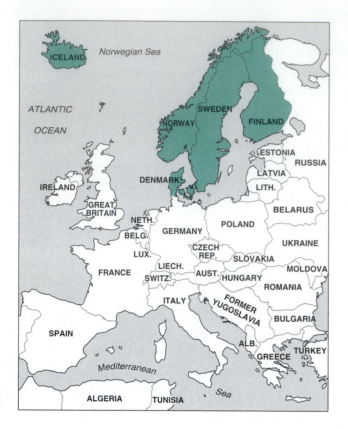

■ Introduction

The native name for the part of Europe we call Scandinavia is *Norden*, literally meaning the North. It encompasses five nations: Denmark, Finland, Iceland, Norway, and Sweden; six cultures: Danish, Faroese, Finnish, Icelandic, Norwegian, and Swedish; seven flags: Denmark, the Faroe Islands, Finland, Iceland, Norway, Sweden, and the Aland Islands; and eight languages: Danish, Dano–Norwegian, Faroese, Finnish, Icelandic, Lappish, Neo–Norwegian, and Swedish. It is therefore not surprising that there is a wide diversity of cultures among the Scandinavians.

Geography, climate, history, lifestyle, and religion all have played a role in the development and acceptance of dance in a given culture. The flat islands of Denmark, the spectacular fjords and mountains of Norway, the rich farmlands and deep woods of Sweden, and the lakes and forests of Finland–each has had an influence on the native music and hence on the traditional dance of the Nordic lands. Of equal if not greater importance is Scandinavia's proximity to other European countries. Germany and the British

*Gordon E. Tracie was founder and director of Skandia Folkdance Society, Seattle, and folklore consultant for the Smithsonian Institution, Washington, D.C.

Isles seem to have been the ultimate source of much material, but Poland and France have also made significant contributions, as has been the case throughout Europe. The cold northern climate has dictated a need for heavy clothes, primarily wool, and for substantial shoes, both of which are reflected in Scandinavian folk costumes.

The pietistic movement of past generations had a devastating effect on dance and dance music in many parts of Scandinavia. Fortunately there were enough "folklore pockets," where musical traditions survived, to be able to pass on a remarkable heritage of true Folk Dances. Today, virtually all dancing in the Northlands is recreational in nature, rather than consciously ceremonial or ritualistic, although remnants of ancient seasonal rites do remain in the Midsummer and Yuletide serpentine dances and in the courting aspects of singing games. In contrast to the Folk Dances in many parts of the world, traditional Scandinavian dancing is almost exclusively coeducational in nature. With but a few exceptions, one always has a partner of the opposite gender with whom to dance. This is true in rings and other formations as well as in couple dances.

Perhaps the single most characteristic feature of Scandinavia's folklore–oriented dances is the predominance of couple rotation. Because this turning is usually relatively fast, factors not present in other types of dancing come into play. The focus is no longer on one or more independent persons, but on a single couple; hence counterbalance and momentum play a vital role. Furthermore, the need for a strong male lead is essential, for it is the man who must "start the wheel turning" and "steer."

It should go without saying that the single most important element in attaining authentic folk spirit in a dance is correct music. Lacking that, a Folk Dance is but a shell without a soul. Proper inspiration and motivation in a given dance can be assured only when the music approximates that with which the dance "grew up." From time immemorial, the dance music of Norway and Sweden has been played on bowed string instruments, usually without the aid of any percussion other than a tapping foot. Predecessors to the violin such as the bowed harp are named in Old Norse literature as far back as the 1300s, and many playing techniques used for instruments predating the violin are still extant in today's Norwegian and Swedish folk fiddling. Open strings characteristically serve as drones, a practice that generates legato rather than a staccato "drive" to the music. In Dalarna, Sweden's folklore district, fiddlers speak of "glued bowing," in which the bow seldom leaves the strings. Norway's Hardanger fiddle and Sweden's keyed fiddle "nyckelharpa" go a step further: Like the viola d'amore, they employ a set of unbowed understrings that vibrate in sympathetic resonance with the bowed strings, thus enhancing the instrument's sonority. All of this contributes to a sustaining legato quality in the music, which is in turn imparted to the dance itself.

The "town orchestra" tradition in Denmark–akin to that in many other parts of Europe–and the predominance of the accordion–an association with Imperial Russia in Finnish tradition–have on the other hand produced a musical style considerably different from that of their Nordic neighbors. Inasmuch as dance naturally reflects music, the variance in dancing style between the Scandinavian countries can be illustrated by a continuum, as follows:

Legato, loose, "springy" (NORWEGIAN) to
Legato, more precise, lilting (SWEDISH) to
Quite precise, smooth (DANISH) to
Staccato, very precise, "crisp" (FINNISH)

The above differences are readily evident in the various Schottische forms:

Norwegian "Reinlander"–Swedish "Schottis"–
Danish "Rheinlaender"–Finnish "Jenkka"

and corresponding Polka forms:

Norwegian "Polka," "Galopp"–Swedish "Polka"–
Danish "Polka"–Finnish "Polkka"

The two most important holidays in Scandinavia are Christmas (Danish, Norwegian, Swedish: "Julen"; Finnish: "Joul") and Midsummer (Danish, Norwegian: "Sankt Hans"; "Jonsok"; Swedish: "Midsommar"; Finnish: "Juhannus"). These are occasions to break out one's traditional folk dress if one is a fiddler, dancer, or participant in a procession, and the time to witness and participate in the most Folk Dancing, short of a specific folk music or dance festival.

■ *Denmark*

DANCE CHARACTERISTICS

Through all Danish Folk Dance shines a distinctly light–hearted, often whimsical quality that is consistent with the convivial Danish temperament. Not infrequently, an element of satire pervades, for the Dane is blessed with a great sense of humor.

The bulk of Danish Folk Dances bear a close kinship to the dances of the British Isles, with which Denmark has had both cultural and economic ties for centuries. Quadrilles, Longways sets, and dances for two or three couples abound. The melodies often sound a lot like English or Scottish dance tunes, and they are obviously cognates. Denmark is the only one of the Nordic lands that has the rollicking Anglo–Celtic 6/8 rhythm, for example, and it has it in abundance. Danish Folk Dance instructions

are organized geographically, the material having been meticulously collected from all parts of the land since around the turn of the century. A distinction is made between "folkedanse," Folk Dances, and "gamle danse," old–time dances. The latter (which include the 19th–century Ballroom Dances, Waltz, Polka, and Mazurka) are not accorded the same reverence as the former. But the Folk Dances exist in Denmark today only through the efforts of organized Folk Dance societies, which limit their origin to the century between 1750 and 1850. Like Danish folk costumes, they are no longer a true living tradition.

During the past several years, there has been an effort, which has met with considerable success among young people's groups, to rekindle an interest in old–time dancing and its music, but in a modern setting (i.e., without "folk" costumes). The traditional Folk Dance ensemble of two violins, clarinet, and bass viol, still the norm for the formal Folk Dance movement, has been augmented by accordions, guitars, mandolins, and even bass saxophones. Needless to say, there is precious little cooperation between the advocates of these two approaches and what we in America lump together as Folk Dance.

■ *Norway*

DANCE CHARACTERISTICS

A folklorist's delight, Norway is without a doubt the most remarkable of the Scandinavian nations when it comes to the retention of native dance forms. In the remote valleys of this rugged land of fjords and mountains are to be found some of the oldest surviving dances in western Europe. Regional dances, "bygdedansar," such as the *Gangar*, *Springar*, *Halling*, and *Pols*, actively learned and danced today, have an unbroken tradition dating back to the 16th century. The formal Folk Dance movement recognizes two other forms: song–dance and figure dances. Song–dance, "songdans," a lyrical dance–song predominant during the Middle Ages, which died out in Norway centuries ago but survived in the Faroe Islands. The form was reintroduced to Norwegian Folk Dancers around 1900 as an adjunct to the promotion of "Nynorsk," the Old Norse–based second language of the land. Figure–dances, "turdansar," consist of Reels, Contras, and Sequence Dances from the 19th century, many of ultimate foreign origin.

Because the Norwegians more than any other Scandinavians have retained the qualities of spontaneity and improvisation in their dancing, the Folk Dances of Norway are the most difficult for foreigners to emulate.

■ *Finland*

DANCE CHARACTERISTICS

The folk music and dance of Suomi/Finland reflects two distinct historical influences: the original Finno-Ugric linguistic heritage and the Scandinavian culture of Russia to the east. Finland is bilingual, with just under 10 percent of the population speaking Swedish. Hence there are two distinct Folk Dance movements, the pure Finnish and the Finland–Swedish, each with its own traditions.

The pure Finnish idiom is quite unlike that of the rest of Scandinavia. A different minor mode gives many Finnish tunes a seemingly melancholy quality. Yet the dance is very often brisk in character, which is, of course, reflected in the dancing. The Finns display a great deal of verve and "snap" in their dancing, giving many Folk Dances an element of "fire." Steps are small and danced with a fast, even bounce. Frequently an abrupt change of tempo or rhythm occurs, making for added variety and interest.

■ *Sweden*

DANCE CHARACTERISTICS

"The Swedish forest," wrote a 19th–century naturalist, "sings in three–quarter time." A romantic but apt description, because the bulk of Sweden's native melodies are in triple meter, mostly "polska," a rhythmic form older than and unrelated to the Waltz and not to be confused with the relatively modern Polka. Long the national dance of Sweden, the "Polska" has survived from the late 1500s right into the 20th century, its most widely known form being the Hambo. Because the bowed strings of the fiddle have traditionally provided the music for Sweden's native dances, the interpretation is legato, a quality befitting the tranquil nature of the Swedish landscape and people. It has been said that the Swede's distaste for excessive display of emotion likely accounts for the relative conservatism of Swedish Folk Dancing. Nevertheless, Swedish dance style is buoyant with the same lightness as found in Denmark, but with an air of dignity and reserve that mirrors a more serious nature.

The dances promulgated for over a century by the formal Folk Dance societies in Sweden are mainly the products of mid–19th century national romanticism, and thus never actually danced by the "folk." It was not until around 1970, concurrent with a remarkable renaissance of interest in Swedish country fiddling, that true dances of the people became a part of the Folk Dance movement. Thanks to the work of a few devoted researchers, an unbelievable number of old dances, mostly "Polska" types, were rescued from oblivion through interviews with elderly fiddlers and folks who had danced them when young. These "bygdedanser," regional dances, have at last reunited the Folk Dancer with the folk fiddler and the vibrant, unbroken tradition of native Swedish music.

Bitte Mand I Knibe

(Little Man in a Fix)
Danish

BITTE *MAND I KNIBE* IS A VERY popular little dance, both in Denmark and all over the United States. *Knibe* means to be in a "spot" or "fix."

Records: EZ 6009; Folk Dancer MH 1054; Viking 400.

Music: Burchenal, E., *Folk Dances of Denmark*, p. 44, and *Folk Dances from Old Homelands*, p. 62; LaSalle, D., *Rhythms and Dances for Elementary Schools*, p. 115.

Formation: Two couples, woman to right of partner. Men hook left elbows and place right arm around partner's waist, women place left hand on man's left shoulder.

Steps: Running step, Tyrolian Waltz, Waltz.

DIRECTIONS FOR THE DANCE

Meter 3/4 • Directions are same for man and woman, except when specially noted.

■ *Measures*

    I. Run Around

1–8   Beginning left, take small running steps forward, moving counterclockwise. Couples lean away from pivot point.

1–8   As running steps are continued, men grasp left hands and raise left arms, holding women's left hand with their right, and two women move under arch and pass each other. Women turn counterclockwise to face center, men lower left arms, and women grasp each other's right hand on top of men's left–hand grasp. All four continue to take small running steps, moving counterclockwise.

    II. Tyrolian Waltz

9–12   Men release left hand, women right. The two couples turn back to back. Each couple takes couple position, inside hands shoulder height, outside arm relaxed at side. Man beginning left, woman right, take four Tyrolian Waltz steps moving in the direction facing. Arms reach forward and draw back with each step. They do not swing forward.

13–16   Closed position. Man beginning left, woman right, take four Waltz steps, turning clockwise, progressing anywhere.

9–16   Repeat action of measures 9–16.

■ **NOTE**

As the dance repeats, each couple dances with another couple. If a couple cannot find a couple for the first figure, they are **in a fix!** They go to the center and dance the running steps alone, with two hands joined. The next time the man will avoid being the **man in a fix** by hooking arms with another couple quickly for the first figure.

Den Toppede Høne (The Crested Hen) Danish

DEN *TOPPEDE HØNE* MEANS "The Crested Hen," referring to the fact that in Denmark the men wore red stocking caps with a tassel representing a rooster comb. The women added to the fun of the dance by trying to pull the man's cap off as he went through the arch. If successful, then the woman became "crested" hen.

Dance A While CD: #15. "Crested Hen (Den Toppede Høne)."

Records: Dancecraft DC 162402 LP; Folkraft 1159, 1194; World of Fun LP 4, Side A–6.

Cassette: Dancecraft 162402.

Music: Burchenal, E., *Folk Dances of Denmark*, p. 49; LaSalle, D., *Rhythms and Dances for Elementary Schools*, p. 150. Neilson, N. P., and Van Hagen, W., *Physical Education for Elementary Schools*, p. 300.

Formation: Set of three, two women and a man, hands joined to form a circle.

Step: Step–hop.

DIRECTIONS FOR THE DANCE

Meter 2/4

■ *Measures*

Part I

1–8	Beginning left, step–hop around circle clockwise, taking a vigorous stamp on first beat. Dancers lean away from center as they circle.
1–8	Jump, bringing feet down sharply on first beat, step–hop around circle counterclockwise.

Part II

9–10	Continuing step–hop, women release joined hands, place free hand on hip, and right–hand woman dances through arch made by man and left–hand woman.
11–12	Man turns under his left arm, following right–hand woman through arch.
13–14	Left–hand woman dances through arch made by man and right–hand woman.
15–16	Man turns under his right arm, following left–hand woman through arch.
9–16	Repeat action of measures 9–16.

■ MIXER

The man may progress forward to the next group at the completion of part II.

Familie Sekstur

Danish

F AMILIE SEKSTUR MEAN'S "FAMILY SIXSOME" and is pronounced *fa-MEEL-yeb SEKS-toor*. This Danish mixer is similar to American Square Dance figures and steps.

Record: Dancecraft DC 74518; Viking 400.

Music: Farwell, Jane, *Folk Dances for Fun*, p. 20.

Formation: Couples in single circle, woman to right of partner, hands joined, held at shoulder height, elbows V–shaped. Dancers stand close to each other.

Steps: Buzz step, walk.

DIRECTIONS FOR THE DANCE

Meter 6/8 • Directions are the same for man and woman except when specially noted.

■ *Measures*

1–8	Introduction. Beginning right, take 16 buzz steps to side (right crosses over left, right knee bending slightly). Circle moves clockwise. Take small light steps, keep circle small with elbows bent, and lean back slightly for better action.

I. In and Out

9–10	Beginning right, take four steps toward center, slowly extending joined hands above head. On fourth step, everyone nods head to greet everyone.
11–12	Beginning right, take four steps backward, to return to original formation, arms gradually lowering to original position (elbows bent, joined hands shoulder height). On fourth step, nod head to partner.
13–16	Repeat action of measures 9–12.

II. Grand Chain

17–24	Face partner and join right hands shoulder high, elbows bent, and continue around circle with grand right and left. Count out loud one to seven for each person met, keeping the seventh person for new partner. This keeps mixers in order. It is especially fun if counted in a Scandinavian language. Danish counting:

one–*en*, pronounced *enn*
two–*to*, pronounced *toe*
three–*tre*, pronounced *tray*
four–*fire*, pronounced *feer*
five–*fein*, pronounced *femm*
six–*sexs*, pronounced *sex*
seven–*syv*, pronounced *syou*.

III. Swing

1–8	Swing position, with man's left arm, woman's right, extended straight out at shoulder level.
	Swing new partner in place, taking 16 buzz steps, ending with woman on man's right. All join hands to form single circle.
	Repeat action of part I–III, measures 9–24, 1–8, until end of record.

Familjevalsen

Swedish

FAMILJEVALSEN MEANS "THE FAMILY WALTZ" and is pronounced *fah-MIL-yeh-vahls-en*. Although this dance may be found throughout the Scandinavian countries, the Swedish version is described here as taught by Gordon E. Tracie, Seattle.

Dance A While CD: #23. "Family Waltz (Familjevalsen)."

Records: Viking Skandia Album 1; any lively Swedish waltz.

Music: Farwell, Jane, *Folk Dances for Fun.*

Formation: Couples in single circle, woman to right of partner, hands joined, held at shoulder height, elbows V–shaped.

Steps: Waltz balance, Waltz.

DIRECTIONS FOR THE DANCE

Meter 3/4 • Directions are for man; woman's part reverse.

■ *Measures*

I. Balance

1   Beginning left, take one Waltz balance turning toward corner.

2   Beginning right, take one Waltz balance turning toward partner.

3–4   Repeat action of measures 1–2.

II. Waltz

5–8   Take closed position with corner. Arms, man's left, woman's right, are extended straight out, shoulder height. Man places left thumb against the palm of the woman's right hand and closes his hand around the back of her hand. Beginning left, take four Waltz steps turning clockwise, progressing in line of direction. On last Waltz step, form circle, man placing partner on right side. Repeat dance from beginning with new corner.

■ STYLE

This should be a very smooth yet lively dance. Be sure to exchange smiles or greetings with corner and partner on the Waltz balance. Remember that the body rises and low–ers during a Waltz balance. The Waltz is light, graceful, and fast.

■ MIXER

Skandia, Seattle, traditionally starts with partner on left, so that first Waltz in closed position (Part II) is with partners.

Hambo

Swedish

THE *HAMBO* (ITS FULL NAME IS *HAMBOPOLSKA*), OFTEN called the national dance of Sweden, is practiced far beyond the borders of its homeland. It is danced in neighboring Scandinavian countries and in Swedish national groups around the world; in the United States it is a top favorite among folk dancers.

The Hambo is the most common living example of the once all–popular Swedish "Polska"–a distinctly Nordic music and dance form dating back to the 16th century. Because the Hambo is a living Folk Dance, yesterday's version is not the same as today's, according to Gordon E. Tracie.* The form most common in the United States is a relatively old style called *nighambo*, referring to the characteristic "dip" on the first beat. It was brought to the United States by Swedish immigrants more than a half–century ago.

Records: Folk Dancer MH 2002, 2003, 2004; Folkraft 1048, 1164; Merit AV 1047 LP; Viking Skandia Album II.

Position: Couple, inside hands joined at shoulder height, outside hands on hip, thumb pointing backwards, fingers forward.

Steps: Step swing or Waltz balance, Polska.

DIRECTIONS FOR THE DANCE

Meter 3/4 • Directions are for man; woman's part reverse, except when specially noted.

■ Measures

I. Introduction

1 Beginning left, take one step swing (dal step) or Waltz balance, turning body slightly away from partner, letting inside hands reach forward.

2 Take one step swing or Waltz balance slightly forward, turning body slightly toward partner, drawing inside hands backward.

3 Take three steps or Waltz step in line of direction.

II. Hambo (Polska) Step

4 Shoulder–waist position.

Man's part: Count 1, beginning right, step (with flat foot and bent knee) forward in line of direction with foot turned outward to start clockwise pivot. Place foot between partner's feet. Count 2, step left slightly forward in line of direction (almost in place) pivoting almost 360° clockwise. Body rises, coming up on ball of left foot. Count 3, touch ball of right foot firmly close behind left heel.

Woman's part: Count 1, beginning left, step almost in place pivoting 180° clockwise, bending left knee slightly. Count 2, right foot describes an arc, skimming floor, and touches toe close behind left heel. Body starts to rise.

Hambo (continued)

*Gordon E. Tracie, the late director of Skandia Folkdance Society, Seattle.

Count *and*, as body continues to rise, push slightly with left foot and leap into air. Count 3, complete 180° turn while both feet are in air, landing on right foot placed forward in line of direction between man's feet.

5–7   Repeat action of measure 4 three times.

8   Beginning right, take three steps almost in place. Take couple position, facing line of direction.

▪ STYLE

1. The Hambo is a very graceful, smooth–flowing dance. The music should be moderate speed, not fast. At the proper tempo, the dancers appear very relaxed and their movements effortless. Extra turns and twirls are to be discouraged.

2. The upper torso is always upright. The torso is lowered, or settles with the bending of the knee to accompany the primary accent (count 1). It rises on count 2. This body movement is subtle.

3. Both dancers should always be in control of their own body weight. The body is well "grounded" by planting each foot firmly in the step pattern. The touch of the man's right foot (count 3) acts to stabilize the body while pivoting. His weight is actually on both feet momentarily.

4. The woman should not let her right lower leg "fly up," or flick in the air, as it describes the arc (count 2).

5. The man guides the woman while in the air. He does not lift her as she receives her impetus for height from her push (count *and*).

6. Once the basic footwork is learned, perfection and styling of the dance takes several years of regular practice and conscious effort to improve one's style.

▪ SUGGESTIONS FOR TEACHING THE HAMBO (POLSKA) STEP

1. Understand basic rhythm.

Man: 3/4				Woman: 3/4			
Step	Pivot	Touch		Step	Touch	Leap	Step
R	L	R		L	R		R
1	2	3		1	2	and	3

2. Men stand single–file, facing a wall; women single–file, facing an opposite wall.
   a. Analyze basic step (without partner) for each group. Practice basic step in place.
   b. Analyze basic step (with turn) for each group. Emphasize exact placement of each foot in relation to line of direction and a specific wall. Face original wall with each Hambo step.

3. Double–file lines, couples in shoulder–waist position.
   a. Practice step with partner.
   b. Practice individually and then together, alternately.

4. Double circle, couples in shoulder–waist position.
   a. Practice step progressing around room.
   b. Then analyze Introduction to Hambo and practice complete dance.

Norwegian Polka (Scandinavian Polka)

THE NORWEGIAN POLKA IS ALSO KNOWN as the *Scandinavian Polka*, *Seattle Polka*, and *Ballroom Polka*. Gordon E. Tracie* suggests that the Americanized version may come from a simplification of the Norwegian dance *Parisarpolka*, meaning "Parisian Polka." The Norwegian immigrants probably brought the Parisarpolka to America, where it changed somewhat in form but retained the original Scandinavian Polka music.

Dance A While CD: #19. "Polka."

Records: Viking V–806,** Viking V–812, Folkraft 1411, Folk Dancer MH 2001, 2004, Norse 45; or any good Scandinavian Polka, eight–measure phrase.

Position: Couple.

Steps: Walk, pivot turn.

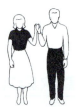

DIRECTIONS FOR THE DANCE

Meter 2/4 • Directions are for man; woman's part reverse.

■ *Measures*

Part I

1–2   Beginning left, take three walking steps in line of direction and stamp.

3–4   Beginning right, take three walking steps in reverse line of direction and clap, clap.

Part II

5   Beginning left, walk two steps in line of direction. Face partner on second step and take shoulder–waist position.

6–8   Beginning left, take a six–step pivot turn clockwise, progressing in line of direction. Partners should lean away from each other in turn. Man should end with back to center of room.

■ VARIATIONS

1. Measures 5–6   Walk four steps in line of direction.
   Measures 7–8   Four-step pivot turn clockwise.

2. Measures 1–2   Take two steps in line of direction and a Two-Step in place, facing partner.
   Measures 3–4   Repeat in reverse line of direction.

3. Measures 1–2   Take three-step turn in line of direction. Clap at end of turn.
   Measures 3–4   Repeat in reverse line of direction.

■ TEACHING SUGGESTIONS

1. For help teaching pivot turn, see p. 59.

2. To simplify dance for the beginner, it is helpful to teach two walking steps in measures 5–8 in couple position, followed by two steps pivoting in shoulder–waist position and repeat. Gradually change the sequence to the regular four– or six–step pivot.

---

*Gordon E. Tracie, late director of Skandia Folkdance Society, Seattle.
**Out of print.

Seksmannsril

Norwegian

*S*EKSMANNSRIL MEANS "SIX PERSONS' REEL" and is pronounced *seks-mahns-REEL*. It is classified as a formal Folk Dance. The dance comes from the region of Asker. Mrs. Helfrid Rudd* taught this dance at the University of Washington, 1951.

Record: Viking V 300. Viking Skandia album.

Formation: Three couples in single circle, woman to right of partner; hands joined with arms outstretched, shoulder height.

Steps: Step–hop.

DIRECTIONS FOR THE DANCE

Meter 2/4 • Directions are same for both woman and man, except where specially noted.

■ *Measures*

	1–4	Introduction: no action.

Figure 1

Ring

A	1–7	Beginning left, take 14 step–hops to left, circle moving clockwise.
	8	Take three stamps (left, right, left), turning to face counterclockwise.
	1–7	Beginning right, take 14 step–hops to right, circle moving counterclockwise.
	8	Take three stamps (right, left, right), clapping hands once on first stamp. Partners face, joining two hands. Arms are outstretched with outside arms slightly higher than inside arms; body leans toward center of circle. Inside hands of all couples almost touch in center of circle.

Two–Hand Hold

B	9–15	Man beginning left, woman right, take 14 step–hops, moving in line of direction; man moves forward, woman backward. As couples are leaning slightly toward center of circle, body has banking effect as traveling.
	16	Clapping hands once, take three stamps turning away from partner to face corner; man turns left, woman right, and join two hands with outstretched arms, still leaning toward center.
	17–23	Continuing to move in line of direction, repeat action of measures 9–15, woman moving forward, man backing up.
	24	Turning back to face partner, (man turns right, woman left) repeat action of measure 16.

Chain

C	25–32	Giving right hand to partner, grand right and left around the ring, step–hopping (beginning left). Continue on meeting partner the first time. Second time facing partner, take three stamps and rejoin hands in single circle.

---

*Mrs. Helfrid Rudd, Norwegian Folk Dance authority, Oslo, Norway.

Figure II

Ring

A | 1–8 | Repeat action of Figure I, A, measures 1–8.

Hand Clapping

B | 9–24 | Repeat action of Figure I, B, measures 9–24; instead of joining hands, clap hands on each step–hop. Action of arms while clapping is vertical: right hand swinging down, left up for clap, right hand coming up, left down for next clap, and alternating thereafter.

Chain

C | 25–32 | Repeat action of Figure I, C, measures 25–32.

■ **NOTES**

1. During Figure I, A, some groups prefer to swing arms in and out while circling.

2. The Reel is a happy dance and must be danced quickly and with abandon. Stamps and claps are very precise. The dancers call "hey" or "ho" as they turn away or toward partners.

Snurrbocken

Swedish

SNURRBOCKEN, PRONOUNCED *SNOOR-BOOK-EN*, MEANS "the whirl and bow." Like the Hambo, it is a form of Swedish Polska. According to Gordon E. Tracie,* the second (bowing) part of the dance is a bit of rustic satire in which the farm folk burlesqued the gentry and their affected mannerisms. Traditionally it was at just this point that the fiddler could have *his* fun with the dancers by setting the timing and tempo of his bow sequence–often with long delays–and it was up to the dancers to follow him!

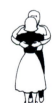

Records: Folk Dancer MH 1047: Viking V 200.

Music: *Svenska Folkdanser och Sallskapsdancer,* Svendska Ungdomsringen, Stockholm.

Position: Shoulder–waist.

Steps: Polska step, running step.

DIRECTIONS FOR THE DANCE

Meter 3/4 • Directions are for man; woman's part reverse.

■ *Measures*

I. Polska Turn

1–8 | Beginning left, take eight Polska steps turning clockwise progressing in line of direction. Analysis of Polska step: Man's part: Count 1, step forward left, pivoting clockwise. Count 2, continue pivoting on left and

Snurrbocken (continued)

*Gordon E. Tracie, late director of Skandia Folkdance Society, Seattle.

place ball of right foot near left foot (weight remains on left foot, right foot helps to maintain balance). Count 3, step forward right. Woman's part: Count 1, step on both feet, preparing to pivot clockwise. Count 2, step right, pivoting clockwise. Count 3, step left, pivoting clockwise.

II. Run

9–16   Conversation position, with free hand on hips (fingers forward, thumb back). Beginning left, take 24 light, small, running steps forward in line of direction.

III. Bows

17   Place hands on own hips fingers forward, thumbs back, and turn slowly toward partner, man with back to center, woman facing the center.

18   Slowly bow low to each other with dignity.

19   Each turn one half–turn, man counterclockwise, facing center, woman clockwise, facing outward.

20   Slowly bow while back to back.

21   Each turns one–half more to face each other. Take shoulder–waist position to repeat dance.

■ NOTES

1. This Polska step, sometimes called Delsbopolska, after a district in the province of Halsingland, is related to the Hambo step but begins with the man's **left** and has a pivot, whereas the Hambo–Polska begins with the man's **right** and has a "dip" (first beat) at the beginning of each step.

2. The recording by Folk Dancer begins with a bow instead of a Polska.

Swedish Varsouvienne   Swedish

ALL OF THE SCANDINAVIAN LANDS HAVE virtually identical Varsouviennes, which are different but related in both music and step pattern to the well–known American Varsouvienne or "Put Your Little Foot."

Records: Folk Dancer MH 1023; Folkraft 1130.

Music: Bergquist, Nils, *Swedish Folk Dances*, p. 12; Herman, Michael, *Folk Dances for All*, p. 32.

Position: Conversation, outside hands on hip, thumb pointing backward, fingers forward.

Steps: Walk, Waltz, Mazurka type.

DIRECTIONS FOR THE DANCE

Meter 3/4 • Directions are for man; woman's part reverse.

■ *Measures*

I. Walk and Heel

1–2 Beginning left, take three steps, man dancing almost in place; the woman takes a full turn counterclockwise and moves across in front of man to his left side. Man places left arm around woman's waist and woman places right arm on man's left shoulder, outside hands on hip. Place right heel with toe raised (woman's left) slightly forward. Outside hand is always on hip.

3–4 Beginning right, repeat action of measures 1–2, woman turning clockwise, returns to original position. Place left heel with toe raised forward.

5–8 Repeat action of measures 1–4.

II. Mazurka

9–10 Beginning left, step forward with slight accent, draw right to left, hop right, sweeping left across right. Repeat.

11–12 Repeat action of measures 1–2.

13–16 Beginning right, repeat action of measures 9–12.

III. Waltz

17–24 Closed position. Beginning left, take eight Waltz steps, turning clockwise, progressing in line of direction.

■ **VARIATION**

Measures 9–10, as in Sweden, instead of sweeping foot across, kick left foot forward and back fast. This is referred to as "fryksdal–step."

Swedish Waltz

Swedish

SWEDISH WALTZ HAS BEEN POPULAR IN THE United States for at least 50 years. Gordon E. Tracie* in his study of dances in Scandinavia in 1948 discovered that such a Swedish Waltz was not danced in Sweden. However, an elderly couple from the country (Dalarna) recognized it as the nearly forgotten *Norsk Vals* (Norwegian Waltz), which they had danced in their youth. Scandinavian immigrants undoubtedly brought the dance to this country at the turn of the century.

Dance A While CD: #23. "Family Waltz (Familjevalsen)."

Records: National 4510. Any good Swedish Waltz in moderately slow tempo with eight-measure phrases.

Position: Couple, inside hands joined at shoulder height.

Step: Waltz, step–swing, or Waltz balance.

Swedish Waltz (continued)

*Gordon E. Tracie, late director of Skandia Folkdance Society, Seattle.

DIRECTIONS FOR THE DANCE

Meter 3/4 • Directions are for man; woman's part reverse.

■ *Measures*

1   Beginning left, take one step–swing (dal step) or Waltz balance (step touch) almost in place turning body slightly away from partner, inside hands reaching forward as arms are extended forward shoulder height.

2   Beginning right, move slightly forward, taking one step–swing of Waltz balance and turn body slightly toward partner, inside hands drawing backward as arms are extended backward shoulder height.

3–4   Beginning left, take two Waltz steps or six steps in Waltz rhythm in line of direction. More advanced dancers make one solo turn, turning away from partner (man left, woman right) while moving in line of direction. This turn is facilitated by man stepping back in line of direction right, woman left, on second waltz step before continuing turn.

5–8   Closed position or shoulder–waist position. Beginning left, take four Waltz steps, turning clockwise. Woman turns out under man's left arm on last Waltz step to assume couple position.

To Ting

Danish

*T*o Ting means "two things." This refers to the two different rhythms, 3/4 and 2/4.

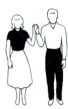

Records: Folk Dancer MH 1018; Viking Skandia Album I.
Music: Herman, Michael, *Folk Dances for All*, p. 52.
Position: Inside hands joined, outside hands on hips.
Steps: Waltz, walk, pivot turn.

DIRECTIONS FOR THE DANCE

Meter 3/4 • Directions are for man; woman's part reverse.

■ *Measures*

Part I

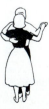

1   Moving forward, beginning left, take one Waltz step turning away from partner, swinging inside arms forward, hands at shoulder level.

2   Moving forward, take one Waltz step, turning toward partner, swinging inside arms back.

3–4   Repeat action of measures 1–2.

5–8   Closed position. Beginning left, take four Waltz steps, turning clockwise, progressing in line of direction.

1–8   Repeat action of measures 1–8.

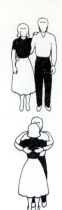

Meter 2/4

Part II

9–12   Conversation position, outside hands on hips. Beginning left, take four walking steps forward.

13–16   Shoulder–waist position. Beginning left, turn clockwise with four steps in a pivot turn.

9–16   Repeat action of measures 9–16.

Variation

9–12   The Danes skip four forward.

13–16   Turn with four step-lifts (svejtril steps) in pivot turn.

Totur*

Danish

TOTUR OR *TWO DANCE* IS A MIXER FROM the district of Vejle in western Denmark. Dancers get new partners at the completion of the "chain" or grand right and left. It is customary to smile at each person you meet in the chain.

Records: Folk Dancer MH 1021; Viking V–401.

Formation: Single circle, couples facing center, woman to right of partner, hands joined, held at shoulder level.

Steps: Walk, Two–Step, Polka.

DIRECTIONS FOR THE DANCE

Music 2/4 • Directions are for man; woman's part reverse, except in the introduction.

■ *Measures*

Introduction

1–8   Beginning left, take 16 walking steps, eight Two–Steps or eight Polka steps clockwise.

1–8   Repeat action of measures 1–8 counterclockwise.

Figure I

9   Single circle. Open position, men facing line of direction, joined hands toward center of circle. Beginning left, take one Two–Step toward center of circle.

10   Continue in same direction with two walking steps.

11–12 Beginning right, moving away from center, repeat action of measures 9–10 back to place in reverse open position or backout.

13–16 Beginning left, take four Polka steps, turning clockwise, progressing in line of direction.

9–16   Repeat action of measures 9–16.

Figure II

1–8   Partners face, grasp right hands and grand right and left around circle with walking, Two–Steps, or polka steps.

1–8   Continue grand right and left. **Note:** At the end of this figure, dancers may have a new partner for repeat of the dance.

Repeat Figures I and II alternately for remainder of record.

---

*This dance was arranged from the dance used in *The Folk Dancer*, Vol. 5, December 1945, pp. 10–11.

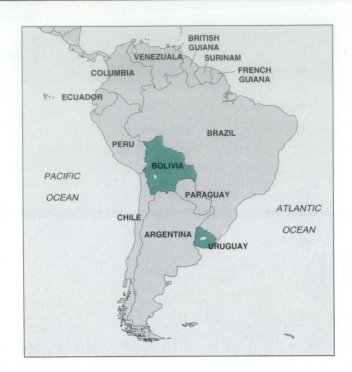

Carnavalito

Bolivia

CARNAVALITO IS A DANCE FROM BOLIVIA. It was presented at Maine Folk Dance Camp by Laura Zanzi de Chavarria from Uruguay.

Just before Lent, while some countries are celebrating Mardi Gras, Latin America is celebrating Tiempo de Carnaval. Several South American countries have their own Carnavalito. This one is one of Bolivia's most popular dances. It is danced at many fiestas, but mainly during the Carnaval festivities–up and down the streets.

Dance A While CD: #1. "Carnavalito."

Record: Folk Dancer LPM MH 004A; High/Scope LC 84–743–253.

Formation: No partner. Lines facing forward, one person behind each other, hands joined.

Steps: Three walking steps forward and hold.

DIRECTIONS FOR THE DANCE

Meter 4/4. Directions are the same for both woman and man.

■ *Measures*

9 measures — Introduction: no action. Slow, slow, quick, quick, slow. Drum beats, followed by seven accented beats.

Part I

1–8 — Leader leads line in a serpentine figure. Beginning right, take three steps forward and hold, bending forward at waist (right, left, right, hold). Take three steps forward and hold, body straightening up (left, right, left, hold). This step is like a schottische, but with a "hold" instead of a "hop."

Part II

1–4 — Leader leads line into a broken circle with 16 step hops.

5–8 — Then the line reverses. Take 16 step hops in the opposite direction with the last person leading the line.

Repeat all in the original direction. In the last repeat, Part I is only half as long.

Ranchera

Uruguay

RANCHERA IS A COUPLE DANCE FROM Uruguay. It was presented by Laura Zanzi de Chavarria at the Maine Folk Dance Camp. *Ranchera* has been danced at all Uruguayan festivities since 1850. It is called "el limpia sillas"–the chair cleaner–because when this music is played, everyone gets up to dance. It is the most popular dance of Uruguay.

Record: Folk Dancer 45 RPM MH 1131–A; Folk Dancer LPM MH 004A.

Formation: Couples scattered, all facing **front,** side by side with woman to right of man, inside hands joined.

Step: Walking Waltz.

DIRECTIONS FOR THE DANCE

Meter 3/4 • Directions are for man; woman's part is the reverse.

■ *Measures*

Part I

1–4 — Starting with outside foot, take one Waltz step forward. Drop hands, turn to face opposite direction with one Waltz step. Join inside hands and take one Waltz step toward the back wall; and one Waltz step to face each other.

Ranchera (continued)

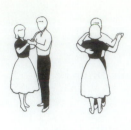

| 5–8 | Balance to side, man's left, woman's right; balance to other side. Turning away from partner (all the way around) take two Waltz steps and clap on count 5 (Counts 1 – 2 – 3 – 4 – clap – 6). |

Part II The Square

1–2	Semi–open position, couple moves forward with two waltz steps.
3–4	Closed position, take two waltz steps, turning clockwise three–fourths around to face left wall.
5–8	Repeat action of measures 1–4 to face back wall, alternating semi–open and closed position.
1–4	Repeat action of measures 1–4 to face right wall, alternating semi–open and closed position.
5–8	Repeat action of measures 1–4, alternating semi–open and closed position, but end up facing back wall, woman on man's left.

Part III

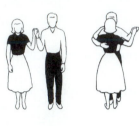

| 1–8 | Repeat action of Part I, towards back wall. |

Part IV

| 1–16 | Closed position, take 16 Waltz steps, turning clockwise, progressing freely around the floor. |

Part V

| 1–2 | Man holding woman's right hand in his left, take one Waltz step to change places, woman going under man's arm. Still holding hands, with one Waltz step, balance away from each other. |

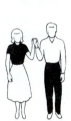

Cue: under and pull back.

| 3–8 | Repeat movement of measures 1–2 three more times, ending in Varsouvienne position with woman on man's left. |

Part VI

| 1–8 | Keeping woman in front, partners exchange sides with one Waltz step; exchange sides again with one Waltz step. Dancers look into partners eyes as they cross sides. Repeat for a total of eight side to sides. This sequence is in place. |
| 1–8 | Repeat action of measures 1–8, moving forward while exchanging places. Move freely around the room. |

Part VII

| 1–8 | Repeat action of Part I, inside hands joined. |

Social Dance

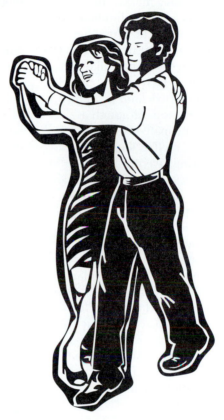

INTRODUCTION

Dance and music are not static forms. They mirror the culture in which they exist by reflecting the past, present, and any intercultural exchanges that have occurred. The everchanging human scene is absorbed and acted out in dance and music forms.

The Renaissance of the 15th and 16th century in Italy and France saw the rebirth of interest in learning, literature, arts, and creative expression in general. The invention of printing made it possible for dance instruction and music notation to be widely distributed. Avid interest in dance and the creation of new musical forms swept through the courts of Europe. The period saw the establishment of dance teaching as a profession. New court dances were developed by professionals for the nobility. Courts used dance as an opportunity to educate courtiers in social graces and deportment. Queen Elizabeth established social dance as an important part of court life. English country dance began to appear in court, and English dancing schools were in vogue. Dances in the latter part of Queen Elizabeth's reign were gay, lively, and extremely popular.

The first half of the 16th century (1500–1550) saw the Basse dance reign as queen of the dance along with caroles, pavanes and turgions. During the last half (1550–1600) brawls (branle), rounds, heys, ring dances, galliards, courantores, La Voltas and allemandes were the dances of the day. Dancing became an everyday adjunct to court life in the palaces of the Renaissance.

In Colonial America, military balls and elaborate cotillions were popular. The hearty pioneers brought dance to the taverns and public dance halls with their western migration. In more modern times, college proms and special festive occasions were the impetus for social dancing. Night clubs became the ballrooms for the dancing public. Clubs often specialized in a particular type of dance such as Country Western Swing of one variety or the other, Latin, or simply an evening of ballroom favorites danced to the "big band" sound. Social Dance has always been a viable part of the social life in America.

■ Phases of Social Dance

Since the 1900s, eight periods have marked the progress of Social Dance, and each was stimulated or motivated by a new style of music. The *Foxtrot* had its beginnings in the early 1900s as a fast trotting step to a new jazz called "ragtime." Novelty dances like the Bunny Hug and the Grizzly Bear were widely popular during World War I. Next came Dixieland jazz and an athletic dance called the Charleston. Although a strenuous dance done to a syncopated beat, it found great favor among those sporting the "flapper style" of dress and look of the Roaring Twenties.

From the 1930s to the 1950s, big band music produced hundreds of tunes that have become classics. The *Lindy*, also called jitterbug and later Swing, made its appearance. Big band music changed the Foxtrot into a smooth dance with many variations. Even the Waltz took on a new, more sophisticated look. The Big Apple, Shag, and Lambeth Walk were the main dance interest of the college crowd. The popularity of dancing to big band music increased the need for and the number of dance studios. The swinging and swaying of big band music also gave rise to large public ballrooms across the country. Although the Swing faded with the demise of the big bands, it returned in the 1980s and 1990s to be danced to a variety of rhythm styles of the period.

The *Tango* was a fad during the 1920s and has remained a ballroom favorite over the years, although at times overshadowed by interest in other Latin dances. Stimulated by an influx of Latin music, the Cuban Rumba started a new trend toward Latin dances in the 1930s. The Brazilian Samba, Mambo, Cha Cha Cha, Calypso, Merengue, and later the Bossa Nova all enjoyed brief but exciting periods of popularity. The Tango, however, has endured as a ballroom favorite.

The beat and sound decibels produced by rock music demanded a dance response that was to characterize the period during and after World War II. Rock and roll was the music of such legends as Elvis Presley, the Beatles, Rolling Stones, and the Beach Boys. Dance movement became unencumbered by pattern or partner except as the dance action was performed facing and gyrating with another person. Dance bands and dance floor space became smaller.

Disc jockeys and recorded music became the norm. Novelty or fad dances such as the Twist, Slop, Mashed Potato, Swim, Monkey, Pony, Bug, Hitch Hiker, Watusi, Hully Gully, and Jerk enjoyed various degrees and length of popularity. Television and videos became the major vehicles for disseminating rock and roll music, dance, manners, and dress.

Country Western had its roots in the music and songs brought by European immigrants to the Appalachian Mountains in the Eastern United States. The mix of people from this region with a wider spectrum of people during World War II led to an explosion of interest in the music and songs of these mountain people. Songs and music of the cowboys from Texas and the Southwest had generally become entrenched after the Civil War. These two music and dance forms coupled with the adaptation of western cowboy dress became what is now known as Country Western. Country Western radio stations have long enjoyed popularity with a loyal listening public.

Swing, Disco Swing, and Country Swing are the basic patterns used in dancing to Country Western music. Line dancing has emerged to take its place alongside Country Western dance. Both enjoy a wide following and are danced to the same music at the same time. While couples dance in the line of direction around the dance floor, line dancers carry on in the center moving forward and back or sideways without interfering with the traditional flow of dancers around the perimeter.

From the inner cities comes Street dance. Break dancing and Hip Hop have roots in African American culture. Break dancing is an acrobatic form coming out of New York's south Bronx. Hip Hop has its roots in rap, but also embraces soul, funk, jazz, and dance hall reggae. The accompanying music is electronic funk with a machine-gun style chanting called rap.

■ Competition

Competition has long been a part of the history of ballroom dance. In England an Open Foxtrot Competition was held in 1920. It was so successful that a later event, the Ivory Cross Competition, featured "heats" held in various provincial centers and in London. Dance teams thus qualified for the Grand Finals, which were held in December of 1921. The success of this type of qualifying led to the first national competition sponsored by the *Daily Sketch*, a London newspaper. In 1922 England held its first major competition to determine the best "all-rounder." Teams competed in three dances: the Waltz, Foxtrot, and One-Step.

The success of these early events led to many big ballroom championships and competitions throughout England well into the 1950s. The Star Championship held since 1920 terminated in the '50s but was replaced in 1953 by the International

Championships held at Albert Hall in London. The latter continues to this day. Undoubtedly the most famous British competition is the internationally renowned Blackpool Dance Festival begun in 1930. This renowned festival draws dancers from around the world and is open to professionals and amateurs alike. Thousands of couples from all over the world convened at the 1998 Blackpool Festival. Some 75 couples from North America competed in one or more competitions. The United States is reported to have enjoyed unprecedented success with the Brigham Young University team securing wins in both the Ballroom and Latin Formation Championships in what is an exclusively amateur division.

In the United States the major venues for ballroom dance competition are the hundreds of dance competitions held annually across the country. In the early 1930s the Harvest Moon Hall was a major venue and at its height in the 1940s was a dance classic!

Of major importance at present is the Ohio Star Ball that began as a one-day event in 1977 designed to attract dancers from the immediate area. Its success led to a two-day and later a three-day competition in the late '70s. By the mid '80s entries had grown from 3,000 to 10,000. Billed as the Championship Ballroom Dance, the Ohio Star Ball has been televised by the Public Broadcasting System (PBS) for 13 years. The viewership is reported to have increased from 9 million in 1991 to more than 13 million at the present. The Ohio Star Ball is a monumental dance spectacular celebrating its 20th anniversary.

In the past decade both amateur and professional dancers have been entering contests in record numbers. The United States Amateur Ballroom Dance Association sponsors a network of contests and reports a rapid rise in member organization from 15 to 40 in the late 1990s. Other major competitions are the United States Ballroom Championships and the Imperial Society of Teachers of Dance. These venues plus hundreds of regional competitions make the ballroom scene one of beauty, skill, and exciting action enjoyed by dancer and spectator alike.

Competitive ballroom dance, whether for the amateur or professional, is a tough world. In a major division, for example, up to 50 couples may be selected from successive rounds lasting less than two minutes. Final selection may then be made from as few as six couples. Judges look for timing, rhythm, hip movements, head control, accuracy of footwork, and the level of difficulty of the routine. These determinations are made in two major divisions: Latin, which includes rumba, samba, cha-cha, paso doble, and jive, and Modern, which includes waltz, tango, foxtrot, quick step, and Viennese waltz. Couples may compete as a amateur, professional, or pro-am status. Although some compete only in one form, many compete in all 10 forms.

Public awareness of ballroom dance has come about through the influence of a number of factors. Ice-dancing uses ballroom dance forms, as does the skating in Ice Capades. Television, of course, has played an enormous role. Observances such as Ballroom Dance, sponsored by the New York Mayor's Office, and a move by Alabama dancers to have their senator help establish a National Ballroom Dance Week help build enthusiasm. College and university campuses have shown renewed interest in ballroom dance. Brigham Young University sports the largest ballroom dance program in the country along with a touring performance group that travels and performs internationally. Other active centers are Wisconsin, Texas, University of California at Berkeley, and New York University. Several have very active dance teams. The attraction of ballroom dance seems to be that it allows a certain intimacy that produces a sense of pride, resulting in greater self-assurance for participants. This is in contrast to the solo type performance of rock and roll.

The reemergence of "touch dancing," or ballroom forms of the early 1900s, seems refreshing and widely welcomed. The likelihood, however, of its comeback matching its earlier popularity depends upon two circumstances: composers writing music for this type of dance and space to accommodate large groups of dancers. In earlier times there were major ballrooms, such as Roseland and the Rainbow Room in New York, especially designed for large crowds. At present there are no great moves by composers or promoters to support the renewed interest in these earlier dance forms.

■ Dancesport

Dancesport is the term given to ballroom dance competition held in the Olympics. It combines the theatrical performance elements of the activity with the aura of a sport. Like swimming, wind surfing, and ice skating, dancesport is an extension of a widely popular recreational activity.

The International Olympic Committee (IOC) provisionally recognized dancesport in June 1995 and gave it full Olympic status in 1998. The International Dance Sports Federation (IDSF) is a nonprofit, nonpolitical organization, founded in 1957, that controls 95 percent of all international competitions, including granting of events governed by IDSF rules. The International Body of Dance Teachers and Promoters controls the remaining group of fully professional dancers.

The worldwide flavor and involvement in IDSF is demonstrated by the fact that between general meetings the affairs are conducted by a presidium composed of members from Germany, Australia, England, Denmark, Japan, Switzerland, Scotland, Russia, and the United States. The formation of the IDSF has greatly increased the interest in dancesport throughout the world. Membership at present consists of 64 countries from five continents. The World Rock 'n' Roll Confederation (WRRC) is an associate member representing some 30 countries.

The five dances used in dancesport competition are: the Modern Waltz, Tango, Viennese Waltz, Slow Foxtrot, and Quickstep. All dances are performed by a couple using the closed hold position. Figures have been standardized and categorized into various levels for teaching. Vocabularies, techniques, rhythms, and tempos have been internationally agreed upon to make instruction uniform.

■ Vintage Dance

Dances through the ages have cast their spell. They are a part of the common culture and a heritage to be borrowed, shared, and re-created. Thus, it is not surprising that there is, at present, considerable interest in reconstructing the ballroom dances of the 19th and early 20th centuries. Staging quadrilles, contras, waltzes, polkas, rags, and tangos provide a rich opportunity for research and re-creation in the areas of costuming, makeup, lighting, sound, and expanding dance skills.

It appears, therefore, that dance and the music that influenced it have come full circle. Big bands and partner or "touch" dancing have reappeared. Live bands playing a variety of rhythms such as Foxtrot, Swing, Latin, Rock, and Jazz are back in demand. Variety in music spawns variety in dance forms. America is dancing, and dancing in style!

TEACHING SOCIAL DANCE

Dealing effectively with inherent variables such as class size, available space, length of unit, and materials to be taught is of prime importance to both the teaching and learning process. The following teaching techniques should be used carefully in relation to these variables.

■ Formations

The line, single line facing one direction or parallel lines with partner couples facing, is a highly effective formation to use in a social dance class. This formation allows students to see and hear the demonstration clearly. It also allows the teacher to face the class for explanations and turn his or her back to the class for demonstration purposes. When there are two teachers, each can work with his or her back to a line in the parallel line formation. In the single line, couples may be side by side. In the parallel line, couples are opposite. The line formations are especially essential when teaching beginning steps.

■ Walk-Through

The teacher should be clearly seen and heard while demonstrating and analyzing the action of a step. On cue, the class should then follow through several times. The walk-through tempo should begin slowly and gradually increase until it is up to the tempo of the music to be used. The step should be tried first to music without a partner, then with a partner and music. A time free of instructional direction should be provided after the walk-through. During this time the teacher should circulate among the dancers giving individual assistance as needed.

■ The Cue

The whole principle of unison practice to develop rhythmic awareness is contingent upon the accuracy of a system of cueing. A signal, such as "ready and," serves to start the dancers in unison. It is important that the cues be given rhythmically! This helps the student to feel the timing. A variety of cues are used to help the student remember the foot pattern and rhythm. For example:

4/4	1–2	3	4
Rhythm cue:	slow	quick	quick
Step cue:	step	side	close
Direction cue:	turn	side	close
Style cue:	down	up	up
Warning cue:	"get ready for the break"		
Foot cue:	right	left	right

A good technique is to change from one cue to the other as needed. Cueing is a help, not a crutch, and should be abandoned as soon as the students appear to be secure in their execution. Cueing at any stage in the learning process is best when done over a sound system that amplifies the voice.

■ Demonstration

The advantages of demonstration are (a) it hastens learning when students see what is to be learned, (b) it facilitates learning the style and flow of dance movement, and (c) teaching requires less talking, so that more practice is available. Demonstration is most helpful at the following times:

1. At the beginning of the lesson with partner and music to give a whole picture of the pattern. This is also a good motivational device.

2. When presenting a new step. Demonstrate the man's and woman's parts separately, then the leads as students take partners.

3. Demonstrate to teach style, leads and partner relationships, and timing.

4. Occasionally demonstrate incorrect form followed by correct form.

5. Demonstrate for clarification.

■ Unison versus Free Practice

The walk–through for a new step should be done in unison responding to teaching cues. The whole motion of the group assists in the learning process and allows the teacher the opportunity to spot problems. Teacher–directed unison practice should be abandoned as soon as a majority have learned the step. Free practice transposes the class into a "natural" situation, more akin to the way it is to be done as a leisure pursuit.

At every level of progress in the teaching and learning process, the student should be made aware of the importance of rhythm and the use of space when moving around the dance floor. Understanding rhythm means that the man can more creatively combine and lead a variety of dance patterns to any given piece of music. Understanding space means that the man can lead his partner around the dance floor in the traditional line of direction and at the same time employ steps and dance positions that allow him to steer his partner through and around other dancers without interrupting his or their movements.

■ Dance Lesson Preparation

Teacher preparation should begin with selecting the basic step to be taught. Next analyze the underlying rhythm and know where the accent is placed in the music. Study the style of the movement used in the step and practice with the music so that it can be accurately demonstrated. One teacher will need to know both the man's and the woman's part and be able to demonstrate them with a student from time to time. Two teachers demonstrating is a more ideal situation, but one well–prepared teacher can lead a good student after a class walk–through usually without out–of–class practice. In addition, the teacher should carefully analyze the position, leads, style, and teaching cues for both the man's and woman's parts and develop routines for practicing the step forward, backward, or in place.

■ Sample Lesson Plan

The daily lesson plan should include learning objective, music selection, background information about the dance, teaching progression, and evaluation. Objectives are the perceived outcomes of the lesson. Example: Dance the magic step in time with the music. Choose several musical selections with moderate tempo to provide sameness of beat, yet variety of sound for class practice. Most dances have backgrounds stemming from a country, region, type of music, or a personality. This is a typical and viable model for creating a good and effective lesson plan.

■ Teaching Progression

The teaching progression is the blueprint of the lesson and should be a supportive guide for the teacher and an effective road map for the students to achieve the objectives of the plan. The lesson should proceed from the known to the unknown. Begin the lesson with a warm–up and review, which means dancing and polishing something already learned. Follow with new material that should constitute the greater portion of the lesson. Then add free practice time and give individual assistance as needed. Throughout the lesson be alert to partner changes so that there is an ample exchange of opportunities for each student to dance with skilled and less skilled dancers. The evaluation (see section on evaluation in Chapter 2, "Effective Group Instruction") should guide the teacher to class needs and provide students with some positive sense of their progress. The most important thing is to teach with enthusiasm and make each lesson a fun–filled occasion.

■ Technology Aids Teaching

Modern audio products such as the variable speed tape deck and CD player, wireless microphone systems, and "Dick Tracy–like" wireless remote wristwatch combine to free dance teachers from the stationary microphone and record player. The wireless microphone system consists of a light wire frame attached to the head and plugged into a belt pack transmitter thus giving the teacher complete mobility and easy vocal command during instruction. Depending on the manufacturer, the equipment has a range of 300 to 1000–plus feet and battery life of 15 to 18 hours. The wireless remote wristwatch makes it possible to control one CD and two tape decks. In addition, it starts and stops the music, adjusts the tempo, rewinds, moves fast forward, and can choose tracks on one or two CD decks.

STYLE OF SOCIAL DANCE

Social style ballroom dancing does not follow the rules of competition or dancesport. American Ballroom Dancing has borrowed steps and dances from many, many countries. Few of these are now done in the authentic style of any country. In most cases, it was the rhythmic quality that was fascinating and not its meaning. Therefore, only a semblance of the original style remains in the Latin American dances done on our dance floors.

Particular consideration needs to be given to the importance of the individual as a person and the development of one's own style. Since all individuals are different, it is folly to try to get them all to perform exactly alike. The individual who likes to dance will work for the right feeling and take a pride in the way it looks. The dance will gradually reflect an easy confidence and become part of the individual's personality.

At the beginning, few students realize the importance of good basic posture and footwork to the beauty and style of any dance. An easy, upright, balanced posture and motion of the feet in line with the body will make the dancer look good regardless of how limited the knowledge of steps. *Style* means the specific way of moving in any one dance as influenced by rhythmic qualities of the music, cultural characteristics of a country, or the current style of the movement. Styles of dances change from time to time with the rising popularity of a new star, a new band sound, or a new promotional venture by the popular dance studios.

■ *Footwork in Social Dance*

Footwork is a term used to discuss the manner of using the feet in the performance of dance steps. With the exception of body posture, it has the most significant bearing on form and style. Far too often the placement of the feet and the action of the legs give a distorted appearance to the dance. The beauty, continuity, and balance of a figure may be lost entirely due to any comic and, at the same time, tragic caricature unintentionally given to the motion.

Some general principles are involved in the application of good footwork to good dance style.

1. The weight should be carried on the ball of the foot for easy balance, alert transfer of weight from step to step, and change of direction.

2. The feet should be pointing straight ahead. When moving from one step to another, they should reach straight forward or backward in the direction of the desired action and in line with or parallel to the partner's feet.

3. Any action will start with feet together. When moving, feet should pass as closely as possible. With a few exceptions, the feet should always come together before reaching in a new direction. This known as a follow-through with the feet, and it is used in the Foxtrot, Waltz, and Tango.

4. The feet are never dragged along the floor from one step to another, but are picked up and placed noiselessly in the new position.

Occasionally, as in the Tango, the foot glides smoothly into place with the two reaching and without a scraping sound on the floor.

5. The legs should reach forward or backward from the hip. The action is initiated by stabilizing the trunk and swinging the leg freely.

6. The faster the rhythm, the shorter the step. The slower the rhythm, the more reaching the step.

7. Changes of direction are more readily in balance and under control if initiated when the feet are close together rather than when they are apart.

8. For the specific actions of reaching with one foot forward or backward, as in a corté or a hesitation step, the arch of the foot should be extended and the toe pointed.

9. Turning and pivoting figures are most effectively executed from a small base of support with the action of the man's and the woman's feet dovetailing nicely. This is possible when the action of the foot is a smooth turn on the ball of the foot with the body weight up, not pressing into the floor.

10. In accordance with the characteristic cultural style of a dance, the footwork will involve specific and stylized placement of the feet. This styling is described with each dance.

■ *One-Step/Dance Walk*

All smooth dances used to have a gliding motion with the ball of the foot. However, change in style now dictated a *dance walk* that is much like a regular walk when moving forward. It is a step forward on the heel of the foot, transferring the weight to the ball of the foot. This action is used by both man and woman when they are moving forward. The backward step is a long reach to the toe, transferring the weight to the ball of the foot.

In closed dance position, the man is reaching forward and the woman backward, simultaneously. There is a tendency for the man to step sideways so as not to step on the woman's foot, but he should step forward directly in line with her foot. The woman consequently must reach backward into her step not only to avoid being stepped on but to give him room for his step. Master dance teachers have been quoted as saying, "If the woman gets her toe stepped on, it is her own fault." This reemphasizes the point that the dance walk is a long reaching step and both man and woman must learn to reach out confidently. It is this reach that makes the style smooth and beautiful and provides contrast to other smaller steps. Taking all small steps gives the style a cramped, insecure feeling. The following points describe the mechanics of the forward dance walk.

1. The body sways forward from the ankles. The weight is on the ball of the foot.

2. The trunk is stabilized firmly. The leg swings forward from the hip joint. The reach results in a long step rather than a short, choppy step. An exaggerated knee bend will cause bobbing up and down.

3. The foot swings forward and the heel is placed on the floor first, followed by a transfer of weight to the ball of the foot. The feet never drag along the floor.

4. The legs are kept close together, with the feet passing closely together. The toes are facing straight ahead.

5. Man and woman dance on the same forward line. One should avoid letting one's feet straddle the partner's feet.

The backward dance walk is not an easy movement because one feels unstable moving backward. It should be practiced particularly by the woman since she will be moving backward a large part of the time.

1. The body weight is over the ball of the foot. One should take care not to lean forward or backward. The woman is pressing against the man's hand at her back.

2. The trunk is stabilized firmly. The leg swing backward from the hip joint with a long, smooth reach. Avoid unnecessary knee bend of the standing leg.

3. The foot is placed backward on the toe with weight transferring to the ball of the foot. The weight remains on the ball of the foot, the heel coming down only momentarily during the next step.

4. The legs and feet pass as closely as possible and in a straight line. One should avoid toeing out, heeling out, and swinging backward outside of the straight line.

DANCE POSITIONS

Successful performance with a dance partner depends on learning how to assume the dance positions* most often used in social dance: *closed position, open* or *conversation position, left parallel position, swing out* or *flirtation position, left parallel position, side car, shine, wrap,*

_____

* Refer to the glossary for descriptions of other positions.

reverse open, and side-by-side position. Dancers should learn how to assume the closed position as soon as they begin working with a partner. The results will lead to good balance, comfort, and confidence in leading and security in following. The closed position is the basic dance position. The others are adaptations of it.

■ *Closed Position*

Each factor in the analysis of the closed position is significant. It is not a mere formality. Those who are learning dance will tend to form better dance habits if they understand specifically how the position aids the dance rather than being left to manage as best they can.

1. **Partners should stand facing each other, slightly offset to their left, with shoulders parallel.** The right foot of each partner should be placed between the partner's feet, near the front of the foot. When bending knees they should not knock together. A comfortable distance should be maintained. The body posture is in good alignment.

2. **The feet should be together and pointing straight ahead.** The weight is over the balls of the feet.

3. **The man's right arm** is placed around the woman so that his arm **gives her security and support. The right hand is placed in the center of the woman's back, just below the shoulder blades.** The man should keep his right elbow lifted to help support the women's left arm. The fingers should be closed and the hand almost flat so that the man can lead with the fingers or the heel of the hand. The man's arm is extended away from his body with the elbow pointing slightly out to the right side. The man's left hand should be no higher than the shortest person's shoulder level. A majority of leads are initiated by the man's shoulders, right arm, and hand.

4. **The woman's left arm rests gently but definitely in contact with the man's upper arm** and the hand should lie along the back of the man's shoulder as is comfortable. The woman's ability to follow is often determined by her response to the action of the man's arm.

5. **The woman should arch her back against the man's right hand and move with it.** All pressure leads for change of step will come from the man's right hand and she will feel them instantly.

6. **The woman's free hand is raised sideways and the man holds the woman's right hand in his left hand approximately between them at a level just above the woman's shoulder.** The man may let her fingers rest on his upturned palm, or he may grasp lightly with his thumb against her fingers and close his fingers around the back of her hand. He should not push with his hand.

7. **Both man and woman should look at each other or over the partner's right shoulder.**

8. **Resistance is essential.** A limp body or a limp hand is the surest indication of insecurity; a poor lead elicits a slow response. Dancers need to understand the difference between tension, which does not allow for easy moving along with one's partner, and relaxation, which cannot respond readily to change. An in-between state of body alertness–called *resistance*–is more desirable.

Some **common errors** in the use of closed position are the following:

1. Partner standing at an angle in a half–open position. This causes diagonal motion of the footwork and is uncomfortable.

2. Partner too far away.

3. Lack of support in the man's right arm.

4. Lack of contact of the woman's left arm.

5. Primary use of man's left hand to lead by a pushing or pumping action.

6. Lack of resistance by either man or woman.

7. Man's right hand too high on woman's back, pulling her off balance.

8. Woman's weight back on heels.

9. Man leaning forward from the waist off balance.

10. Man pulling back with his left shoulder and hand, causing an awkward angle of motion.

11. Woman leaning heavily on partner's arm.

■ *Trends in Vocabulary and Leading*

The closed dance position is presently being referred to as the *frame*. The term conjures a body position of substance, firmness, or presence as opposed to "limp" or "just there." In addition, the terms "man and lady" or "man and woman" are being replaced by "lead" and "follow." Further, the traditional "women follow–men lead" notion is being reversed, but not because of gender imbalance! The reversal is used to stimulate sensitivity to a partner's responsibilities. Switching roles, albeit temporarily should improve a dancer's ability to lead or to follow.

■ *Techniques of Leading and Following*

Leading is done primarily by the use of the body, arms, and hands. The man sets the rhythm, decides what steps are to be used, and controls the direction and progression around the floor. The woman is completely dependent upon her partner. Therefore, an alert yet easy posture should be assumed to allow dancers to move as a unit. The firmness of the man's hand on the woman's back is an important pressure lead for changes in dance position and direction. Through the use of gentle yet firm leads, the man can make dancing a mutually pleasant experience.

The woman's responsibility is to follow her partner and adapt to any rhythm or style. She should maintain an easy resistance to give the man an alert, movable partner to lead. The woman should always maintain contact with her partner's upper right arm and shoulder and give firm resistance to his hand on her back. Should the man be a poor leader, the woman must then pay close attention to his body movement, particularly the shoulders and chest, in order to follow. When in a position apart from a part-ner, following requires a firm controlled arm that responds to a lead by simultaneous action of the body. In the challenge position, the woman's only lead is visual. She must be alert and follow her partner's action by watching him. Some general rules for fol-lowing are: (a) keep the man's rhythm and be alert to his leads; (b) support one's own weight; (c) step straight back with a reaching motion to give partner room to step straight ahead; (d) pass feet close together; (e) know the basic steps and leads; (f) try not to anticipate partner's action; and (g) work on maintaining proper body alignment and good easy posture.

SPECIFIC DIRECTIONS FOR LEADING

1. **To lead the first step,** the man should precede the step off with the left foot by an upbeat, forward motion of the body.

2. **To lead a forward moving pattern,** the man should give a forward motion in the body, including the right arm, which will direct the woman firmly in the desired direction.

3. **To lead a backward moving pattern,** the man should use pressure of the right hand. This will draw the woman forward in the desired direction.

4. **To lead a sideward moving pattern in closed position,** the man should use pressure of the right hand to the left or right to indicate the desired direction.

5. **To lead a box step,** the man should use a forward body action followed by right–hand pressure and right–elbow pull to the right to take the woman into the forward sequence of

the box. Forward pressure of the right hand followed by pressure to the left side takes her into the back sequence of the box.

6. **To lead a box turn,** with slight pressure of the right hand, the man should use the right arm and shoulder to guide or bank her into the turn. The shoulders press forward during the forward step and draw backward during the backward step.

7. **To lead into an open position,** or conversation position, the man should use pressure with the heel of the hand to turn the woman into open position. The right elbow lowers to the side. The man must simultaneously turn his own body, not just the woman, so that they end facing the same direction. The left arm relaxes slightly and the left hand sometimes gives the lead for steps in open position.

8. **To lead from open to closed position,** the man should use pressure of the right hand and raise the right arm up to standard position to move the woman into closed position. She should not have to be pushed, but should swing easily into closed position as she feels the arm lifting. She should come clear around to face the man squarely.

9. **To lead into right parallel position** (left reverse open position), the man should not use pressure of his right hand, but rather should raise his right arm, rotating her counter-clockwise one–eighth of a turn while he rotates counterclockwise one–eighth of a turn. This places the man and the woman off to the side of each other, facing opposite directions. The woman is to the right of him but slightly in front of him. The man should avoid turning too far so as to be side by side as this results in poor style and awkward and uncomfortable motion. The man's left hand may assist the lead by pulling toward his left shoulder.

10. **To lead from right parallel position to left parallel position,** the man should pull with his right hand, lowering the right arm, and push slightly with his left hand causing a rotation clockwise about a quarter turn until the woman is to the left of him but slightly in front of him. They are not side by side.

11. **To lead a hesitation step,** the man should use pressure of the right hand on the first step and sudden body tension to control a hold of position as long as desired.

12. **To lead all turns,** the man dips his shoulder in the direction of the turn, and his upper torso turns before his leg and foot turn.

13. **To lead into a pivot turn,** clockwise, the man should hold the woman slightly closer, but with sudden body tension. Resistance is exerted outward by both the man and woman leaning away from each other in order to take advantage of the centrifugal force of the circular motion. The right foot steps between partner's feet, forward on the line of direction, while the left foot reaches across the line of direction and turns on the ball of the foot about three–quarters of the way around.

14. **To lead into a corté** (dip) the man should use firm pressure of the right hand with sudden increased body tension going into the preparation step. Then the man should draw his partner forward toward him as he steps back into the dip. The left foot taking the dip backward should carry the weight, and careful balance of the weight should remain over that foot. Pressure is released as they recover to the other foot.

15. **Finger pressure leads and arm control** are important. Many times the man's only contact with his partner is with one hand or changing from hand to hand. A soft, gentle hand hold and a limp arm make it impossible to lead the variations of Swing, Cha Cha Cha, or Rumba. It is necessary that the woman exert slight resistance to the man's grasp so that pressure in any direction is reacted to instantly. Both man and woman should maintain elbow control by holding the arm firmly in front of the body with elbows down and always slightly bent. The arm is seldom allowed to extend in the elbow as this destroys the spring action needed to move out and in and under without jerking. The fingers often need to slip around the partner's without actually losing contact, in order to maintain comfortable action of the wrist and arm.

16. **To change the rhythm pattern,** the man exerts extra pressure with the right hand and pushes a little harder from the chest.

17. **Visual lead.** When partners are apart, as in the shine position of Cha Cha Cha, the woman watches her partner closely.

■ *Following*

The woman's responsibility in dancing is to follow her partner and adapt to any rhythm or style he dances. She should maintain an easy resistance, not rigidity or tension, throughout the body. This is referred to as having *tone*. If there is no tone and the woman is too relaxed or stiff, leading becomes very difficult. The man's ability to lead his partner will be enhanced when she has tone. In other words, it takes cooperation for two people to dance well, the same way it takes two people for a satisfactory handshake. The woman should always maintain contact with her partner's upper right arm and shoulder and give resistance against his hand at her back, moving with it as it guides her. If the man is a poor leader, then the woman must pay close attention to his body movement, particularly his chest and shoulder movement, in order to follow. Following, when in an apart position, requires a firm, controlled arm that responds to a lead by simultaneous action of the body. A limp arm with no resultant body response makes leading difficult in Swing, Rumba, and Cha Cha Cha. In the challenge position, the woman's only lead is visual. She must be alert and follow her partner's action by watching him. The good dancer will aim to dance with beauty of form. The woman can make a poor dancer look good or a good dancer look excellent. She can also cramp his style if she takes too small a step, has poor control of balance, dances with her feet apart, dances at an awkward angle, or leans forward.

GENERAL RULES FOR FOLLOWING

1. Keep the man's rhythm.
2. Be alert to partner's lead
3. Support one's own weight. Arch the back and move with the partner's hand.
4. Step straight backward with reaching motion so as to give the partner room to step straight ahead.
5. Pass the feet close together.
6. Know the basic steps and basic leads.
7. Try not to anticipate partner's action, just move with it.
8. Give careful thought to proper body alignment and good posture.

Foxtrot

THE *FOXTROT*, AS A present–day form, is of relatively recent origin. The only truly American form of Ballroom Dance, it has had many steps and variations through the years. The Foxtrot gets its name from a musical comedy star, Henry Fox, of the years 1913–1914 (Hostetler 1952), who danced a fast but simple trotting step to ragtime music in one of the Ziegfeld shows of that time. As an additional publicity stunt, the theater management requested that a star nightclub performer, Oscar Duryea, introduce the step to the public but found that it had to be modified somewhat, because a continuous trotting step could not be maintained for long periods without exhausting effort. Duryea simplified the step so that it became four walking steps alternating with eight quick running steps. This was the first Foxtrot.

Since that time, under the influence of Vernon and Irene Castle and a series of pro–fessional dancers, the Foxtrot has been through a gradual refining process and has developed into a beautifully smooth dance. It claims considerable popularity today.

Music from ragtime through the blues on down to modern jazz and swing has had its effect on the Foxtrot. The original Foxtrot was danced to a lively 2/4 rhythm. Its two parent forms were the One–Step, 2/4 ––––– quick quick quick quick rhythm; the other was the Two–Step, 2/4 |–––|–––| quick quick slow or step–close–step. Both of these forms are danced today but have given way to a slower, smoother 4/4 time and a more streamlined style. The Foxtrot is danced in three tempos (slow, medium, and fast) and can be adapted to almost any tempo played in the music.

The basic Foxtrot steps can be used together in any combination or sequence. A dancer who knows the basic steps and understands the fundamentals of rhythm can make up his or her own combinations easily and gradually develop the possibilities for variation in position, direction, and tempo.

FOXTROT RHYTHM

The modern Foxtrot in 4/4 time, or cut time, has four quarter beats or their equivalent to each measure. Each beat is given the same amount of time, but there is an accent on the first and third beats of the measure. When a step is taken on each beat (1–2–3–4), these are called *quick beats*. When steps are taken only on the two accented beats (1 and 3), they are twice as long and are called *slow beats*.

4/4	— — — —		4/4	— — — —	
	Q Q Q Q	One-step		Q Q Q Q	One-step
	1 2 3 4			1 2 3 4	

4/4	—— ——		4/4	—— ——	
	S S	Dance walk		S S	Dance walk
	1–2 3–4			1–2 3–4	

A use of these quick and slow beats and a combination of them into rhythm pat–terns form the basis for all of the modern Foxtrot steps. There are two patterns used predominantly: the magic step and the Westchester box step.

Foxtrot (continued)

■ Magic Step

The magic step pattern represents broken rhythm as it takes a measure and half of music and may be repeated from the middle of the measure. It is an uneven rhythm pattern, slow slow quick quick.

```
        /    /          /
4/4 |  S    S    |   Q  Q
       __   __       __  __
    |   1  2  3  4  |  1  2    |
```

uneven rhythm
Magic step

■ Westchester Box Step

The Westchester box step is a one–measure pattern, but it takes two measures to complete the box. The rhythm is uneven, slow quick quick. The rhythm may also be played in cut time, but it is still slow quick quick. Beats 1 and 2 are put together to make 1 beat. Beats 3 and 4 are put together to make 1 beat. The time signature for cut time is ¢. It is played faster and feels very much like 2/4 time.

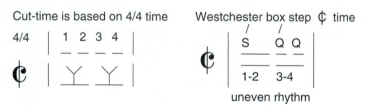

Cut-time is based on 4/4 time

```
4/4  |  1  2  3  4  |
      __ __ __ __
 ¢   |   Y     Y    |
```

Westchester box step ¢ time

```
            /       /
        S    Q  Q
 ¢      __   __ __
      |  1-2    3-4   |
```

uneven rhythm

FOXTROT STYLE

Foxtrot style truly reflects its American origin. It is the least affected of any of the Ball–room Dances. Completely without stylized or eccentric arm, foot, head, or torso movement, the Foxtrot is a beautifully smooth dance. The body is held easily erect and follows the foot pattern in a relaxed way with little up and down or sideward movement. The good dancer glides normally along the floor and blends the various steps together without bobbing or jerking. This effect is accomplished by long, reaching steps with only as much knee bend as is needed to transfer the weight smoothly from step to step. It gives the Foxtrot a streamlined motion and a simple beauty of form that can be enjoyed without strain or fatigue, dance after dance. As one becomes more and more skillful at putting together steps for the Foxtrot, there will be increasing joy derived from the tremendous variety of quick and slow combinations.

FUNDAMENTAL FOXTROT STEPS

Directions are for man, facing line of direction; woman's part is reversed, except when noted.

- ## *Introductory Steps*

- ### ONE-STEP

(Closed position)

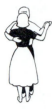

STEPS	4/4 COUNTS	RHYTHM CUE
Step L forward	1	quick
Step R forward	2	quick
Step L forward	3	quick
Step R forward	4	quick

STYLE: It is like a regular walk, heel first.

Step L backward	1	quick
Step R backward	2	quick
Step L backward	3	quick
Step R backward	4	quick

STYLE: Reach straight back with toe of foot.

NOTE: Refer to detailed analysis of One-Step, pp. 372–375.

- ### TURN

Counterclockwise (L) step on each beat (L, R, L, R) in place.

VARIATION: Alternate 4 quick and 4 slow. Try different combination of rhythms, moving forward, backward, turning, and sideward.

- ### DANCE WALK

(Forward or backward*) (Closed position)

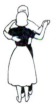

STEPS	4/4 COUNTS	RHYTHM CUE
Step L forward	1–2	slow
Step R forward	3–4	slow
Step L forward	1–2	slow
Step R forward	3–4	slow

STYLE: It is like a regular walk, heel first, but should be a long, smooth, reaching motion.

Step L backward	1–2	slow
Step R backward	3–4	slow
Step L backward	1–2	slow
Step R backward	3–4	slow

STYLE: It is a long, smooth, reaching motion to the toe of the foot, straight back.

LEAD: A basic position that gives security and support.

NOTE: Refer to detailed analysis of Dance Walk, pp. 372–373

---

*Check the lead indication, p. 374.

Fundamental Foxtrot Steps (continued)

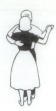

▪ SIDE CLOSE

(Chasse; a sideward–moving step) (Closed position)

STEPS	4/4 COUNTS	RHYTHM CUE
Step L sideward	1	quick
Step R to L, take weight on R	2	quick

STYLE: Steps should be short, smooth, sideward motion, on the ball of the foot.

LEAD: Knowledge of cues used to lead specific positions or directions.

NOTE: Repetition of this step will continue action to man's left.

■ *Magic Step Series*

Magic Step (Basic step)   Right and Left Parallel   Pivot Turn

Open Magic Step   The Conversation Pivot

Magic Left Turn   The Corté

The magic step series was created by Arthur Murray (1954). It is called by this name because it can be varied in a surprising number of ways. The pattern is uneven rhythm and requires a measure and a half for one basic step. This is called broken rhythm.

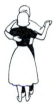

▪ MAGIC STEP

(Basic Step) (Closed position)

STEPS	4/4 COUNTS	RHYTHM CUE
Step L forward	1–2	slow
Step R forward	3–4	slow
Step L sideward, a short step	1	quick
Close R to L, take weight on R	2	quick

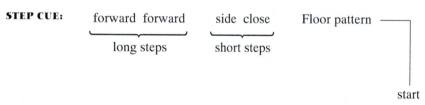

STEP CUE: forward forward   side close   Floor pattern

long steps   short steps

start

STYLE: The forward steps should be long, smooth, walking steps, straight ahead. The woman, moving backward, takes a long step reaching from hip to toe.

LEAD: A body and right arm lead forward.

VARIATIONS ON THE MAGIC STEP PATTERN: The following three techniques are used for maneuvering in a closed dance position.

1. Forward or backward–the man may maneuver forward or backward if he is aware of the traffic around him. The lead to move backward is a pressure lead at the woman's back during the quick quick beats and then a step into the backward direction on the next slow beat. Generally the man will not have room to move backward more than one or two consecutive patterns.

2. Right or left–the man may maneuver to the right or to the left to go around another couple. He will change direction on the quick quick beats by use of a pressure lead with his right hand and turn his body at the same time one-eighth of a turn to the right so as to travel diagonally outward or one-eighth turn to the left so as to travel diagonally inward beginning with the next slow beat. The

right turn is particularly handy in leading a partner out of a crowded situation away from the center of the floor. Closed position is retained throughout.

3. Dance in place–used on a crowded dance floor. Closed dance position:

STEPS	4/4 COUNTS	RHYTHM CUE
Step sideward L, slide R to L, no weight change	1–2	slow
Step sideward R, slide L to R, no weight change	3–4	slow
Step sideward L	1	quick
Close R to L, take weight R	2	quick

STEP CUE: Step slide, step slide, quick quick.

STYLE: The steps are very small.

LEAD: Increase pressure with the right hand to keep the woman from stepping back. Indicate sideward action.

NOTE: The man may maneuver this in–place pattern into a turn counterclockwise by the use of the right hand and elbow.

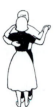

■ OPEN MAGIC STEP
(Closed position)

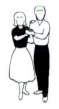

STEPS	4/4 COUNTS	RHYTHM CUE
Step L forward	1–2	slow
Step R forward	3–4	slow
Step L forward a short step, turning to open dance position	1	quick
Close R to L, take weight R	2	quick
Step L forward in open position	3–4	slow
Step R forward	1–2	slow
Step L forward a short step	3	quick
Close R to L, take weight R	4	quick
Step L forward	1–2	slow
Step R forward	3–4	slow
Step L forward a short step, turning to closed position	1	quick
Close R to L, take weight R	2	quick

STEP CUE: Slow slow quick quick.

STYLE: It is a heel lead on the slow beats in open position for both the man and woman.

LEAD: To lead into an open position or conversation position, the man should use pressure with the heel of the right hand to turn the woman into open position. The right elbow lowers to the side. The man must simultaneously turn his own body, not just the woman so that they end facing the same direction. The left arm relaxes slightly and the left hand sometimes gives the lead for steps in the open position.

LEAD: To lead from open to closed position the man should use pressure of the right hand and raise the right arm up to standard position to move the woman into closed position. The woman should not have to be pushed but should swing easily into closed position as she feels the arm lifting. She should move completely around to face the man squarely.

Fundamental Foxtrot Steps (continued)

LEAD: The man may wish to return to closed position on the quick beats following the first two slows in open position.

NOTE: It is possible to maneuver when going into open position so that the couple opens facing the line of direction and afterward closes with the man still facing the line of direction, starting from closed position as follows:

STEPS	4/4 COUNTS	RHYTHM CUE
Step L forward	1–2	slow
Step R forward	3–4	slow
Step L, R moving around the woman on the L side while turning her halfway around to open position	1–2	quick, quick
Step L forward in open position moving in line of direction	3–4	slow
Step R forward	1–2	slow
Step L, R in place, bringing the woman around to face the closed dance position	3–4	quick quick

STEP CUE: Slow slow come around/slow slow in place.

STYLE: The woman must be sure to swing around, facing the man, into a correct closed dance position while taking two quick beats.

LEAD: The man must start bringing his right elbow up to indicate to the woman that he is going into closed position on the first quick beat.

NOTE: Any number of open magic steps may be done consecutively when traveling in the line of direction without fear of interfering with the dancing of other couples.

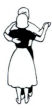

■ MAGIC LEFT TURN

(Closed position)

STEPS	4/4 COUNTS	RHYTHM CUE
Step L forward a short step	1–2	slow
Step R backward, toe in and turn counterclockwise one-quarter	3–4	slow
Step in place L, toeing out L, and turning one-quarter counterclockwise	1	quick
Step R to L, take weight R, and finish the one-half turn	2	quick
Repeat to make a full turn.		

STEP CUE: Rock   rock   step   close.
           S   S   Q   Q

STYLE: The slow steps forward and backward are like short rocking steps, but the body is straight, not leaning.

LEAD: The man must strongly increase pressure at the woman's back on the first step so that she will not swing her left foot backward. Then he uses his firm right arm to turn her with him counterclockwise. As the woman reacts to these two leads, she will step in between the man's feet and pivot on her left foot as he guides her around.

NOTE: The pattern may be reduced to a quarter–turn at a time, or it may be increased to make a full turn at a time. This variation provides a means of turning in place or of turning to maneuver into position for another variation or for recovering the original line of direction. Because of this, it is often used to tie together all types of Foxtrot variations.

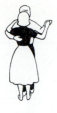

■ RIGHT AND LEFT PARALLEL MAGIC STEP

(Closed position)

This is a delightful variation involving right and left parallel position.

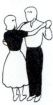

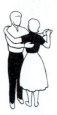

STEPS	4/4 COUNTS	RHYTHM CUE
Step forward	1–2	slow
Step R forward	3–4	slow
Step L sideward a short step, turning to R parallel position	1	quick
Close R to L, take weight on R	2	quick
Step forward L, diagonally in R parallel position	3–4	slow
Step forward R	1–2	slow
Step in place L, turning in place one-quarter clockwise into L parallel position	3	quick
Close R to L, take weight on R	4	quick
Step forward L in L parallel position	1–2	slow
Step forward R	3–4	slow
Step in place L, turning to R parallel	1	quick
Close R to L, take weight on R	2	quick
Step L forward in R parallel position	3–4	slow
Step R forward	1–2	slow
Step L in place, turning to closed position	3	quick
Close R to L, take weight on R	4	quick

STEP CUE: Slow slow quick quick.

STYLE: The woman in parallel position must reach back parallel to the man's forward reach.

LEAD: To lead into right parallel position the man should not use pressure of his right hand but rather should raise his right arm rotating the woman counterclockwise one–eighth of a turn while he rotates counterclockwise one–eighth of a turn. This places the man and woman off to the side of each other facing opposite directions. The woman is to the right of the man but slightly in front of him. The man should avoid turning too far so as to be side by side as this results in poor style and awkward and uncomfort-able motion. The man's left hand may assist the lead by pulling toward his left shoulder.

LEAD: To lead from right parallel position to left parallel position, the man should pull with his right hand lowering the right arm and push slightly with his left hand causing a rotation clockwise about a quarter of a turn until the woman is to the left of him but slightly in front of him. They are not side by side.

NOTE: The couple should move forward in a zigzag pattern, down the floor, changing from one parallel position to the other. The man must be careful to take the quick beats in place as he is changing position in order to make a smooth transition. A more advanced use of this variation is to make a half–turn clockwise in place on the quick beats as the man changes from right parallel position to left parallel position so that the man would then travel backward in the line of direction and the woman forward. A half–turn counterclockwise in place would then turn the couple back to right parallel position. Innumerable combinations of this variation will develop as dancers experiment with changes of direction.

Fundamental Foxtrot Steps (continued)

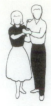

■ THE CONVERSATION PIVOT

(Open position)

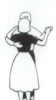

STEPS	4/4 COUNTS	RHYTHM CUE
Step L forward	1–2	slow
Step R forward	3–4	slow
Step L around the woman clockwise going into closed position	1–2	slow
Step R between woman's feet and pivot on the R foot, turning clockwise	3–4	slow
Step L forward a short step, taking open position again	1	quick
Close R to L, taking weight R	2	quick

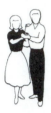

NOTE: Two extra slow beats have been added for this variation, S S S S Q Q.

STEP CUE: Step step pivot pivot quick quick.

STYLE: Couples must hold the body firmly and press outward to move with the centrifugal force of the motion on the pivot turn. The woman will step forward in between the man's feet on the third slow beat and then around him with her left foot on the fourth slow beat, followed by a quick quick to balance oneself in place.

LEAD: See lead indication above. The pivot turn is only the third and fourth slow beats. Then the man will lead into open position and take the quick beats.

NOTE: Following this variation it is usually wise to dance one more magic step in open position before leading into the basic closed position. Note details on pivot turn, pp. 388–390.

■ THE CORTÉ

(A fascinating dip step in magic step rhythm) (Closed position)

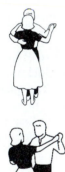

STEPS	4/4 COUNTS	RHYTHM CUE
Step L forward	1–2	slow
Step R forward	3–4	slow
Step L sideward a short step	1	quick
Close R to L, take weight on R	2	quick
Dip L backward	3–4	slow
Transfer weight forward onto R foot	1–2	slow
Step L sideward, a short step	3	quick
Close R to L, take weight R	4	quick

STEP CUE: Slow slow   quick quick   dip   recover quick quick.
              (preparation   (corté)   (weight forward)
               beats)

STYLE: *Man*—The weight is transferred onto the left foot as the man steps backward into the dip. The left knee is bent, the back is straight, the right toe extends forward. *Woman*—Her weight is transferred onto the right foot as she steps forward into the dip. The right knee is bent and directly over her foot. The back is arched, keeping her straight up and down. The left leg is extended strongly from the hip through the knee of the pointed toe. Her head should be turned left to glance at the extended foot. For additional style details, see Tango, The Corté pp. 422–423.

LEAD: To lead into a pivot turn clockwise, the man should hold the woman slightly closer, but with sudden body tension. Resistance is exerted outward by both man and woman leaning away from each other in order to take advantage of the centrifugal force of the circular motion. The right foot steps between partner's feet, forward on line of direction, while the left foot reaches across the line of direction and turns on the ball of the foot about three-quarters of the way around. The man must take care not to step too long backward or to dip too low as it is difficult for both man and woman to recover in good style.

NOTE: The exciting part about the corté is that it may be used as a variation in the dance or it may be used as a finishing step at the end of the music. It is perfectly acceptable to end a beat or two in advance and hold the position to the end of the music. It is also acceptable to corté after the music has finished. There is no pressure to get the corté on the last note of the music.

■ *Box Step Series—Westchester*

Westchester Box Step	Cross Step	Grapevine Step
Box Turn	Twinkle Step	

The Westchester box is based on slow quick quick rhythm in 4/4 or cut time. It is a one-measure pattern–but it takes two measures to complete the box–with uneven rhythm in a smooth style. It is a combination of dance walk and side close.

■ WESTCHESTER BOX STEP

(Closed position)

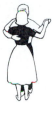

STEPS	4/4 COUNTS	RHYTHM CUE
Step L forward	1–2	slow
Pass R alongside of L, no weight change; step R sideward	3	quick
Close L to R, take weight on L	4	quick
Step R backward	1–2	slow
Pass L alongside of R, no weight change; step L sideward	3	quick
Close R to L, take weight on R	4	quick

STEP CUE: (a) Forward   side   close.
                S   Q   Q
      (b) Backward side   close
         long steps short steps.

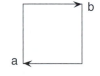

Floor pattern

STYLE: The forward step is a heel step. Both forward and backward steps should be long reaching steps. Dancers must not lose a beat by pausing as they slide alongside the standing foot.

LEAD: To lead a box step the man should use a forward body action followed by right-hand pressure and right elbow pull to the right to take the woman into the forward sequence of the box. Forward pressure of the right hand followed by pressure to the left side takes the woman into the back sequence of the box.

NOTE: The man must understand the concept of the forward side close as being the forward sequence of the box and the backward side close as being the back sequence of the box. It is important because this terminology will be used in future patterns and leads.

Fundamental Foxtrot Steps (continued)

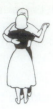

■ BOX TURN

(Left) (Closed position)

STEPS	4/4 COUNTS	RHYTHM CUE
Step L forward, toe out; turn one-quarter to L	1–2	slow
Step R sideward	3	quick
Close L to R, take weight on L	4	quick
Step R backward, toe in; turn one-quarter to L	1–2	slow
Step L sideward	3	quick
Close R to L, take weight on R	4	quick
Step L forward, toe out; turn one-quarter to L	1–2	slow
Step R sideward	3	quick
Close L to R, take weight on L	4	quick
Step R backward, toe in; turn one-quarter to L	1–2	slow
Step L sideward	3	quick
Close R to L, take weight on R	4	quick

STEP CUE: Turn side close, turn side close.

STYLE: The woman is taking the reverse of this pattern except that, when the woman steps forward with her left foot, instead of toeing out as described for the man, she steps forward between man's feet. This style for the woman greatly facilitates the turn.

LEAD: Refer to lead indications above. A cue for the lead might be bank side close, draw side close.

NOTE: The man may use this turn to maneuver himself into any direction he may wish to use next.

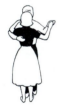

■ CROSS STEP

(Closed position)

This is a simple but pretty step turning to open dance position momentarily on the forward sequence.

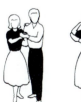

STEPS	4/4 COUNTS	RHYTHM CUE
Step L forward	1–2	slow
Step R sideward, turning to open position	3	quick
Close L to R, take weight on L	4	quick
Step R forward in open position	1–2	slow
Step L forward, turning on L foot to face partner in closed position	3	quick
Close R to L, take weight R	4	quick

STEP CUE: Forward side close, cross side close.

STYLE: The man and woman do not open up to a side to side position but open just enough to step forward on the inside foot, which feels like a crossing step. It should be accented by a long reaching step on the heel but not a dipping knee or body action.

LEAD: To lead into an open position or conversation position, the man should use pressure with the heel of the right hand to turn the woman into open position. The right elbow lowers to the side. The man must simultaneously turn his own body, not just the woman so that they end facing the same direction. The left arm relaxes slightly and the left hand sometimes gives the lead for steps in the open position.

LEAD: To lead from open to closed position, the man should use pressure of the right hand and raise the right arm up to standard position to move the woman into closed position. She should not have to be pushed but should swing easily into closed position as she feels the arm lifting. She should move completely around to face the man squarely.

NOTE: It is possible to go into this step when the man is facing out so that the cross step may travel into the line of direction.

■ TWINKLE STEP

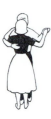

(Closed position)

This is a slow quick quick rhythm using right and left parallel positions, led from the forward sequence of the box pattern.

STEPS	4/4 COUNTS	RHYTHM CUE
Step L forward	1–2	slow
Step R sideward	3	quick
Close L to R, take weight on L	4	quick
Step R diagonally forward in R parallel position	1–2	slow
Step L sideward, turning from R parallel to L parallel position	3	quick
Close R to L, take weight on R	4	quick
Step L diagonally forward in L parallel position	1–2	slow
Step sideward R, turning from L parallel to R parallel position	3	quick
Close L to R, take weight on L	4	quick
Step R diagonally forward in R parallel position	1–2	slow
Step L sideward turning to closed position	3	quick
Close R to L take weight on R	4	quick

STEP CUE: Slow quick quick.

STYLE: The quick steps are small. Changing from one parallel position to the other is done in a very smooth rolling manner. The woman needs lots of practice alone to learn the back side close pattern because it is on the diagonal backward parallel to the man.

LEAD: To lead into right parallel position the man should not use pressure of his right hand, but rather should raise his right arm rotating the woman counterclockwise one-eighth of a turn while he rotates counterclockwise one-eighth of a turn. This places the man and woman off to the side of each other facing opposite directions. The woman is to the right of the man but slightly in front of him. The man should avoid turning too far so as to be side by side as this results in poor style and awkward and uncomfortable motion. The man's left hand may assist the lead by pulling toward his left shoulder.

LEAD: To lead from right parallel position to left parallel position, the man should pull with his right hand lowering the right arm and push slightly with his left hand causing a rotation clockwise about a quarter of a turn until the woman is to the left of him but slightly in front of him. They are not side by side.

NOTE: Progress is a zigzag pattern down the floor. The parallel part of the steps may be repeated as many times as desired before going back to closed position.

Fundamental Foxtrot Steps (continued)

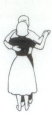

◾ GRAPEVINE STEP

(Closed position)

It is a beautiful pattern in slow quick quick time with four quick steps added to make the grapevine design, using parallel position.

STEPS	4/4 COUNTS	RHYTHM CUE
Step L forward	1–2	slow
Step R sideward, turning into R parallel position	3	quick
Close L to R, take weight on L	4	quick
Step R diagonally forward in R parallel position	1	quick
Step L sideward, turning to L parallel position	2	quick
Step R diagonally backward in L parallel position	3	quick
Step L sideward, turning to R parallel position	4	quick
Step R forward in R parallel position	1–2	slow
Step L sideward turning to closed position	3	quick
Close R to L, take weight on R	4	quick

STEP CUE: slow quick quick   quick quick quick quick   slow quick quick

forward sequence   grapevine pattern   transition back to
of box   closed position

STYLE: Practice on the grapevine step alone will help dancers get this pattern smoothly and beautifully. Cue man: forward side back side (R, L, R, L) on the grapevine step. Cue woman: back side forward side (L, R, L, R) on the grapevine step.

LEAD: To lead into right parallel position the man should not use pressure of his right hand, but rather should raise his right arm rotating the woman counterclockwise one–eighth of a turn while he rotates counterclockwise one–eighth of a turn. This places the man and woman off to the side of each other facing opposite directions. The woman is to the right of the man but slightly in front of him. The man should avoid turning too far so as to be side by side as this results in poor style and awkward and uncomfortable motion. The man's left hand may assist the lead by pulling toward his left shoulder.

LEAD: To lead from right parallel position to left parallel position, the man should pull with his right hand lowering the right arm and push slightly with his left hand causing a rotation clockwise about a quarter of a turn until the woman is to the left of him but slightly in front of him. They are not side by side.

LEAD: The lead is from the forward sequence of the box.

NOTE: The man should maneuver to face out before he starts this step so that the grapevine step may travel in the line of direction. He may maneuver into this by use of a three–quarter turn or a hesitation step.

◾ The Pivot Turn

The continuous pivot turn is a series of steps turning clockwise as many beats as desired. The man should be careful that he has room to turn, as the pivot turn pro–gresses forward in the line of direction if done properly, and he should not turn so many steps as to make his partner dizzy. The principle involved in the footwork is the dovetailing of the feet, which means that the right foot always steps between partner's feet and the left foot always steps around the outside of partner's feet. The pivot turn described here has two slow beats as a preparation followed by four quick beats turn–ing and comes out of it into the box step.

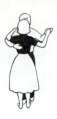

■ THE PIVOT TURN

(Closed position)

STEPS	4/4 COUNTS	RHYTHM CUE
Step L forward	1–2	slow
Step R forward, starting to turn the body clockwise increasing the body tension	3–4	slow
Step L, toeing in across the line of direction and rolling clockwise three-quarters of the way around on the ball of the L foot	1	quick
Step R, between partner's feet forward in the line of direction, completing one turn	2	quick
Step L, toeing in and reaching forward but across the line of direction, turning clockwise three-quarters as before	3	quick
Step R, between partner's feet forward in the line of direction, completing the second turn	4	quick
Step L forward in the line of direction, not turning but controlling momentum	1–2	slow
Step R sideward	3	quick
Close L to R, take weight on L	4	quick
Step R backward	1–2	slow
Step L sideward	3	quick
Close R to L, taking weight R	4	quick

STEP CUE: Step ready
    S   S
    turn turn turn turn
    Q Q Q Q
    forward side close
      S   Q   Q
    back side close
     S   Q Q

slow quick quick
L   R   L

quick R

quick L

quick R

quick L

slow R

slow L

start

LOD

THE WOMAN: On the second slow beat, the woman receives the lead as the man increases body tension. She does the same. Then, on the first quick beat, she has been turned far enough to place her right foot forward in between his feet on the line of direction, left foot across the line of direction, right foot between, left across, and into the box step.

STYLE: They both must lean away, pressing outward like "the water trying to stay in the bucket." The concept of stepping each time in relation to the line of direction is what makes it possible to progress while turning as a true pivot turn should do.

Fundamental Foxtrot Steps (continued)

LEAD: To lead all turns, the man dips his shoulder in the direction of the turn and his upper torso turns before his leg and foot turn.

LEAD: To lead into a pivot turn clockwise, the man should hold the woman slightly closer, but with sudden body tension. Resistance is exerted outward by both man and woman leaning away from each other to take advantage of the centrifugal force of the circular motion. The right foot steps between partner's feet, forward on line of direction, while the left foot reaches across the line of direction and turns on the ball of the foot about three-quarters of the way around.

FOXTROT COMBOS

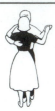

The Foxtrot routines are listed here merely as examples to show how the various steps can be used in combination for practice routines. They are listed from simple to complex. (Closed position, unless otherwise indicated.)

1. *Dance Walk*
   4 dance walk forward
   4 dance walk backward
   4 dance walk forward
   4 dance walk, travel left
   in a circle
2. *Dance Walk*
   4 dance walk forward
   2 pen magic step
   conversation pivot

3. *Magic Step*
   2 magic steps
   2 open magic steps
   conversation pivot
4. *Magic Step—Box*
   2 magic steps
   1 box step
   2 magic steps (open)

5. *Magic Step/Corté*
   1 magic step (open or closed)
   corté (recover)
   1 side close
   1 box turn
   corté (recover)
6. *Advanced Combo*
   1 magic step
   1 single twinkle to open
   1 single twinkle to left parallel
   1 single twinkle to open
   1 single twinkle to close

Disco Dance

DISCO STANDS TO THE SEVENTIES as Rock stood to the sixties. *Disco* comes from the word *discotheque*, which in France is a place where records and disques are stored. In the United States, a discotheque is a place where records are played and one can listen or dance to rock music. Disco Dance has become a descriptive term that encompasses a wide variety of dance steps to many musical rhythms. Originally the partners did not touch and the patterns were simple, characterized by (1) stationary base, (2) response to a steady beat—predominantly 4/4 time, (3) action in the upper torso (this is styling of hands and movement of body above the hips), and (4) not following the lead of a partner.

What began as fury and inspiration became fashion. How to keep the momentum going became a major concern as record sales declined and disco attendance dropped. Two events occurred that increased the desire of the whole nation for dance. Studio 54 in New York City proved that a discotheque could work on a grand scale. People wanted an opportunity to exhibit themselves. Gone were the glitter balls; they were replaced by video screens with computer graphics. The disc jockey continued to be in the driver's seat. The dance floor was more spacious. The music and the atmosphere for overstimulation was shared with a profusion of lights, sound, rhythm, and spectacles that could be interpreted as the formula for "pleasure and high times."

The other event was the movie *Saturday Night Fever*. John Travolta strutted and presented a virile young man's need to be assertive, seeking a stage on which to perform.

"Touch dancing" was the new phrase for holding one's partner. The Hustle is credited with bringing people together again on the dance floor. One of the common tunes for dancing was "Feelings"–the dance included body contact, dancing in one spot, responding to the music, and a 4/4 rhythm.

Clubs reopened and new ones arrived to meet the new disco interest. With the Hustle, partners touching once again, the dance studios were back in business. Many of the old forms, like the Lindy and the Latin Dances, and the closed dance position or variations, reappeared. Disco in the '90s refers to dance. The music is rock or a blend of soul, reggae, and disco–an irresistible mix of sounds. The music may be live or recorded.

Disco Swing

DISCO SWING FOLLOWS the syncopated rhythm of rock and roll. Many are dancing 4–count swing (even rhythm, Single Lindy) or 6–count swing (uneven rhythm, the Double Lindy). The dance is smoother and glides more like Country Western than Jitterbug. The turns are the same as Swing, but perhaps with different names. The approach to Disco Swing is more casual as the dancers explore one move after another; the feet pause or ignore the step pattern while turns or twirls are in progress; when the maneuvers are completed, the dancers pick up the beat and resume the step pattern. In the discos, with today's social climate and the advent of assertive feminism, it is acceptable for the woman to lead the moves.

Whoever knows the leads, leads. The leads may be pressure from the hands, or eye or verbal contact. Refers to Swing for 6–counts (Double Time Swing) pp. 399–400. Follow the directions for the many turns of the Double Time Swing.

Hustle with Partner

THE PARTNER HUSTLE WAS popular during the "Disco" dance era, (the late '70s). In the mid '90s, the partner hustle resurfaced as part of several "night club" dance styles. Music, ranging from 160–190 B.P.M., may be used. There is also a Hustle line dance, the California Hustle p. 447.

4/4	rock	step	step	____		step	____
	___	___	___	___		___	___
	1	2	3	4		1	2

Directions are for the man; the woman's part is reversed, except when noted.

Basic Step, Clockwise

(Two Hands joined, man's hands palm up)

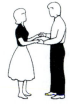

	4/4 COUNTS	RHYTHM CUE	STEP CUE
Step L backward, a little behind R heel	1	quick	rock
Step R in place	+	quick	step
Step forward L, pivots clockwise 180°	2	slow	step forward
Step back R	3	slow	step back

NOTE: Four basics step equals three measures of music.

STYLE: Keep steps small

LEAD: The man pulls down with both hands on count 2, to initiate the partner turn.

STYLE: The forward and back steps are almost in a straight line. The style is very smooth, be careful not to bounce with the "rock step."

Social Basic Step, Counter Clockwise

(Semiopen position with women at right angle to partner, man left hand lowered. Man is pointing left foot to side, women is pointing right foot forward)

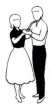

	4/4 COUNTS	RHYTHMIC CUE	STEP CUE
Man's Part			
Step L side	1	quick	side
Step R in place	+	quick	check
Step forward L, crossing in front of right, pivot counter-clockwise 90°	2	slow	cross
Step back R, pivoting counter-clockwise 90°	3	slow	back

NOTE: On count 2, the man's crossing step is placed in between the women's feet. He follows her around.

Women's Part

Step R back, next to left	1	quick	together
Step L forward, pivot counter-clockwise 90°	+	quick	forward
Step R side, pivot counter-clockwise 90°	2	slow	side
Step L back	3	slow	back

COMBINATION OF BASIC STEPS

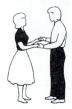

The couple moves from *social swing position* to *two hands joined position*, than back to *social*.

HUSTLE VARIATIONS

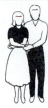

Many of the swing moves are used in the Partner Hustle. Refer to Single Time Swing.

Charleston

THE ROARING TWENTIES SAW the advent of Dixieland jazz and the *Charleston*. Definitely a fad dance, the Charleston comes and goes, only to reappear again. The dance, with its fancy footwork and carefree abandon, is a challenge to young and old. Black dock workers of Charleston, South Carolina, are credited with performing the dance steps eventually referred to as the Charleston. In 1923, the Ziegfeld Follies popularized the step in a show called "Running Wild." Teachers toned the kicking steps down and interspersed them with the Two–Step and Foxtrot, and the United States had a new popular dance. The *Varsity Drag* was one of many dances that incorporated the basic Charleston step. The dance permitted individuals to express their ability with many Charleston variations, independent of their partner.

Charleston (continued)

CHARLESTON RHYTHM

The Charleston rhythm is written in 4/4 time. The bouncy quality of the music occurs in the shift of accent, becoming highly syncopated rhythm.

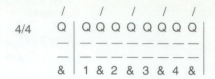

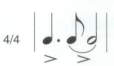

The rhythm is an even beat pattern of quicks counted "*and* 1, *and* 2, *and and* 3, *and* 4." The knee bends on the *and* before the step. It is the *and* that gives the Charleston its characteristic bounce. Rhythmically, the beats are:

The accent shifts from the first beat to the eighth note tied to the third beat, which gives punch to the rhythm. The rhythm is jerky, staccato, and syncopated.

CHARLESTON STYLE

The twisting of the feet and the bending of the knees before each step, then the straightening of the leg, are basic. The arms move in opposition to the feet: For example, step left, point right and swing both arms across to the left, step right, point left, and swing arms across right. The Charleston may be danced as a solo; in a line with a group; or with a partner, side by side, on the same foot, or facing each other, hands joined or closed position.

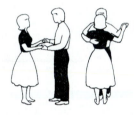

■ *Charleston with Partner*

Partners may be side by side, on the same foot or facing each other, hands joined or closed position. The lead is visual. The man starts with his L, woman R. Any step changes start with man's L. Man and woman stop together.

TEACHING SUGGESTIONS

1. Practice rhythm first. Feet slightly apart and parallel, bend knees (*and*), straighten legs (count 1). Repeat the action of "*and* 1, *and* 2, *and* 3, *and* 4." Then add the music.

2. Practice pivot on balls of feet. Heels out (*and*), heels in (count 1). Repeat.

3. *Charleston Twist.* Combine **1** and **2**. Bend knees and heels out (*and*), straighten legs and heels in (count 1). Repeat.

4. Add arm movement, swinging arms in opposition to feet. Swinging arms helps to maintain balance.

5. If balance and timing are difficult, try sitting on the edge of a chair to establish the rhythm; then stand behind the chair, holding onto the back for support.

6. Teach all figures in place. Then move forward and backward. Practice without music, slowly. If record player has a variable speed, introduce music as soon as possible. Gradually increase tempo until the correct tempo is reached.

FUNDAMENTAL CHARLESTON STEPS

RECORD: "The Golden Age of the Charleston," EMI Records LTD., GX 2507; or any good recording of the 1920s.

FORMATION: Free formation, all facing music.

■ POINT STEP

(Feet together, weight on R)

STEPS	4/4 COUNTS	DIRECTION CUE
Bend R knee	and	and
Step forward L	1	step forward
Bend L knee	and	and
Point R toe forward, straighten knees	2	point forward
Bend L knee	and	and
Step back R	3	step back
Bend R knee	and	and
Point L toe back, straighten knees	4	point forward

ARMS: Swing arms in opposition to legs. R toe forward, L arm swings forward, R arm swings back; L toe forward, R arm swings forward, L arm swings back.

■ SINGLE KICK STEP

(Feet together, weight on R)

STEPS	4/4 COUNTS	DIRECTION CUE
Bend R knee	and	and
Step forward L	1	step forward
Bend L knee	and	and
Kick R leg forward, straighten knees	2	kick forward
Bend L knee	and	and
Step back R	3	step back
Bend R knee	and	and
Kick L leg back	4	kick back
Straighten knees	and	and

ARMS: Swing arms in opposition to the kick. Kick R leg forward, L arm swings forward, R arm swings back; kick L leg forward, R arm swings forward, L arm swings back.

■ *Variations*

1. *Double Kick.* Step forward left; kick right forward, then backward; step right in place. Repeat kicking left forward, then backward; step left.
2. *Single Diagonal Kick.* Step sideward left, kick diagonally forward across left leg, step sideward right, kick diagonally forward across right leg.

■ THE CHARLESTON TWIST

(Weight on the balls of both feet, heels touching, toes pointing out)

1. The twist comes from pivoting on balls of feet, heels turned out, then pivoting on balls of feet, heels turned in. Heels are slightly off the floor to allow the pivot action.

STEPS	4/4 COUNTS	DIRECTION CUE
Bend knees, pivot in on balls of feet	and	heels out
Pivot out, straighten knees	1	heels in
Repeat over and over.		

Charleston (continued)

2. Twist and snap (heels touching, toes pointing out, weight on R).

STEPS	4/4 COUNTS	DIRECTION CUE
Bend R knee, pivot in on ball of foot, lifting L leg up, knee turned in	*and*	heel out
Pivot out on ball of R foot; straighten knees; place L foot by heel of R, toe pointed out; L takes weight	1	heel in
Bend L knee; pivot in on ball of foot, lifting L leg up, knee turned in	*and*	heel out
Pivot out on ball of L foot, straighten knees, place R foot by heel of L, toe pointed out; R takes weight	2	heel in

■ JUMP

STEPS	4/4 COUNTS	DIRECTION CUE
Bend both knees together	*and*	bend
Jump forward diagonally L, both arms swing L, shoulder height	1	jump
Bend both knees	*and*	bend
Jump back, both arms swing down	2	jump
Repeat jump and arms forward and back	*and* 1 *and* 2	
Bend both knees together	*and*	
Jump forward diagonally R, both arms swing R, shoulder height	1	jump
Bend both knees together	*and*	
Jump back, both arms swing down	2	jump
Repeat jump and arms forward and back	*and* 1 *and* 2	jump jump
Alternately jump L R L R, arms swing L R L R	*and* 1 *and* 2	jump

■ SWIVEL

Weight on heel, pivot toes R (count *and*); weight on toes, pivot heels R (count 1). Continue to move R, heel, toe, heel, toe. Arms swing L and down, repeating with heel, toe. Travel on counts *and* 1 *and* 2. Reverse movement to travel L.

■ SUZY Q

Pivoting on L heel and R toe simultaneously (count *and*), then pivoting on L toe and R heel simultaneously (count 1). Continue alternating, traveling R. Hands in front of chest, elbows out as heels are apart; drop elbows as toes are apart; alternate elbows out and dropped with foot movement. Reverse footwork to travel L.

■ TWELFTH STREET RAG

Composed Charleston Dance p. 116.

Swing (Jitterbug)

SWING IS AN UMBRELLA TERM for a wide variety of dance, such as West Coast Swing, East Coast Swing, Jive, Jitterbug, Shag, and Lindy Hop. With the advent of Dixieland jazz during the Roaring Twenties, a variety of dances appeared, including the *Lindbergh Hop.* Cab Calloway is credited with referring to the Lindy hoppers as "jitterbuggers." The dance went through a fad period of being extremely eccentric with its wild acrobatics inspired by the rising popularity of boogie woogie. The Big Apple, the Shag, and the Swing were all products of that period. They changed after World War II to a more syncopated rhythm called rock and roll with the Double Time Swing pattern and to the Swing with the smooth, sophisticated triple rhythm, which came in a short time later. All during the Rock period, both Double and Triple Time Swing could be seen on American Bandstand. A softer sound called boogie, but no relation to boogie woogie, has greater synthesization of electronic equipment.

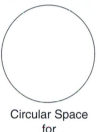

Circular Space
for
Swing Dance

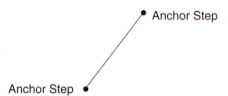

Anchor Step

Anchor Step

Narrow Space
for
West Coast Swing Dance

Swing is danced to a wide variety of music and reflects the dance style of the particular music–Big Band music of the '40s, rock and roll, rhythm and blues, Salsa, Reggae, Country Western, and Cajun–all written in 4/4 or cut time. Swing includes the rhythm of Lindy Hop, Single Time, Double Time, and Triple Time. Some refer to these as Jitterbug. The term *Swing* is also applied to myriad of figures as the couple covers a *circular space* in one area. There is wide variation in the footwork and figures.

East Coast Swing and *Triple Time* are synonymous. *West Coast Swing* is a more difficult and sophisticated dance. West Coast Swing is referred to as a *slot dance* because the couple moves back and forth in a narrow space, always the same space. The dance evolved in the '50s on the West Coast in the small clubs where dance space was limited.

We will continue to use the term *Swing* for Single, Double, and Triple Time Swing. Circular Space for Swing Dance Narrow Space for West Coast Swing Dance

SWING RHYTHM

Swing is written in 4/4 or cut time. It is extremely adaptable to fast or slow rhythm or to 4/4 time from Foxtrot to hard rock in quality. The Shag was actually the first dance to be called Jitterbug, and its slow slow quick quick rhythm set the pattern for all of the others. The Single Time Swing has the same rhythm.

Swing (Jitterbug) (continued)

It was not really in use much in recent years. It is shown here to demonstrate the transition into the more active Swing patterns.

4/4	/ step	step	/ rock	step
	S	S	Q	Q
	1	2 3	4 1	2

uneven rhythm

Single Time

Double Time is very adaptable to slow or fast music. This style was very popular in the '50s. Accent is on the offbeat.

4/4	dig	/ step	dig	/ step	rock	/ step
	Q	Q	Q	Q	Q	Q
	1	2	3	4	1	2

even rhythm

Double Time

Triple Time is more often danced to the slow, mellow, sophisticated tempos.

4/4	/ step	close	step	step	close	step	/ rock	step
	Q	Q	S	Q	Q	S	S	S
	1	and	2	3	and	4	1	2

triple   triple

uneven rhythm

Triple Time—East Coast Swing

SWING STYLE

Exciting styles and positions are in use for Swing. It is a matter of taste for the individual dancers whether they use a dig step, a step–hop, or a kick step. However, the basic rhythm must be maintained by both man and woman to coordinate the pattern together, unlike Discotheque (dancing apart), in which the step or rhythm pattern of each partner is unstructured. The man is able to lead the dance because of the magnificent body alertness of both partners. A firm body and tone in the arm and fingers enable quick response in any direction. The space between partners is controlled by a spring tension in the elbow, which never extends fully but allows the pull away and the spring back smoothly and with control. The woman uses her arm as a pivot center. The elbow is down and the hand is up for the underarm turns, and she turns around her arm but does not let it fly in the air. There should never be the appearance of arms flying loose or entangled. The fingers slip easily around one another without losing contact. Even the free arm is bent and remains close to the body.

Swing steps tend to cover a circular space in one area of the floor. The footwork is at all times small and close together, with rolling and turning on the ball of the foot. The turning action for beginner steps is always on the first step (count 2) of the pattern when the woman is on her right foot and the man is on his left. The rhythm pattern is generally the same over and over but the changes of position and direction and the constant subtle smooth roll to offbeat rhythm generates a fabulous excitement for both dancer and observer.

WEST COAST SWING RHYTHM

West Coast Swing Rhythm is 6 or 8 beats. It is a slower rhythm than East Coast Swing (120–130 B.P.M.).

All Uneven Rhythm

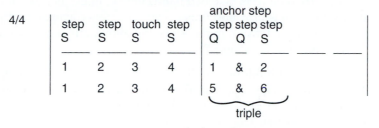

uneven rhythm—6 count

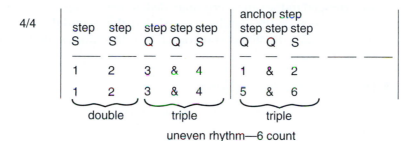

uneven rhythm—6 count

uneven rhythm—8 count

FUNDAMENTAL SWING STEPS

Directions are for the man; the woman's part is reversed, except when noted.

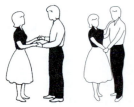

- **DOUBLE TIME SWING**

(Beginners–two hands joined; experienced–social swing position)

STEPS	4/4 COUNTS	RHYTHM CUE
Touch L to instep of R	1	quick
Step L in place	2	quick
Touch R to instep of L	3	quick
Step R in place	4	quick
Step L backward, a little behind R heel	1	quick
Step R forward	2	quick

Swing (Jitterbug) (continued)

STEP CUE: Dig step, dig step, rock step.

STYLE: The body takes a *slight* motion, tipping forward from the waist and dipping the outside shoulder (man's L, woman's R) on the first dig step like an upbeat. Take care not to exaggerate this motion. It is very subtle. The dig is a touching of the toe lightly to the instep of the other foot. It should not be a tap step that makes noise on the floor. The feet are close together for this beat. The weight is carried on the ball of the foot and the steps are small throughout the step. The amount of knee bend depends on individual preference as to style; however, the action should be smooth and rolling rather than bouncy.

NOTE: Beginners must learn this pattern alone until they can move accurately with the rhythm. Then dancers take two hands joined, man's hands palm up. The elbow is down, forearm is firm, and fingers exert resistance against partner's. On the rock step there is a spring tension in the arms that allows an "apart–together" action that is smooth and has arm control.

LEAD: The man holds both of their hands close together and dips slightly with his left shoulder on the first dig step. The woman pushes slightly against his hands on the first dig step so as to receive his lead. This technique teaches the woman to give the necessary resistance for all future leads.

NOTE: The above progression provides instant success with Swing. The variations listed are arranged in the order recommended. In describing the variations, the analysis will refer to action on the first dig, the first step, the second dig, the second step, the rock step or the first dig step, second dig step, or the entire pattern, rather than by counts as in other dances.

■ *Double Time Variations*

All Double Time swing moves may be danced in single time rhythm by taking out the dig steps.

Collegiate	Swing Out Break	Wrap
Break to Semiopen Position	Continuous Underarm Turns	Double Brush Off
Semiopen Basic	Brush Off	Dish Rag
Basic Turn	Tuck Spin	Overhead Swing

■ COLLEGIATE (TURNING BASIC)

(Two hands joined, man's hands palm up)

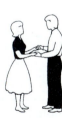

STEPS	STEP CUE
Man brings both hands close together and dips the left shoulder	first dig
Man steps L forward close to the L of the woman, pivots clockwise at close range on the L foot	first step
Woman steps R diagonally forward across to the R of the man at close range and pivots clockwise on the R foot	first step
Both take dig and step in place	second dig step
Both rock out and in using arm control	rock step

STEP CUE: Dig turn, dig in place, rock step.

STYLE: Resistance in the arms and fingers hold the couple in a tight, close–facing position on the pivot turn. Each needs to step in close to partner on the pivot foot (man's L woman's R). The steps are small.

LEAD: The man can help the woman pivot by the pull of his hands and body. He dips the left shoulder on the first dig to give her the cue for this turn. When used in combination with other variations, the man will take or release hands on the rock steps. (a) An optional lead is to reach sideways with each hand shoulder high on the first step and bring the hands back together on the second step. This creates a butterfly turn effect. (b) A second optional and more advanced lead is the man may pivot to right parallel position on the first dig and to left parallel on the first step. It is a quick change of position like a cock turn and is led by a push and pull action in the hands. The second dig step and rock step are the same as before.

■ BREAK TO SEMIOPEN POSITION

(Two hands joined)

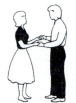

STEPS	STEP CUE
Dig in place, the man preparing to pull the woman toward him	first dig
Man and woman step toward each other, the man pulling the L hand downward and placing R arm around her waist	first step
Both take dig step, pivoting to semiopen position	second dig
Both step backward a short step in semiopen position	second step
Rock step in same position	rock step

STEP CUE: Pull down, come together, rock step.

STYLE: The steps are small.

LEAD: The man pulls down on her hand so that, as they come into semiopen position, the man's left hand holding the woman's right hand ends up in the correct position for basic.

■ SEMIOPEN BASIC

(Social Swing position)

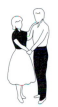

STEPS	STEP CUE
Dig in place, L to instep of R	first dig
Step forward a short step L	first step
Dig R to instep of L	second dig
Step backward a short step R	second step
Rock step	rock step

STEP CUE: Dig step, dig step, rock step.

STYLE: Dancers remain in social swing position throughout. All steps are small. The hand grasp is low with a straight elbow and held in close to the body. The man's fingers reach around the little-finger side of the woman's hand.

■ BASIC TURN

(Social Swing position)

The basic turn is used in social swing position as previously described. When repeated over and over, it should be done turning the couple around in place clockwise. The man makes the step turn by taking the first step with his left foot on a clockwise curve toward the woman and pivoting about a quarter-turn on the ball of the left foot. He finishes the remainder of the pattern from that new direction. Repeat as desired. As the dancers become skillful at this turn they will find they can turn a half-turn or more each time by pivoting a greater degree on the stepping beat.

STEP CUE: Dig turn, dig-step, rock step.

STYLE: The woman will have no trouble adjusting to this turning action. She will roll on the ball of her foot.

LEAD: A dip of the man's left shoulder and a slight pull of his right arm around her waist take her along easily into the turn.

Swing (Jitterbug) (continued)

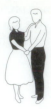

■ SWING OUT BREAK (ARCH OUT)

(Social Swing position)

The man takes the entire pattern in place once as he turns the woman out under his left arm to face him.

STEPS	STEP CUE
Man moves his L hand from the low position to a position in close at waist level	first dig
Man raises his L hand above her head and turns her under to face him.	first step
Woman on R foot pivots clockwise halfway around to face him	
Both take a dig step in place facing partner	second dig step
Both rock away and together using elbow control	rock step

STEP CUE: Dig turn, dig step, rock step.

STYLE: Woman keeps the R elbow level with shoulder and forearm at right angles, and turns around her own arm, not under it. His arm is high enough so that she does not have to duck to get under. The woman's pivot step is short so that they do not get too far apart. They must have room to take the rock step with elbow control.

LEAD: The man leads the starting motion by bending his left elbow to bring his hand in to waist level on the first dig. This cues the woman. She is waiting with her right foot in dig position and with the lead she can step with him into the first step. His arm must be raised high enough on the first step to clear her head as she turns under.

NOTE: The face-to-face position is called swing out position–dancers will have one hand joined (man's L, woman's R). The man should bring her back to position by using the break to social swing position.

■ CONTINUOUS UNDERARM TURNS (INSIDE TURN)

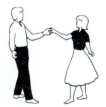

(Swing out position)

The man and woman exchange places as he turns her counterclockwise across to his position and steps around her to her position.

STEPS	STEP CUE
Man increases pressure on woman's hand	first dig
Both man and woman take a short step forward. Man turns clockwise on his L foot while turning woman under counterclockwise on her R foot	first step
Take dig and step in place	second dig step
Rock step out and in, controlling with firm arm	rock step

STEP CUE: Dig turn, dig step, rock step.

STYLE: Both turn halfway around on the first step but stay in close so that there is room for the remainder of the basic step. They have exactly exchanged places after one complete pattern.

LEAD: The man turns his hand knuckles up, fingers down, so that the woman's fingers can slip around his fingers as she turns. Then he brings his hand down palm up.

NOTE: This underarm turn can be repeated over and over. It will serve as a connecting step to any other variation. The man may lead back to social swing or reach for the woman's other hand for any of the two-hands-joined variations that follow.

■ BRUSH OFF (WALK THROUGH)

(Also called flirtation pass) (Swing out position)

This step begins with the woman in swing out position after one underarm turn, leaving the man's hand in palm–up position. It is basically a man's left turn.

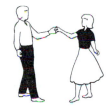

STEPS	STEP CUE
Take dig in place	first dig
Man steps forward toward L side of the woman, shifting her R hand into his R hand, while he turns counterclockwise one-quarter on his L foot until his back is to the woman. She steps diagonally forward, pivoting on her R foot clockwise as in the collegiate and moving around behind the man.	first step
Take dig in place, continuing to turn	second dig
Man brings both of his hands behind his back. He steps on the right foot, turning counterclockwise one-quarter more to face the woman, and changes her R hand into his L hand. The woman steps on the L foot, turning clockwise to face the man	second step
Rock step out and in, using arm control	rock step

STEP CUE: Man turns and turns rock step.

STYLE: While doing this pattern, the couple have exchanged places, each turning a half-turn. The woman can control the space factor because she can stay in close to him as she goes around him.

LEAD: The transfer of hands should be done smoothly and without losing contact.

NOTE: It is especially fun to follow the brush off with an underarm turn. The man should be prepared to lead into it immediately after the rock step.

■ TUCK SPIN

(Swing out position)

STEPS	STEP CUE
Man moves both of woman's hands to his R (woman turns slightly to her L), pulls woman toward himself in a sharp action	first dig
Man steps in place, releasing her hands; he pushes her in the opposite direction with a quick flip, spinning her clockwise once around on her R foot	first step
Woman catches her balance with the digging foot, man resumes joined-hand position	second dig
They step in place together	second step
Rock step out and in	rock step

STEP CUE: Tuck spin, dig step, rock step.

STYLE: The woman must spin smoothly a full–turn around in place on right foot without losing her balance.

LEAD: There must be firm arm and finger control for the woman to respond to this with the proper timing. Woman offers arm resistance. Man catches her left hand in his left, then changes to swing out position.

NOTE: The man may also spin at the same time. His turn will go counterclockwise on the left foot.

Swing (Jitterbug) (continued)

■ WRAP (CUDDLE)

(Two hands joined)

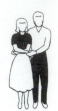

STEPS	STEP CUE
Take dig, man lifts his L arm and prepares to turn the woman counterclockwise	first dig
Step forward a short step, and, without releasing hands, the man will move his raised L hand across in front of her and up over her head as she is turning counterclockwise one-quarter on her R foot	first step
Dig in place still turning.	second dig
Step backward, as the woman finishes in a position close to him on his R side. His R arm is around her waist and her arms are crossed in front as they finish in the wrap position (his R joins her L)	second step
Rock step back and forward together	rock step

STYLE: A smooth roll is important.

NOTE: To unwrap, the man initiates a reverse roll, turning the woman clockwise back to starting position and assisting with a gentle right–arm push. Another variation on the unwrap is for the man to release with his left hand and pull with the right hand, rolling the woman out to his right. Again this should be taken on the two dig steps and they finish off with the rock in face–to–face position.

■ DOUBLE BRUSH OFF

(Swing out position)

The couple must know how to do a single brush–off step. The double brush–off step is twice through the rhythm pattern. Starting position is swing out position (man's L, woman's R hand joined).

First time through the rhythm pattern (dig step, dig step, rock step):

STEPS	STEP CUE
Man starts first brush–off step, turning L one-half, woman steps forward slightly	first dig step
He reaches out palm up with his L hand to take her L hand, they are side by side, the woman on the L; the woman's step is in place	second dig step
The man releases her R hand behind his back and reaches around in front under their L hand to take her R hand	rock step

Second time through the rhythm pattern (dig step, dig step, rock step):

STEPS	STEP CUE
Man raises L hand, pulling the woman under with the R and turning her counterclockwise as both hands go up over her head	first dig step
He releases the L hand, as he begins to turn his second brush off, turning counterclockwise as his R arm comes down behind his back	second dig step
He changes her R hand into his L as he finishes his turn to face the woman	rock step

STYLE: This must have the look of a complete flowing action. The woman must stay in close to the man. Both must keep the dig step, dig step, rock step pattern going in their feet. Steps are small.

LEAD: The most important lead is when the man reaches out palm up to take her left hand. The second lead is when he pulls with the right hand and both hands go over her head.

Swing (Jitterbug) (continued)

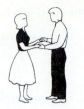

- **DISH RAG**

(Two hands joined)

The couple rolls to the man's left, woman's right, turning back to back and rolling on around face to face. They must keep the footwork of the Double Time Swing going. It is one complete pattern.

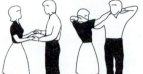

- **OVERHEAD SWING (OCTOPUS)**

(Two hands joined) (octopus)

The couple steps forward right side to right side. Each swings the right arm over partner's head, behind the neck and slides the right hand down the right arm of partner to a right-hand grasp. The dancers must keep the basic footwork going. It is one complete pattern.

Triple Time–East Coast Swing

T RIPLE TIME IS LOVELY AND pleasant to do to a nice swingy Foxtrot. It should be smooth and relaxing.

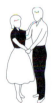

- **TRIPLE RHYTHM**

(Social Swing position) (Three little steps to each slow beat; these are similar to a fast Two–Step.)

STEPS	4/4 COUNTS	RHYTHM CUE
Step L forward		
Close R to L, take weight R	1 *and* 2	quick quick slow
Step L forward		
Step R backward		
Close L to R, take weight L	3 *and* 4	quick quick slow
Step R backward		
Rock Step		
Step L backward, a little behind R heel	1	slow
Step R in place	2	slow

STEP CUE: Triple step, triple step, rock step.

STYLE: The triple rhythm should be small shuffling steps, keeping the feet close to the floor. Weight is on the ball of the foot. Basic style is that of Double Time Swing.

LEAD: The man cues the woman for the triple steps by increasing the tension in his right hand as he starts the shuffle step forward. Other leads are the same as for the Double Time Swing.

NOTE: Any of the variations for Double Time Swing can be done in triple rhythm, and dancers frequently change from one rhythm to another during one piece of music.

Triple Time–East Coast Swing (continued)

▪ TRIPLE TIME SWIVEL STEP

(Social Swing position and traveling in line of direction, forward; rhythm pattern changes)

STEPS	4/4 COUNTS	RHYTHM CUE
Man's Part (woman's part is the reverse)		
Step L forward		
Close R to L	1 *and* 2	quick quick slow
Step L forward		
Step R forward		
Close L to R	3 *and* 4	quick quick slow
Step R forward		
Pivot on R foot to face partner, and bring L foot alongside of it, shifting weight to L foot	1	slow
Pivot on L foot to face open position, bring R foot alongside of it, shifting weight to R foot	2	slow
Repeat pivot on R foot	3	slow
Repeat pivot on L foot	4	slow
Step L forward		
Close R to L	1 *and* 2	quick quick slow
Step L forward		
Step R backward		
Close L to R	3 *and* 4	quick quick slow
Step R backward		
(turning woman out clockwise in an underarm turn)		
Rock step (in swing out position)	1, 2	slow slow

STEP CUE: Triple step, triple step
swivel 2 3 4
triple step, triple step, rock step.

STYLE: The swivel steps are tiny, crisp, and neatly turning, just a quarter turn on each pivot. The body turns with the foot closed, open, closed, open.

LEAD: The man must lead the swivel step by turning the woman from open to closed, and so forth.

NOTE: The couple progresses along the line of direction as the pivot turn is being done in four quick steps.

SWING COMBOS

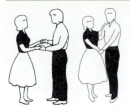

The Swing routines are combinations for practice, which are listed from simple to complex. They may be used for either Shag, Single Time, Double Time, or Triple Time. (Two hands joined or social swing position, unless otherwise indicated.)

1. *Basic Swing Out and Close*
   1   basic
   single underarm break
   break to original position
2. *Basic–Swing Out–Underarm Turn Close*
   1   basic
   single underarm break
   break to original position
3. *Swing Out and Collegiate*
   2   basics
   single underarm break
   3   collegiate steps
   underarm turn
   original position

4. *Swing Out and Brush Off*
   2   basics
   single underarm break
   brush off
   underarm turn
   original position
5. *Collegiate–Brush Off*
   2   basic
   single underarm break
   underarm turn
   3   collegiate steps
   underarm turn
   brush off
   underarm turn
   original position

6. *Collegiate–Tuck–Spin*
   2   collegiate steps
   tuck spin
   underarm turn
7. *Collegiate–Wrap*
   2   collegiate steps
   wrap
   unwrap
8. *Wrap–Unwrap Spin*
   2   collegiate steps
   wrap
   unwrap
   tuck spin
   underarm turn

West Coast Swing

■ WEST COAST SWING STYLE

The woman's step is different from the man's; partners do not mirror each other. The step is like the Cuban walk (p. 474). Little kicks and toe touches on the beat give flair for a sophisticated look. The anchor steps (quick, quick, slow) occur at the end of the slot. The couples move in a narrow space. Refer to West Coast Swing definition, diagram, p. 397 and West Coast Rhythm page 399.

■ SUGAR PUSH

(Basic step) (Two hands joined)

STEPS	COUNTS	STEP CUE
Man's Part		
Step back L	1	step
Step R to L	2	together
Touch L	3	touch
Step forward L	4	step
Step R behind L (hook) in place and release man's R, woman's L hand (swing out position)	5	hook
Step L in place, pushing off	*and*	step
Step R in place	6	step
Woman's Part		
Step forward R	1	step
Step forward L	2	step
Touch R to L instep	3	touch

West Coast Swing (continued)

Turning R towards partner, step back R (continue to travel in slot)	4	step
Step L behind R (hook) and release woman's L man's R hand	5	hook
Step R in place	*and*	step
Step L in place	6	step

STEP CUE: The cue "walk" may be used for counts 1, 2, 4.

STYLE: The footwork and hips are like the Cuban walk (refer to p. 474). Dig, pressing the foot into the floor while moving forward.

LEAD: The arms need to be firm (give weight) as the woman moves forward, the man pulling toward him. On count 3 the woman leans a little more forward, body rising to receive the *push*. On count 4 the man *pushes* as the woman moves backward. Both dancers must offer resistance. The man initiates the *pull* and *push*.

NOTE: The steps on counts 5 and 6 are the "anchor steps." The woman may choose to do a "coaster step" for counts 5 and 6. Coaster step is step back L, close R to L, step forward L.

VARIATION: Triple step. Counts 3, 4 become "3 and 4" (QQS). Instead of Touch Step, man steps LRL, woman steps RLR.

■ UNDERARM TURN

(Swing out position)

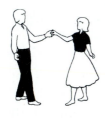

Woman passes the man's R side, turns under her arm to face opposite direction.

STEPS	COUNTS	STEP CUE
Man's Part		
Moving to L side, step L	1	step
Step forward R	2	step
Moving toward slot, step L, pivoting clockwise	3	side
Step R, still turning	*and*	step
Raising L arm, step L into the slot. Now facing opposite direction	4	step
Step R behind L	5	hook
Step L	*and*	step
Step R in place	6	step
Woman's Part		
Step forward R	1	step
Step forward L	2	step
Take 3 running steps (R, L, R) to the end of slot, turning counterclockwise under R arm, on count 4	3 *and* 4	run, run, turn
Step L behind R	5	hook
Step R	*and*	step
Step L in place	6	step

LEAD: Man pulls the woman forward, left hand down, raises arm for turn on count 4.

NOTE: Alternate one Sugar Push sequence with one Underarm Turn. Woman may use "coaster step" for counts 5 and 6.

■ LEFT SIDE PASS

(Swing out position)

Woman passes man's left side.

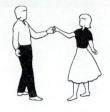

STEPS	COUNTS	STEP CUE
Man's Part		
Moving to R side, step L across R	1	step
Pivoting counterclockwise on L, step R near L (now facing slot)	2	step
Following woman, take 3 steps (L, R, L)	3 *and* 4	step, step, step
Facing opposite direction, step R behind L	5	hook
Step L	*and*	step
Step R in place	6	step
Woman's Part		
Step forward R	1	step
Step forward L	2	step
Passing partner (man's left side), traveling in the slot, take 3 short running steps (R, L, R) pivoting counterclockwise on last run	3 *and* 4	run, run, turn
Facing opposite direction, step L behind R	5	hook
Step R	*and*	step
Step L	6	step

NOTE: The Left Side Pass is usually preceded by one Sugar Push.

STYLE: Woman holds L arm, elbow bent, to chest as she passes partner and turns.

LEAD: On count 4 man drops L shoulder, pulls his L hand down as woman passes.

■ WHIP

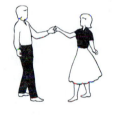

(Swing out position)

Starting in Swing out position, couple moves into closed position, makes one complete turn clockwise as a couple at the center of the slot, separates into Swing out position, and ends in original position.

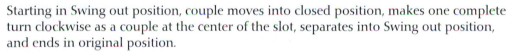

STEPS	COUNTS	STEP CUE
Man's Part		
Step back L	1	step
Moving to L side, step R across L and move into closed position	2	cross
Step L forward, pivoting clockwise as a couple	3	turn
Continuing to turn, step R in place	*and*	and
Step L across slot (L and R feet straddle slot)	4	step
Step R behind L (hook), continuing to turn as a couple	5	hook
Releasing man's R, woman's L hand and separating, step L forward into slot. Now facing original direction	6	step
Step R behind L, step L, step R in place	7 *and* 8	hook, step, step
Woman's Part		
Step forward R toward partner	1	step
Moving into closed position step L pivoting clockwise to face partner	2	pivot
Step back R	3	back
Close L to R	*and*	together
Step R forward between the man's two feet	4	step
Continuing to turn clockwise as a couple, step L	5	step
Release woman's L, man's R hand and step back R	6	step
Step L behind R, step R, step L in place	7 *and* 8	hook, step, step

NOTE: Woman's Part, counts 3 and 4, is a *coaster step*. It may be cued as "coaster step" (3 and 4) (QQS).

Lindy Hop

THE *LINDY HOP* EMERGED IN the late 1920s to a sound of a new style of music being played in Harlem. The African American jazz musicians of that day called this new rhythm "swinging the beat."* The music was swinging and so were the dancers. The name *Lindy Hop* came from a dancer named Shorty Snowden. During a dance marathon in the '20s, a reporter asked him what he was doing, and in honor of Charles Lindbergh's recent "hop" over the Atlantic, he said, "Lindy Hop." The Lindy Hop is considered the granddaddy of all the American swing forms.

The Lindy Hop incorporated many moves from a previous dance fad, the Charleston. Many other steps, often theatrical, were created for dance contests in Harlem. An example is *Air Steps*, or putting the women in the air with a flip.

The Lindy Hop's popularity was driven by many events of the day. Whitey's Lindy Hopper, a dance troupe from Harlem, toured the United States and Europe. Popular movies, such as *Day at the Races* and *Hellzapoppin*, included Lindy Hop dance scenes. These factors helped the Lindy Hop continue to gain popularity as it moved into middle class America. A *Life* magazine article in 1943, marking a high point of popularity, called the Lindy Hop "America's true Folk Dance." After World War II, the Lindy Hop's popularity declined.

In the Mid '80s, dancers from California (Erin Stevens and Steve Mitchell), Sweden (founding members of the Rhythm Hot Shots), and England (the Jiving Lindy Hoppers) went to New York seeking the guidance of some original Lindy Hoppers. These people wanted to learn more than what they had seen in old movies or magazines.** Frankie Manning, an original member of Whitey's Lindy Hoppers, had just started dancing again, after retiring from the post office. These dancers worked with Frankie and other original Lindy Hop dancers and used this new knowledge to revive the Lindy Hop.

More recently, the Lindy Hop has exploded onto the dance scene. Movies like *Swing Kids* and *Malcolm X* have Lindy Hop dance sequences. TV commercials are using the Lindy Hop (the most notable is the spring 1998 Gap Khaki "Swings" ad campaign). Bands are playing music in the style of the '30s and '40s swing bands (Big Bad Voodoo Daddy). The Lindy Hop revival is in full swing!

STYLE: Knees are bent and there is a constant gentle bounce throughout the movements. Bend over slightly from the waist. Women are slightly more upright than men. Self-expression is encouraged.

MUSIC: Normal tempo is 140–160 BPM

▪ FULL LINDY BASIC

(Swing Out–Lindy position)

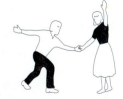

Starting in Swing Out–Lindy position, couple moves into closed position, makes one complete turn clockwise as a couple, and separates into Swing Out position.

STEPS	COUNTS	STEP CUE
Man's Part		
Step back L, bending slightly forward, look at partner. Leave R foot in place	1	rock
Step in place R	2	step

---

* Refer to: Michael Wagner, "Swing Dance," p. 8, *Viltis*, September/October 1997

** Personal communication from Erin Stevens

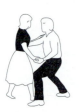

Steps	Counts	Step Cue
Pivoting one-quarter clockwise, step forward L	3	three
Right hand moves to social position		
pivoting one-eighth clockwise step R behind left (leave left foot in place)	*and*	and
pivoting one-eighth clockwise step left in place, left knee bent	4	four
Face Off Position		
Step R behind L (hook) in place, release right hand	5	hook
pivoting one-quarter clockwise on R, step side L on L	6	step
pivoting one-quarter clockwise on L, step back R	7	step
Step L in place	*and*	in
Step R in place	8	place

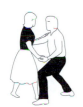

Woman's Part

Steps	Counts	Step Cue
		swivel
Step swivel R, wave left hand in the air	1	swivel
Step swivel L, wave left hand in the air	2	swivel
Step forward R	3	three
pivoting one-quarter clockwise, step side L with L (leave right foot in place)	*and*	and
pivoting one-quarter clockwise, step R in place	4	four
Face Off Position		
Pivoting one-quarter clockwise, step side L	5	run
Remove left hand from man's shoulder		
Step side L with R, crossing R in front	6	run
Step side L with L	7	step
Pivoting one-quarter clockwise, step R in place	*and*	in
Step L in place	8	place

STYLE: Always keep eye contact with partner. On counts 1 and 2, the man is mimicking "bowing down" to the woman. On Counts 1 and 2 the woman may vary her arm movement.

LEAD: On count "3 *and*," man leans forward with left shoulder. Man releases right hand on Count 5, allowing the woman to move away.

VARIATIONS: On counts 1 and 2, either the man or the women may change their footwork: for example, a heel drop or a kick away may be substituted. These variations are executed independent of the partner.

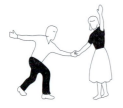

■ BASIC TO A JOCKEY

(Swing Out–Lindy position)

Starting in Swing Out–Lindy position, man makes one complete turn clockwise (women, one and a half), bringing the women to his right side, ending in the Jockey position.

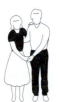

STEPS	COUNTS	STEP CUE
Repeat count 1–4 for Full Lindy Basic		
Man		
Step in place R. Do not release right arm as in the basic, with right arm, reach around to partner's right side, starting to bring her into the Jockey position.	5	

Lindy Hop (continued)

Pivoting one-half clockwise on R, Step side L	6
Step back R	7
Step L in place (next to R)	and
Step back R	8

Woman

Pivoting one-quarter clockwise on R, step side L	5
Pivoting one-quarter clockwise on L, step forward R	6
Pivoting one-quarter clockwise on R, step side L	7
Step R in place (next to L)	and
Pivoting one-quarter clockwise on R, step back L	8

■ LINDY CHARLESTON

(Jockey position)

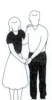

Direction are for the man. The women's footwork is reversed.

STEPS	COUNTS	STEP CUE
Step back L	1	rock
Step in place R	2	step
Kick L forward	3	kick
Step L	4	step
Kick R forward	5	kick
Swing R foot back to place	6	and
Kick R back	7	kick
Step R	8	step

NOTE: This step is usually repeated two to three times.

STYLE: Man releases his left hand, woman's right hand. Free arms swing forward and back during the Charleston footwork. A constant bounce is maintained during the step.

■ JOCKEY TO A SWING OUT

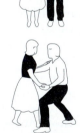

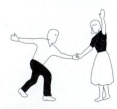

STEPS	COUNTS	STEP CUE
Man's Part		
Repeats the footwork of the basic	1–8	
Woman's		
Step back R	1	rock
Step in L	2	step
Step R forward	3	step
Step L together	and	together
Step R forward (now in face off position)	4	step
Repeat count 5–8 of Lindy Basic, ending in swing out–Lindy position	5–8	

LEAD: Man rejoins his left hand with woman's right hand on counts 7 and 8 of the previous measure. By Count 4, the man's right hand has returned to the middle of the woman's back.

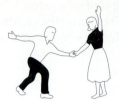

■ SHINE

(Swing Out–Lindy position)

Man stays in place, bringing his knees together and apart as the women swivel steps clockwise around him, waving her left hand in the air, *Shining*.

STEPS	COUNTS	STEP CUE
Man's Part (wobbly knees)		
With feet together, weight on L, both knees go to the side	*and*	and
Step in place R and bring knees together	1	in
Both knees go to the side	*and*	and
Step in place L and bring knees together	2	in
Repeat counts: *and 1 and 2*	*and 3–8*	
Repeat count 1–8		
Woman's Part		
Starting with R, women takes 16 swivel steps to move clockwise around the man		

STYLE: Women is trying to attract attention, waving and smiling as she moves around the man.

LEAD: On approximately count 5 of a basic, the man would say "Hey Baby, do you want to Shine?" During the next basic he waits for a yes or no answer from the woman. When he hears a "yes," at the end of that basic, the shine starts. He continues to hold on to the women's right hand with his left as she moves around him.

Cajun Dance

CAJUN DANCE MUSIC, and food are very popular. In the 1980s Chef Paul Prudhomme of New Orleans attracted nationwide attention with his Cajun cooking and references to Cajun culture. Cajun culture suddenly bounced all over the United States. It exemplifies a true spirit of *joie de vivre*. The Cajun heritage is keyed to family, music, and the French language.

The word "Cajun" evolved from the word "Acadian" with the loss of an unstressed syllable (*cf.* Injun from Indian). The Acadians originally came from the French provinces of Normandy and Picardy along the English Channel. The first French colony, Acadie,* was established in 1604 in Nova Scotia, Canada. For political reasons the British deported the Acadians in 1755. Some migrated south, finally settling in the flatlands and bayous of Louisiana with other French. This coastal area, actually 22 of the 64 parishes of Louisiana, is referred to as Acadia, Acadiana, or Evangeline country.

From France the Acadians brought their 17th–18th century culture to the New World. Their culture evolved and adapted with that of the French, English, Spanish, and African Americans. The white French–speaking people of Acadia are referred to as Cajuns; the black French–speaking people are Creoles. (These are not the same Creoles who settled New Orleans.)

Cajun Dance (continued)

---

*Acadie, which the French called their settlement, was a descriptive word of the Micmac Indians, members of the Algonquin tribe.

Families have always gathered together for social occasions, first at homes and later at barns and dance halls. Music, French ballads, dancing, cards, and of course food were enjoyed. These gatherings were called *fais-dodo* ("go to sleep") because the children were bedded down in another room while the parties lasted till the wee hours. When the halls became night clubs, the children were excluded.

■ Music

Originally the fiddle was the primary instrument and someone sang old French ballads. The interaction of the Acadians and Creoles influenced the music. The singing became less important as two fiddles played, one melody, one rhythmic backup. More French songs were lost in the 1880s when the German immigrants introduced the button accordion. By the 1920s, the accordion had displaced the fiddles. But during the '30s and '40s fiddles returned as the Cajun musicians were influenced by their Texas neighbors' Country Western music. Later Bob Wills's western swing, Nashville Country Western music, and rock and roll all touched Cajun music too. After World War II Cajuns returned home with a sense of pride and a rebirth of Cajun music took place. The folk festivals also encouraged traditional Cajun musicians to come forward. Michael Doucet is to be credited with his leadership in restoring interest in traditional Cajun music, encouraging acoustic playing, and playing outside the lounges.

Today the button accordion is the lead instrument and the accordion player also sings French songs. The fiddle and small triangle make up the band. In larger bands there are guitars, spoons, drums, bass, and sometimes brass. Of course there is electric amplification. Cajun music, sometimes referred to as "Chanky Chank" sounds, is a mix of sounds, styles, and cultural history.

A relatively new offshoot of Cajun music is *Zydeco*, a combination of Cajun and rhythm and blues with a Caribbean musical pulse. Eighty years ago a song was written. "Zydeco es Pas Salee," which means "the snap beans have no salt." Zydeco is Cajun slang for the French words "Les Haricots" which means "green snap beans." Today Zydeco means snappy music. Bands include a piano, accordion, and a rubboard (metal washboard or steel vest) strapped on the musicians who wear metal casings on the fingers to produce a myriad of sounds. The songs are in English or French. The rhythm is 4/4 with a strong 1–2, 1–2 beat.

■ Records

Cajun: *Parlez Nous á Boire* (Two-step, swing, blues, waltz), CD 322; *Allon á Lafayette, Bayou Boogie*, Beausoleil; *Stir Up the Roux*, Bruce Daigrepont Zydeco: *Louisiana Blues and Zydeco*. Clifton Chenier. CD 329; *Louisiana Zydeco Music*, Boo Zoo Chavis. *Motordude Zydeco*, A–2 Fay Records; *Pick Up On This*, CD 2129; and *My Name is Beau Jocque*, Beau Jocque, PCD–1031.

■ Dance

The Acadian dance repertoire included the Quadrille, Lancer, Polka, Mazurka, Play party types referred to as *Danserond*, and Contredanse. Many dances were performed without instrumentation during the 40 days before Lent, so they sang in French, which helped to keep the language alive. Young and old danced, especially those of a "marrying age." The contredanse was more like the Appalachian Big Circle, a country dance. In the late '40s the Cajun round dance scene was very similar to that in Texas. It is almost a step back in time to watch the Cajuns dance the Waltz, Two-Step, and One-Step. Jitterbug is danced to Two-Step music. Zydeco is the latest dance. There are Two-Steps, One-Steps, and a few Waltzes. Zydeco and Cajun music affect the dancing styles. Cajun dance is smoother, more precise. Dancers circle the floor with more turns and the movement is horizontal. Zydeco dancers move in one spot with greater hip action. The syncopated Zydeco beat generates a bouncy vertical style with few turns. The dancers move subtly, upright with bent knees and lower to the floor. The dance is flavored with small kicks.

Cajun Waltz

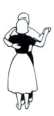

METER: 3/4. Directions are for man; woman's part reverse.

FORWARD WALTZ: Closed position. The man pulls the woman close, wrapping most of his right forearm around the woman's shoulder blades. Moving in the line of direction, step on each beat (left, right, left). The first step is longer, followed by a shuffle, shuffle. The man travels forward, woman backward, most of the time; minimal turning. Two measures (6 steps) to turn in place counterclockwise; may turn clockwise.

WOMAN TURN: Couple travels forward. Man releases right hand and steps slightly to left side (count 1) and forward (count 2, 3) as woman turns clockwise under his left arm, 3 steps. As she turns, she places her left bent arm behind her back. As she completes the turn, the couple resumes the closed position.

DOUBLE TURN: Couple travels forward and man releases right hand. Man takes three steps forward as woman turns with three steps clockwise under his left arm, places her left arm behind her back; woman continues to travel backward as the man turns counterclockwise three steps under his left arm; resumes the closed position.

STYLE: The dance is smooth as if gliding on ice. A fluid movement is achieved by dancing on the balls of the feet and absorbing the movement with bent knees.

Cajun Two-Step

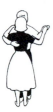

METER: 2/4 OR 4/4. Directions are for man; woman's part reverse.

Closed position. The man pulls the woman close, wrapping most of his right forearm around the woman's shoulder blades. Progressing forward, the couple turns slowly counterclockwise, strep–close–step touch. Step to the left side, and slightly forward, close right to left, step left in place, touch right to left instep (4 counts). May turn clockwise.

STYLE: The dance is smooth. In some areas, dancers rock slightly side to side.

Cajun One-Step

METER: 4/4. Directions are for man; woman's part reverse.

Closed position. Travel forward stepping side to side on each beat (side touch, side touch). Turning counterclockwise, step side touch near instep, step side touch near instep, step side touch near instep, step side touch near instep.

Transition One–Step to Two–Step or vice versa. The change of pattern is made when the feet are together.

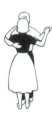

Cajun Jitterbug

CAJUN *JITTERBUG* IS frequently danced to Two–Step music. The steps are smooth with many variations.

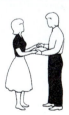

METER: 2/4. Directions are for man; women's part reverse.

Two hands joined. The basic step appears to be a "slight limp" with weight on right foot. Step left and lightly drag the right to the left, accent the second and fourth beats as the body drops (knees bend) ever so slightly. Step is smooth, not a jerk or bounce. Step–close, step–close, (one *and* two *and*). The lead may change to right close, right close or during the moves, step alternately left, right on each beat like Four Count Swing, coming back into step close, step close. The arms push–pull like a parallelogram; arms held chest–high push to right side, pull left arm back, shift right side to right side and pivot clockwise using side close, side close or buzz step. Reverse to left side by side without losing a beat. The arms are never straight, sometimes referred to as "noodle arms."

The man leads the moves. All the figures are smooth, one leading to the next as the dancers cover a circular space. Refer to Swing, pages 397–405, for different figures. Additional figures resemble Bavarian Laendler.

Zydeco Two-Step

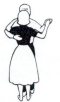

METER: 2/4. Steps based on eight counts. Directions are for man, woman's part reversed.

MUSIC: "Paper in My Shoe" by Boozoo Chavis; "Railroad Blues" by Lynn August; "Johnie Billie Goat" by Boozoo Chavis.

(Closed position)

STEPS	COUNTS	RHYTHM CUE
Moving in place, step left	1	slow
Bend knee (slight bounce)	2	
Step right	3	quick
Step left	4	quick
Step right, bend knee (slight bounce)	5–6	slow
Step left	7	quick
Step right	8	quick

STEP CUE: Step, drop, step, step; step, drop, step, step.

NOTE: Move in place. Travel forward in line of direction, stepping forward on counts 1 and 5. Turn clockwise or counterclockwise on counts 1 and 5.

STYLE: Keep steps small and controlled. Keep body accented downward, knees slightly bent, feet relatively flat on the floor with weight over the balls of the feet. Shoulders and arms are relatively still and parallel with the floor. The movements and gestures are smooth and subtle. The emphasis is more on the rhythm and footwork.

TEACHING SUGGESTIONS

Bounce in place 8 or 16 counts before starting step. Start with slow music. Repeat any variations 2 or 3 times to establish the pattern. Increase tempo. Steps are quick and light.

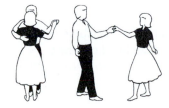

■ Variations

1. Closed position, 1 basic step. Repeat basic step, counts 1–6, then as man pushes left hand against woman's right hand (woman pushes right hand against man's left) man steps left foot behind his right, steps right in place and relaxes right hand, (counts 7–8). Woman steps right behind her left, steps left in place.

2. From closed position, move into Swing Out position and continue basic step. Keep joined hands and arms firm as basic step continues. Return to closed position on count 1.

3. Step on the toe, pivot or twist the heel in and out on counts 2 and 6. This is sometimes called "eat a beat."

Zydeco Two-Step (continued)

4. Brush (kick forward). Step left, brush right forward, step right, step left. Step right, brush left forward, step left, step right.

5. Closed position: step left turning clockwise, step right, left (slow, quick, quick). Open position: step right, brush left forward, step left, step right (quick, quick, quick, quick). Turn on the first step. Take two sets to make one complete turn.

Tango

HE *TANGO* BEGAN as a raw, sensuous dance born on the Rio de la Plata in Buenos Aires amid the slums in a multiracial setting. In its earliest form, the name *tangoo*, an onomatopetic rendition of the sounds of drums, strongly suggest its African origin. As with all dance forms, the Tango has passed through many evolutions. During its formative stages, it was a combination of *Candombe*, a syncopated African dance, the *Habanera*, an 18th century European dance, and the *Milango*, an indigenous Argentine dance.

The Tango and its music was introduced to Paris and the Riviera by wealthy South Americans after World War I. It became the rage of Paris, and it is from this setting and refinement that it spread throughout Europe and came to North America.

The 1990s have become the new age of the Tango. *Tangueros* are found in major cities around the world. Devotees attend workshops, organize weekly dances, and practice to improve their skills while exchanging feelings and excitement about danc–ing the Argentine Tango. While maintaining its smooth, sophisticated, and suave style, the Tango's new charm lies in its improvised nature that relies on communication between partners rather than executing prelearned step routines.

TANGO RHYTHM

The modern Tango is written in both 2/4 and 4/4 time. Here it will be presented 2/4 time.

2/4	S	S	Q Q S		2/4	S	Q Q		2/4	Q Q S
	1	2	1 and 2			1	2 and			1 and 2

uneven rhythm   uneven rhythm   uneven rhythm

Basic tango rhythm   Box step rhythm   Twinkle rhythm

The Tango rhythm is a deliberate accented beat that is easily distinguished. Few dancers have trouble following the Tango rhythm. There is a calculated contrast between the slow promenade beats of the first measure and the staccato of the Tango break in the second measure.

TANGO STYLE

The Tango is characterized by a deliberate glide, not sliding the foot on the floor, but a long reach from the hip with a catlike smoothness and placement of the ball of the foot on the floor. The knees remain straight. The break, which is quick quick slow, is a sudden contrast ending in the subtle draw of the feet together. It is this combination of slow gliding beats and the sharp break that makes the Tango distinctive. Restraint is achieved by the use of continuous flow of movements and a controlled, stylized break presenting disciplined and sophisticated style, instead of a comic caricature. The dancer should strive to effect the idea of floating. Care should be taken to avoid the look of stiffness. Since the long reaching glide is used, the feet should pass each other close together. The draw in the Tango close is executed slowly, taking the full length of the slow beat to bring the feet together and then sweep quickly into the beginning of the basic rhythm again. The woman should synchronize the action of her drawing step with that of the man. The body and head are carried high and the woman's left hand, instead of being on the man's shoulder as in other dances, reaches around the man at his right shoulder–blade level. The fingers of the hand are straight and the arm is in a straight line from the elbow to the tip of the fingers.

Once in a while, deliberately move the shoulders forward in opposition to the feet. For example, stepping left, the right shoulder moves forward. The fan steps, most glamorous of all Tango patterns, turn, whip, or swirl in an exciting, subtle way. The fan style is described in detail with the variations used.

FUNDAMENTAL TANGO STEPS

Directions are for the man, facing the line of direction; the woman's part is reversed, except as noted.

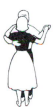

■ BASIC TANGO STEP

(Closed position)

A combination of the promenade or walking step and the break.

STEPS	2/4 COUNTS	RHYTHM CUE
Step L forward	1	slow
Step R forward	2	slow
Step L in place	1	quick
Step R sideward abruptly	*and*	quick
Draw L to R, weight remains on R	2	slow

STEP CUE: Slow slow Tango close.
      S   S   QQ   S

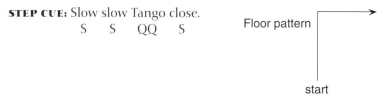

Floor pattern

start

STYLE: The slow beats are long, smooth, gliding steps. The feet pass each other closely. The break quick quick slow is in place or slightly forward.

LEAD: Man must draw to the right with right hand and elbow to guide the woman in the break step.

NOTE: This step repeats each time from the man's left foot, because there is no change of weight on the draw. This pattern will tend to carry the couple outward toward the wall. It immediately becomes necessary to know how to vary the step in order to counteract this action. Open position, right parallel position, or quarter–turn all may be used for this purpose.

Fundamental Tango Steps (continued)

Open Position Basic Tango	Half-Turn Clockwise	Right Parallel Basic Tango
The Box Step	Quarter-Turn	The Corté
Cross Step and Quarter-Turn	Open Fan	Half-Turn Counterclockwise

■ OPEN POSITION BASIC TANGO

(Closed position)

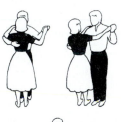

STEPS	2/4 COUNTS	RHYTHM CUE
Step L into open position, turning abruptly	1	slow
Step R forward, in open position	2	slow
Step L forward, a short step, pivoting on L foot abruptly to face partner in closed position	1	quick
Step R sideward, in closed position	*and*	quick
Draw L to R, no change of weight	2	slow

STEP CUE: Open step close side draw.

STYLE: The abrupt turning to open position on the first slow step and the turn back to closed position are sharp and only a firmness in the body can accomplish this.

LEAD: Refer to leads 7 and 8, p. 375. The lead is sudden and on the first slow beat.

■ RIGHT PARALLEL BASIC TANGO

(Closed position)

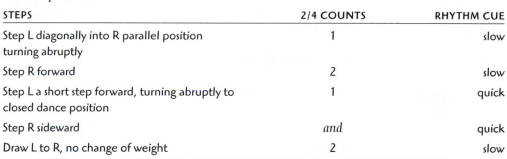

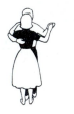

STEPS	2/4 COUNTS	RHYTHM CUE
Step L diagonally into R parallel position turning abruptly	1	slow
Step R forward	2	slow
Step L a short step forward, turning abruptly to closed dance position	1	quick
Step R sideward	*and*	quick
Draw L to R, no change of weight	2	slow

STEP CUE: Parallel step close side draw.

STYLE: Right parallel travels diagonally forward; woman's foot reaches parallel to man's left foot. The second slow is an exaggerated reaching step forward.

LEAD: To lead into right parallel position (left reverse open position) the man should not use pressure of his right hand, but rather should raise his right arm rotating the woman counterclockwise one-eighth of a turn while he rotates counterclockwise one-eighth of a turn. This places the man and woman off to the side of each other facing opposite directions. The woman is to the right of the man, but slightly in front of him. The man should avoid turning too far so as to be side by side as this results in poor style and awkward and uncomfortable motion. The man's left hand may assist the lead by pulling toward his left shoulder.

■ QUARTER-TURN

(Closed position)

STEPS	2/4 COUNTS	RHYTHM CUE
Step L forward	1	slow
Step R forward	2	slow
Step L, turning one-quarter counterclockwise	1	quick
Step R sideward	*and*	quick
Draw L to R, no change of weight	2	slow

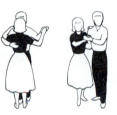

■ CROSS STEP AND QUARTER-TURN

(Closed position)

STEPS	2/4 COUNTS	RHYTHM CUE
Step L sideward	1	slow
Step R across in front of L, take weight R	2	slow
Step L sideward, turn toe out, turn one-quarter counterclockwise	1	quick
Step R sideward	*and*	quick
Draw L to R, no change of weight	2	slow

STEP CUE: Side cross turn side close.

STYLE: All of this pattern is taken in closed position. The turn actually begins by a pivot on the crossing foot at the end of the second slow beat.

LEAD: Refer to Lead 12, p. 375.

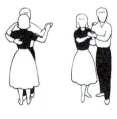

■ HALF-TURN COUNTERCLOCKWISE

(Closed position)

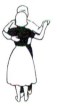

STEPS	2/4 COUNTS	RHYTHM CUE
Step L into open position, turning abruptly	1	slow
Step R forward, a short step, pivoting one-quarter counterclockwise on the R foot; bring up R arm and turn the woman around the man a three-quarter turn to closed position	2	slow
Step L bringing L foot next to R foot	1	quick
Step R sideward	*and*	quick
Draw L to R, no weight change	2	slow

STEP CUE: Step pivot break side draw.

STYLE: The woman pivots counterclockwise on her left foot (second slow beat) around the man a three–quarter turn into closed position. The woman's step on this beat was a longer step than the man's, giving her freedom to pivot. She must bring her first quick step with R foot alongside of left foot.

LEAD: Man must bring up his right arm and elbow firmly, almost lifting her so that she can pivot easily on her left foot on the second slow beat.

■ HALF-TURN CLOCKWISE

(Closed position)

STEPS	2/4 COUNTS	RHYTHM CUE
Step L into open position, turning abruptly	1	slow
Step R forward, a long step, pivoting one–half clockwise on the R foot around the woman into closed position	2	slow
Step L sideward, a short step apart from where R foot is at the end of the pivot	1	quick
Step R sideward	*and*	quick
Draw L to R, no weight change	2	slow

Fundamental Tango Steps (continued)

STEP CUE: Step pivot break side draw.

STYLE: The man smoothly pivots on his right foot clockwise about halfway around the woman. The woman turns clockwise in place on her left foot. This step is very easy for the woman.

LEAD: Refer to lead indications 7 and 8, p. 375, for open and closed position. The main lead is increased resistance in hand, arm, and body as the man pivots halfway around the woman.

■ DOUBLE CROSS

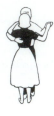

(In twinkle rhythm closed position)

STEPS	2/4 COUNTS	RHYTHM CUE
Step L sideways	1	slow
Step R across in front of L	2	slow
Point L sideways, take weight slightly	1	quick
Pivot hips to R with a slight push off with L, take weight R	*and*	quick
Swing L across in front of R, take weight L	2	slow
Point R to side	1	quick
Pivot hips to L with slight push off with R, take weight L	*and*	quick
Swing R across in front of L, take weight R	2	slow

STEP CUE: Side cross pivot and cross pivot and cross.
            S   S   Q   Q   S   Q   Q   S

STYLE: Stay in closed position throughout. Woman crosses in front, also.

LEAD: Firm body and arm control are needed to hold closed position.

NOTE: Finish with break side draw quick quick slow. This could also be done with the woman crossing behind.

■ THE BOX STEP

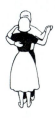

The rhythm of the Tango box step is like that described in the Foxtrot–slow quick quick–forward side close, back side close. The Tango gliding action will be used on the first slow beat. The box step variations for Foxtrot may also be used here, including the box turn and the grapevine step. Refer to pp. 385, 386, and 388.

■ THE CORTÉ

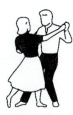

The corté is a dip, most often taken backward on the man's left or right foot. It is a type of break step used to finish off almost any Tango variation and is used as an ending to the dance. The skilled dancer will learn to use the corté in relationship to the music of the tango so that the feeling of the corté will correspond to the climax or the phrase of the musical accompaniment.

    The left corté will be described here. A right corté may be taken by starting on the right foot and reversing the pattern. A preliminary step is nearly always used as a preparation for going into the corté. It is described here as a part of the rhythm of the corté.

STEPS	2/4 COUNTS	RHYTHM CUE
Step forward L, a short step	1	quick
Shift weight back onto R	*and*	quick

Corté

STEPS	2/4 COUNTS	RHYTHM CUE
Step L backward, take weight, and bend L knee slightly	2	slow
Recover forward, take weight R	1	slow
Step L in place beside R	2	quick
Step R in place beside L	*and*	quick

STEP CUE: Rock and dip recover quick quick.

         Q   Q   S   S   Q   Q

STYLE: As the *man* steps backward into the corté, the weight is all taken on the standing foot with a bent knee. The man should turn his bent knee slightly outward so that the woman's knee will not bump his as they go into the dip. His left shoulder and arm move forward (the left leg and left shoulder are in opposition). His back should remain straight. He should avoid leaning either backward or forward. His right foot should be extended (arched) so that the toe is only touching the floor.

The *woman* should step forward on the right, arch her back, and place all of her weight over the forward right foot. The right knee is bent. The left leg is extended behind and should be a straight line from hip to toe. A bent line makes the whole fig–ure sag. The left arch of the foot should be extended so that the toe is pointed and remains in contact with the floor. If the woman steps forward too far or does not bend the forward knee, she will be forced to bend at the waist, which destroys the form of the figure. She may look back over her left shoulder. The execution of the dip should be as smooth as any slow backward step.

The man should avoid leaping or falling back into the dip.

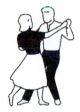

LEAD: The left shoulder leads forward as the man goes into the preparation step on the first beat. There is an increase of tension of the man's right arm and hand also on the first beat, plus general resistance throughout the upper body. The man will draw the woman with his right arm when stepping into the dip and release on the recovery step. The lead is essential for the corté as the pattern cannot be executed correctly unless both man and woman are completely on balance and ready for it.

NOTE: The recovery step is followed by two quick steps left right, which finish count 2 and complete the measure of music. These may be omitted when they follow a variation that takes up those extra counts. Learn the footwork first, then work on the style.

■ *Fan Step*

The *fan* is a term used to describe a manner of executing a leg motion, in which the free leg swings in a whiplike movement around a small pivoting base. This should not be a large sweeping movement in a wide arc but rather a small subtle action initiated in the hip and executed with the legs close together. The balance is carefully poised over the pivoting foot at all times. When the man and woman take the fan motion, the action is taken parallel to partner; that is, the right leg, which is free, swings forward. When it reaches its full extension, just barely off the floor, the right hip turns the leg over, knee down, while pivoting on the standing foot to face the opposite direction. The right leg then swings through forward and the weight is taken on the right foot. This action usually is done in slow rhythm. Accompanying the hip action there is also a lift and turn on the ball of the standing foot. This lift permits the free leg to swing through gracefully extended and close in a beautiful floating style.

Fundamental Tango Steps (continued)

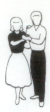

▪ OPEN FAN

(Open position)

STEPS	2/4 COUNTS	RHYTHM CUE
Step L forward	1	slow
Step R forward	2	slow
Step L in place, releasing R arm around woman, and turn halfway around to the right to a side-by-side position with woman on man's L	1	quick
Step R sideward, a short step	*and*	quick
Draw L to R, no weight change (the man's L hand is holding the woman's R)	2	slow
Step forward L	1	quick
Swing the R leg forward, pivoting on L foot while fanning the R, coming halfway around to open position	*and*	quick
Step forward R in open position	2	slow
Step L forward, pivoting toward the woman into closed position	1	quick
Step R sideward	*and*	quick
Draw L to R, no weight change	2	slow

STEP CUE: Slow slow open side draw/fan through break side draw

STYLE: When the man releases his arm around her, the woman turns halfway around to the left. On the fan, the woman steps right, swings left leg forward, hip turns over, knee faces down. Foot is kept close to the floor and sweeps through pivoting clockwise to open position, and weight is transferred forward onto left foot. She then goes into break step with partner.

LEAD: The man drops his right arm and pulls away from the woman to side–by–side position. Then, with his left hand, he pulls in as he fans through to open position and from there lifts his right arm into closed position for Tango close.

NOTE: This is an easy beginner step in fan style and gives them the thrill of the Tango.

▪ GRAPEVINE FAN

(Starting in open position)

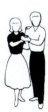

STEPS	2/4 COUNTS	RHYTHM CUE
Step L forward	1	slow
Rock forward and back R, L	2 *and*	quick quick
Step R backward rising on R toe and lifting L leg just off the floor	1	slow
Step L backward, turning toward partner	2	quick
Step R sideward, turning to face reverse open position	*and*	quick
Step L forward in reverse open position	1	quick
Fan R leg forward and through to open position	*and*	quick
Step R forward, in open position	2	slow
Step L forward, a short step, turning to closed position	1	quick
Step R sideward	*and*	quick
Draw L to R, no weight change	2	slow

STEP CUE: Step rock and back grapevine step fan through break side close.

S   Q   Q   S   Q   Q   Q   Q   S   S   Q   Q   S

STYLE: The couple should not get too far apart or lean forward to maneuver this grapevine pattern. They should stand upright and keep carefully balanced over standing foot. The fanning leg swings in line with the travelling and facing action, not in a side arc. The legs are kept close together.

LEAD: This is a pattern man and woman must know together but the man cues the woman by use of both hands and use of his body in turning from one position to another.

NOTE: This is a beautiful pattern when used following the forward and open rock.

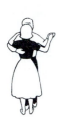

■ PARALLEL FAN

(Fan style in parallel position; starting in closed position)

STEPS	2/4 COUNTS	RHYTHM CUE
Man's Part: Starts and ends in closed position. Starting L, take one basic Tango step, slow slow quick quick slow		
Step L forward	1	slow
Step R sideward turning to open position	2	quick
Step L to R, taking weight L	and	quick
Step R forward, turning woman to R parallel position	1	slow
Rock backward onto L, turning woman to open position	2	slow
Rock forward onto R, turning woman to R parallel position	1	slow
Rock back onto L, turning woman to open position	2	slow
Step R forward in open position	1	slow
Take Tango–close step, turning to closed position	2 and 1	quick quick slow
Woman's Part: Starting right, take one basic tango step, slow slow quick quick slow.		
Step R backward	1	slow
Step L sideward, turning to open position	2	quick
Step R to L, taking weight on R	and	quick
Step L forward (fan), pivoting to R parallel position	1	slow
Step R forward (fan), pivoting to open position	2	slow
Step L forward (fan), pivoting to R parallel position	1	slow
Step R forward (fan), pivoting to open position	2	slow
Step L forward (fan), pivoting to R parallel position	1	slow
Step R forward (fan), pivoting to open position	2	slow
Step L forward, turning to closed position	1	slow
Take Tango close	2 and 1	quick quick slow

STEP CUE: With slow and quick rhythm except for the fan: rock rock rock rock/forward break side draw.

STYLE: The steps are small in the fan part of the step so that the woman may turn without reaching for the step. The man in the fan part of the step rocks forward, back, forward, back in place, as he turns the woman. She takes her fan, pivoting alternately on the left, right, left, right, swinging the free leg forward a short distance until the toe just clears the floor and then turning the hip with her pivot to the new direction and reaching through for the next step. The woman should rise slightly on her toe as she pivots. This smooths out the turn and makes one of the most beautiful movements in Tango.

Fundamental Tango Steps (continued)

LEAD: Man's first lead will be to lower right arm into open position. He then guides her forward with his right hand, moving her alternately from right parallel position to open position until the end when he raises his right arm and turns her to closed position.

NOTE: A corté may be added to this figure instead of the Tango close by stepping through to open position on the R (count 1), turning the woman quickly to closed position, rocking forward and back (counts 2 *and*); corté (count 1), recover onto the L foot (count 2) and finish with Tango close (counts 1 and 2).

TANGO COMBOS

The Tango routines are combinations for practice, listed from simple to complex. (Closed position, unless otherwise indicated.)

1. *Basic*
   2 basic steps
   1 basic step (open position)
2. *Basic, Cross Step*
   2 basic steps
   4 cross steps and quarter–turn
3. *Box, Basic, Cross Step*
   2 box steps
   1 basic step
   1 cross step and quarter–turn

4. *Basic, Cross, Corté*
   2 basics
   1 cross step, quarter–turn
   1 corté
5. *Advanced Combo*
   2 box steps
   1 basic
   1 cross step
   open fan

6. *Advanced Combo*
   2 basics
   open fan
   half-turn clockwise
   corté
   1 basic

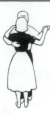

Waltz

ALTHOUGH A MAJORITY of the middle European countries lay some claim to the origin of the *Waltz*, the world looked to Germany and Austria, where the great Waltz was made traditional by the beautiful music of Johann Strauss and his sons. It has a pulsating, swinging rhythm, which has been enjoyed by dancers everywhere, even by those who dance it only in its simplest pattern, the Waltz Turn. Its immediate popularity and its temporary obscurity are not unlike other fine inheritances of the past, which come and go with the ebb and flow of popular accord. Early use of the Waltz in America was at the elegant social balls and cotillions. Its outstanding contribution to present–day dancing is the Waltz position. Even in its early stages, it was quite some time before this position was socially acceptable. Now the closed position is universally the basic position for Ballroom Dancing.

The Waltz music is played in three different tempos–slow, medium, and fast. The slow or medium Waltz is preferred by most people. However, the fast Waltz is a favorite of those who know the Viennese style. The slower American style is danced for the most part on a box pattern, but the use of other variations has added a new interest.

WALTZ RHYTHM

The Waltz is played in 3/4 time. It is three beats per measure of music, with an accent on the first beat. The three beats of Waltz time are very even, each beat receiving the same amount of time. The three movements of the Waltz step pattern blend perfectly with the musical tempo or beat of each measure. The tempo may be slow, medium, or fast.

```
        /
3/4 | slow    slow    slow
    | ____    ____    ____
    | ____    ____    ____
    |  1       2       3
          even rhythm
       Slow  box rhythm
```

Canter rhythm in Waltz time is a means of holding the first and second beats together so the resultant pattern is an uneven rhythm, or slow quick slow quick. It is counted 1, 3, 1, 3.

```
        /                        /
3/4 | _____  ____  ____ | _____  ____  ____
    | _____  ____  ____ | _____  ____  ____
    |  1  -  2       3    |  1  -  2       3
               uneven rhythm
               Canter rhythm
```

The Viennese Waltz is an even three–beat rhythm, played very fast. It is a turning pattern. There is only one step on the first beat of the measure and a pivot of the body on that foot for the two remaining counts of the measure.

```
        /
3/4 | step     pivot
    | ____  ____  ____
    | ____  ____  ____
    |  1     2     3
         even rhythm
       Viennese rhythm
```

WALTZ STYLE

The Waltz is a smooth dance with a gliding quality that weaves an even pattern of swinging and turning movement. The first accented beat of the music is also accented in the motion. The first step of the Waltz pattern is the reaching step forward, back–ward, sideward, or turning. Because it is the first beat that gives the dance its new impetus, its new direction, or a change of step, there evolves a pulsating feeling, which can be seen rather markedly and is the chief characteristic of the beauty of the Waltz. This should not be interpreted as a rocking or bobbing motion of the body. On count 1, the man steps *flat* on the sole of the foot; on counts 2–3, the body rises stepping on the ball of the foot. The rising action is sometimes described as a *lift*. The "fall and rise" action of the body is seen in every step. The footwork is most effective when the foot taking the second beat glides past the standing foot as it moves into the sideward step. The feet should never be heard to scrape the floor, but should seem to float in a silent pattern. In closed position, it is important for the woman to be directly in front of the man, their shoulders parallel.

Waltz (continued)

FUNDAMENTAL WALTZ STEPS

Directions are for the man, facing line of direction; woman's part is reversed, except as noted.

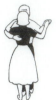

■ BOX STEP

(Closed position)

STEPS	3/4 COUNTS	STYLE CUE
Step L forward	1	flat
Step R sideward, passing close to the L foot	2	lift
Close L to R, take weight L	3	lift
Step R backward	1	flat
Step L sideward, passing close to the R foot	2	lift
Close R to L, take weight R	3	lift

STEP CUE: Forward side close/back side close.

STYLE: The forward step is **on the heel.** Follow through on the second beat, moving the free foot closely past the standing foot, but do not lose a beat by stopping. Body rises on counts 2, 3 as stepping on ball of foot. The floor pattern is a long narrow rectangle rather than a square box.

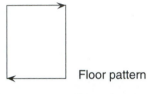

Floor pattern

LEAD: To lead a box step the man should use a forward body action followed by right–hand pressure and right elbow pull to the right to take the woman into the forward sequence of the box. Forward pressure of the right hand followed by pressure to the left side takes the woman into the back sequence of the box.

NOTE: The man must understand the concept of the forward side close as being the forward sequence of the box and the backward side close as being the back sequence of the box. This terminology will be used in future patterns.

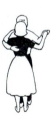

■ BOX TURN

(Left)–(Closed position)

STEPS	3/4 COUNTS	STYLE CUE
Step L forward, toe out, turning one-quarter L	1	flat
Step R sideward, gliding past the L foot	2	lift
Close L to R, taking weight L	3	lift
Step R backward, toe in, turning one-quarter L	1	flat
Step L sideward, gliding past the R foot	2	lift
Close R to L, taking weight R	3	lift
Step L forward, toe out, turning one-quarter L	1	flat
Step R sideward, gliding past the L foot	2	lift
Close L to R, taking weight on L	3	lift
Step R backward, toe in, turning one-quarter L	1	flat
Step L sideward, gliding past the R foot	2	lift
Close R to L, taking weight R	3	lift

STEP CUE: Turn side close, turn side close.

WOMAN: The woman is taking the reverse pattern, except that, when the woman steps forward with the left foot, instead of toeing out as described for the man, she steps forward between the man's feet, her left foot next to the instep of the man's left foot. This style greatly facilitates the turn.

MAN: A common error is that the man tries to step around his partner. The woman must be directly in front of her partner.

STYLE: Accent the first step by reaching with a longer step. However, man must be careful not to overreach his partner. There is no unnecessary knee bending or bobbing up and down.

LEAD: To lead a box turn with slight pressure of the right hand, the man should use the right arm and shoulder to guide or bank the woman into the turn. The shoulders press forward during the forward step and draw backward during the backward step.

NOTE: For the right turn, start with the right foot. Follow the same pattern with opposite footwork.

■ *Teaching Strategy for Changing Leads—Turn Right, Turn Left*

It is important to learn to turn counterclockwise and clockwise. The foot must be free to *lead* in the direction of the turn: left lead for left turn; right lead for right turn. There are several ways to change the lead. With the left, step balance or a hesitation step, then start the box with the right foot (right side close, left side close). Another is to take two Waltz steps forward, take the third Waltz step backward; right foot is now free to turn right. To return to the left lead, either step (R) balance or take two Waltz steps forward and the third one backward; then the left foot leads again. Once the student can turn left and right, the teacher should present a definite routine that drills this change. When students learn this concept for the Waltz, they will be able to transfer the principle to other rhythms.

■ *Waltz Step Variations*

Hesitation Step	Weaving Step	Streamline Step
Cross Step	Twinkle Step	Viennese Waltz

■ HESITATION STEP

(Closed position)

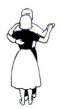

STEPS	3/4 COUNTS	STYLE CUE
Step L forward	1	flat
Bring R foot up to the instep of L and hold, no weight change	2, 3	lift
Step R backward	1	flat
Bring L foot up to the instep of R foot, no weight change	2, 3	lift

STEP CUE: Step close hold.

STYLE: Smooth.

LEAD: To lead a hesitation step the man dips his shoulder in the direction of the turn, and his upper torso turns before his leg and foot turn.

NOTE: As in the Foxtrot, a beautiful combination is to dance two hesitation steps, then the first half of the box turn, two hesitation steps and then the second half of the turn. The hesitation step repeated may also be done turning either counterclockwise or clockwise and may be useful in maneuvering for the next step.

Fundamental Waltz Steps (continued)

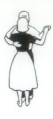

■ **CROSS STEP**

(Closed position)

STEPS	3/4 COUNTS	STYLE CUE
Step L forward	1	flat
Step R sideward, turning to open position	2	lift
Close L to R, taking weight L	3	lift
Step R forward, in open position	1	flat
Step L forward, turning on L foot to face partner in closed position	2	lift
Close R to L, taking weight R	3	lift

STEP CUE: Forward side close, cross side close.

STYLE: The position is opened to semiopen position, just enough to step forward on the inside foot, which feels like a crossing step. It should be accented by a long, smooth, reaching step on the heel, not a dipping or bobbing action.

LEAD: To lead into an open position or conversation position, the man should use pressure with the heel of the right hand to turn the woman into open position. The right elbow lowers to the side. The man must simultaneously turn his own body, not just the woman so that they end facing the same direction. The left arm relaxes slightly and the left hand sometimes gives the lead for steps in the open position.

LEAD: To lead from open to closed position the man should use pressure of the right hand and raise the right arm up to standard position to move the woman into closed position. The woman should not have to be pushed but should swing easily into closed position as she feels the arm lifting. She should move completely around to face the man squarely.

NOTE: When man is facing out in closed position, he can go into this step and the cross pattern will travel in line of direction.

■ **WEAVING STEP**

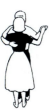

Same as cross step but crossing from side to side. (Closed position)

STEPS	3/4 COUNTS	STYLE CUE
Step L forward	1	flat
Step R sideward, turning to open position	2	lift
Close L to R, taking weight L	3	lift
Step R forward in open position	1	flat
Step L forward, turning to side-by-side position facing the reverse line of direction	2	lift
Close R to L, taking weight R	3	lift
Step L forward, in side-by-side position	1	flat
Step R forward, turning to open position	2	lift
Close L to R, taking weight L	3	lift
Step R forward in open position	1	flat
Step L forward, turning to closed position	2	lift
Close R to L, taking weight R	3	lift

STEP CUE: Forward side open/cross side reverse/cross side reverse/cross side close.

STYLE: Reach into crossing step on the heel. It is a long reaching step on the accented beat.

LEAD: Turn woman to semiopen position for first cross step and then drop right arm and lead through with the left hand to side-by-side position, facing the reverse line of direction. Next time, as they reverse direction, the man puts his arm around her in open position and follows standard procedure for returning to closed position.

NOTE: The weave pattern may be repeated back and forth, crossing as many times as desired, but should go back to closed position as described above.

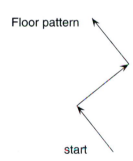

■ TWINKLE STEP

(Closed position)

It is led from the back sequence of the box step.

STEPS	3/4 COUNTS	STYLE CUE
Step L forward	1	flat
Step R sideward turning into R parallel position	2	lift
Close L to R, taking eight L	3	lift
Step R, diagonally forward in R parallel position	1	flat
Step L sideward, turning from R parallel to L parallel position	2	lift
Close R to L, taking weight R	3	lift
Step L diagonally forward in L parallel position	1	flat
Step R sideward, turning from L parallel position to R parallel position	2	lift
Close L to R, taking weight on L	3	lift
Step R diagonally forward in R parallel position	1	flat
Step L sideward turning to closed position	2	lift
Close R to L, taking weight on R	3	lift

Floor pattern

start

STEP CUE: Step turn close. The second beat has a short step and a smooth roll from one position to another. The woman reaches parallel to the man's step, except that she is stepping diagonally backward, which takes a lot of practice for the woman to do it well.

LEAD: To lead into right parallel position the man should not use pressure of his right hand, but rather should raise his right arm rotating the woman counterclockwise one-eighth of a turn while he rotates counterclockwise one-eighth of a turn. This places the man and woman off to the side of each other facing opposite directions. The woman is to the right of the man but slightly in front of him. The man should avoid turning too far so as to be side by side as this results in poor style and awkward and uncomfort-able motion. The man's left hand may assist the lead by pulling toward his left shoulder.

LEAD: To lead from right parallel position to left parallel position the man should pull with his right hand lowering the right arm and push slightly with his left hand causing a rotation clockwise about a quarter of a turn until the woman is to the left of him but slightly in front of him. They are not side by side.

NOTE: Progress is in a zigzag pattern down the floor in the line of direction and may repeat over and over as desired.

■ *Suggestions for Variations*

Any student or teacher who has followed these directions this far should be prepared to make use of the advance twinkle, corté, and pivot turn described under the Foxtrot by transposing a slow, quick, quick in 4/4 time into slow, slow, slow in 3/4 time. Refer to corté p. 384, Twinkle p. 387, Pivot Turn p. 389.

Fundamental Waltz Steps (continued)

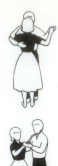

■ **STREAMLINE STEP**

(Closed position)

An advanced step seen in the International Style and competition. Dancers travel in the line of direction and need a lot of space to move. Step on every beat, each step forward. The feet are never together, always moving forward! Step flat on the first beat; body rises on counts 2–3. The floor pattern, although forward, zigs and zags. In addition to moving forward, the dancers may rock or grapevine.

ROCK: Forward, backward, forward; backward, forward, backward.

GRAPEVINE: Semiopen position, travel in line of direction.

■ **VIENNESE WALTZ**

The **rhythm** is three even, quick beats now instead of slow. The Viennese Waltz music is fast and it is hard to keep one's balance on the pivot step when it is slowed down, so that students get discouraged learning the step. An experiment of a half-Viennese has proved successful in getting students to learn the pivot step by doing it first on the right foot and then taking a regular Waltz step on the left sequence.

3/4	step	side	cross	step	pivot	
	1	2	3	1	2	3
	quick	quick	quick	right	pivot	

Half-Viennese step

Half–Viennese Step:

1. Both man and woman need to practice this pattern alone, traveling down line of direction.

STEPS	3/4 COUNTS	RHYTHM CUE
Step L forward, turning one-quarter counterclockwise	1	quick
Step R sideward, turning one-quarter counterclockwise	2	quick
Slide the L foot, heel first, in across R to the R of the R foot. Transfer weight to L foot. Both toes are facing the reverse line of direction, feet are crossed	3	quick
Step R backward and pivot one-half counterclockwise on the R foot	1	quick
Bring the L foot up to the instep of the R foot and with the L toe help balance on the R foot	2, 3	quick quick

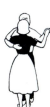

2. Closed position, the man facing the line of direction.

Starting L, the man takes the step side cross while the woman, starting R, takes the back pivot	1, 2, 3	all quick
Starting R, the man takes the back pivot while the woman, starting L, takes step side across	1, 2, 3	all quick

STYLE: The couple remains in closed position throughout. The steps are small as the woman is turning on a small pivot base while the man takes step side cross. Since the man turns one–quarter on his forward step, his second step is in line of direction, a small step and cross on third beat. Then he steps back a short step and pivots while woman takes the step side cross. The dancers always progress in the line of direction. Use two Waltz steps for one complete turn. The body resistance is firm for both man and woman. They must lean away, pressing outward but keeping the center of gravity over the pivoting feet. The shoulders tilt slightly in one direction and then the other; tilt left as the left foot leads, right as the right foot leads. Do not resist the momentum of body weight, but rather give into the momentum.

LEAD: Firm body and arms in correct position. The momentum comes from the rapid transfer of the body forward in the line of direction every time on count 1.

CUE: 1, 2, 3, 1, 2, 3.

Viennese Step:

3. The true Viennese with a step pivot repeated over and over is in closed dance position. Man starting L forward, woman R backward.

STEPS	3/4 COUNTS	RHYTHM CUE
Step L forward, pivoting on the ball of the foot one-half counterclockwise; the right foot coming up to the instep of the L and with the R toe, helps to balance on the L foot	1, 2, 3	all quick
Step R backward, pivoting on the ball of the foot one-half counterclockwise; the L foot coming to the instep of the R helps to balance on the R foot	1, 2, 3	all quick

STEP CUE: Step pivot, step pivot.

STYLE: There is a lift of the body going into the pivot, which lifts the body weight, momentarily allowing the feet to pivot with less weight. Take care not to throw the weight off balance.

LEAD: Same as above.

VARIATIONS: The hesitation step as given under the box pattern is very helpful in giving a rest from the constant turning. Also, by using an uneven number of hesitation steps, the right foot is free and the whole Viennese turn may be changed to a clockwise turn starting with the right foot and applying the pattern with opposite footwork.

WALTZ COMBOS

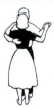

These Waltz routines are combinations for practice, listed from simple to complex. (Closed position, unless otherwise indicated.)

1. *Balance and Box*
   2 balance steps
   (forward, backward)
   4 box steps
2. *Waltz Box*
   1 box step
   2 forward Waltz steps
   1 box turn
3. *Cross Box and Turn*
   2 cross steps
   1 box turn

4. *Hesitation and Box Turn*
   2 hesitation steps
   (forward, backward)
   1 box turn
5. *Cross Step and Weaving*
   2 cross steps
   1 weaving step
6. *Advanced Combo*
   1 box turn
   4 twinkle steps
   2 hesitation steps
   2 pursuit Waltz steps
   1 corté
   1 forward Waltz step

7. *Advanced Combo*
   6 streamline steps (18 beats)
   2 twinkle steps
   4 streamline steps
   2 hesitation steps

Country Western

COUNTRY WESTERN DANCE has been around for a long time; it is definitely a grassroots dance. As country western music has increased in popularity so has Country Western Dance. Country western music, a twangy honky–tonk sound as played by Bob Wills and his Texas Playboys in the late 1930s, was just the beginning. The music is influenced by spirituals, Dixieland jazz, and the big band sound. The fiddle, steel guitar, and deep bass give country western music its character. The fiddle was part of the band. Wherever country western music is played, people dance. The dances are based on old Folk Dances, Square Dances, and Social Dances, topped off with a new look, called Country Western. *Swing, One-Step, Two-Step, Schottische, Waltz,* and *Line Dances* are all part of the repertory.

COUNTRY WESTERN STYLE

The Country Western look starts with cowboy or roper boots. Tight fitting jeans are worn by both men and women. Large belt buckles adorn the dancers. Cowboy hats are commonly seen on the dance floor, though, for the last few years, younger men have been switching to baseball hats. In some settings, women may wear a western skirt instead of jeans. When dancers have a free hand, they hook the thumb near the belt buckle or into the closest pocket.

DANCE HALL ETIQUETTE

At Country Western Dances, several types of dancing may take place simultaneously. The perimeter of the dance floor is for round dances; the slower ones dance in the inside lane. Fast and slow dancers move counterclockwise around the floor. The Swing Dancers and Line Dancers split the center area, with line dancers closer to the band.

The man takes the woman's hand or arm or offers his arm to escort her onto or off the dance floor and to return her to her seat.

In Western and Cajun dancing it is customary to leave the dance floor and return to your table or side of the room, even if you plan to dance the next dance with the same partner. The man still takes the woman's hand or arm and offers his arm to escort her onto and off the dance floor and to return her to her seat.

Traditional Country Western Swing

TRADITIONAL COUNTRY WESTERN SWING RHYTHM

Traditional Country Western Swing is danced to a faster 4/4 time song, between 170 and 200 B.P.M. At times the traditional "cowboys" dance faster than the music, dancing with the music, not to the beat of the music. On popular country music TV programs and at many dance studios, the style of country swing performed is the East Coast Swing. The only difference from ballroom style is the music played.

COWBOY SWING STYLE

The cowboys have a very smooth style. They slide their feet along the floor, almost never picking them up for a step. The emphasis of the dance is on the arm movements and the figures that are performed more so than the footwork. During many figures, the feet may not move at all.

Steps are small and arms are kept bent and close to the body. Two factors figured in the development of this style: (1) the fast tempo of music does not allow for large gestures, and (2) traditional dance floors were very small. Large steps or movement would cause a couple to bump into another couple.

Although from a distance, this style may look wild, with a good partner, the moves are very controlled and flow smoothly from one variation to another. There is a constant counterbalance between partners, allowing a "leaning" away (with a bend at the elbow joint) that is the characteristic mark of Cowboy Swing.

POSITION: Two hands joined

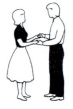

■ *Basic Step*

*4/4 counts

RHYTHM		CUE
Step L, diagonal L forward	*1 and*	slow
Women: Step R, diagonal L forward (crossing in front of her L foot)		
Step R forward	*2 and*	slow
Pivot 180° counterclockwise on R foot	3	quick
Slide L to R foot, *keep weight on R foot*	*and*	quick
Begin again	4	

*The Basic must be done four times to start at the beginning of the next measure.

Traditional Country Western Swing (continued)

STEP CUE: One, Two, Together.

STYLE: The Basic Step is performed moving in a clockwise motion. Knees slightly bent and forearms at the side with elbows bent. The man and women lean away from each other (counterbalance). Letting go would cause a partner to fall backwards. Shoulders are slightly back and hips are over the heels. On the *together* step of the Basic, some cowboys will touch their left foot to the side or slightly lift it off the floor for a little extra flair.

LEAD: On count *1 and*, the man pulls the left side of his body back, guiding his partner to his right side. On count 3, the man brings both hands in front of him for a counterbalance with his partner.

COWBOY SWING VARIATIONS

The man's hands must be able to rotate easily in woman's hands during any variation.

Cowboy Arch   Cross   Cuddle   Hammer–Lock

Octopus   Pretzel   Walk Through

■ COWBOY ARCH

POSITION: Two hands joined

The man lifts up his left arm (forming the "arch") and goes under as woman goes behind him, trading places. Prep: Man releases his right hand

STEPS	STEP CUE
Man steps diagonally left forward on L while raising L arm.	one
Man steps R forward while turning one-quarter L (L shoulder back).	two
Man lowers L arm and leans back over R foot, counterbalancing with his partner in a swing out position	together
Finish move with women's inside turn, page: 402	

STEP CUE: Man, Goes, Under.

STYLE: As the man goes under his arm, he bends his knees so that he does not knock off his hat.

In the swing out position, the man is not facing his partner, but looks at her with his peripheral vision. "Real cowboys" look at their partners out of the corner of their eye.

LEAD: Man's left hand guides women to his right side.

■ COWBOY CROSS

POSITION: Two hands joined

The man lifts up both hands. Keeping them together, he leads the women to his right side going under his hands, ending with arms in a "crossed" position.

STEPS	STEP CUE
Cross	one
Man steps forward on L while raising both hands	
Man moves over his L foot and turns one-quarter R (R shoulder back) while taking both hands over the woman's head	two
Woman on R foot pivots counterclockwise one-half turn	
Man lowers both hands and leans back over L foot, counterbalancing with partner	together

Uncross (feet do not move)

Man lifts both hands up, brings woman in front of him, turning her clockwise	one
Man lowers both hands to belt level and leans over his R foot, counterbalancing with partner	two
Man repeats cross and uncross	
Finish move with women's inside turn, page: 402	

STEP CUE: Cross, Lady, Under.
Uncross, Cross, Uncross, Turn through

STYLE: After the first step is taken, both the man and woman's feet remain in place, pivoting on both feet to face toward partner. Both man and woman must keep their elbows bent on all counterbalances.

LEAD: Man lifts both hands up and together and gently pulls the woman toward his right side to the cross position. The woman must allow the man's hand to twist in hers, as she goes under his hands.

■ COWBOY CUDDLE

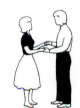
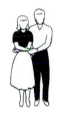

POSITION: Two hands joined

STEPS	STEP CUE
Cuddle In	one
Man Steps forward on L while raising his L hand	
Without releasing hands, the man will move his raised L hand across in front of her and up over her head as she is turning counterclockwise one-half on her R foot	two
Man lowers L hand as the woman finishes in the cuddle position close to him on his R side. Man leans forward over L foot, counterbalancing with his partner as she leans back over her L foot	together
Cuddle Out (feet do not move)	
Man lifts L hand up and gently pushes with his R forearm against her back to start her turning clockwise one-half	one
Man lowers L hands to belt level and leans back over his R foot, counterbalancing with partner	two
Man repeats Cuddle In and Cuddle Out	
Finish move with women's inside turn, page: 402	

STEP CUE: Cuddle, In Cuddle, Out Cuddle, In Cuddle, Out Cuddle, Through

STYLE: After the first step is taken, both man and woman's feet remain in place. The woman pivots on her feet to turn. Both man and woman must keep their elbows bent on the Cuddle Out counterbalance.

LEAD: Man lifts left hand up and gently pulls the woman toward his right. The woman must allow the man's hand to twist in hers, as she goes under his hands. In the Cuddle position, the man must be sure that his hands are at her waist level.

Cowboy Swing Variations (continued)

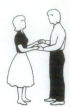

▪ WALK THROUGH (BRUSH OFF)

POSITION: Two hands joined

PREP: Let go of your right hand

The man moves through the space where the woman's left arm is, seemingly walking through the arm.

STEPS	STEP CUE
Man steps diagonally left forward on L foot while turning counterclockwise (L shoulder back)	one
Man continues to turn and steps side on R foot. Release L hand when it is pulled against R side	two
Man leans back over R foot. Bring L hand to L side (palm facing back) to catch woman's R hand	together
Woman leans back over L foot and slides R hand along his waist to reconnect with his L hand (woman's palm up)	
Finish move with women's inside turn, page: 402	

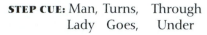

STEP CUE: Man, Turns, Through
Lady Goes, Under

STYLE: This move is often used at the end of a combination or to finish off a variation that has ended in the swing out position.

LEAD: Man using left hand, pulls partner forward toward right side.

▪ OCTOPUS

POSITION: Two hands joined

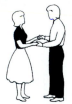

STEPS	STEP CUE
Part I	one
Man steps diagonally L forward on L foot	
Woman steps diagonally L forward on R foot, ending R hip to R hip	
Man swings both arms up and over both heads. Lowering L hand behind your head and your R hand behind your partner's head. Octopus position	two
Man lets go with both hands, and R hands slide along partner's right arm. Turn one-eighth to R and lean away catching R hands. (Keep R elbow bent.)	together
Part II	
Man raises R elbow and pulls partner to R side. Woman steps side R on R.	one
Man turns woman L (clockwise) under R arm. Man turns one-quarter counter clockwise (L shoulder back) (woman is behind man) and step side R on your R. He folds R arm behind his back and brings L hand to L side.	two
Man puts her R hand into his L hand (behind his back). Continue turning one-quarter clockwise (right shoulder back). Man leans back over R foot. Woman leans back over L foot. Man's L hand is holding woman's R hand.	together
Finish move with women's inside turn, page: 402.	

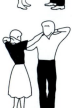

STEP CUE: Up and Over
Change Hands
Turn the lady

LEAD: Pull your partner to your right side by raising both arms.

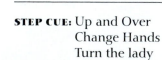

■ PRETZEL

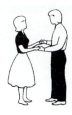

POSITION: Two hands joined; the man's hands must be able to rotate easily in woman's hands.

The man moves through three different position in one continuous move.

STEPS	STEP CUE
Part I: Man's Hammer–Lock	one
Man steps diagonally L forward on L foot while raising left arm.	
Man steps forward on R foot while turning clockwise one-quarter (L shoulder back) and goes under L arm. (Man must lower L elbow so he does not hit partner in the face.) Man folds R forearm to back in a hammer-lock position.	two
Man pivots on both feet, continuing turning clockwise. Extend L arm to L and in front of woman's waist.	together
Woman steps back onto R foot while turning clockwise one-quarter.	
Part II: Back to Back	one
Man raises L arm. Pulling woman behind him with R arm while stepping L on L foot to a slightly wider stance.	
Man continues pulling partner to R. While passing back to back man raises R arm and lowers L arm.	two
Partners are now R hip to R hip, with L arms behind the back.	together
Part III: Man turns, pulls partner from behind	one
Man bends right elbow 90°.	
Woman turns clockwise one-eighth while moving over R foot.	
Man pivots on both feet counterclockwise one-quarter (L shoulder back). At the same time man brings R forearm over his head and lowers it to chest level, keeping L hand behind. Woman is behind man.	two
Woman steps on L foot by man's L side while turning clockwise one-quarter.	
Man releases his R hand while pulling L hand and partner from behind his back. Man raises L arm to pull partner under his arm and in front of him.	together
Woman steps forward on R foot while passing under partner's arm.	
She pivots counterclockwise one-half (L shoulder back) and steps back on L foot.	
End in swing out position	

Finish move with women's inside turn, page: 402.

STEP CUE:
Man,	Goes,	Under
Back	To,	Back
Over Man's Head,	Pull Lady From Behind	

STYLE: This move must flow from one part to the next effortlessly. Once the man begins the Pretzel he does very little, if any, stepping. The woman must move around him as needed. This step is usually performed very quickly. Total control must be achieved before speed is increased.

LEAD: In Part I, Man pulls right hand (palm facing back) back and down guiding the woman to right side. Man continues to pull gently with right hand to turn woman's left shoulder to man's left shoulder.

Texas Two-Step Swing

POSITION: Two hands joined.

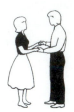

Directions are for the man; the woman's part is reversed.

STEPS	4/4 COUNTS	STEP CUE
Step L in place	1	step
Touch R to L	2	touch
Step R in place	3	step
Touch L to R	4	touch
Step L backward, a little behind R heel	1	rock
Step R forward	2	step

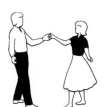

FIGURES: Swing out position. The variations occur on the first 4 counts.

1. Woman turns clockwise under her R arm, in place.
2. Man turns clockwise under his L arm in place.
3. Man and woman exchange places as he turns her counterclockwise across to his position and steps around her to her position.

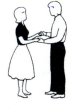

4. Two hands joined. Man raises L arm, woman steps R toward partner, turning counterclockwise under his arm, steps L as she is side by side on his R. Lower man's L, woman's R arms. Now in Cuddle position (Wrap). Rock, step. In this position, dancers may go forward, travel clockwise or counterclockwise in place dancing the Texas Two–Step. To unwrap, the man initiates a reverse roll, turning the woman clockwise back to starting position. Refer to page 404.

Ten-Step

TEN–*STEP IS ALSO* known as the *Ten-Step Polka.* A similar dance, 8 beats, is the Jessie Polka. Country western dancers call the Jessie Polka the *Eight-Step Shuffle,* or *Cowboy Polka.*

METER: 2/4 fast or 4/4 slow. Directions are presented in beats.

RECORD: Grenn 25371.

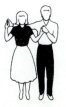

MUSIC: Fiddle music; suggested tunes: "Uncle Pen," "Cajun Moon," "New Cut Road," "On the Road Again," "East Bound and Down."

POSITION: Couples in Varsouvienne position; woman's right–hand fingertips touch man's right for ease of turn; man's left hand reaches over (fingers down) woman's left, holding just above waist.

DIRECTIONS FOR THE DANCE

■ *Beats*

Part I

1–2 Beginning left–right knee bent–touch left heel forward, left foot turned to a 45° angle, and return. Shift weight to left.

3 Touch right toe backward.

4 Brush (scuff) right heel as returning (no weight).

5 Touch right heel forward, right foot turned to a 45° angle.

6 Sweep right, heel leading, across in front of left.

7–8 Touch right heel forward, right foot turned to a 45° angle, and return, taking weight.

9 Touch left heel forward, left foot turned to a 45° angle.

10 Sweep left, heel leading, across in front of right.

Part II

11–18 Beginning left, take four Two–Steps forward in line of direction (quick, quick, slow–four times).

STYLE: Review Line Dance style, p. 447. Knees are slightly bent, keep the dance smooth.

■ *Variations for Part II*

Part I is referred to as "think steps" because the leader decides what variation to do. During Part II partners may improvise with a wide variety of maneuvers. The number of Two–Steps may be increased by an even number.

1. Woman turns under man's left arm once or twice while moving forward.

2. Man lifts right hand over woman's head, woman taking four Two–Steps turns toward the man, and moves to his left side to face line of direction in promenade position. Repeat Part II; then man raises his right arm over his head like a lariat and woman taking four Two–Steps travels behind the man. She starts to turn counterclockwise 360° (third Two–Step); her right shoulder comes to his right shoulder; man lifts his left arm up and extends his right arm down at his side, shoulder to shoulder; she pivots to face forward in original position (fourth Two–Step).

3. *The Train.* Taking four Two–Steps, woman moves in front of man, two hands still joined and resting on her shoulders. Repeat Part II in this position. Woman Two–Steps back to place.

4. Take two Two–Steps forward; on the next two Two–Steps, the man raises his right arm over her head, and the woman travels in front of man to face him. Arms are crossed, extended and firm, with right hand on top. Repeat Part II. Pivoting counterclockwise, take four Two–Steps. Repeat Part II. Man lifts right arm over his head as she travels around behind him, turning 360° as in variation 2 to face original position.

5. *Wheel Around.* In Varsouvienne position, take four Two–Steps; the couple turns counterclockwise, the man dancing almost in place as the woman travels forward. Or turn clockwise, the woman dancing almost in place, as the man travels forward.

Traditional Two-Step

THE *TRADITIONAL TWO-STEP* is also known as the *Shuffle*. The dance is done in a smooth, flowing style. The rhythm–slow, slow, quick, quick, exactly like the Fox Trot Magic rhythm–is known as a *shuffle* beat.

Different Two-Step rhythms, noteworthy for their many regional variations, exist. The Texas Two-Step is an example. Although most common in Texas, this dance is popular throughout the United States and Canada. Texas Two-Step rhythm is quick, quick, slow, or step-together step. The Traditional Two-Step is normally danced to music between 75 and 95 B.P.M. The Texas Two-Step may be danced to faster music, up to 120 B.P.M.

In the mid 1990s, Country Western dance competitions became popular. A modern style Two-Step, used for competitions, has a reversed rhythm; quick quick, slow, slow. This style is favored in urban dance studios. Beginning variations on the first "quick" creates a snappier look. In rural areas of the country, where dance is considered a social activity, the traditional rhythm is maintained.

TWO-STEP RHYTHM

The music is written in 4/4 time. The step pattern takes a measure and a half of music. It is an uneven rhythm pattern–slow, slow, quick quick.

```
4/4  |  S         S       |  Q    Q
     |  ___       ___     |  __   __
     |  ___       ___     |  __   __
     |  1    2    3    4  |  1    2
              uneven rhythm
```

TWO-STEP STYLE

The dance has smooth, controlled steps; there is no pumping of arms or bouncing. The closed dance position has several variations. The body has good posture alignment, with a straight back and knees slightly bent. Quite a bit of space should be left between partners in variations of the closed position. Man's left palm faces up and woman's right palm faces down, resting lightly in man's left; man's right arm may be straight, right hand folding over woman's left shoulder. The position of the woman's left arm varies. The woman may fold her left hand over his right elbow; her elbow is down, her arm is limp, which gives a "careless look." Her left arm may be extended to rest on top of man's right arm. Or she may hook her thumb into one of the man's belt loops on his right side. They face each other squarely, shoulders parallel.

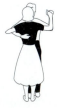

The dancers glide around the floor in a counterclockwise direction and cover a lot of territory. Although there are many variations, most dancers relax and move forward, with an occasional turn, or the man dances backward, but always they move in the line of direction.

MUSIC: Suggested tune, "Mercury Blue."

POSITION: Closed.

Directions are for the man; the woman's part is reversed.

STEPS	4/4 COUNTS	RHYTHM CUE
Step L forward	1–2	slow
Step R forward	3–4	slow
Step L forward	1	quick
Step R forward	2	quick

STYLE: The forward steps should be long, smooth, gliding steps, straight ahead. The woman moving backward, takes a long step, reaching from hip to toe. If the music is slow, for balance on the slow steps, dancers may step forward L, touch R to L (for balance), step forward R, touch L to R.

LEAD: The body leads forward.

■ *Variations*

Over the past several years, many different variations have been added to the Two–Step repertoire. Some couples appear to be *swinging* as they move around the dance floor.

The basic footwork is maintained while executing the variations, which usually start on the first *slow*. Hands stay joined, except when noted. The man's hands must always be able to rotate easily in the woman's hands. Once in position, the lead may decide to travel for a few Basics before moving on to the next position.

■ VARSOUVIENNE (Starting from Closed position)

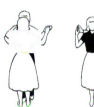

RHYTHM	CUE
S	Man lifts L hand up and begins to turn woman counterclockwise 180°.
S	Man changes her R hand to his R hand continuing turning the woman 180°.
QQ	Man steps to woman's L side continuing turning her 180° (During the SSQQ the woman has turned one and one half times)
	Man shakes L hands with the woman ending in Varsouvienne position.
S	Man lifts L hand and pulls down with R, causing the woman to turn clockwise 180°.
S	Man guides woman behind him.
QQ	Man lowers his L hand in front of woman. She steps up to his L side into a reverse Varsouvienne.
S	Man guides woman in front of him with L hand, starting to turn her clockwise 180°.
S	Man releases L hand and continues turning woman with his right hand 180°.
QQ	Man changes her R hand to his L, turning her 180° back to social position.

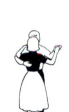
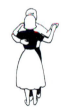

■ LITTLE WINDOWS (Starting from Varsouvienne position)

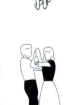
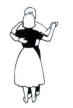

S	Keeping R hand high, man raises L hand over woman's head, turning her clockwise 180°.
S	Man continues turning woman clockwise 180° with both hands.
QQ	Bring R arm to a 90° angle, man finishes turning woman clockwise 180°, ending in Little Windows. R hips together, man facing line of direction, woman facing reverse line of direction.
	This position may be reversed by turning the woman counter clockwise two and a half times, until the left hips are together, man facing reverse line of direction and woman facing line of direction.
	Return to closed position by turning the woman clockwise one and one-half turns.

Traditional Two-Step (continued)

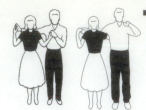

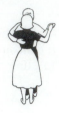

■ **YOKE** (Starting from Varsouvienne position)

S	Man lifts his L hand up and over woman's head, gently turning her clockwise 180°.
S	Keeping L hand high, man moves R hand clockwise over woman's head, continuing turning her 180°.
QQ	Man lowers both hands behind necks, into a yoke position
	This position may be reversed by turning the woman counterclockwise two turns in front of the man, guiding her to his left side
	Return to closed position by turning the woman clockwise two turns.

Traveling Cha Cha

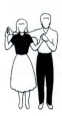

METER: 4/4. Directions are printed in beats.

BEATS:

1	2	3	&	4
Slow,	Slow,	Quick,	Quick,	Slow

MUSIC: "I Like It, I Love It" by Tim McGraw, "Big Heart" by The Gibson Miller Band, "I'm Not Strong Enough to Say No" by Blackhawk.

POSITION: Varsouvienne Position.

DIRECTIONS FOR THE DANCE

■ *Beats*

1–2	Beginning left, rock forward and backward right.
3 & 4	Cha Cha. Shuffle backward left, right, left.
5–6	Rock backward right, rock forward left.
7 & 8	Cha Cha. Shuffle forward right, left, right.
1–4	Repeat action of beats 1–4 above.
5–8	Repeat action of beats 5–8 above. On beats 7–8 raise right hands over woman's head while she turns one–half left to face man.
1–4	Man rocks forward left, backward right, cha, cha, cha; woman rocks forward left, backward right and on beats 3–4 cha, cha, cha turning one–half right under right hands to Varsouvienne position.
5–8	Man rocks backward right, forward left, cha, cha, cha; woman rocks backward right, forward left, and on beats 7–8 cha, cha, cha turning one–half left to face man.
1–4	Man rocks forward left, backward right, cha cha, cha; woman rocks backward left, forward right, cha, cha, cha turning one–half right on beats 3 & 4 to Varsouvienne position.
5–8	Both rock backward right, forward left, cha, cha, cha.

1–4	Rock forward left, backward right turning one–half right, beats 1–2, cha, cha, cha, facing reverse line of direction.
5–8	Rock forward right, backward left turning one–half left, beats 5–6, cha, cha, cha, facing line of direction.
1–8	Repeat action of beats 1–8 above.
1–2	Walking forward, step left, right, woman making full turn right under right hands.
3 & 4	Cha, cha, cha forward, left, right, left.
5–6	Walking forward, step right, left, woman making full turn left under right hands.
7 & 8	Cha, cha, cha forward, right, left, right.
1–8	Repeat action of beats 1–8 above.
1–2	Step left, right, woman crossing in front of man to his left side.
3–4	Beginning left, cha, cha, cha in place, dropping right hands, woman backs under man's left arm. Rejoins right hands behind man.
5–6	Step right, left, woman crossing behind man to his right side.
7 & 8	Beginning right, cha, cha, cha in place, dropping left hands, woman moves forward under man's right arm. Rejoin left hands in front of man.
1–8	Repeat action of beats 1–8 above.

Sweetheart Schottische

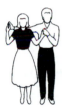

METER: 4/4. Directions are presented in beats.

MUSIC: "Queen of Memphis" by Confederate Railroad or any country song with a steady 4/4 beat.

POSITION: Varsouvienne position.

DIRECTIONS FOR THE DANCE

■ *Beats*

Starting position: Feet together, weight on right.

1–2	Beginning left, step forward, scuff right foot.
3–4	Step right forward, scuff left foot.
5–8	Step backward, left, right, left, scuff right foot.
9–10	Step right side with right foot, scuff left foot.
1–4	Grapevine left. Step side left, behind right, side left, scuff right foot.
5–8	Man: grapevine right, scuff left foot, lifting left hand to turn woman one–half clockwise.
	Woman: step right, left, right, scuff left foot, turning one–half clockwise in front of man. End facing reverse line of direction and slightly to the left of man.

Sweetheart Schottische (continued)

1–4	Man: lifting both hands to turn woman full turn counterclockwise, grapevine left and scuff right foot.
	Woman: making full turn counterclockwise in front of partner step left, right left, scuff right foot. Ending facing reverse line of direction and slightly to the right of man.
5–8	Drop left hands.
	Man: walk forward right, left, right, scuff left foot turning woman clockwise under joined right hands.
	Woman: turning clockwise once and a half under joined right hands, step right, left, right, scuff left foot. End facing line of direction on man's right in Varsouvienne position.

NOTE: The action does not divide evenly into 8 counts; therefore, the pattern will not follow 8 count phrases.

Line Dance

LINE DANCE AS A specific dance form has become widely popular. It flourishes with equal enthusiasm in schools, dance halls, clubs, and senior centers. Its chief attraction lies in the fact that since a partner is not required, everyone can participate. Formations are equally unencumbered, ranging from dancers simply scattered about the floor all facing one direction to lines and circles.

Line dancing, or nonpartner dance, has enjoyed an extensive and rich history. In addition to its longevity as a dance form, line dancing also facilitates beginning dance instruction. Its value is particularly apparent when starting a unit with line dances and *then* moving to partner dances. The major benefits of line dancing are:

- Everyone is dancing.
- Dancers have a chance to learn and practice uninhibited by a partner.
- Many basic movements may be introduced to the students as a line dance.

Many of the popular novelty and fad dances of the past such as Bunny Hop, Big Apple, and Hokey Pokey are nonpartner line dances. If all the nonpartner dances from various world cultures were added to this mix, we would have to say, without a doubt, that the line dance is the grand dame of dance!

TEACHING TIPS FOR LINE DANCING

1. When applicable, having students move to the colored lines on the gym floor helps organize the class.
2. Students need to be an "arms distance" apart. This allows them enough space to move and discourages roughhousing.
3. When facing the class, the instructor's movement should be a mirror image to the students' movement. When the students move to their right, the instructor should move to the left.

4. Rotate lines often. The front row moves to the back and all other lines move forward. Rotating lines provides several benefits:
   - All students will have a chance to be in the front row with a clear view of the instructor and the demonstration of steps.
   - The instructor has an equally good view of all student reactions and progress.
   - Rotation prevents troublemakers from lingering in the back row and creating a disruption.

5. In a large class, the instructor can watch one line at a time and assist as needed. For this technique, after a line has been reviewed by the instructor, the students sit down while maintaining their lines.

6. Many line dances face a different direction or wall on each repetition and are known as *four-wall line dances*. When the dance is repeated facing a new direction, the instructor should move to maintain a position in front of the students. This effort tends to reduce student disorientation. Once the class knows the dance, cueing the steps should be sufficient.

Line dances can be flexible enough to fit a variety of musical tastes and trends catered to class interest. In the mid–1990s line dancing was generally a country west–ern phenomenon, though not all line dancing has a country western character. Dances such as Macarena gained popularity well beyond country western dancers.

LINE DANCE STYLE

The dance reflects the style of music played: Country Western, Disco, Rap, or Pop. In Country Western Line dancing, when the hands are free, the thumbs are hooked near the belt buckle or both hands are overlapped behind the back with palms facing out.

California Hustle

THE *HUSTLE IS WRITTEN* in 4/4 time. The accent is on the first beat of each measure. Traditionally the Hustle is danced to 6 counts of music (one and half measures). The tap (touch) step is characteristic of all Hustles.

4/4	/ tap	step	tap	step	/ step	step
	Q Q S		Q Q S		S	S
	1	2	3	4	5	6

CALIFORNIA HUSTLE

There are many Hustles, some for no partners, others for couples. The *California Hustle* is also called the *Los Angeles Hustle* and, in New York, *Bus Stop*.

METER: 4/4. Directions presented in beats.

RECORDS: High/Scope RM9; DC 74528.

CASSETTE: High/Scope RM9.

MUSIC: Betty White Records, How to Hustle D115.

FORMATION: Free formation, all facing music. No partners.

California Hustle (continued)

■ *Beats*

Starting position: feet together, weight on left.

Back and Forward Steps

1–3	Beginning right, take three steps backward.
4	Tap left foot to right foot or point left toe backward. Weight remains on right.
5–7	Beginning left, take three steps forward.
8	Tap right foot to the left foot or point left toe forward. Weight remains on left.
9–12	Repeat steps 1–4.

Grapevine to Side

1	Step left to left side.
2	Step right, crossing in front of left.
3	Step left to left side.
4	Tap right toe to left foot. Weight remains on left.
5	Step right to right side.
6	Step left, crossing in front of right.
7	Step right to right side.
8	Tap left toe to right foot. Weight remains on right.
9–10	Step left to left side; tap right to left–no weight.
11–12	Step right to right side; tap left to right–no weight.

Take a quarter–turn to left to face a new direction and repeat dance.

Cowboy Boogie

C OWBOY BOOGIE, also called *Country Boogie,* is a Country Western Line Dance.

METER: 4/4. medium to fast. Directions are presented in beats.

MUSIC: "Friends in Low Places," or popular 4/4 country western tune.

FORMATION: Scattered, all facing music.

DIRECTIONS FOR THE DANCE

■ *Beats*

1–4	Grapevine. Beginning right, step sideward, cross left behind right, step sideward right, scuff left heel forward and clap.
5–8	Repeat grapevine beginning left.

9–10	Step right in place, scuff left heel.
11–12	Step left in place, scuff right heel.
13–16	Moving backwards, step right, left, right, and lift left knee up (hitch).
17–18	Rock forward left, touch right in back.
19–20	Rock backward right, touch left in front.
21–24	Rock forward left, rock back right, rock forward left, pivoting on left foot, one-quarter turn left and swing right knee up (hitch).

El Tango Sereno*

EL TANGO SERENO (Sair AY no) (Serene) has been composed as a Line Dance by Henry, "Buzz" Glass, February 1994. The composer was granted a fellowship to study in Mexico in 1954–55. He also taught Social Dance for a major dance studio in the United States. The dance may be adapted to a "Four Corners" dance or a partner or mixer dance.

RECORDS: Hoctor 45–H–640 or other Tangos as El Choclo, La Cumparsita, or Adios Muchachos. See Round Dance labels as Grenn (Top), Windsor, or others.

FORMATION: Form lines facing forward. Hands may be gracefully extended sideward. Woman may move skirts to the flow of the dance.

DIRECTIONS FOR THE DANCE

METER: 4/4

■ Measures

Introduction

| 1–4 | Wait in place two measures. Step sideward left (count 1), step right in place (count 2), step left next to right (count 3), step right in place (count 4). Repeat the above (4 counts). Note: Adapt to individual introduction. |

Part I Point and Draw, Walk 2 3

| 1–2 | Point left foot sideward (toes down) (count 1), hold (count 2), draw left foot to right (count 3), hold (count 4). Moving sideward left, take 3 walking steps (left, right, left) making a half-turn right on the third step to face right (3 counts) and point right foot down (count 4). |
| 3–4 | Repeat action of measures 1–2, beginning right. End making a quarter turn left to face front. |

Part II Step–Together Cross/Side Break

| 1 | (Like a Twinkle step or Yemenite Three) |
| | Step sideward left (count 1), step right beside left (count 2), step left across right (count 3) and hold (count 4). Maneuver on hold to face front. |

El Tango Sereno (continued)

_____

* El Tango Sereno included by permission of Henry "Buzz" Glass, Oakland, California.

2	Step sideward right (count 1), step left beside right (count 2), step right across left (count 3), hold (count 4).
3	Repeat action of part II, measure 1. End facing front, weight on left.
4	Side–Break: Step sideward right (count 1), step left in place (count 2), step on right beside left (count 3), and hold (count 4).

Part III Clockwise Circle

1	Moving clockwise in a circle (abut 4 feet in diameter) step left diagonally forward (sideward) (count 1) and hold (count 2). Step right forward and in front of left (count 3) and hold (count 4). Slow Slow.
2	Beginning a series of "quick steps," step left on top of circle (count 1), step backward on right (count 2), step back–sideward on left (count 3), step backward on right (count 4). Quick, Quick, Quick, Quick.
3–4	Follow circular pattern, repeating action of part III, measures 1–2.

Part IV Temptation Two–Step

The Temptation Two–Step has a feeling of "step–close–step" and "down up down" with a gentle thrust of bent elbow.

1	Facing sideward left, step left forward (count 1), bending knees, close right to left straightening (count 2), step left forward bending knees (count 3). Maneuver on both feet making a half–turn right and straightening (count 4) to face right side.
2	Repeat action of part IV, measure 1 stepping right, left, right and end facing front again.

Part V Get Down Step

1	Beginning left, take a short step forward (count 1), step right backward in place (count 2), and straightening step left beside right (count 3), step right beside left (count 4).
2	Repeat action of part V, measure 1.

VARIATION: One may use the Get Down Step to maneuver to face a new wall for the repetition of the dance. This makes it a Four Corners dance.

Electric Slide

Electric slide was first danced in 1990 to a pop song, "Electric Boogie." Soon after, the Electric Slide also gained popularity in Country Western Line Dance circles.

METER: 4/4, medium to fast. Directions are presented in beats.

MUSIC: "Electric Boogie" or any popular song.

FORMATION: Lines of dancers, all facing front.

DIRECTIONS FOR THE DANCE

■ Beats

1–4	Beginning right, step sideward right, close left to right, step sideward right, close left to right, step touch.
5–8	Repeat same action to left
9–12	Moving backward, step right, close left to right, step right and touch left heel to right foot.
13–14	Rock forward left, touch right (dig) in place. May swing right arm in arc, bending over, and touch floor in front of left foot on the "dig."
15–16	Rock backward right, touch left (dig) in place.
17–18	Step left (count one), pivoting on left one–quarter turn left and brush right foot forward (count two).

■ *Variations*

1–4	Take three fast slides to right, letting left foot drag, step right, touch left. Repeat to left
1–4	Or grapevine right (right, left, right), touch left heel. Repeat left.

STYLE: Bend knees on grapevine.

■ ELECTRIC SLIDE TO FUNK MUSIC

MUSIC: Any popular Funk tune.

STYLE: Bring knees up high. Bend elbows and work arms like a hammer alternately. On the rock, twist shoulders and torso forward and back. Add hops, at every opportunity. Whole body makes exaggerated moves to the music.

freeze

*F*REEZE IS A Country Western Line Dance.

METER: 4/4, medium fast. Directions presented in beats.

RECORD: MH 37.

CASSETTE: MH C37.

MUSIC: Suggested tunes: "Tulsa Line," "Swingin,'" "Elvira."

FORMATION: Line of dancers, all facing forward.

Freeze (continued)

■ *Beats*

1–4	Grapevine: beginning left, step left sideward; step right behind left; step sidewards left; lift right knee turned out, crossing right heel in front of left, then kick right foot out.
5–8	Grapevine: beginning right, repeat action of measures 1–4 to the right.
9–12	Traveling backward, step back left, right, left; lift right knee turned out, crossing right heel in front of left, then kick right foot out.
13–14	Rock. Step forward right, touch left to right. Step backward left, touch right to left.
15–16	Turning one–quarter turn right, pivot on right foot with left knee bent, foot off the floor, touch left to right. Weight remains on right. Left foot is free.

STYLE: Review Line Dance style, p. 447.

■ *Variations*

1. Funky or Hip Hop music. Use upper body and arms, turning shoulders left and right. Lift knees high.
2. Zydeco Music. Upper torso quiet, footwork subtle. Merengue step and body action.

four Corners

FOUR CORNERS IS A Country Western Line Dance.

METER: 4/4 medium to fast. Directions presented in beats.

RECORD: MH 35.

CASSETTE: MH C35.

MUSIC: Suggested tunes: "Tulsa Line," "Swingin,'" "Elvira."

FORMATION: Free formation, all facing music.

DIRECTIONS FOR THE DANCE

■ *Beats*

1–2	Swivel heels to left and return.
3–4	Swivel heels to right and return.
5	Touch right heel forward, foot turned out to 45° angle.
6	Sweep right heel in front of left.

7–8	Touch left heel forward, foot turned out to 45° angle, and return. Weight on right.
9	Touch left heel forward, foot turned out to 45° angle.
10	Sweep left heel in front of right.
11	Touch left heel forward, foot turned out to 45° angle.
12	Touch left toe backward.
13–14	Step left forward, chugging with right knee raised.
15	Step backward right.
16–19	Repeat action of beats 12–15.
20	Touch left toe backward.
21–22	Turning foot slightly left, step left forward, chugging while turning a quarter-turn left with right knee raised.
23–26	Grapevine: step right, crossing in front of left; step left sideward; step right behind left; touch left toe to left side.
27	Return left to right, stepping on left
28–29	Touch right toe to right side and return right to left. Weight on both feet.

STYLE: Review Line Dance style, p. 447.

Para Bailar*

PARA BAILAR (IN ORDER to Dance) presents an easy line dance as choreographed by Henry "Buzz" Glass, January 1997. It uses Caribbean rhythms with a dose of Latin patterns to form a delightful dance recalling a deep blue sea and sculptured palm trees with a splash of greenness.

RECORD: Limbo Rock, Challenge #45–9131

FORMATION: Lines of dancers all facing front, may be done "four wall style" or facing front and back wall alternately.

DIRECTIONS FOR THE DANCE

METER: 2/4

■ Measures

Part I Beguine Basic/Samba Balance

1–2	Beguine Basic: stand with feet about a foot apart. Bending slightly forward, step left in place (count 1), leaning sideward left, touch right ball of foot sideward about a foot apart (count and) step left in place (count 2). Now step

Para Bailar (continued)

---

* *Para Bailar* included by permission of Henry "Buzz" Glass, Oakland, California.

right directly under body (count 1), lean sideward right and touch left ball of foot left sideward (count and), then step right in place (count 2). There is an easy sway and accent of hip movement.

3–4   Samba Balance: balance forward with a Two–Step (flat–toe–flat), left, right, left (counts 1 and 2) and then backward, right, left, right (counts 1 and 2).

5–8   Repeat action of measures 1–4.

Part II Cross Step

1–4   With body bent forward, move sideward right with 7 steps crossing left (flat foot) over the ball of right foot with short rapid steps (left, right, left, right, left, right, left) (2 measures). Reverse direction, move sideward left with right (flat) in front of left (2 measures). Movement has the feeling of a buzz step with slight movement in hips and knees.

Part III Twisty Two–Step

5–8   Accenting movement with the sway of arms at waist level, move forward with twisty Two–Step (left, right, left) (flat–toe–flat) (counts 1 and 2), then right, left, right (counts 1 and 2). Making a quarter turn left, use the same pattern left, right, left and right, left, right (2 measures) to face a new wall Four Corners.

Saturday Night Fever Line Dance

THIS DANCE CONTAINS many of the disco dance steps that were made popular by the Movie *Saturday Night Fever.*

METER: 4/4

MUSIC: "Staying Alive"

FORMATION: Lines of dancers, all facing front.

DIRECTIONS FOR THE DANCE

■ *Beats*

Walks forward & back

1–4   Walk back. Beginning right, step back right, left, right, touch left foot to right and clap.

5–8   Repeat walking forward, beginning left.

9–16   Repeat actions of counts 1–8.

Walks side, turns side

1–4   Walk side. Beginning right, walk to the right, right, left, right, touch left foot to right and clap.

5–8	Repeat walking left, beginning left.
9–12	Three step turn to the right. Beginning right, turn 90° to right, step forward right, pivoting 90° clockwise, on right foot, step side left on left. (end facing back wall). Pivoting 180° clockwise on left foot, step side right on right. End facing front. Touch left foot to right and clap.
13–16	Three step turn to the left. Repeat action of counts 9–12 to the left.

Roll It (feet are shoulder width apart)

1–2	With hands at waist level, roll them around in a counterclockwise motion.
3–4	Reach behind the back and clap twice.
5–8	Repeat actions of counts 1–4.

Style: Move hips to the right on counts 1–2 and left on counts 3–4

Point

1	Lift right arm, side high right, pointing up with index finger.
2	Cross the right arm in front of the body, pointing side left low.
3–6	Repeat actions of count 1 and 2 twice.

Funky Chicken

Arms are raised, with hands in a fist by shoulders, elbows are dropped to the side, in a wing flapping motion on counts 7 and 8.

| 7 | Rise up on ball of the feet, toes together and heels out. Click heel together |
| 8 | Repeat action of count 7. |

Heel Toe

1	Touch right heel in front.
2	Repeat.
3	Touch right toe behind.
4	Repeat.
5	Touch right heel in front.
6	Touch right toe behind.
7	Step forward on right (leaving left in place).
8	Pivoting on right foot 90° counterclockwise, slide left foot to right.

Slappin' Leather

SLAPPIN' LEATHER IS A Country Western Line Dance choreographed by Gayle Brandon.

METER: 4/4, medium to fast. Directions presented in beats.

MUSIC: Suggested tunes: "Elvira," "Tulsa Times," "Swingin,'" "Baby's Got Her Blue Jeans On."

FORMATION: Line of dancers, all face front.

Slappin' Leather (continued)

■ *Beats*

1–4	Swivel, weight on balls of feet; spread heels apart, heels together; spread heels apart, heels together.
5–8	Touch right heel forward, step right in place. Touch left heel forward, step left in place.
9–12	Repeat action of beats 5–8.
13–14	Tap right heel in front twice, foot turned out.
15–16	Tap right toe in back twice.
17–20	Star. Touch right toe forward, to right side, behind left, and to right side.
21	Slap leather! Weight remains on left. Swing right foot behind left and slap right boot with left hand.
22	While turning a quarter turn left (pivot on left foot), swing right foot to right side and slap right boot with right hand.
23	Swing right foot in front of left and slap right boot with left hand.
24	Swing right foot to right side and slap right boot with right hand.
25–28	Grapevine: Beginning right, step right, step left behind right, step sideward right, chug (scoot) right, lifting left knee up (hitch), and clap hands.
29–32	Beginning left, repeat action of beats 23–26 to the left.
33–36	Traveling backward, step right, left, right, chug (scoot) right, lifting left foot behind right leg and slap left heel with right hand.
37–38	Step forward left, close right next to left. Weight on both feet.
39–40	Step forward left, stomp on right foot next to left, weight on both feet.

STYLE: Review Line Dance style p. 447.

Watermelon Crawl

ATERMELON CRAWL IS A line dance choreographed by Sue Lipscomb.

METER: 4/4. Directions are presented in beats (40 beats).

MUSIC: "Watermelon Crawl," Tracy Byrd, Atlantic.

FORMATION: Line of dancers all facing front.

DIRECTIONS FOR THE DANCE

■ *Beats*

1–2	Beginning right, touch right toe to left toe, pointing right toe and knee diagonally left. Touch right heel to left toe, pointing right toe and knee diagonally right.
3–4	Step right beside left (beat 3), step left beside right (ball of foot) (beat and), step right beside left (beat 4).
5–6	Touch left toe beside right toe, pointing left toe and knee diagonally right, touch left heel beside right toe, pointing left toe and knee diagonally left.
7–8	Step left beside right, step right beside left (ball of foot) (beat and), step left beside right.
9–10	Charleston: beginning right, step forward right, kick left foot forward and clap (all kicks are about 4 to 6 inches high).
11–12	Step back left, touch right toe back and clap.
13–14	Repeat action of beats 11–12.
15–16	Step back left, touch ball of right foot beside left and clap.
17–18	Grapevine: beginning right, step side right, step left behind right.
19–20	Step right side, kick left foot forward diagonally right.
21–22	Step left side, cross right foot behind left.
23–24	Step left side, pivoting one-quarter turn left, touch ball of right foot beside left foot and clap.
25	Take a long step forward right (both knees bent).
26–27	Slide left foot forward toward right foot, continuous motion (2 beats) ending left beside right.
28	Straighten up and clap (weight remains on right foot).
29	Take long step back left (both knees bent).
30–31	Slide right foot back to left foot, continuous motion (2 beats) ending right beside left.
32	Shift weight to left foot, straighten up and clap.
33–34	Raise left heel as weight shifts to right foot and push right hip to right side (beat 33) (right leg straight, left knee bent). Raise right heel as weight shifts to left foot and push left hip to left side (beat 34) (left leg straight, right knee bent).
35–36	Repeat action of beats 33–34.
37–38	Step forward right (beat 37) (left leg extended back with left toe touching floor), turn counterclockwise one-half turn (beat and), shift weight forward to left foot (beat 38).
39–40	Repeat action of beats 37 and 38.

Western Wind*

WESTERN WIND IS A Country Western Line Dance choreographed by Kathy DuBois, La Crosse, Wisconsin, in 1995.

METER: 4/4. Directions presented in beats.

MUSIC: "Any Way the Wind Blows" by Brother Phelps.

FORMATION: Lines of dancers, all facing front.

DIRECTIONS FOR THE DANCE

■ Beats

Rock and Cross

1–2	Beginning right, rock onto right to right side, rock onto left in place.
3–4	Step right across in front of left, hold.
5–6	Rock onto left to left side, rock onto right in place.
7–8	Step left across in front of right, hold.

Stamp, Clap

1–2	Stamp forward right, clap.
3–4	Stamp forward left, clap.
5	Stamp forward right (weight remains on left).
6–7	Clap, clap.
8	Hold.

Hips Right, Left

1–2	Shift weight to right foot and bump hips right twice.
3–4	Shift weight to left foot and bump hips left twice.
5–6	Step forward right, turning one–quarter counterclockwise, step left in place.
7–8	Step forward right, turning one–quarter counterclockwise, step left in place.

Step, Scuff, Hitch

1–2	Step forward right, scuff left.
3–4	Hitch left knee scooting forward on right, step forward left.
5–6	Hook right foot behind left ankle, turn one–quarter counterclockwise (weight on left).
7–8	Stamp right next to left twice (weight on left).

Grapevine

1–2	Step right to right side, step left behind right.
3–4	Step right to right side, touch left next to right turning one–quarter counterclockwise.
5–6	Step left to left side, step right behind left.
7–8	Step left to left side, scuff right foot, turning one–quarter counterclockwise.

Grapevine

1–8	Repeat action, Grapevine 1–8.

---

* *Western Wind* included by permission of Kathy DuBois of La Crosse, Wisconsin.

Cha Cha Cha

A CUBAN INNOVATION of the old basic Latin form (danson), the *Cha Cha Cha* is said to be a combination of the Mambo and American Swing. A close look shows its rhythm to be that of a Triple Mambo, its style that of the Rumba, and its open swingy variations that of the Triple Time Swing. It does not have as heavy a quality or as large a foot pattern as the Mambo; nor has it the smooth sophistication or the conservative figures of the Rumba. It reflects a light, breezy mood, a carefree gaiety, and a trend in the challenge steps for dancers to ad–lib variations to their heart's content. Consequently one sees variations in almost every known position.

CHA CHA CHA RHYTHM

In 4/4 time, the catchy rhythm and delightful music of the Cha Cha Cha have brought dancers and musicians alike a new treat in the undeniably Latin flavor. The rhythm has been a controversy. Originally it was done on the offbeat of the measure, and then there was a widespread acceptance of the onbeat rhythm, which is the easier way, but again the trend is to go back to the offbeat rhythm. Analysis in this edition will be done with the offbeat rhythm.

```
4/4    /              S    S      Q  Q  | /
                                         S

              2    3      4 and   1
                   uneven rhythm
```

The rhythm is an uneven beat pattern of slow slow quick quick slow and will be counted 2 3 4 *and* 1, with the 4 *and* 1 being the familiar Cha Cha Cha triple. Rhythmically the beats are as follows:

```
4/4    |  —   ♩ ♩  ♪♪♩  ♩
              cha cha  cha
```

Note that the last beat of the triple is a quarter note, not an eighth note as is sometimes misinterpreted.

CHA CHA CHA STYLE

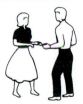

The Cha Cha Cha is seen danced in a variety of positions as it moves in and out of the variations. However, the three basic positions are closed position, face–to–face position, and challenge position (which is completely apart from but facing partner). Beginners like the facing position with two hands joined. The woman holds her arms up with the elbows just in front of her body. The hands are up, fingers pointing inward. The man

Cha Cha Cha (continued)

reaches over the top of the woman's forefingers and grasps her fingers with his fingers and thumb. The woman exerts a little resistance against his fingers. Both man and woman hold the forearms firm so that the man can push, pull, or turn her, and she responds, not with arm motion or shoulder rotation, but with body motion forward, back, or turning. The arm and hand, when free, are held up parallel to the floor in bent–arm position, and they turn with the body as it moves.

The Cha Cha Cha, with its light bouncy quality, is delightfully Latin as it carries with it some of the subtleness of the Rumba movement. The forward foot should be placed nearly flat on the floor. The knee is bent over the stepping foot. The back step (instead of a flat step that tends to give the appearance of a sag) is a toe step, holding the body firmly so as to avoid the sag. The Cha Cha Cha triple is taken with very small steps in place or traveling but is kept close to the floor. The upper body is held comfortably upright and the head focuses on one's partner in a typical gracious Latin manner. The eye contact brings the dance to life.

FUNDAMENTAL CHA CHA CHA STEPS

Directions are for man, facing line of direction; woman's part is reverse, except as noted.

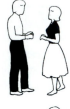

■ BACK BASIC STEP

(Challenge or Two hands joined)

STEPS	4/4 COUNTS	RHYTHM CUE
Step L sideways (preliminary step)	1	slow
Step R backward	2	slow
Step L forward in place	3	slow
Step R in place next to L	4	quick (cha)
Step L in place	*and*	quick (cha)
Step R in place	1	slow (cha)

NOTE: There is a side step on the accented first beat to begin the dance only and it is not used again.

■ FORWARD BASIC STEP

STEPS	4/4 COUNTS	RHYTHM CUE
Step L forward	2	slow
Step R back in place	3	slow
Step L in place next to R	4	quick (cha)
Step R in place	*and*	quick (cha)
Step L in place	1	slow (cha)

STEP CUE: Back forward Cha Cha Cha/forward back Cha Cha Cha.

STYLE: The back basic has the toe step, the forward basic has the flat style (see Cha Cha Cha style). Dancers have a tendency to pound the feet on the floor for the Cha Cha Cha. It should be neither a pounding nor scuffing sound.

LEAD: The man leads by pulling with his right hand going into the back basic or pushing with the left hand going into the forward basic. If arm and elbow are firm, finger resistance aids in getting the message across. The body should respond by moving backward or forward.

POSITION: The basic Cha Cha Cha may be done in closed, facing, or challenge position.

NOTE: This is the basic step of Cha Cha Cha. The forward half is also called the "forward break"; the back half is the "back break." They may be used with either foot leading when called for in a particular variation. Sometimes the Cha Cha Cha part of the step is used to travel rather than being in place.

■ *Cha Cha Cha Step Variations*

Open Break	Cross Over Turn	Jody Break	Kick Swivel
Cross Over	Chase Half–Turn	Reverse Jody	Kick Freeze
	Full Turn	Shadow	

■ OPEN BREAK

(Two hands joined or Latin social position)

The purpose of the break is to change position from face to face to side by side. The couple may open to either right or left. The right break is described next.

■ RIGHT BREAK

STEPS	4/4 COUNTS	RHYTHM CUE
Step R backward, releasing R hand hold with woman	2	slow
Step L forward in place	3	slow
Step R in place, turning one-quarter clockwise to face R in a side-by-side position	4	quick
Step L in place	*and*	quick
Step R in place	1	slow

STEP CUE: Break open turn Cha Cha Cha.

STYLE: The released hand and arm remain up in place and turn with the body.

LEAD: The man releases right hand or right turn, left hand for left turn, and guides through to the side–by–side position with the other joined hand. As the man does this, the woman should exert slight resistance against his arm with her arm or wrist to facilitate following forthcoming leads in side–by–side position.

NOTE: The left break will start forward with the left foot and turn one-quarter left.

■ CROSS OVER

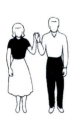

(Side–by–side position, having taken the open break to the right)

Man's left is holding woman's right hand. Start with the inside foot (man's left, woman's right).

STEPS	4/4 COUNTS	RHYTHM CUE
Step L forward	2	slow
Step R back in place	3	slow
Step L in place, turning to face woman, and release her R hand	4	quick

Fundamental Cha Cha Cha Steps (continued)

Step R in place, still turning on around, take woman's L hand	*and*	quick
Step L in place, finishing a half-turn to face opposite direction in side-by-side position	1	slow

Repeat, starting with the inside foot (man's right, woman's left) and turning back to starting position.

STEP CUE: Forward turn Cha Cha Cha.

STYLE: On the forward step, the inside foot should step straight ahead. The body is upright and the head is looking over the inside shoulder at partner. The free hand is up. Avoid bouncing, leaning forward, turning back on partner, or looking at the floor.

LEAD: The man's inside hand guides forward into the forward step and pulls back to start the turn. If the arms of both man and woman remain up when turning, the arms are ready to receive the lead when changing from one hand to the other.

NOTE: If the open break was taken to the left side, then the cross over step will begin with the inside foot (man's right, woman's left). The cross over step may be repeated from side to side any number of times.

■ RETURN TO BASIC

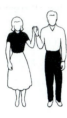

(Side–by–side position, facing right starting with the inside foot)

STEPS	4/4 COUNTS	RHYTHM CUE
Step L forward	2	slow
Step R backward in place, turning to face partner	3	slow
Step L, R, L in place taking both of the woman's hands	4 *and* 1	quick quick slow
With R foot now free, go into a back basic		

■ RETURN TO BASIC

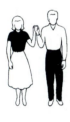

(Side–by–side position, facing left starting with the inside foot)

STEPS	4/4 COUNTS	RHYTHM CUE
Step R forward	2	slow
Step L backward in place, turning to face partner	3	slow
Step R, L, R, in place taking both of the woman's hands	4 *and* 1	quick quick slow
With the L foot now free, go into a forward basic		

LEAD: If the man uses pressure against the woman's fingers of the hand he holds just before he takes both hands, she will recognize the intent to go back to basic and will facilitate the transition.

■ CROSS OVER TURN

(Side by side, facing left, starting with the inside foot [man's right, woman's left])

STEPS	4/4 COUNTS	RHYTHM CUE
Step R forward, turning counterclockwise away from the woman about halfway around	2	slow
Step L in place, continuing to turn counterclockwise, completing the turn around to face the woman	3	slow
Bring feet together and hold	4 *and* 1	quick quick slow
Free the L foot and step into a forward basic on count 2		

STEP CUE: Out around *hold* Cha Cha Cha/forward step Cha Cha Cha.

STYLE: A smooth spin on the ball of the foot is taken on counts 2 and 3 and then a sudden hold during the Cha Cha Cha part gives this variation a bit of special pizazz. It is necessary to count the timing carefully so as to step forward into basic again on count 2. The lady is turning clockwise.

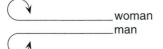
woman
man

LEAD: The man, knowing he is going into the cross over turn, will not grasp the woman's hand as he comes through from the other side but will place the heel of his hand against the back of her hand and push out slightly into the turn. He must then direct her into a back basic as he steps into his forward basic.

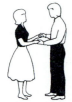

NOTE: Of course, the turn may be taken from either side. The man may use this variation as a lead into challenge position, in which case he will not rejoin hands with partner but will remain apart, facing partner.

■ CHASE HALF-TURN

(Challenge position or Two hands joined)

It is a turning figure in which the man is always one turn ahead of the woman. He will start the turn while she takes a back basic. On her next forward basic she starts the turn. After the desired number of turns he will finish with a forward basic while she completes her last turn to face him. The forward break is used with alternating feet for all turns.

STEPS	4/4 COUNTS	RHYTHM CUE
Man's Part		
Step L forward, turning clockwise on both feet halfway around with back to woman	2	slow
Take weight on R foot	3	slow
Step L, R, L in place	4 *and* 1	quick quick slow
Step R forward, turning counterclockwise a half turn, on both feet, to face woman's back	2	slow
Take weight on L foot	3	slow
Step R, L, R in place	4 *and* 1	quick quick slow
Woman's Part		
Step R backward	2	slow
Step L forward in place	3	slow
Step R, L, R in place	4 *and* 1	quick quick slow
Step L forward, turning clockwise on both feet halfway around with back to man	2	slow
Take weight on R foot	3	slow
Step L, R, L in place	4 *and* 1	quick quick slow

STEP CUE: Turn about Cha Cha Cha.

STYLE: The turn about is called a swivel turn and is done with both feet in an apart position. The step is forward, the swivel turns toward the back foot, with the weight on the balls of the feet. There is a cocky manner as man and woman look over the shoulder at partner.

LEAD: The man drops both hands when stepping forward left foot, and the rest is a visual lead for the woman. She keeps turning if he does. When the man wishes to go back to basic, he will take a forward basic while she does her last turn and then rejoin hands and go into a back basic on the right foot.

NOTE: The half turn may be done again and again. A familiar styling is to tap partner's shoulder when facing partner's back.

Fundamental Cha Cha Cha Steps (continued)

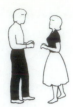

▪ FULL TURN

(Challenge position)

Step L forward, pivoting clockwise a half turn. Step right in place, again pivoting clock–wise a half turn. Take Cha Cha Cha in place, facing partner.

LEAD: The lead is a visual one, having let go of hands to start the turn and taking the hands to finish it.

STYLE: The manner is a bit cocky as each looks over the shoulder at partner. The pivoting steps are small and on the ball of the foot for good balance and smoothness.

NOTE: The man will make a complete turn while she does a back basic, and then she follows with a complete turn while he does a back basic.

▪ JODY BREAK

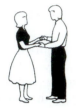

(Two hands joined)

STEPS	4/4 COUNTS	RHYTHM CUE
Step L backward, and at the same time changing hands from a two-hand grasp to a right-hand grasp	2	slow
Step R forward, and at the same time pull with the R hand to guide the woman into a counterclockwise turn	3	slow
Take Cha Cha Cha (L, R, L) in place, guiding the woman into Varsouvienne position	4 *and* 1	quick quick slow
Step R backward in Varsouvienne position	2	slow
Step L forward in place and, at the same time, release the left hand and guide the woman with the R hand to turn clockwise	3	slow
Take Cha Cha Cha (R, L, R) in place, guiding the woman back out to original position, facing man completing half turn clockwise	4 *and* 1	quick quick slow

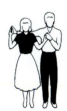

NOTE: This may be repeated over and over without changing the right–hand grasp. When the man desires to go back to regular basic, he will change to two–hand grasp and forward basic when the woman returns to facing position.

Woman's Part: Starting right foot into regular back break.		
Step R backward, allowing man to change from two-hand grasp to a R-hand grasp	2	slow
Step L forward, toeing out and pivoting on L counterclockwise, being guided by man's lead toward Varsouvienne position	3	slow
Take Cha Cha Cha (R, L, R), finishing the turn into Varsouvienne position beside the man	4 *and* 1	quick quick slow
Step L backward in Varsouvienne position	2	slow
Step R forward, toeing out and pivoting on the R clockwise, being guided by the man's lead towards the original facing position	3	slow
Take Cha Cha Cha (L, R, L) in place finishing the turn to face partner	4 *and* 1	quick quick slow

STEP CUE: Back forward Cha Cha Cha.

STYLE: Both man and woman should keep steps small and not get too far apart. Large steps and big movement spoil the beauty of this lovely figure and make it awkward to maneuver.

LEAD: Arm tension control makes it possible for the man's lead to guide the woman smoothly in and out of Varsouvienne position.

■ VARIATIONS FROM JODY POSITION

(Also called Varsouvienne position)

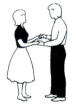

1. **Reverse Jody:** While in Varsouvienne position, both break back on the inside foot, and while stepping forward turn one–half clockwise in place to reverse Varsouvienne, with the woman on the left of the man, and take Cha Cha Cha in place. Repeat, starting with the inside foot, and turn counterclockwise to end up in original position. This may be repeated any number of times. Steps are very small. Both partners are using back break continuously.

2. **Shadow:** While in Varsouvienne position, both break on the inside foot, then releasing the Varsouvienne grasp, step forward, the man guiding the woman across in front of him. Take the Cha Cha Cha, finishing the cross over, and catch inside hands. Woman is to left of man. Repeat, starting with the inside foot and crossing the woman in front of the man to a hand–grasp position on his right. This may be repeated any number of times. Return to Varsouvienne position with the woman on the right when ready to go back to a facing position and back to a regular basic.

STYLE: In the shadow, couples do not get farther apart than a bent-elbow control. The footwork in the apart position changes on count 2 to a back–cross style; that is, the inside foot crosses behind the standing foot. The action of the changing sides with partner is done on the Cha Cha Cha beats like a running motion.

STEP CUE: Cross step Cha Cha Cha.

LEAD: The man leads with his fingers, pulling her on count 4.

NOTE: The man may lead the woman across in front of him or in back of him.

■ KICK SWIVEL

(Two hands joined)

STEPS	4/4 COUNTS	RHYTHM CUE
Step L sideward	2	slow
Kick R across in front of L	3	slow
Put both feet together and swivel both toes to the R and then both heels to the R	4 *and* 1	slow slow
Repeat stepping R sideward	2	slow
Kick L across in front of R	3	slow
Put both feet together and swivel both toes to the L and then both heels to the L	4 *and* 1	slow slow
Return to basic from either side by using the free foot, if left to lead a forward basic, if right to lead a back basic.		

STEP CUE: Step kick swivel swivel.

STYLE: Dancers should take small steps. Keep the kick low and take the swivel steps with the feet and knees close together. One may bend the knees slightly. The man and woman kick in the same direction.

Fundamental Cha Cha Cha Steps (continued)

LEAD: The man pulls both of the woman's hands in the direction of the step kick, and then he puts the hands close together and gives a push–pull action for the swivel. Part of the lead the woman picks up visually.

NOTE: The two swivel steps take the place of the three cha cha cha steps and are even rhythm, being the equivalent of counts 4 and 1.

■ KICK FREEZE

(Facing position or Latin social position)

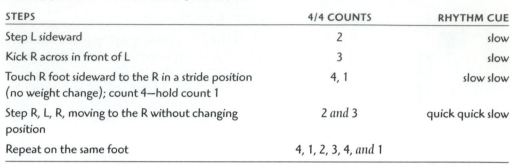

STEPS	4/4 COUNTS	RHYTHM CUE
Step L sideward	2	slow
Kick R across in front of L	3	slow
Touch R foot sideward to the R in a stride position (no weight change); count 4—hold count 1	4, 1	slow slow
Step R, L, R, moving to the R without changing position	2 and 3	quick quick slow
Repeat on the same foot	4, 1, 2, 3, 4, and 1	

STEP CUE: The posture on the freeze straightens to be extra firm and holds with the leg extended sideward. Arms extend sideward to butterfly position. The body may turn slightly to the right during the Cha Cha Cha but should end up facing partner.

LEAD: The man pulls both of the woman's hands in the direction of the kick and then suddenly increases tension as arms and legs swing to freeze position. They hold the position 1 beat. Then he releases pressure and leads sideward for the quick slow beats.

NOTE: The freeze is on counts 4, 1. These are two extra counts added to the regular pattern. It is best to take the kick freeze twice to make it fit rhythmically with the music. Return to basic by leading into a back basic with the right foot.

CHA CHA CHA COMBOS

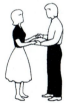

The Cha Cha Cha routines are combinations for practice, listed from simple to complex. (Partners facing, unless otherwise indicated.)

1. *Open Break and Cross Over*
   2 forward and back basics with open break
   4 cross overs
2. *Cross Over With Turn*
   2 basics with open break
   3 cross overs and turn
   repeat
3. *Cross Over and Freeze*
   2 basics with open break
   2 cross overs
   2 freeze
   1 cross over and turn

4. *Basic and Chase*
   2 basics
   4 half turns
   2 full turns
5. *Basic and Jody*
   2 basics
   4 jody breaks

6. *Jody Variations*
   2 basics
   jody break
   2 double jody
   2 shadow
7. *Basic and Kick Freeze*
   2 basics (closed position)
   2 kick freeze

Mambo

THE *MAMBO* IS A Cuban Dance that appeared on the ballroom scene in the United States shortly after World War II. It is a very free dance allowing for individual interpretation and innovation. Probably due to its difficult rhythm, it became less popular in the 1950s than the Cha Cha Cha. However, it did survive and finds renewed interest among dancers in the United States, especially the advanced dancer. Over the years it has become more sophisticated and conservative. It is most often done in closed position.

MAMBO RHYTHM

The rhythm is difficult and has spurred controversy as to whether the rhythm is off–beat or onbeat, that is, quick, quick slow or slow quick quick. Because of its highly syncopated beat, it has been a difficult rhythm to learn. The rhythm pattern described here will be in 4/4 time, that is, quick quick, slow.

4/4   —— —— —— ——
         4   1   2   Hold

A preparation step on the first two beats of the measure is helpful in getting started with the Mambo beat.

4/4   —— —— ——   —— —— —— ——
         1   2   Hold   4   1   2   Hold
          Preparation   Mambo Rhythm

MAMBO STYLE

The sultry rhythm and oddly accented beat gives the dance a heavy jerky quality, which may be interestingly thought of as a "charge." Basically, the style is Rumba movement, but as one steps forward on the accented fourth beat, it is with the sud–denness of a quick lunge, but immediately pulling back for the second quick beat, giv–ing the jerky quality to the dance. The "charge" movement is further accented by a slightly heavier step and the action of the shoulders, which move forward alternately in opposition to the stepping foot. The arms and hands are carried in a bent elbow position parallel to the floor, palms down. The arms move the shoulders and thus the Mambo presents a more dynamic body movement than any of the other Cuban dances.

FUNDAMENTAL MAMBO STEPS

Only the basic step will be given here since all variations may be taken from the Cha Cha Cha. The relationship between the Mambo and the Cha Cha Cha will also be

Fundamental Mambo Steps (continued)

noted. Cha Cha Cha variations may be found on pages 461–466. Directions are for the man, facing the line of direction; woman's part is reverse, except as noted.

Preparation Step (Used only at the beginning of the dance to get started on the Mambo beat)

STEPS	4/4 COUNTS	RHYTHM CUE
Step L in place	1	Quick
Step R in place	2	Quick
Hold	3	Hold
THE BASIC STEP		
Step L diagonally forward to R	4	Quick
Step R back in place	1	Quick
Step L sideward L	2	Slow
Hold, closing R to L	3	No weight change
Step R diagonally backward to L	4	Quick
Step L back in place	1	Quick
Step R sideward R	2	Slow
Hold closing L to R	3	No weight change

STEP CUE: Cross back side, cross back side.

STYLE: Dancers should avoid taking too large a step. The sideward step tends to increase the size of the total pattern and may look very awkward if taken too wide. The quality is sultry.

LEAD: The man's lead is a sharp shoulder action as his shoulder moves forward in opposition to the stepping foot. The woman should merely follow the action of his leading shoulder and not try to figure out which shoulder to move.

POSITION: Latin social position

NOTE: The first half of this step is referred to as the "forward break" and the back half as the "back break." It may be used as in the Cha Cha Cha.

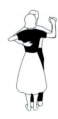

■ *Mambo Variations*

These variations are fully described in the Cha Cha Cha found on pages 461–466. Also refer to Cha Cha Cha Combos on page 466.

Open Break	Cross Over and Cross Turn
Chasse	Jody Break and Double Jody
Shadow	

NOTE: In making the transition from Cha Cha Cha to Mambo one must keep in mind the relationship between the two rhythms.

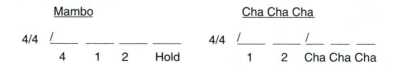

Merengue

T

HIS CLEVER LITTLE DANCE from the Caribbean could very well be a favorite with the young adult set if they really had a chance to explore it. The music is a peppy, pert, marchlike rhythm, and the dance patterns are the most simple of all the Latin dances. There are two styles: the original "limp step" from the Dominican Republic and the more even, smooth Haitian style. The Haitian style will be described here.

MERENGUE RHYTHM

In 4/4 time, there is a very pronounced beat of the music, which has an exciting uneven beat in the rhythm pattern, but the dance follows the basic beats of the measure and is in even rhythm.

```
4/4   | Q      Q      Q      Q
      |_____
      |_____
      | 1      2      3      4
         even rhythm
```

MERENGUE STYLE

Perhaps Merengue style could be described as a combination of the Rumba movement and a majorette swagger step. The feet are placed flat, but the weight is on the ball of the foot for easy balance. It is a controlled hip movement resulting from the bent-knee action with each step as in the Rumba, but it has the almost sassy quality and breezy manner of the majorette. A slight rock sideways with the shoulders to accompany the foot pattern is optional. It is not meant to be an exaggerated body movement, but the lively music and the character of the step give this dance a delightful touch of humor.

With a simple step, the footwork must be disciplined or it may look sloppy. The feet face squarely forward and close tightly together. The step is small.

FUNDAMENTAL MERENGUE STEPS

Directions are for the man; woman's part is reversed, except as noted.

■ BASIC SIDE STEP

(Latin social position)

STEPS	4/4 COUNTS	RHYTHM CUE
Step L sideward	1	quick
Close R to L, take weight on R	2	quick
Step L sideward	3	quick
Close R to L, take weight on R	4	quick

Fundamental Merengue Steps (continued)

STEP CUE: Side close.

STYLE: Steps are small, head high, focus on partner. Rock body left, right with the step.

LEAD: To lead a sideward moving pattern in closed position, the man should use pressure of the right hand to the left or right to indicate the desired direction.

NOTE: Could travel sideways any number of side steps. Should travel in line of direction.

▪ BOX STEP

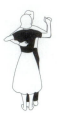

(Latin social position)

STEPS	4/4 COUNTS	RHYTHM CUE
Step L forward	1	quick
Close R to L, take weight on R	2	quick
Step L backward	3	quick
Close R to L, take weight on R	4	quick

STEP CUE: Forward together back together.

STYLE: The same foot leads each time. The shoulders lead the rock from side to side.

LEAD: To lead a box step the man should use a forward body action followed by right–hand pressure and right elbow pull to the right to take the woman into the forward sequence of the box. Forward pressure of the right hand followed by pressure to the left side takes the woman into the back sequence of the box.

▪ BOX TURN

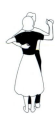

(Latin social position)

STEPS	4/4 COUNTS	RHYTHM CUE
Step L, toeing out to a L one-quarter turn counterclockwise	1	quick
Close R to L, take weight on R	2	quick
Step L backward	3	quick
Close R to L, take weight on R	4	quick

STEP CUE: Turn close back close.

STYLE: A shoulder rock on the turn makes it very easy to lead.

LEAD: See lead indication 6, p. 375.

NOTE: Repeat three times to make a full turn.

▪ CROSS STEP

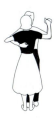

(Latin social position)

STEPS	4/4 COUNTS	RHYTHM CUE
Step L sideward, turning to open position	1	quick
Step R forward, in open position	2	quick
Step L sideward, turning to closed position	3	quick
Close R to L, take weight on R	4	quick

STEP CUE: Open step side close.

STYLE: Each step must be precisely taken in the closed or open position. If the footwork is not square with each position, the merengue loses all of its distinctive character.

LEAD: To lead into an open position or conversation position, the man should use pressure with the heel of the right hand to turn the woman into open position. The right elbow lowers to the side. The man must simultaneously turn his own body, not just the woman, so that they end facing the same direction. The left arm relaxes slightly and the left hand sometimes gives the lead for steps in the open position.

LEAD: To lead from open to closed position the man should use pressure of the right hand and raise the right arm up to standard position to move the woman into closed position. The woman should not have to be pushed but should swing easily into closed position as she feels the arm lifting. She should move completely around to face the man squarely.

VARIATION: The flick is like the cross step, except that there is a *leap* onto the left foot in open position, bending the right knee and flipping the right foot quickly up in back, and then right foot steps forward and side close as above. The man raises his right elbow as he turns to open position into the leap.

■ SWIVEL

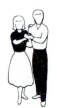

(Open and closed traveling in line of direction)

STEPS	4/4 COUNTS	RHYTHM CUE
Leap L forward in open position flick R foot	1	quick
Step R forward in open position	2	quick
Pivot on R foot to face partner, bringing L foot alongside of R, shift weight to L	3	quick
Pivot on L foot to open position, bringing R foot alongside of L, shift weight to R	4	quick
Repeat pivot on R	1	quick
Repeat pivot on L	2	quick
Step L, turning to closed position	3	quick
Close R to L, taking weight R	4	quick

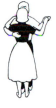

STEP CUE: Leap step, swivel, swivel, swivel, swivel, side close.

STYLE: Steps are tiny and neat, turning exactly a quarter turn each time. The body turns with the foot.

LEAD: To lead into an open position or conversation position, the man should use pressure with the heel of the right hand to turn the woman into open position. The right elbow lowers to the side. The man must simultaneously turn his own body, not just the woman, so that they end facing the same direction. The left arm relaxes slightly and the left hand sometimes gives the lead for steps in the open position.

LEAD: To lead from open to closed position the man should use pressure of the right hand and raise the right arm up to standard position to move the woman into closed position. The woman should not have to be pushed but should swing easily into closed position as she feels the arm lifting. She should move completely around to face the man squarely.

■ LADDER

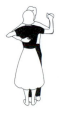

(Latin social position)

STEPS	4/4 COUNTS	RHYTHM CUE
Step L sideward	1	quick
Close R to L, take weight on R	2	quick
Step L forward	3	quick
Close R to L, take weight on R	4	quick

Fundamental Merengue Steps (continued)

STEP CUE: Side close forward close.

STYLE: Footwork small and neat. Face partner squarely.

LEAD: Moving squarely into position helps lead the body. Since there are a lot of direction changes in the Merengue, the woman must be extremely alert to the action of his right arm and shoulder.

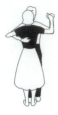

■ **SIDE CLOSE AND BACK BREAK**

(Latin social position)

STEPS	4/4 COUNTS	RHYTHM CUE
Step L sideward	1	quick
Close R to L, take weight on R	2	quick
Step L sideward	3	quick
Close R to L, take weight on R	4	quick
Step L sideward	1	quick
Step R, in place, turning to open position	2	quick
Step L backward, in open position	3	quick
Step R, in place, turning to closed position	4	quick

STEP CUE: Side close side close side open back step.

STYLE: There is a rather sudden swing to open position on count 2 of the second measure and then immediately back to closed position on count 4.

LEAD: Man uses his left hand to push woman out quickly to open position.

MERENGUE COMBOS

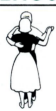

(Closed position)

1. 4 basic steps
   4 box steps
   4 basic steps
   4 box turns
2. 4 basic steps
   4 cross steps
   8 box steps

3. 4 basic steps
   4 box turns
   4 swivels
4. 4 basic steps
   4 ladder
   4 box turns
   4 side close and back break

Rumba

THE LATIN AMERICAN DANCES are to American dancing what garlic is to the good cook. Used sparingly, they can add a tangy interest to our dancing. The *Rumba* is a Cuban dance (along with the Mambo, Bolero, and Cha Cha Cha) but it has enjoyed greater popularity than any of the others, probably because of its slower, more relaxed, smoother style. The music is usually identified by the tantalizing rhythms of the percussion instruments known as the maracas, which carry the continuous quick beat, and the sticks or bongo drum, which beat out the accented rhythm of the dance.

RUMBA RHYTHM

The Rumba is written in 4/4 time and is played both fast and slow. Many Americans prefer the slower Bolero–type tempo, but actually in the Latin American countries the rumba is danced considerably faster. The rhythm is tricky as it is a 1 2 3, 1 2 3, 1 2 count in 4/4 time.

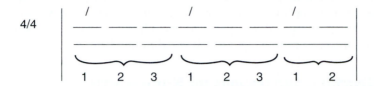

It was taught in the United States for many years as a quick quick slow rhythm, but it has gradually shifted over to a slow quick quick beat with the accent on the first and third beats of the measure. This is the rhythm that will be used in this text.

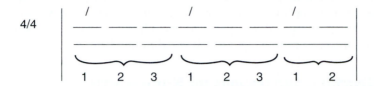

Rumba music has a subtle, beautiful melody with a rolling quality that requires the subtle rolling Rumba movement. It is seldom mistaken for the Cha Cha Cha or mambo music because of its smoothness and continuity.

RUMBA STYLE

Naturally, in the transition, the Rumba lost a lot of its original character. The style has been greatly exaggerated and distorted at times. Some people dance it like the Foxtrot, without attempting to get any of the Cuban flavor. It is hoped that dancers will feel sufficiently challenged to put in a little extra time to get the feeling of the subtle, con-tinuous, rolling motion. Three characteristics make it different from other dances:

1. The action is in the feet and the knees.
2. There is a delayed shift of weight.
3. The upper body is upright and quiet, with a focus on one's partner.

The step itself is comparatively short and flat–footed, with the knee leading. The weight tends to be maintained over the heel of the foot more than in any other dance. The Cuban Rumba movement is a springlike action, resulting from placing the left foot on the floor first, without taking weight but with a bent knee. This is followed by pressing the weight into the floor and straightening the left knee. Accompanying this press into the floor a smooth roll of the weight is shifted to that left foot. The right knee begins to bend and leads the right foot, then free of weight, into its new position. The roll is completed as the weight is transferred gradually to the newly placed right foot. Then the entire action is repeated by pressing the weight into the right foot and straightening the right knee rolling smoothly. As the left foot is freed of weight, the knee leads, shifting the left foot to its new position with the weight coming over it, completing the roll.

The knees should be bent directly over the foot, and the feet should be placed with the toes pointing straight ahead. A pigeon–toed effect should be avoided. As the feet

Rumba (continued)

pass each other, the steps are small and close together, with the toes pointed straight ahead in the line of direction. The movement of the hips is merely the subtle result of the specific action of the feet and the knees. There should be no intentional swinging of the hip from side to side. There needs to be a stabilization of the upper trunk at the waist to keep it easily upright and the shoulders straight.

The head is held with the focus constantly on one's partner. The arm and hand, when free from partner, are held in a bent–elbow position, waist level, palm down. The man does not hold his partner close. There is seldom any body contact.

The Rumba, with its open and encircling patterns, is generally danced within a small space and reflects a dignified, although flirtatious, quality.

■ Teaching Suggestions for Rumba Style

First, practice the motion described above, moving forward in a slow, slow rhythm, working to achieve the feeling of the roll. Practice in front of a mirror is usually help-ful. Second, practice the same motion forward in a slow quick quick rhythm (Cuban walk). Third, practice the motion as in the box step. Finally, practice with partner in closed dance position.

FUNDAMENTAL RUMBA STEPS

Directions are for the man, facing line of direction; woman's part is reversed, except as noted.

■ Basic Rumba Steps

■ CUBAN WALK

STEPS	4/4 COUNTS	RHYTHM CUE
Place L forward, roll weight slowly onto L	1–2	slow
Place R forward, roll weight quickly onto R	3	quick
Place L forward, roll weight quickly onto L	4	quick

STEP CUE: Place–roll roll roll.
       1 – 2 3 4

STYLE: The roll is the springlike action of pressing into the floor. The knee of the free foot bends and leads the foot into its new position, followed by the transfer of weight to that foot.

NOTE: The Cuban walk step is used for all moving variations when not in closed position. It may move forward, backward, or in a circle.

■ BOX STEP

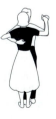

(Latin social position)

STEPS	4/4 COUNTS	RHYTHM CUE
Place L forward, roll weight slowly onto L	1–2	slow
Place R sideward, roll weight quickly onto R	3	quick
Place L close to R, roll weight quickly to L	4	quick
Place R backward, roll weight slowly onto R	1–2	slow
Place L sideward, roll weight quickly onto L	3	quick
Place R close to L roll weight quickly onto R	4	quick

STEP CUE: Forward side close/back side close.

STYLE: The knee leads each step. The feet are placed flat on the floor, in a small box pattern.

LEAD: To lead a box step the man should use a forward body action followed by right-hand pressure and right elbow pull to the right to take the woman into the forward sequence of the box. Forward pressure of the right hand followed by pressure to the left side takes the woman into the back sequence of the box.

NOTE: Students need to understand that this forward, side, close constitutes the forward sequence or forward basic and that back, side, close constitutes the back sequence or back basic. These will be referred to in the variations.

Floor pattern

start

■ *Rumba Step Variations*

Box Turn	Circular Turn	Bolero Break	Varsouvienne Break
Flirtation Break	Parallel Turn	Walk Around	
Side by Side		Parallel Turn	
		Circular Turn	

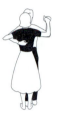

■ BOX TURN

(Latin social position)

The Rumba box step is the same foot pattern as the Westchester box step in the Fox-trot. The box turn will follow the same pattern as the Foxtrot box turn, p. 386. The style is different and one needs to shorten the step and add the Cuban movement.

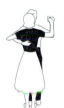

■ FLIRTATION BREAK

(Latin social position)

Starting from Latin social position, dancers will change to flirtation position and travel with the Cuban walk either forward or backward.

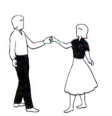

STEPS	4/4 COUNTS	RHYTHM CUE
Step L forward	1–2	slow
Step R sideward	3	quick
Close L to R, roll weight L	4	quick
Step R backward, a larger step changing to flirtation position, removing his R arm from around partner	1–2	slow
Step L sideward	3	quick
Close R to L, roll weight to R	4	quick
Step L forward	1–2	slow
Step R forward	3	quick
Step L forward	4	quick
Step R forward	1–2	slow
Step L forward	3	quick
Step R forward	4	quick

STEP CUE: Slow quick quick.

STYLE: In flirtation position, the dancers use the Cuban walk step, all forward or all back. The man steps back a little larger step when he is changing to flirtation position. Finger pressure and arm control are essential as they are the only way the man has to lead. The free arm is held up, elbow bent, parallel to the floor.

Fundamental Rumba Steps (continued)

LEAD: To lead all turns, the man dips his shoulders in the direction of the turn and his upper torso turns before his leg and foot turn. The man's left–hand position changes to palm up, finger grasp in flirtation position. Man may lead with fingers to push the woman backward, or to pull to bring her forward. Pressure should come on the quick beats, so that change of direction actually occurs on the next slow.

NOTE: The man may lead as many steps in either direction as desired. To return to closed position and basic Rumba box step, the man will be moving the woman forward in flirtation position. During a back sequence on the right foot, the man will go into closed position as follows:

STEPS	4/4 COUNTS	RHYTHM CUE
Step R backward, pulling the woman into closed position	1–2	slow
Step L sideward, changing L-hand position	3	quick
Close R to L, roll to R	4	quick
Step L forward into the forward sequence		

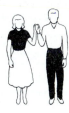

▪ SIDE BY SIDE

(Flirtation position)

Starting from flirtation position with the couple traveling either forward or backward in flirtation position, the man turns one-quarter to the right (woman to the left), to side-by-side position, woman on the man's left.

LEAD: On the quick quick beats, his left hand guides her into side-by-side position. She must then press with her arm against the man's arm or wrist to follow the leads in this position. The man may direct them forward or backward in this position, changing on the quick beats.

▪ CIRCULAR TURN

(Side–by–side position)

Starting from side-by-side position, the couple is traveling forward. The man on the quick beats will change his direction so as to move backward, pulling with his lead hand toward himself to direct the woman to continue forward. This will result in a turn clockwise, side by side. They should focus on each other over the shoulder.

a. Side by side position   ○ - - - - →   b. Circular turn (man moves backward)

□ - - - - →

NOTE: The man may return to basic box when he is on a back sequence with the right foot by facing the woman, taking Latin social position, guiding into the quick quick beats sideward left, and starting the forward sequence on the left foot.

▪ PARALLEL TURN

(Starting from circular turn)

When traveling in circular turn, the man backward, the woman forward, the man on the quick beats will turn suddenly one–half counterclockwise into right parallel position and, turning clockwise, both man and woman will be moving forward, around each other. Return to basic box as noted above.

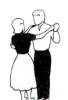

a. Circular turn:
man moving backward
woman forward

b. Parallel turn:
both man and woman
move forward

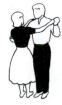

■ BOLERO BREAK

(Latin social position)

Starting in closed dance position, the dancers execute the forward sequence of the box step. Then, as the man starts the back sequence, he turns the woman clockwise under his left arm. The man continues to take the box step in place while the woman travels in a circular pattern clockwise until she faces him again at arm's distance. He has maintained hand contact (his left, her right) during this time and he finally guides her forward toward him back into Latin social position.

STEP CUE: Slow quick quick.

STYLE: The woman will use the Cuban walk when moving around clockwise and keep the man's rhythm until back in closed position. She should keep the body upright, outside arm up and focus on her partner.

a. 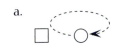   b.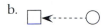

LEAD: The man gives the lead by lifting his left hand high enough so that the woman does not have to duck her head to get under his arm. He also guides her under with his right hand. His left hand guides her around clockwise and finally draws her toward him to Latin social position.

NOTE: Any number of basic sequences (slow quick quick) may be taken, and, if the partners both keep the pattern going, they can move right back into the box step when they come together in closed position.

■ VARIATIONS OF BOLERO BREAK

1. *Walk Around.* As the woman comes around from Bolero break, instead of going into closed position, the man with his left hand will lead the woman toward his right side and past his right shoulder, bringing her around behind him and toward his left side. He then turns one–half left to face her, and they move into Latin social dance position.

STEP CUE: Slow quick quick.

STYLE: The woman will use Cuban walk and keep her circle in close to the man. The man will keep the box step going until she passes his right side, and then he will go into the Cuban walk on a forward sequence and come around to his left to meet her. Both focus on each other. From closed position:

a. Bolero break      b. Walk around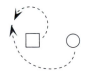

LEAD: The man should raise his left arm high enough so that he does not have to duck his head as she goes around. He will move under his own left arm and turn left to meet the woman.

NOTE: When the man and woman meet, they should go back into Latin social position and box step on whichever foot is free.

2. *Parallel Turn.* As the woman comes around in her wide arc at arm's distance, the man will move in toward her, coming into right parallel position, and they will

Fundamental Rumba Steps (continued)

turn clockwise as far as desired. The man may then lead woman to closed position or twirl the woman clockwise once around in place to finish in Latin social position. The lead for the twirl should come as the man steps into the forward basic sequence with the left foot so that the woman may turn on one basic step starting with her right foot. They finish together in the back part of the box step in Latin social position.

STEP CUE: Slow quick quick.

STYLE: They use the Cuban walk. Focus on each other.

a. Bolero break   b. Man moves forward to parallel position   c. Parallel turn

3. *Circular Turn.* Immediately after the man turns the woman under his left arm to start the Bolero break, he brings his left arm down to a pressure position against her right elbow and turns one-quarter right to be in a side–by–side position. Then the man moves backward, the woman forward, turning in place clockwise. To get out of this turn, the man turns to face the woman and steps back with his right foot into the back basic sequence, taking closed dance position.

STEP CUE: Slow quick quick.

STYLE: They must be in a tight side–by–side position. They will use the Cuban walk. Focus should be on the partner, outside arm up.

LEAD: Firmness in the arm is necessary by man and response to this firm pressure is needed by the woman.

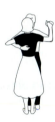

▪ VARSOUVIENNE BREAK

(Latin social position)

This is a delightful series of turns with the couple rolling from one to the other all the while keeping the basic Cuban walk rhythm, slow quick quick, going in the feet. There are four changes of position that should be practiced before the rhythm is added.

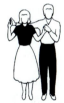

1. *Turn into the Varsouvienne position:* The man releases the woman's right hand and reaches across in front of his right shoulder to take her left hand, pulling it across in front of him, causing the woman to turn clockwise a half turn until she is by his right side, facing in the same direction. The man now holds the woman's left hand in his left and has his right around her waist to take her right hand at her right side. They circle clockwise one complete turn. To do this effectively, the man moves forward, the woman backward to turn in place.

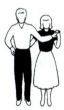

2. *Turn into reverse Varsouvienne position:* The man releases the woman's right hand and turns to his own right, bringing their joined left hands across in front of woman as she turns left until she is by his left side and slightly behind him, facing in the same direction. She reaches around behind him with her right hand to take his right hand at his right side. They continue to circle clockwise another complete turn, the man now moving backward, the woman forward.

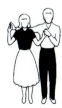

3. *Return to Varsouvienne position:* The man releases the woman's right hand and, turning to his left, brings their joined left hands across in front of him, turning the woman halfway around clockwise until she is to the right of the man. His right arm is around her waist, holding her right hand. They continue turning clockwise, the man again moving forward, the woman backward, one full time around.

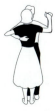

4. *Turn back to Latin social position:* The man releases the woman's left hand and by pulling with his right toward him he turns the woman clockwise halfway around

into closed dance position. He changes her right hand into his left and the man leads into the basic box step, usually on the back sequence with his right foot.

STEP CUE: Slow quick quick or change quick quick.

STYLE: Although this is described in four parts, the transitions into each part should be smooth so as to make the entire maneuver blend into one figure rather than four disconnected parts. There is no set number of Cuban walk steps to be taken for each part. The couple should turn continuously clockwise throughout the figure. Dancers should be careful to maintain good Rumba style throughout.

RUMBA COMBOS

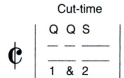

The Rumba routines are combinations for practice, listed from simple to complex. (Latin social position, unless otherwise indicated.)

1. *Cuban Walk and Box*
   4 Cuban walks
   2 box steps
2. *Box and Bolero Break*
   2 box steps
   Bolero break
3. *Box and Flirtation Step*
   2 box steps
   flirtation break forward
   and back

4. *Bolero Break and
   Walk Around*
   2 box steps
   Bolero break and
   walk around
5. *Bolero Break and
   Parallel Turn*
   2 box steps
   Bolero break
   parallel turn

6. *Flirtation Break and
   Reverse Turn*
   2 box steps
   flirtation break
   side by side
   parallel turn

Salsa

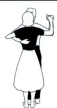

Cut-time

$$\mathcal{C} \quad \frac{Q \quad Q \quad S}{1 \quad \& \quad 2}$$

SALSA MUSIC ENTERED the dance scene in the mid–1960s when the Cubans settled in Miami and southern Florida. Their Latin music became a blend of Afro–Cuban jazz. *Salsa* is the Spanish word for *sauce* and, as the Spanish sauces are spicy, the name seems appropriate.

The Salsa is written in 4/4 cut time. The rhythm is quick, quick, slow. It is counted 1 and 2 of the cut–time beat. The music is fast and lighthearted.

SALSA STYLE

The style is very similar to the rumba: bent knees, small flat footsteps (weight over the heel), hip action of the Cuban walk as it rolls, and upper body held firmly poised, never sagging, rib cage moving subtly side to side, following the action of the feet.

Salsa Style (continued)

◼ Salsa Steps

Directions are for the man, woman's part reversed, except as noted.

◼ BASIC STEP

(Latin social position)

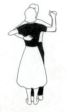

STEPS	COUNTS	RHYTHM CUE
Step L forward	1	quick
Step R backward	*and*	quick
Step L beside R	2	slow
Step R backward	1	quick
Step L forward	*and*	quick
Step R beside L	2	slow

Use basic step to turn L or R in place.

◼ SIDE STEP

(Latin social position)

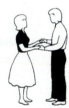

Step sideways L	1	quick
Close R to L	*and*	quick
Step sideways L	2	slow
Reverse to R	1 *and* 2	quick, quick, slow

◼ CROSS STEP

(Two hands joined)

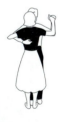

Cross L over R (with exaggeration)	1	quick
Step back R	*and*	quick
Step L close to R	2	slow

Repeat crossing R.

◼ THROW OUT

(Latin social position)

2 Basic Steps (LRL, RLR).

Man releases his right hand, gives the woman a slight push, and takes 2 more Basic Steps in place.

The woman moves away from partner (R, L, R) and comes back (L, R, L) to closed position.

Samba

T HE *SAMBA*, FROM BRAZIL, is the most active of the Latin American dances. It was introduced to the United States about 1929. It is interesting to discover how similar it is to some of the native dance rhythms of Africa. The Samba is sensitive and smooth. The music is fiery, yet lyrical; and the dance is characterized by tiny, light footwork, and the rise and fall of the body (always turning and at the same time swaying back and forth at a most deceiving pendular angle).

SAMBA RHYTHM

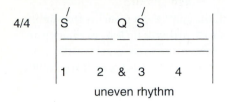

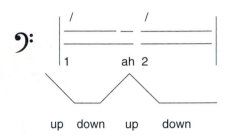

Samba is written in 4/4 cut time and may be either slow or fast, although it is generally preferred at the faster tempo. The rhythm is slow quick slow, an uneven rhythm pattern. It has a double accent, one on each of the two major beats, and these downbeats are represented by the down movements of the dance. It will be counted as 1 *ah* 2 of the cut-time beat.

The execution of the up down weight change is the secret to the smooth, springing rhythm. There is a change of weight from one foot to the other on each of the three beats, down up down, but a preliminary uplift of the body on the upbeat of the music sets the rhythmical swing in motion. The music is fast and lighthearted.

SAMBA STYLE

In contrast to the Rumba, which has a lower body movement, the Samba has a total body action. The easy springing motion comes from the ball of the foot, the flexible ankle, and the easy relaxed knees. The upper body is held firmly poised, never sagging, and it seems to sway forward and back about an axis that centers in the pelvic area. The arm, when not in contact with partner, is held out from the body, a little above waist level, bent at the elbow, parallel to the floor, palm down. The first accented step, count 1, is the largest of the three steps, the other two being like a quick-change weight step. It has been called a "step-ball-change" in the language of tap dancing. It is important to get the correct rhythm and foot pattern before working on the body sway. However, having that mastered, the body sways backward as the feet take the forward basic and forward as the feet take the back basic. Always the pattern is small and on the ball of the foot.

FUNDAMENTAL SAMBA STEPS

Directions are for man; woman's part reversed, except as noted.

■ BASIC STEP

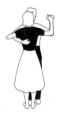

(Forward and back; Latin social position)

STEPS	4/4 COUNTS	RHYTHM CUE
Step L forward	1	slow
Step R forward next to L	*ah*	quick
Step L in place	2	slow
Step R backward	1	slow
Step L backward beside R	*ah*	quick
Step R in place	2	slow

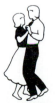

STEP CUE: Forward change weight/back change weight.

STYLE: The steps are small. Feet are close together on the change step. The rise and fall of the body begins on the upbeat with the rise of the body. This is the preparatory motion for each step. With the first step, the down motion is executed on the first slow

Fundamental Samba Steps (continued)

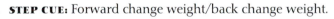

beat, followed by an up motion on the quick beat and down again on the slow beat. The body is controlled. It does not bend at the waist.

LEAD: With the increased pressure of his right hand, the man sways backward slightly when stepping forward with his left foot and sways forward when stepping backward with his right foot. The woman sways forward when the man sways backward, backward when he sways forward, so that the appearance is a rocking action parallel to each other.

■ SAMBA STEP VARIATIONS

Basic Turn	Slow Side Close	Copa Step
Forward Progressive Step	Sideward Basic	

■ BASIC TURN

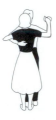

(Latin social position, counterclockwise)

STEPS	4/4 COUNTS	RHYTHM CUE
Step L forward, turning one-quarter counterclockwise	1	slow
Step R forward beside L	*ah*	quick
Step L beside R	2	slow
Step R backward, toe in, and turn one-quarter counterclockwise	1	slow
Step L backward beside R	*ah*	quick
Step R beside L	2	slow

STEP CUE: Turn step step.

STYLE: Keep the down up down motion going. Sway backward and then forward.

LEAD: Bank right arm in direction of turn, and pull into the back step.

NOTE: It is important to turn on a small base, turning on the ball of the foot, not trying to step sideward around partner.

■ FORWARD PROGRESSIVE STEP

(Latin social position)

STEPS	COUNTS	RHYTHM CUE
Step L forward	1	slow
Step R beside L	*ah*	quick
Step L beside R	2	slow
Step R backward, changing from closed position to two hands joined with partner	1	slow
Step L beside R	*ah*	quick
Step R beside L, drop L hand	2	slow

Into Forward Progressive Step (Side-by-side position)

Step L forward and diagonally outward to the L (woman R)	1	slow
Step R beside L	*ah*	quick
Step L beside R	2	slow
Step R forward and diagonally inward toward partner (woman L)	1	slow
Step L beside R	*ah*	quick
Step R beside L	2	slow

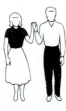

Back to Latin Social Position

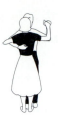

Step L, turning diagonally outward	1	slow
Step R beside L	*ah*	quick
Step L beside R	2	slow
Step R, turning diagonally inward, and take Latin social position	1	slow
Step L beside R	*ah*	quick
Step R beside L	2	slow
Into basic, step forward on the left foot		

STEP CUE: Forward step step change step step/out step step in step step/out step step close step step/forward step step back step step.

STYLE: The couple turns only diagonally away from each other and back, not back to back. When they come in, the outside hand, which is up turning with the body, touches partner's hand, palm to palm. Arm when free stays up.

LEAD: The man's right hand controls the motion and the diagonal position by reaching forward and back with the hand as he turns.

NOTE: The diagonal step should reach in the line of direction each time, so that the couple will progress down the floor. The progressive step may be repeated over and over as desired.

▪ SLOW SIDE CLOSE

(Latin social position)

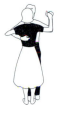

A resting step.

STEPS	COUNTS	RHYTHM CUE
Step L sideward	1	slow
Close R to L, take weight R	2	slow

Repeat three times moving left. The last time, do not take weight right but be ready to go back the other direction. Take four side–close steps to the right.

STEP CUE: Side close side close.

STYLE: The sway of the Samba is discontinued as is the down up down motion. The rhythm is an even–beat step close.

LEAD: Following a basic Samba step forward and back, the man has his left foot free. Stopping the sway and motion by control of his body and right arm, he steps left sideward into the pattern. Check lead indication 4, p. 374.

NOTE: Many beginners find the Samba basic step very tiring, so this step may be used to permit the dancers a resting variation.

▪ SIDEWARD BASIC

(Latin social position)

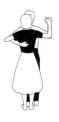

STEPS	COUNTS	RHYTHM CUE
Step L sideward	1	slow
Step R behind L heel	*ah*	quick
Step L in place	2	slow
Step R sideward	1	slow
Step L behind R heel	*ah*	quick
Step R in place	2	slow

Fundamental Samba Steps (continued)

b ⟶

⟵ a

Floor pattern

STEP CUE: Side back step/side back step.

STYLE: Both man and woman may rock the body and turn the head in the direction away from the leading foot. The steps are small. A long step is awkward.

LEAD: The man directs the sideward step with his right arm, but the body leans in the opposite direction.

NOTE: For variation, the man may (1) turn the woman one-quarter counterclockwise as he steps to the left side, so that she turns her back on the direction they are traveling. As he repeats the step to the right, he turns her a half turn clockwise. (2) They may both turn from reverse open position to open position.

■ **COPA STEP**

(Open position)

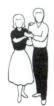

STEPS	COUNTS	RHYTHM CUE
Step L forward	1	slow
Step R back in place on ball of foot, leaving the L foot forward	*ah*	quick
Drag L foot back half the distance, taking weight on L	2	slow
Step R forward	1	slow
Step L back in place on ball of foot, leaving R foot forward	*ah*	quick
Drag R foot back half the distance, taking weight R	2	slow

STEP CUE: Down up drag.

STYLE: The left step forward is flat with the knee bending, and the body leans backward slightly. The right step backward on the ball of the foot is accompanied by a raise of the body, which stays up during the drag of the left foot backward.

LEAD: The man leads into the open position on the back right sequence of the basic step and then starts the copa with the left foot in open position. The man leads the copa action by a back lean and down up up action in the body.

NOTE: Dragging the foot only halfway back allows the copa step, when repeated over and over, to progress forward in open position. If the man opens in reverse open position, the copa will begin on the inside foot.

SAMBA COMBOS

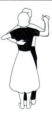

The Samba routines are combinations for practice, listed from simple to complex. (Latin social position, unless otherwise indicated.)

1. *Basic Slow Side Close*
   8 basic (forward and backward)
   8 side close (4 left, 4 right)
2. *Basic Step and Turn*
   4 basic steps
   4 turning left
   8 side close (4 left, 4 right)
3. *Basic: Forward and Sideward*
   8 basic (forward and backward)
   4 sideward steps

4. *Basic Turn–Copa*
   4 basic turn
   4 slow side close
   4 copa steps
5. *Advanced Combo*
   4 basic
   4 sideward basic
   8 forward progressive
   8 copa steps (open)

6. *Advanced Combo*
   4 basic
   8 copa steps
   8 basic turn
   4 slow side close

Periodicals

The following periodicals are of two types. The first type is an association or federation publication dealing with news and current dance events aimed at a particular geographic area. The second type is a more traditional publication that specializes in one dance form and gives in-depth coverage of the social and cultural background of that particular dance form.

Allons Danser. Rand Speyrer, ed., Acadian Music and Dance Co., P.O. Box 15908, New Orleans, LA 70175–5908; (504) 899–0615. Dedicated to preserving Cajun music and culture.

The American Dance Circle. Enid Cocke, 2924 Hickory Court, Manhattan, KS 66503; (913) 539–6306. The Lloyd Shaw Foundation quarterly.

American Squaredancer Magazine. Jon Sanborn, ed., 661 Middlefield Road, Salinas, CA 93906; (408) 443–0761; Fax (408) 443–6402. Covers Square and Round Dances.

Ballroom Dancing Times. Clerkenwell House, 45–47 Clerkenwell Green, London, England ECIR OEB.

Bridges. Lithuanian American News Journal, 2715 E. Allegheny Ave., Philadelphia, PA 19134–5914.

Contralab Quarterly. Howatt, 4155 Carpenter Road, Carlisle, KY 40311; (606) 484–3886.

Country Dance and Song Society News. Country Dance and Song Society, 132 Main Street, P.O. Box 338, Haydenville, MA 01039; (413) 268–7426; Fax (413) 268–7471; e-mail: office@cdss.org.

Country Dance Lines (Country Western). P.O. Drawer 139, Woodacre, CA 94973; (415) 488–0154.

The Dance Gypsy. 57 Sleepy Hollow Road, Essex Junction, VT 05452; (802) 899–2378. Publishes monthly calendar and sponsors dance events in northern New England.

Dancesport Magazine. P.O. Box 13, Boca Raton, FL 33429–0013; (800) ADO-8211. Publication of the American Dancesport Organization.

Dancing USA. DUSA Dept., USABDA, 10600 University Avenue, N.W., Minneapolis, MN 55448–6166; (612) 757–4414; Fax (612) 757–6605.

The Double Toe Times. Jeff Driggers, Ed. Monthly. P.O. Box 1352, St. Albans, WV 25177–1352; (304) 727–9357; Fax (304) 727–9568.

Ethnomusicology. Society of Ethnomusicology, Morrison Hall 005, Indiana University, Bloomington, IN 47405; (812) 855–6672; Fax (812) 855–6673. Good folklore and music dealing with dance.

Flop-Eared Mule. Publication of C.L.O.G. (770) 925–1475.

Folk Dance Scene. Published monthly by the Folk Dance Federation of California So., Inc., 22210 Miston Dr., Woodland Hills, CA 91364.

Footnotes. Square and Folk Dance Federation of Washington, Box 26, Puyallup, WA 98371.

Gotta Dance Magazine. P.O. Box 265, Southeastern, PA 19399–0265; (215) 695–0430. Ballroom, Country Western, Folk, Polka, Swing–New York City to northern Virginia.

Laografia. A newsletter of the International Greek Folklore Society, 6 Golden Star, Irvine, CA 92714; (714) 559–8579.

Let's Dance. Folk Dance Federation of California, Inc., P.O. Box 1282, Alameda, CA 94501.

Northwest Folkdancer. c/o Linda Caspermeyer, 1023 NE 61st St., Seattle, WA 98115–6601.

Round Dancer Magazine. Brian E. Bassett, publishing ed., RR 1 Box 843, Petersburg, PA 16669–9304; (814) 667–2530. An integral part of Round Dance legacy.

Slovakia. A Slovak Heritage newsletter of the Slovak Heritage and Folklore Society of North America, 151 Colebrook Dr., Rochester, NY 14617–2215; (716) 342–9383.

Step-In-Time. Texas Clogging Council. Quarterly. Ethel E. Wilmesmier, ed., 410 Highland Mist Circle, Houston, TX 77015; e-mail: clogdance@ix.netcom.com.

Swing Your Partner Where? Box 1750, Seattle, WA 98111; (206) 624–9699.

The Texas Clogger. Texas Clogging Council. Quarterly. 410 Highland Mist Circle, Houston, TX 77015; e-mail clogdance@ix.netcom.com.

Viltis. International Institute of Wisconsin, 1110 N. Old World Third Street, Suite 420, Milwaukee, WI 53203–1102; (414) 225–6220; Fax (414) 225–6235.

Organizations and Resources

Ballroom Dance Camps, Conferences, and Workshops. 155 Harman Building, Brigham Young University, Provo, UT 84602; (801) 378–4851.

Caller Lab. Standardization of dance programs, accreditation of callers, liability insurance, guidelines for buildings, and foundation for preservation and promotion of Square Dancing. International Association of Square Dance Callers, 829 3rd Ave., S.E., Rochester MN 55904; (507) 288–5121. Fax (507) 288–5827.

College Ballroom Dance Association. Newsletter, Suzanne Zelnik-Geldys, Editor. HPERD–116 Warner Hall, Eastern Michigan University, Ypsilanti, MI 48197; (313) 487–4388.

Contralab. International Association of Contra Callers. c/o Glen Nickerson, 606 Woodland Way, Kent, WA 98031.

Country Dance and Song Society. Promotes the preservation of American Country Dance. English Country Dance also included. Publishes *Country Dance and Song Society News* six times a year, books, and a *Group and Membership Directory;* produces records; sells records, cassettes, videos, books; sponsors dance camps. 132 Main Street (Route 9), P.O. Box 338, Haydenville, MA 01039–0338; Fax (413) 268–7471; E-mail: sales@cdss.org; Web address: www.cdss.org.

Country Dance and Song Society Library and Archives. This collection is located with the Ralph Page Collection, Dimond Library, University of New Hampshire, Durham, NH 03824.

Ethnic Folkarts Center (EFAC). Aims to visually record world leaders who have contributed to the folk music and folk dance scene. 325 Spring Street, Room 314, New York, NY 10013; (212) 691–9510.

Flying Cloud Academy of Vintage Dance. Richard Powers, Director, 3623 Herschel Avenue, Cincinnati, OH 45208; (513) 321–4878.

Folk Alliance. Sponsors annual conferences and coordinates those involved with performing arts. Music is primary focus, dance is included. Division of North American Folk Music and Dance Alliance. 1001 Connecticut Avenue, N.W., #501, Washington, DC 20036; (202) 835–3655. Fax (202) 835–3656; E-mail: fa@folk.org.

Folk Arts Center of New England. Promotes traditional dance, music, and related arts of many cultures. Quarterly newsletter; Folk Dancing Round Boston bi-monthly calendar; Folk-Fone (recording) in Boston area. 1950 Massachusetts Avenue, Cambridge, MA 02140; (617) 491–6084.

Folk Dance Federation of California, Inc. Encourages the study and advancement of Folk Dancing and related arts. Publishes *Let's Dance* and books; sponsors festivals, institutes for teacher training and research in dances, music, and costumes. P.O. Box 1282, Alameda, CA 94501.

Folkmoot. P.O. Box 523, Waynesville, NC 28786; (704) 452–2997.

Historical Dance Foundation, Inc. 31 Union Square West, Suite 15D, New York, NY 10003.

Library of Congress. Largest collection of dance books in the United States. 10 First Street, S.E., Washington, DC 20540. Information: (202) 707–2905; E-mail: lcweb@loc.gov.

1. American Folklife Center. Goal is to preserve and present programs relating to folklife and cultural heritage in the United States. Publishes quarterly newsletter. (202) 707–2905.
2. Archive of Folk Culture. Founded by the Lomaxes in 1978. Archives include dance material in tape recordings, documentaries. Available for research. (202) 707–5510.
3. International Folk Culture Center. Located on campus of Our Lady of the Lake University, 411 S.W. 24th Street, San Antonio, TX 78207–4689; (210) 436–8888. Fax (210) 436–8889 (weekdays). E-mail: ifolkcultu@aol.com.
4. Research. Will respond to questions *only* relating to material held by the Library of Congress. *Will not* respond to questions that local libraries can answer. Write to National Reference Service, Library of Congress, Washington, DC 20540–5570. (202) 707–6500.

The Lloyd Shaw Foundation. Preserves and promotes American Square and Round Dance. The Lloyd Shaw Foundation publishes *The American Dance Circle,* quarterly, Diane Ortner, Editor, 419 NW 40th Street, Kansas City, MO 64116; also sponsors camps and workshops, publishes books, and produces records, videos, cassettes. **WEB address:** http://www.flinthills.com/~lsf. **Membership:** c/o Ruth Ann Knapp, 2124 Passolt, Saginaw, MI 48603. **Archives:** c/o Dr. Wm. Litchman, 1620 Los Alamos SW, Albuquerque, NM 87104. **Sales:** P.O. Box 11, Macks Creek, MO 65786; (573) 363–5868. Fax (573) 363–5820.

National Clogging and Hoedown Council (NCHC). C.L.O.G. merged with N.C.H.C. 507 Angie Way, Lilburn, GA 30247–5239; (770) 925–1475. Fax (770) 717–0918. E-mail: clogibbs@mindspring.com.

National Dance Association. Division of AAHPERD, 1900 Association Drive, Reston, VA 22091–1502 (703) 476–3436. Fax (703) 476–9527.

National Folk Organization of U.S.A. (NFO). Networking with national groups, performing and recreational, is primary focus through exchange of information and resources for folk arts and cultural heritage. Publishes quarterly newsletter. Coordinates with international folk organizations. c/o L. DeWayne Young, 359 S. Cleveland Avenue, Blackfoot, ID 83221; (208) 785–2427.

The National Folk Organization of United States of America. c/o Ms. Lola Walker, 72 North First E., Rexburg, ID 83440.

National Square Dance Directory. Directory includes 10,000 Square, Round, Clogging, and Contra dance clubs in United States, Canada, and around the world. P.O. Box 880, Brandon, MS 39043; (601) 825–6831 or (800) 542–4010.

National Teachers Association (Country/Western Dance) Ms. Kelly Gillette, President, 1817 Lamp Lighter Lane, Las Vegas, NV 89104.

New England Folk Festival Association (NEFFA). Sponsors annual New England Folk Festival. 1950 Massachusetts Avenue, Cambridge, MA 02140; (617) 491–6083.

New England Square Dance Caller. New England Square Dance Information. New England Caller Association, Box 8069, Lowell, MA 01853; (508) 452–3222 or (800) 33DOCDO.

New York Public Library for Performing Arts Dance Collection. Holdings include 40,000 books, plus films, videotapes, oral history tapes. The *Complete Catalogue of Dance Collections of the New York Public Library* is available. Located at the Lincoln Performing Arts Center, 111 Amsterdam Avenue, New York, NY 10023; (212) 870–1657; E-mail: dance@nypl.org; WEB address: www.nypl.org.

1. Published directory in reference section of large libraries.
2. CD–ROM–copy of disc at large libraries.

North American Federation of German Folk Dance Groups. Karin P. Gottier, Editor, 48 Hilltop Road, Tolland, CT 06084.

Orff–Schulwerk Association. National association that promotes the Orff–Schulwerk approach to understanding rhythm. P.O. Box 391089, Cleveland, OH 44139–8089; (216) 543–5366.

People's Folk Dance Directory. P.O. Box 8575, Austin, TX 78713.

Ralph Page Collection. Ralph Page's personal collection of dance and music books is available for research. Special Collections Room, Dimond Library, University of New Hampshire, Durham, NH 03824.

Smithsonian Institution. 1000 Jefferson Drive, S.W., Washington, DC 20560; (202) 357–2139.

1. Smithsonian Center for Folklife Programs and Cultural Studies promotes the understanding and continuity of contemporary grassroots cultures in the United States and abroad. Produces Smithsonian Folklife Festival, Smithsonian Folkways Recordings, exhibitions, documentary films, videos, etc.; 955 L'Enfant Plaza, S.W., Suite 2600, MRC 914, Smithsonian Institution, Washington, DC 20560–0914; (202) 287–3424. Fax (202) 287–3699; E-mail: info@folklife.si.edu.
2. Film Archives. Anthropological films from around the world, dance included.

Society of Folk Dance Historians. Publishes *Folk Dance Phone Book*, sponsors dance opportunities, and preserves history and practice of international folk dancing. 2100 Rio Grande Street, Austin, TX 78705–5513.

United States Amateur Ballroom Dancers Association (USABDA). 1427 Gibsonwood Road, Baltimore, MD 21228 (800) 447–9047. Fax (717) 235–4183 Mary Schaufert, USABDA Central E-mail: usabdacent@aol.com.

The world wide web has many dance related sites. A few addresses are listed below.

1. Balkan Tunes: www.armory.com/~cope/balkantunes/
2. Eastern European Folk Center: www.cnct.com/~ginbirch/eefc/
3. Henry Neeman Dance Hotlist (Country Western, Ballroom, and Square): http://zeus.ncsa.edu:8080/~hneeman/dance_hotlist.html
4. Yahoo Recreation (Folk Dance): www.yahoo.com/Recreation/Dance/Folk/

Record, Cassette, Video Sources: Distributors and Producers

RECORD, CASSETTE, VIDEO SOURCES

The sources listed are of two types: producers who make recordings and distributors who supply retailers. Ordering from a nearby distributor is not only convenient and time-saving but, more important, it alerts the distributor to the dance records and supplies most commonly used in that area. Producers can supply catalogs of their products and suggest sources from which they may be obtained.

Alcazar Records. Excellent source for Bluegrass, Folk, Country Western, Celtic, Cajun and Zydeco, R & B Blues, Jazz, Rock, traditional dance, and British recordings on LPS, CDS, and cassettes. P.O. Box 429, South Main Street, Waterbury, VT 05676–0429; (802) 244–8657; (800) 541–9904; Fax (802) 244–6128.

American Alliance for Health, Physical Education, Recreation and Dance. Publications, products, and services catalogs. Country Western and Line Dance books and videos. Order from AAHPERD: P.O. Box 385, Oxon Hill, MD 20750–0385; (800) 321–0789. Fax (301) 567–9553.

Andy's Front Hall. Folk, traditional, acoustic music store. Books, records, cassettes for American Country Dance, including Contra, New England and West Virginia squares, English Country Dance. Many folk instruments. P.O. Box 307, Voorheesville, NY 12186; (518) 765–4193; (800) 759–1775; Fax (518) 765–4344.

Blue Ribbon. Square, Round Dance and Clogging, DJ Square Dance Records and HI HAT Square Dance Records. Producer: Ernie Kinney Enterprises. 3925 N. Tollhouse Road, Fresno, CA 93726; (209) 227–2764; Fax (209) 224–2163.

BRS Square Dance Records & Engraving. Square and Round Dance Records. Ronda & Bert Swerer, P.O. Box 319, Pinole, CA 94504; Phone/Fax (510) 724–7712.

Can–Ed Media Ltd. Publishers of Dancecraft recordings and books, folk and square dance cassettes and CDs. 43 Moccasin Trail, Don Mills, Ontario, Canada, M3C 1Y5; (416) 445–3990; Fax (416) 445–9976.

Circle 8. North 2030 Hamilton, Spokane, WA 99207; (509) 489–1364.

Country Dance and Song Society, Inc. 132 Main Street, P.O. Box 338, Haydenville, MA 01039–0338; (413) 268–7426. Fax (413) 268–7471.

Dance Plus. Over 500 strict time ballroom CDs. New releases and music list available. 2018 Granby Drive, Oakville, Ontario, Canada, L6H 3X9; (905) 849–4122. Fax (905) 849–7085.

Dance Trax International. CDs for International style, American style, and showcase dancing. 2217 N. Woodbridge, Saginaw, MI 48602; Phone/Fax (517) 799–0349; Orders: (800) 513–2623.

Dance Vision USA. Catalogue of instructional videos, tapes, and CDs. 4270 Cameron Street, Ste. 3A, Las Vegas, NV 89103; (800) 851–2813; Fax (702) 365–6644.

Educational Frontiers. Distributes software, filmstrips, videos, records, cassettes, and CDs. 132 West 21st Street, New York, NY 10011; (212) 675–8567.

Elite Records. 3350–A Highway 6 South, Suite 547; Phone/Fax (713) 980–8339.

Ewers and Mine Software. CD–ROM multimedia interactive dance instruction. 3702 S.W. Court Avenue, Ankney, IA 50021.

Festival Records. Foreign and Folk Dance records, cassettes, videos, books, and folklore imports. 2773 West Pico Boulevard, Los Angeles, CA 90006; (323) 737–3500; Fax (323) 737–3500.

Folk Arts Center of New England. Distributors of Folk Dance records, CDs, cassettes, videos, sheet music, and books. 1950 Massachusetts Avenue, Cambridge, MA 02140; (617) 491–6083.

Folk Circle Association Incorporated. Russell Acton Folk Recreation Center, P.O. Box 488, Berea, KY 40403; (606) 986–8033.

Folk Dancer Record Center. Distributing center for The Michael Herman Record Series. Single records, 45s, 33-10, and albums. CDs also available. 6290 Olin Road, Brandenburg, KY 40108; (502) 422–3655; Fax (502) 422–3655.

Folkraft Records and Tapes. Produces Folkcraft products. P.O. Box 414, Florham Park, NJ 07932; (973) 377–1847.

Gold Star Video Productions. Square, Round, Ballroom videos. P.O. Box 1057, Sisters, OR 97759.

Grenn, Inc. Producer of Grenn Records for Recreational Dancing. Square, Round, Line, and Clogging. 2775 Yellow Creek Road, Akron, OH 44333; (330) 836–5591.

Hendrickson Group. Country Dance books, music, and cassettes. P.O. Box 766, Sandy Hook, CT 06482; (203)426–9266.

High/Scope. Produces High/Scope books, records, CDs, cassettes, and videos. 600 N. River Street, Ypsilanti, MI 48198–2898; (713) 485–2000; Fax (734) 485–0704.

Hilton Audio Products, Inc. 1033 – E. Shavy Circle, Concord, CA 94518; (925) 682–8390; Fax (925) 682–8497; E-mail: HiltonAudio@aol.com.

Hoctor Products for Education. Produces and retails compact discs, records, cassettes, and videos. P.O. Box 38, Waldwick, NJ 07463; (201) 652–7767; Fax (201) 652–2599.

Human Kinetics Publishers. Social Dance cassettes. P.O. Box 5076, Champaign, IL 61825–5076; (800) 747–4457; Fax (217) 351–1549.

International Folk Rhythms, Ltd. Folk dance records, CDs, cassettes, ethnic and educational music and books, electronic equipment, imported clothing and specialties. P.O. Box 1402, Northbrook, IL 60065; (847) 564–2880.

Kentucky Dance Foundation. Folk Dancer Record Center. 6290 Olin Road, Brandenburg, KY 40108; (502) 422–3655; Fax (502) 422–3655 or Phone/Fax (502) 422–3655.

Kimbo Educational. Producers of a wide variety of dance and musical play activities, videos, cassettes, and records for school and recreational use. P.O. Box 477, Long Branch, NJ 07740; (908) 229–4949; Fax (908) 870–4440.

Lamon Records. Singing Calls, Hoedowns, Round Dances, Clogging, Waltz, Line Dancing. Lamon Studios, P.O. Box 25371, Charlotte, NC 28229; (704) 573–8999.

Living Traditions. *Roll up the Rug, Triple-time Swing, Volume 1, and Rhythm & Blues. Roll up the Rug, Triple-time Swing, Volume 2, and Rhythm & Blues & Beyond. Really Swingin' - Frankie Manning's Big Band Favorites. Cascade of Tears, 15 Romantic Dances. Popular Vintage Dances.* Cajun Music. Zydeco Music. 2442 N.W. Market Street, #168, Seattle, WA 98107; (206) 781–1238; (800) 500–2364.

Lloyd Shaw Foundation, Inc. P.O. Box 11, Macks Creek, MO 65786; (573) 363–5868; Fax (573) 363–5820. E-mail: Audio@mail.usmo.com.

Melody House Publishing Co. World of Fun records and cassettes. Collection includes American Play Party Games, American Square Dances, and many International dances. 819 N.W. 92nd Street, Oklahoma City, OK 73114; (404) 840–3383; Fax (405) 840–3384.

Musical Services. Helmut Licht–Variety cassettes and CDs of ballroom favorites. 409 Lyman Avenue, Baltimore, MD 21212; (800) 892–0204; Fax (410) 433–7948.

Norsk, Ltd. Carries Scandinavian folk music, primarily Norwegian and Swedish. LP, CDs, and cassettes. Jofrid Sodal, 770 Linden Avenue, Boulder, CO 80304; (303) 442–6452.

Palomino Records. 1404 Weavers Run Road, West Point, KY 40177; (800) 328–3800.

Perry's Place Records and Supplies, Inc. 1155 Lexington Road, Nicholasville, KY 40356; (606) 885–9440.

Princeton Book Company Publishers. Source for dance books and videos. 614 Route 130, Hightstown, NJ 08520; (609) 426–0602; (800) 220–7149; Fax (609) 426–1344.

Pro Dance. CDs for class practice or home use all in international dance rhythm (BPM). Suite 201, 1152 Victoria Street, Lemoyne QC, J4R 1R1, Canada.

Reeves Records, Inc. Square, Round, Clogging, Books, Manuals. P.O. Box 17668, Dallas, TX 75217–0668; (214) 398–7508; Fax (214) 398–4081.

Roper Records. Produces a wide variety of Social Dance records, 45s, LPs, and cassettes. CDs include ballet, tap, jazz for class use. 45–15 21st Street, Long Island City, NY 11101; (718) 786–2401.

Square Dance Record Roundup. Dealer in square, folk, line, round, and clogging records. 957 Sheridan Boulevard, Denver, CO 80214; (303) 238–4810.

Starlight Dance Studio. Ballroom Dance Videos; 6506 El Cajon Boulevard, San Diego, CA. 92115; (619) 287–9036.

Supreme Audio, Inc. Distributor of square dance and round dance records. Large collection of Square, Clogging, Country Western, Texas, East Coast Swing, and West Coast Swing videos. Source for audio equipment for instructors. P.O. Box 50, Marlborough, NH 03455–0050; (800) 445–7398; Fax (603) 876–4001.

Wagon Wheel Records and Books. Excellent source for folk, square, and clogging dance records, cassettes and teaching materials. Paul Jones, 17191 Corbina Lane, #203, Huntington Beach, CA 92649; (714) 846–8169.

Wagon Wheel/Windsor Records. Records and CDs. P.O. Box 5576, Whittier, CA 90607–5576; (562) 698–6557.

Wanna Dance Records. Saving Music. P.O. Box 69, Brookline, MA 02146; (888) 938–4700; www Wannadance.com.

Worldtone Music, Inc. Distributes Folk, Square, Ballroom, Jazz, Contra, Clogging. Producers of Worldtone Folk Music. 230 Seventh Avenue, New York, NY 10011; (212) 691–1934. Fax (212) 691–2554.

Instructional Aids: Records/Cassettes and Videos

■ AMERICAN COUNTRY DANCE

American Country Dances (1775–95). Eight Tunes. Cassette. George A. Fogg, 40 Gray Street, Boston, MA 02116-6210

Dances from Appalachia, Series I, II, III. Berea College, Box 287, Berea, KY 40404

■ CAJUN

Cajun Dancing, Step by Step Instruction. Waltz, Two-Step, One-Step, Cajun Jitterbug. **Introduction to Cajun Dancing, Vol. I & II.** (Video) Speyrer, Cynthia, and Randy Speyrer. Gretna, LA: Pelican Publishing Co., 1993. **Allons Dancer!** Randy Speyrer, P.O. Box 15908, New Orleans, LA 70175-5908 (504) 899-0615.

Floyd's Record Shop. Cajun mail order. P.O. Box 10, 434 E. Main Street, Ville Platte, LA 70586 (318) 363-4893; (800) 738-8668.

Louisiana Catalog. Cajun mail order. 148959 W. Main Street, Cut Off, LA 70345-9436 (318) 632-4100; (800) 375-4100; Fax (504) 632-4129.

Modern Music Center. Cajun mail order. P.O. Box 856, 413 N. Parkerson, Crowley, LA 70526 (318) 783-1601.

Savoy's Music Center. Cajun mail order. P.O. Box 941, Eunice, LA 70535 (318) 457-8490; (318) 457-7389.

■ CLOGGING

Any musical selection with a 2/4 time signature may be used for clogging. Square Dance music without calls (hoedown music) is a good choice when the tempo is appropriate for the skill level of the dancers. Many musical selections can be made more appropriate if the instructor uses a variable-speed record player. The following are examples of records with music of a moderate tempo.

Appalachian Clog Dance Steps (Video). Duke Publishing Co. Jerry Duke, 14 Ardenwood Way, San Francisco, CA 94132 (415) 338-1850.

Bar Clogging in St. Louis (Video). Rush McAllister, 1109 S. Taylor Avenue, St. Louis, MO 63110.

Chinese Breakdown/Rockabout, Sets In Order 2123. **Phase Craze/Pavalon Stomp,** Sets in Order 2114.

Clog Dancers' Choice, Old Time Fiddle Tunes for Clogging Practice. Bob Dalsemer. Cassette.

Clogging Appalachian Free-Style Techniques and **Line Dancing Video for Seniors.** Video Vacation, 306 West Avenue, Lockport, NY 14094.

Clogging and Buck Dancing, Dances of the World: Appalachia. Clogging groups with history and commentary. **Talking Feet,** Solo Southern Dance, Buck Flatfoot and Tap by Mike Seeger and Ruth Pershing. Country Dance and Song Society, 17 New South Street, Northampton, MA 01060 (413) 584-9913.

Dixie on My Mind, Rhythm Records RR 157. **I'm Just a Redneck in a Rock and Roll Bar;** Rhythm Records RR 118. **Trucking Fever,** Rhythm Records RR 151.

Dueling Banjos/Pitter Patter, Wagon Wheel WW 125. **Rain/Timber,** Wagon Wheel WW 134.

Gladys Stomp/Clogging Down Yonder, Red Boot Records RB 301.

Louisiana Saturday Night, Chaparral Records C-311.

Melody Hoedown, Lamon Records LR 10076.

Minstrel Man, Jay-Bar-Kay Records JBK 6018.

Ragtime Annie/Sasafrass, Blue Star BS 1612.

Talking Feet is also available from Flower Films and Video, 10541 San Pablo Avenue, El Cerrito, CA 94530; (415) 525-0942.

Ten Toe Percussion: Clog, Tap, and Step Dancing (Irish step dancing, French-Canadian step dancing, Cape Breton step dancing, Appalachian flatfooting, English clogging and rhythm tap dancing). Ira Bernstein, 179 Flint Street, Asheville, NC 28801 (704) 255-9393; Fax (704) 255-9291; E-mail: IraTenToe@aol.com.

■ CONTRA

Contra Dance Music from Western Massachusetts, Fourgone Conclusions. Record FHR 029L.

Eight American Contras and Squares as called by the dean of New England callers. Cassette. George A. Fogg, 40 Gray Street, Boston, MA 02116-6210.

Farewell to the Hollow, New England Tradition. Cassette CSWM 9860 C.

Fluke Hits, The Fish Family Dance Band. Reels and jigs, couple dances from Scandinavia, a few Cajun tunes. Cassette MAR 9012C.

Hold the Mustard, Hold the Mustard. Contra music for dancing and listening. Record HTM IL.

Kitchen Junket, Yankee Ingenuity. Traditional New England Square Dances, suitable for Contra. Cassette ALC 200A/BC. Side 1–music only, Side 2–Tony Parkes's calls.

Live from Contrafornia, The Glasnotes. Spirited collection of Bay Area favorites. Cassette AVO 103C.

Mistwold, Canterbury Country Orchestra. Traditional dance tunes. Record F&W 5L.

New England Chestnuts, Vol. 1 & 2, Randy and Rodney Miller. Tunes for New England Contras. Cassette ALC 203/4C.

Southerners Plus Two Play Ralph Page, The English Folk Dance and Song Society, RP 500.

■ COUNTRY WESTERN

Kicker Dancin' Texas Style: How to Do the Top Ten Country and Western Dances like a Texas Cowboy. 1982. Rushing Productions, 5149 Blanco Road, #214, San Antonio, TX 78216.

Let's Do It Productions. Country Western, Line Dance Videos and Manuals. P.O. Box 5483, Spokane, WA 99205 (509) 235–6555; Fax (509) 235–4445.

National Association of Country Dances. P.O. Box 9841, Colorado Springs, CO 80932.

Texas Dance Styles by Valerie Moss and Scott Schmitz. **Texas Two-Step, Down and Dirty** (Jerk, Twist, Stroll, Monkey, Hustle, etc.) PPI Parade Video, 88 St. Francis Street, Newark, NJ 07105.

Texas Two Step. Coffey Video Productions, 3300 Gilbert Lane, Knoxville, TN 37920 (800) 423–1417.

28 Country Swing Moves and Combinations. National Association of Country Dances, P.O. Box 9841, Colorado Springs, CO 80932.

■ FOLK DANCE

Single records are recommended as a primary music source for instruction. Multiband, long–playing records arranged in a series are useful and economical. Records or cassettes packaged in series form offer a variety of basic steps, nationalities, and formations. They are usually graded easy to difficult; thus they are adaptable to all ability levels. These would also be suitable for One–Night Stands. Single records or audio cassettes make it less expensive to upgrade dance selections, thus keeping dance materials current.

Easy American Dances #105 and **Easy Israeli Dances,** Yehuda Emanuel of Israel. **Favorite Folk Dances of Kids and Teachers,** Sanna Longden. **High Scope Dances.** Phyllis Weikart. Worldtone Music, Inc., 230 Seventh Avenue, New York, NY 10011 (212) 691–1934; Fax (212) 691–2554.

Easy Folk Dance Lessons for Children, Dancecraft Cassette Series. A series of six cassettes supervised by

Jack Geddes, lecture at MacMaster University School of Physical Education (Canada). The series contains graded dnaces from a number of nationalities based on locomotor skills. Dance directions accompany each cassette. Series numbers are DC 387, 487, 587, 687, 787, 887.

Folk Dances from 'Round the World, Merit Audio Visual. A seven–album series containing twelve or more dances each from the United States and abroad. Each album presents steps for dancers of increasing ability. Well–illustrated manuals of dance instructions accompany each album. It is especially useful to beginning folk dance teachers. (Formerly the RCA Victor Series supervised by Michael and Mary Ann Herman.)

Folkdances 1, 2, 3, 4. High/Scope Videos, 600 N. River Street, Ypsilanti, MI 48190–2898.

International Dance Discovery. Publishes a Folk/Ethnic Dance Video catalogue. 1025 South Minor Road, Bloomington, IN 47401 (313) 485–0704; Fax (313) 485–2000.

Michael Herman Record Series. Folk Dancer Record Center, 6290 Olin Road, Brandenburg, KY 40108. Phone/Fax (502) 422–3655.

Pericles in America. Video of Greek dance and Pericles Halkias, Greek clarinet player. **Salute to Immigrant Cultures.** Film, three days of folk dance in Manhattan. Ethnic Folkarts Center (EFAC), 325 Spring Street, Room 314, New York, NY 10013 (212) 691–9510.

■ LINE DANCE

Brentwood House Video. 5740 Corsa Avenue, Suite 102, Westlake Village, CA 91362.

Country Line Dancing for Kids. Country Line Dancing. More Country Line Dancing. Diane Horner. Quality Video, Inc., 7399 Bush Lake Road, Minneapolis, MN 55439.

Fun and Funky Freestyle Dancing. Line Dancing. Line Dancing, Vol. 2. New Line Dancing. Christy Lane. Brentwood House Video, 5740 Corsa Avenue, Suite 102, Westlake Village, CA 91362.

Line Dancing for Seniors, Vol. I. Grant F. Longley. New England Caller, Inc., P.O. Box 8069, Lowell, MA 01853.

■ ONE-NIGHT STANDS

Suggested One–Night Stands Records/Cassettes: Lloyd Shaw–Elementary Kit. Melody House (World of Fun).

When the Work's All Done. A Square Dance Party for Beginners and Old Hands. Bob Dalsemer. TC 125C (with), TC 126 (without).

■ SOCIAL DANCE

Music for Social Dance or Ballroom Dance is subject to the particular "sound" in vogue in each generation. "Standards" are records that are recognized by musicians and public alike as favorites and do, indeed, survive several generations. In addition to local distributors, the four most extensive sources are: Grenn, Hoctor, Roper, and Windsor. Refer to Appendix C for distributors.

Amuse-A-Mood Co. Catalogue of books, manuals, instructional tapes, and videos. Booklets covering dance steps (beginner to advanced), history of swing and music fundamentals. 128 Hancock Place N.E., Leesburg, VA 22075.

Arthur Murray Dance Magic Series: Waltz, Tango, Swing, Samba, Merengue, Night Club, Rumba, Salsa, Cha Cha, Dancin' Dirty, Fox Trot, Mambo. Princeton Book Co., 12 West Delaware Avenue, Pennington, NJ 08534 (800) 220-7149; Fax (609) 737-1869.

B & M Dance Productions (AD). American Social Dance instructional videos–beginner to advanced. "How-To" tapes teach beginner to advanced steps. 6804 Newbold, Bethesda, MD 20817.

Betty White Reocrds. **Foxtrot** D101; **Waltz** D102; **Cha Cha Cha** D103; **Rumba** D104; **Mambo** D105; **Tango** D106; **Charleston** D107; **Lindy** D109; **Merengue and Samba** D110.

Windsor Ballroom Dance Records, 45s, LPs.

Charleston. Hip Hop. Hoctor Products for Education, P.O. Box 38, Waldwick, NJ 07463 (201) 652-7767; Fax (201) 652-2599.

Club Salsa, Vol. 1. Moves for salsa and mambo, variations with turn combinations. Video, 46 minutes. **Club Salsa, Vol. 2.** Longer turn combinations, added step patterns, tips on leading and following. Video, 54 minutes. **Dance Time.** Video, 45 minutes. **Dance with Me, Vol. 1.** Foxtrot, Waltz, Tango, and Rumba. **Dance with Me, Vol. 2.** Mambo, Cha–Cha, and Swing. **Let's Lindy Hop, Vol. 1.** Video, 45 minutes. **Let's Lindy Hop, Vol. 2.** Video, 51 minutes. Mad Degrees Productions, P.O. Box 2945, Beverly Hills, CA 90213-2945 (800) 326-4997.

Complete Guide to Party Dance. Christy Lane's new video of most requested party dances: Electric Slide, YMCA, Macarena, Chicken Dance, Stroll, Conga, Hand Jive, Swing, etc. National Dance Association, Attn: Millie Puccio, 1900 Association Drive, Reston, VA 20191-1598.

Dance Lovers. VHS videos, music, and tapes. P.O. Box 7071, Asheville, NC 28802.

Dancing Times Limited. Extensive stock of Ballroom Dancing Times books and videos. 45–47 Clerkenwell Green, London, EC1R OEB, England.

Fred Astaire Dancing: Ballroom (Foxtrot, Waltz), **Latin** (Cha Cha, Salsa). Best Film and Video Corp., Great Neck, NY 11021.

Not Strictly Ballroom: Social Dance Library of Video Tapes. Eight tapes cover Fox Trot, Waltz, Tango, Viennese Waltz, Rumba, Cha Cha, East Coast Swing, Samba, Mambo, Merengue, West Coast Swing and Country Western Dances: Two-Step, Waltz, Polka, Cha Cha, Eastern Swing, Western Swing, Country Line Dances, the "B.C." Vance Productions, c/o Colortech Video Productions, 4501 College Boulevard, Suite 110, Shawnee Mission, KS 66211-9989.

Pattern Ballroom Dances for Seniors. Video of 27 Dances, 1992. Mary J. Sarver, 1224 S.W. Normandy Terrace, Seattle, WA 98166.

Rhythm Dances (Polka and Regional dances, Samba, Merengue, Swing, Mambo, Cha Cha and Rumba). **Smooth Dances** (Fox Trot, Waltz, Tango). Myrna Martin Schild, SIU Box 1126, Edwardsville, IL 62026.

Savoy-Style Lindy Hop, Levels 1, 2, 3 (Video). **Shim Sham** (Video). Swing/Tap line from the '30s and '40s. Other videos, CDs and cassettes. Living Traditions, 2442 N.W. Market Street, #168, Seattle, WA 98107 (206) 781-1238; (800) 500-2364.

Supreme Audio, Inc. Large collection of Square, Clogging, Country Western, Texas, East Coast Swing, and West Coast Swing videos. P.O. Box 50, Marlborough, NH 03455-0050; (800) 445-7398; Fax (603) 876-4001.

Tango–Argentine Style. Instructional video by Alberto Toledano and Loreen Arbus. Tanguero Productions, 5351 Corteen Place, Code AD11, North Hollywood, CA 91607.

West Coast Swing: International Dancing in America Series. Skippy Blair. R & R Video–International Dancing in America Series, 3649 Whittier Boulevard, Los Angeles, CA 90023.

■ SQUARE DANCE

Records without calls should be chosen for musical key, beat, and overall good phrasing. Callers and teachers who specialize in patter calls will find a welath of instrumentals or Hoedowns available. Instructors should listen to and select their own background music.

Records with calls are excellent supplementary instructional aids. Videos add a visual as well as an auditory dimension during the beginning learning stages.

Smoke on the Water. Square Dance Classics, Bob Dalsemer. TC 123C (with), TC 124C (without).

Square Dance Party for the New Dancer, No. 1. Bob Ruff, Wagon Wheel Cassette or LP 1001. Includes eight singing calls, 1 Contra, and 1 Hoedown. Callerlab movements 1–22.

Square Dance Party for the New Dancer, No. 2. Bob Ruff, Wagon Wheel Cassette or LP 1002. Includes eight singing calls, 1 Contra, 1 Hoedown. Callerlab movements 1–34.

Square Dance Videos, A Division of Tra Bien, Inc. Mainstream, Basic, and Plus. P.O. Box 1350, Maplewood, NJ 07040.

Suggested Hoedown Records:

Banjo Plucking/The Other Side. Wagon Wheel 126.

Bill John/Freddies Fancy. Wagon Wheel 121.

Dueling Banjo/Pitter Patter. Wagon Wheel 125.

Get Down Number One/Long Journey. Windsor 4167.

Golden Reel/Chordex. Windsor 4166.

Rock Island Ride/Mt. Mist. Windsor 4185.

Sherbrooks. Grenn 12204.

Sugarfoot Rag. Grenn 12201.

Yellow Creek. Grenn 12209.

VIDEOS

Allons Danser! Randy Speyrer, P.O. Box 15908, New Orleans, LA 70175–5908; (504) 899–0615. "Cajun Dancing" step by step instruction. Waltz, Two-Step, One-Step, Cajun Jitterbug.

Best Film and Video Carpo., Great Neck, NY 11021. "Fred Astaire Dancing: Ballroom (Fox Trot, Waltz), Latin (Cha Cha, Salsa)."

Brentwood House Video. 5740 Corsa Ave., Suite 102, Westlake Village, CA 91362. "Line Dancing," "New Line Dancing," "Fun and Funky Freestyle Dancing,"

Coffey Video Productions. 3300 Gilbert Lane, Knoxville, TN 37920; (800) 423–1417. "Texas Two Step."

Country Dance and Song Society. 17 New South Street, Northampton, MA 01060; (413) 584–9913. "Clogging and Buck Dancing," "Dances of the World: Appalachia." Clogging groups with history and commentary. "Talking Feet" Solo Southern Dance, Buck Flatfoot and Tap by Mike Seeger and Ruth Pershing.

Duke Publishing Co. Jerry Duke, 14 Ardenwood Way, San Francisco, CA 94132; (415) 338–1850. "Appalachian Clog Dance Steps."

Ethnic Folkarts Center (EFAC). 325 Spring St., Room 314, New York, NY 10013; (212) 691–9510. "Pericles in America" video of Greek dance and Pericles Halkias, Greek clarinet player; "Salute to Immigrant Cultures" film, three days of folk dance in Manhattan.

Flower Films and Video. 10341 San Pablo Avenue, El Cerrito, CA 94530; (415) 525–0942. "Talking Feet" Solo Southern dance: buck, flatfoot, and tap by Mike Seeger and Ruth Pershing.

Folk/Ethnic Dance Videos Catalogue. Published by International Dance Discovery, 1025 South Minor Road, Bloomington, IN 47401.

High/Scope Videos. 600 N. River Street, Ypsilanti, MI 48198–2898; (313) 485–2000; Fax (313) 485–0704. "Folk-dances" 1, 2, 3, 4.

Hoctor Products for Education. P.O. Box 38, Waldwick, NJ 07463; (201) 652–7767; Fax (201) 652–2599. "Hip Hop," "Charleston."

National Association of Country Dances. P.O. Box 9841, Colorado Springs, CO 80932. "28 Country Swing Moves and Combinations."

New England Caller, Inc. P.O. Box 8069, Lowell, MA 01853. "Line Dancing for Seniors, Vol. I," Grant F. Longley.

PPI Parade Video. 88 St. Francis St., Newark, NJ 07105. "Texas Dance Styles" by Valerie Moss and Scott Schmitz; "texas Two–Step," "Down and Dirty" (Jerk, Twist, Stroll, Monkey, Hustle, etc.).

Princeton Book Co. 12 West Delaware Avenue, Pennington, NJ 08534. "Arthur Murray Dance Magic Series." Waltz, Tango, Swing, Samba, Merengue, Night Club, Rumba, Salsa, Cha Cha, Dancin' Dirty, Fox Trot, Mambo.

Quality Video Inc. 7399 Bush Lake Road, Minneapolis, MN 55439. "Country Line Dancing for Kids," "Country Line Dancing," "More Country Line Dancing," Diane Horner.

R & R Video International Dancing in America Series. 3649 Whittier Blvd., Los Angeles, CA 90023. "West Coast Swing," Skippy Blair.

Rushing Productions. 5149 Blanco Rd., #214, San Antonio, TX 78216. "Kicker Dancin' Texas Style." How to do the top ten Country and Western Dances like a Texas cowboy, 1982.

Sarver, Mary J. 1224 SW Normandy Terrace, Seattle, WA 98166. "Pattern Ballroom Dances for Seniors," 27 dances, 1992.

Schild, Myrna Martin. SIU Box 1126, Edwardsville, IL 62026. "Smooth Dances" (Fox Trot, Waltz, Tango). "Rhythm Dances" (Polka and Regional Dances, Samba, Merengue, Swing, Mambo, Cha Cha, and Rumba).

Supreme Audio, Inc. P.O. Box 50, Marlborough, NH 03455–0050; (800) 445–7398; Fax (603) 876–4001. Large collection of Square, Clogging, Country Western, Texas, East aCoast Swing, and West Coast Swing videos.

Video Vacation. 306 West Ave., Lockport, NY 14094. "Line Dancing Video for Seniors," "Clogging Appalachian Free-Style Techniques."

Wagon Wheel Records and Books. Bob Ruff, 8459 Edmaru Ave., Whittier, CA 90605; (310) 693–6976. "The Fundamentals of Square Dancing," Parts I & II.

Worldtone Music, Inc. 230 Seventh Avenue, New York, NY 10011; (212) 691–1934; Fax (212) 691–2554. "High Scope Dances," Phyllis Weikart; "Favorite Folk Dances of Kids and Teachers," Sanna Longden; "Easy American Dances #105" and "Easy Israeli Dances," Yehuda Emanuel of Israel.

Bibliography

GENERAL

Armstrong, Alan. *Maori Games and Hakas.* Wellington, New Zealand; St. Paul, Auckland, New Zealand and Sidney, Australia: A. H. & A. W. Reed, 1971.

Bandem, I. Made, and Fredrik Eugene deBoer. *Kaja and Kelod Balinese Dance in Transition.* Oxford, New York, Melbourne, Kuala Lumpur: Oxford University Press, 1981.

Beliajus, Vyts F. "Choson–Korea, Land of the Morning Calm," *Viltis*, vol. 31, no. 5, Jan.–Feb. 1973, pp. 5–16. "Traditional Korean Dance," pp. 7–10; "Musical Instruments of Korea," pp. 10–11; "Korean Folk Mask Drama," pp. 12–15.

Basso, Keith H. *The Gift of Changing Woman.* Anthropological Papers, No. 76. Smithsonian Institute, Bureau of American Ethnology. U.S. Government Printing Office, Washington, D.C., 1966.

Bauer, Marion, and Ethel R. Peyser. *Music Through the Ages: An Introduction to Music History.* 3rd ed. Revised by Elizabeth E. Rogers, ed. New York: G. P. Putnam's Sons, 1967.

Botkin, B. A. "The Play–Party in Oklahoma," *Follow the Drinkin' Gou'd.* J. Frank Dobie, ed. Publications of the Texas Folk–Lore Society, no. VII. Austin, TX: Texas Folk–Lore Society, 1928.

Bowers, Faubion. *Theatre in the East, A Survey of Asian Dance and Drama.* New York: Thomas Nelson & Sons, 1956.

———. *The Dance in India.* New York: Columbia University Press, 1953.

Campbell, Joseph. "The Ancient Hawaiian Hulas," *Dance Observer*, vol. 13, no. 3, 1946, pp. 32–33.

Chapline, Claudia. "Dance and Religion," *Journal of Health, Physical Education and Recreation*, vol. 28, no. 8, November 1957, p. 39.

Costa, Mazeppa King. "Dance in the Society and Hawaiian Islands Presented by Early Writers 1767–1842." Master of Arts thesis, University of Hawaii, 1951.

Craddock, John R. "The Cowboy Dance," *Coffee in the Gourd.* J. Frank Dobie, ed. Publications of the Texas Folk–Lore Society, no. II. Austin, TX: Texas Folk–Lore Society, 1925. (Reprint edition, 1935.)

Damon, S. Foster. *The History of Square Dancing.* Barre, MA: Barre Gazette, 1957.

Daniel, Ana. *Bali Behind the Mask.* New York: Alfred A. Knopf, 1981.

Dansley, Harry and Kenneth and Jean Bigwood. *The New Zealand Maori in Color.* Wellington, New Zealand, St. Paul, Auckland, New Zealand, and Sidney, Australia: A. H. & A. W. Reed, 1963.

deZoete, Beryl, and Walter Spies. *Dance and Drama in Bali.* London: Faber and Faber Ltd., 1988.

Emery, Lynne Fauley. *Black Dance in the United States from 1619 to 1970.* Palo Alto, CA: National Press Books, 1972.

Ericson, Jane Harris (ed.). *Focus on Dance VI.* Washington, D.C.: American Association for Health, Physical Education and Recreation, 1972.

Fisher, James S. *Geography and Development, A World Regional Approach*, 4th ed. New York: Macmillan Publishing Company, 1992.

Haskins, Samuel. *African Image.* London: The Bodley Head, 1967.

Hill, Kathleen. *Dance for Physically Disabled Persons. A Manual for Teaching Ballroom, Square and Folk Dances to Users of Wheelchairs and Crutches.* Washington, D.C.: American Alliance for Health, Physical Education and Recreation, 1976.

Holy, Ladislav. *The Art of Africa Masks and Figures from Eastern and Southern Africa.* London: Paul Hamlyn, 1967.

Howard, Alan. *Polynesian Readings on a Cultural Area.* Bernice P. Bishop Museum, Honolulu: Chandler Publishing Co., 1971.

Howard, Alan and Robert Borofsky. *Developments in Polynesian Ethnology.* Honolulu: University of Hawaii Press, 1989.

Kaepplu, Adrienne L. "Folklore as Expressed in the Dance in Tonga," *Journal of American Folklore* 80(316): 160–168, 1967.

———. "Tonga Dance: A Study in Cultural Change," *Ethnomusicology* 14(2): 266–277, 1970.

Kealünohomoku, Joann Wheeler. "Dance History Research: Perspectives from Related Disciplines." Warrenton, VA: Proceedings of the Second Annual Conference on Research in Dance of the Committee on Dance Research, July 4–6, 1969.

———. "A Court Dance Disagrees with Emerson's Classic Book on the Hula," *Ethnomusicology* 8(2): 161–164, 1964.

———. "Hopi and Polynesian Dance–A Cross Cultural Comparison," *Ethnomusicology* 11:343–58, 1967.

Kennedy, Douglas. *English Folk Dancing Today and Yesterday.* London: G. Bell and Sons, 1964.

Kraus, Richard. *History of the Dance in Art and Education.* Englewood Cliffs, NJ: Prentice–Hall, 1969.

———. "Mexican Moriscas: A Problem in Dance Acculturation," *Journal of American Folklore*, vol. 62, no. 244, April–June 1949, pp. 87–106.

Lawler, Lillian B. *The Dance in Ancient Greece.* Middletown, CT: Wesleyan University Press, 1964.

Lawson, Joan. *European Folk Dance: Its National and Musical Characteristics.* New York: Pitman Publishing Co. 1953.

Mason, Kathleen Griddle (ed.). *Focus on Dance VII.* Washington, D.C.: American Association for Health, Physical Education and Recreation, 1974.

Meerloo, Joost A. M. *The Dance: From Ritual to Rock and Roll—Ballet to Ballroom.* New York: Chilton Co., 1960.

Parrinder, Geoffrey. *African Mythology.* London: Paul Hamlyn, 1967.

Pollenz, Phillippa. "Change in Form and Function of Hawaii Hulas," *American Anthropologist*, 52: 225–234, 1950.

———. "The Puzzle of Hula," *American Anthropologist*, 50:647–656, 1948.

Poort, W. A. *The Dance in the Pacific.* Katwijk, Netherlands: Van Der Lee Press, 1975.

Sachs, Curt. *World History of the Dance.* New York: W. W. Norton and Co., 1937.

Segy, Ladislas. *African Sculpture.* New York: Dover Publications, Inc., 180 Varick Street, 1958

Shapiro, Harry. *The Peopling of the Pacific Rim.* The Thomas Burke Memorial Lecture, 1964.

Stearns, Marshall Winslow, and Jean Stearns. *Jazz Dance.* New York: Macmillan Pub. Co., 1968.

Thorpe, Edward. *Black Dance.* New York: Overlook Press, 1989–90; Reprint, 1994.

Tierou, Alphonse. *Dooplé, The Eternal Law of African Dance.* Translated from the French by Dierdre McMahon. USA: Harward Academic Publishers, 1992.

Van Zile, Judy. *Dance in Africa, Asia, and the Pacific.* New York: MSS Information Corporation, 1976.

Wallace, Carol McD., et al. *Dance: A Very Social History.* New York: The Metropolitan Museum of Art, 1986.

Wang, Kefen. *The History of Chinese Dance.* Translated into English by Ke Ruibo. Beijing, China: Foreign Languages Press, 1985.

Youmans, John Green. "History of Recreational and Social Dance in the United States," University of Southern California, Ph.D. dissertation (Microcard), 1966.

MOVEMENT AND RHYTHM

Burton, Elsie C. *Introduction to Movement Fundamentals.* Minneapolis, MN: Bureau of Artistry, 1971.

Cusimano, Barbara E. "Teaching Tips: Rhythmic Activities," *Journal of Health, Physical Education and Recreation*, vol. 60, no. 4, April 1989, p. 11.

Gilbert, Anne Green. *Creative Dance for All Ages.* Reston, VA: American Alliance for Health, Physical Education, Recreation and Dance, 1992.

H'Doubler, Margaret. *Dance: A Creative Art Experience.* Madison, WI: The University of Wisconsin Press, 1957.

Lockhart, Aileen, and Esther E. Pease. *Modern Dance Building and Teaching Lessons.* Dubuque, IA: Wm. C. Brown Co., 1966.

Murray, Ruth Lovell. *Dance in Elementary Education: A Program for Boys and Girls.* New York: Harper & Row, 1963.

Pangrazi, Robert P. *Dynamic Physical Education for Elementary School Children*, 12th ed. Boston: Allyn and Bacon, 1998.

AMERICAN DANCE SAMPLER

Boyd, Neva. L., and Tressie M. Dunlavy. *Old Square Dances of America.* Chicago: H. T. Fitzsimmons Co., 1932.

Brewster, Mela Sedillo. *Mexican and New Mexican Folk Dances.* Albuquerque: University of New Mexico Press, 1938.

Burchenal, Elizabeth. *American Country Dances.* New York: G. Schirmer, 1918.

Casey, Betty. *Dance Across Texas.* Austin, TX: University of Texas Press, 1985.

Czarnowski, Lucille. *Dances of Early California Days.* Palo Alto, CA: Pacific Books, 1950.

———. "Spanish Mexican Dance: California and the Southwest," *Focus on Dance VI.* Jane Harris Erickson, ed. Washington, D.C.: American Association of Health, Physical Education and Recreation, 1972, p. 23.

Damon, S. Foster. *A History of Square Dancing.* Barre, MA: Barre Gazette, 1957.

Demille, Agnes. *The Book of the Dance.* New York: Golden Press, 1963.

Duggan, Anne Schley, Jeanette Schlottmann, and Abbie Rutledge. *Folk Dances of the United States and Mexico.* The Folk Dance Library, vol. 5. New York: Ronald Press, 1948.

Duke, Jerry. *Dance of the Cajuns.* San Francisco, CA: Duke Publishing Co., 1987.

———. *Clog Dance in the Appalachians.* San Francisco, CA: Duke Publishing Co., 1984.

Ericson, Jane Harris (ed.). *Focus on Dance VI.* Washington, D.C.: American Association for Health, Physical Education and Recreation, 1972.

Evanchuk, Robin. "Cajun–Sight, Sound and Movement," *Ethnic and Recreational Dance: Focus on Dance VI.* Dance Division of American Association for Health, Physical Education, and Recreation, Washington, D.C., 1972, pp. 43–46.

Ferrero, Edward. *The Art of Dancing.* New York: Dick Fitzgerald, 1859.

Ford, Henry, and Mrs. Henry Ford. *Good Morning,* 4th ed. Dearborn, MI: Dearborn Publishing Co., 1943.

Greene, Hank. *Square and Folk Dancing.* New York: Harper and Row Pub., 1984.

Hendrickson, Charles Cyril. *Early American Dance and Music: John Griffiths, Dancing Master. 29 Country Dances.* 1788. No. 1 in the Series. Sandy Hook, CT: The Hendrickson Group, 1989.

Keller, Kate Van Winkle. *If the Company Can Do It!: Techniques in Eighteenth-Century American Social Dance.* Sandy Hook, CT: The Hendrickson Group, 1990.

Keller, Kate Van Winkle, and Genevieve Shimer. *The Playford Ball. 103 Early Country Dances 1651–1820 As Interpreted by Cecil Sharp and His Followers.* Chicago: The Country Dance & Song Society, 1990.

Keller, Robert. *Dance Figures Index: American Country Dances, 1730–1810.* Sandy Hook, CT: The Hendrickson Group, 1989.

———. *Dance Figures Index: Eighteenth-Century English Country Dances, 1708–1800.*

———. *British-American Country Dance Title Index.* (In preparation).

Longley, Grant F. *Line Dance Manual, Vol. I.* Lowell, MA: New England Caller, Inc., 1987.

———. *Solo (Line) Dance Manual, Vol. II.* Lowell, MA: New England Caller, Inc, 1979, 1985.

———. *Solo (Line) Dance Manual, Vol. III.* Lowell, MA: New England Caller, Inc., 1990.

McDowell, William. *Tennessee Play Party.* Delaware, OH: Cooperative Recreation Service, 1960.

McIntosh, David Seneff. *Singing Games and Dances.* New York: Association Press, 1957.

Mayo, Margot. *The American Square Dance.* New York: Sentinel Books, 1948.

Melamed, Lanie. *All Join Hands: Connecting People Through Folk Dance.* Montreal: Lanie Melamed, 1977.

Meyers, Rick. *Traditional American Dance Book.* Published 1983. Available from: Rick Meyers, 1827 S.E. 76th, Portland, OR 97215.

Millar, Jolen Fitzhugh. *Country Dances of Colonial America.* Williamsburg, VA: Thirteen Colonies Press, 1990.

Morrison, James. *Twenty-Four Early American Country Dances, Cotillions and Reels.* New York: Country Dance and Song Society, 1976.

Nevell, Richard. *A Time to Dance: American Country Dancing from Hornpipes to Hot Has* New York: St. Martin's Press, 1977.

Ray, Ollie M. *A Fun Encyclopedia of Solo and Line Dances: The Steps That Came and Stayed* Whitewater, WI: Siddall and Ray Research Foundation, Publications for Dance, 1987.

Rohrbough, Lynn. *Handy Play Party Book.* Delaware, OH: Cooperative Recreation Service, 1940.

———. *Play Party Games of Pioneer Times.* Delaware, OH: Cooperative Recreation Service, 1939.

———. *Quadrilles, Thirty American Square Dances.* Delaware, OH: Cooperative Recreation Service, 1941.

Ryan, Grace L. *Dances of Our Pioneers.* New York: A. S. Barnes Co., 1939.

Sharp, Cecil J., and Maud Karpeles. *The Country Dance Book.* London: Novello and Co., 1918 (Reissued, 1946.)

Shaw, Lloyd. *Cowboy Dances.* Caldwell, ID: Caxton Printers, 1939.

———. *The Round Dance Book.* Caldwell, ID: Caxton Printers, 1948.

Spizzy, Mable Seeds, and Hazel Gertrude Kinscella. *La Fiesta: A Unit of Early California Songs and Dance.* Lincoln, NE: The University Publishing Co., 1939.

Theriot, Marie del Norte, and Catherine Blanchet. *Les Danses Rondes: Louisiana French Folk Dances.* Abbeville, LA: R. E. Blanchet, distributor, 1955.

Tolman, Beth, and Ralph Page. *The Country Dance Book.* Weston, VT: Countryman Press, 1937. Brattleboro, VT: The Stephen Greene Press, 1976.

Wakefield, Eleanor Ely. *Folk Dancing in America.* New York: J. Lowell Pratt and Co., 1966.

Werner, Robert. *The Folklore Village Saturday Night.* Dodgeville, WI: Folklore Village Farm, Inc., 1981.

CLOGGING

"American Clogging Abbreviations," *American Clogging,* vol. 2, no. 5, October 1984, pp. 22–31.

Austin, Debra E., and Diana L. Callahan. *Modern Clogging:* n.p.: The Tennessee Moonshine Cloggers, 1977.

Austin, Debra, and Diana Hatfield. *Modern Clogging II.* n.p.: The Tennessee Moonshine Cloggers, 1981.

Bernstein, Ira. *Appalachian Clogging and Flatfooting Steps.* Malverne, NY: Ten Toe Percussion, 1992.

Bonner, Frank X. *Clogging and the Southern Appalachian Square Dance.* Acworth, GA: Bonner Publishing Company, 1983.

Doss, Jane. "A Prospective on Dance in the South," *GAHPERD Journal,* vol. 23, no. 2, Spring 1989, pp. 10–11.

Duke, Jerry. *Clog Dance in the Appalachians.* San Francisco: Duke Publishing Co., 1984.

March, Stephen, and David Holt. "Chase That Rabbit," *Southern Exposure Long Journey Home,* vol. 5, nos. 2–3 Summer & Fall 1977, pp. 44–47.

Meyers, Rick. *Traditional American Dance Book.* Portland, OR: Rick Meyers, 1983.

Nieberlein, Judy. "Step Dancing, Clogging's First Cousin," *Flop-Eared Mule,* March/April 1986, p. 4.

Popwell, Sheila. *Almost Everything You Always Wanted to Know About Teaching Clogging Except How You Ever Let Yourself Get Talked Into Doing This in the First Place!* Huron, OH: Burdick Enterprises, 1980.

Rhodes, Sally. *Fontana Fall Jubilee Clogging.* n.p.: Fontana Village Resort, 1979.

Schild, Myra Martin. *Square Dancing Everyone.* Winston–Salem, NC: Hunter Textbooks Inc., 1987.

Seeger, Mike. *Talking Feet.* Berkeley, CA: North Atlantic Books, 1992.

Smith, Steve. "The History of Clog Dancing," *Rock-Step Gazette,* vol. 2, no. 2, August/ September 1983, p. 8. "The Clog Shoe," *American Clogging,* vol. 2, no. 11, April 1985, p. 15. "The Great Ones," *Clogging,* July/August/ September 1984, p. 8. "The History of Clog Shoes," *American Clogging,* vol. 2, no. 12, May 1985, pp. 16–17. "Traditional Terminology," *Flop-Eared Mule,* January/February 1987, pp. 29–35. "The Revival of Folk Dance," July/August 1986, pp. 10–11.

CONTRA DANCE

Armstrong, Don. *Contra.* Lakewood, CO: The Lloyd Shaw Foundation, 1960.

———. *The Caller-Teacher Manual for Contras.* Los Angeles: American Square Dance Society, 1973.

Briggs, Dudley T. *Thirty Contras from New England.* Burlington, MA: Dudley T. Briggs, 1953.

Brundage, Al, and Reuben Merchant. *Contras Are Fun.* 1952.

Burchenal, Elizabeth. *American Country Dances.* New York: G. Schirmer, 1918. *Community Dance Manual.* Numbers 4 (1954) and 5 (1957). New York: Country Dance Society, Inc.

Dart, Mary. *Contra Dance Choreography: A Reflection of Social Change.* New York: Garland Publishing, Inc., 1995.

Fix, Penn. *Contra Dancing in the Northwest.* Spokane, WA: Penn Fix, 1991.

Ford, Henry, and Mrs. Henry Ford. *Good Morning,* 4th ed. Dearborn, MI: Dearborn Publishing Co., 1943.

Fuerst, Michael, ed. *Midwest Folklore, A collection of Contras, Squares, and other. Dances from Expanded Midwest.* Urbana, IL: Michael Fuerst, 1992.

Gadd, May. *Country Dances of Today: Vol. 2.* New York: Country Dance Society of America, 1951.

Gaudreau, Herbie. *Modern Contra Dancing.* Sandusky, OH: American Square Dance Magazine, 1971.

Henrickson, Charles Cyril. *A Colonial Dancing Experience: Country Dancing for Elementary School Children.* Sandy Hook, CT: The Hendrickson Group, 1989.

Hinds, Tom. *Dance All Night* and *Dance All Night 2.* Arlington, VA: Tom Hinds, 1991.

———. *Dance All Night III.* Virginia: Tom Hinds, 1992.

———. *Dance All Day Too.* Virginia: Tom Hinds, 1995.

Holden, Rickey. *The Contra Dance Book.* Newark, NJ: American Squares, 1956, 1997.

Hubert, Gene. *Dizzy Dances Volumes I and II.* Bethseda, MD: Gene Hubert, 1986.

———. *More Dizzy Dances: Volume III.* Bethseda, MD: Gene Hubert, 1990.

Hutson, James, and Jeffery Spero. *(Southern) California Twirls: A Collection of Contra Dances and Three Community Histories.* Haydenville, MA: The Country Dance and Song Society, 1996.

Jennings, Larry. *Zesty Contras.* Cambridge, MA: The New England Folk Festival Association, 1983.

Kaynor, David A. *Calling Contra Dances for Beginners by Beginners.* Montague Center, MA: David A. Kaynor, 1991.

Keller, Kate Van Winkle and Ralph Sweet. *A Choice Selection of American Country Dances of the Revolutionary Era.* New York: Country Dance and Song Society, 1975.

Kennedy, Douglas, ed. *Community Dance Manual, Books 1–7, 130 Traditional English and American Contras, Squares, Big Circles, Mixers, Waltzes, Polkas, and Marches.* Princeton, NJ: Princeton Book Co. Publishers, 1986.

Kitch, Jim. *To Live Is To Dance: A Collection of Uncommon and Enjoyable Contra Dances.* Phoenixville, PA: Jim Kitch, 1995.

Knox, Roger, ed. *Contras as Ralph Page Called Them.* Ithaca, NY: Roger Knox, 1990.

Nevell, Richard. *A Time to Dance. American Country Dancing from Hornpipes to Hot Hash.* New York: St. Martin's Press, 1977.

Page, Ralph. *An Elegant Collection of Contras and Squares.* Denver, CO: The Lloyd Shaw Foundation, Inc., 1984.

———. *Heritage Dances of Early America.* Colorado Springs, CO: Lloyd Shaw Foundation, 1976.

———. *The Ralph Page Book of Contras.* London: English Folk Dance and Song Society, 1969.

Parkes, Tony. *Contra Dance Calling, A Basic Text.* Bedford, MA: Hands Four Books, 1992.

———. *Shadrack's Delight.* Bedford, MA: Hands Four Books, 1988.

———. *Son of Shadrack.* Bedford, MA: Hands Four Books, 1993.

Richardson, Mike. *Crossing the Cascades, Contra Dances and Tunes from the Pacific Northwest.* Seattle, WA: Mike Richardson, 1992.

Sannella, Ted. *Balance and Swing.* New York: Country Dance Society, Inc., 1982.

———. *Swing the Next.* Northampton, MA: Country Dance and Song Society of America, 1996.

Shacklette, Stew. *Contra Calling Made Easy.* Bradenburg, KY: Kentucky Dance Institute, 1980.

Twork, Eva O'Neal. *Henry Ford and Benjamin B. Lovett: The Dancing Billionaire and the Dancing Master.* Detroit: Harlo Press, 1982.

INTERNATIONAL FOLK DANCE

Beliajus, V. F. *Dance and Be Merry.* Vols. I and II. Evanston, IL: Summy–Birchard Co., 1940.

Beliajus, Vyts. "Jews from Bukhara." *Viltis,* May, 1962.

———. "The Study of Jewish Dance." *Viltis,* October–November 1968.

Bergquist, Nils W. *Swedish Folk Dances.* Cranbury, NJ: Thomas Yoseloff, 1928.

Berk, Fred. *Ha-Rikud, The Jewish Dance.* American Zionist Youth Foundation, Union of American Hebrew Congregations, United States of America, 1972, 1975.

Brehthnach, Breandan. *Folk Music and Dances of Ireland.* Dublin, Ireland: Mercier Press, 1986.

Bryans, Helen L., and John Madsen. *Scandinavian Dances.* Toronto: Irwin Clarke and Co., 1942.

Burchenal, Elizabeth. *Folk Dances from Old Homelands,* 1922; *Folk Dances and Singing Games,* 1922; *National Dances of Ireland,* 1929; *Folk Dances of Germany,* 1938; *Folk Dances of Denmark,* 1940. New York: G. Schirmer, Inc.

Butenhof, Ed. *Dance Parties for Beginners.* Mack Creek, MO: Lloyd Shaw Foundation, 1990.

Casey, Betty. *International Folk Dancing U.S.A.* Garden City, NY: Doubleday & Co., Inc., 1981.

Cavalier, Debbie, Ed. *Canadian Folk Dances.* Miami, FL: Warner Bros. Publications, Inc., 1995.

Chapru, Doleta. *A Festival of the English May.* Dodgeville, WI: Folklore Village Farm, Inc., 1977.

Cwieka, R. *The Great Polish Walking Dance, Volume I; The Polish Running Dance, Volume II; The Polish Figure Dance Book, Volume III: The Krakowiak Dance Workbook, Volume IV; The Kujawiak Dance Workbook, Volume V; The Oberek Dance Workbook, Volume VI; The Zakopane Mountain Dance Workbook, Volume VII.* Copyright © 1983. Order from R. Cwieka, 1375 Clinton Avenue, Irvington, NJ 97111.

Dalsemer, Bob. *Folk Dance Fun for Schools and Families.* Brasstown, NC: John C. Campbell Folk School, 1995.

Duggan, Anne Schley, Jeanette Schlottmann, and Abbie Rutledge. *The Teaching of Folk Dance, Volume I; Folk Dances of Scandinavia, Volume II; Folk Dances of European Countries, Volume III; Folk Dances of the British Isles, Volume IV; Folk Dances of the United States and Mexico, Volume V.* The Folk Dance Library. New York: Ronald Press, 1948.

Dunlay, Kate, and David Greenberg. *Traditional Celtic Violin Music of Cape Breton.* Mississauga, Ontario, Canada: DunGreen Music, 1996.

Dunsing, Gretel and Paul Dunsing. *A Collection of the Descriptions of Folk Dances,* 1972; Second Collection, 1976; Third Collection, 1977.

———. *German Folk Dances.* Vol. 1, Leipzig: Verlag Friedrich Hofmeister, 1936.

———. *Dance Lightly.* Delaware, OH: Cooperative Recreation Service, 1946.

Dziewanowska, Ada. *Polish Folk Dances and Songs.* New York: Hippocrene Books, Inc., 1987.

Eisenberg, Helen, and Larry Eisenberg. *The World of Fun Series of Recreation Recording.* Nashville, TN: Board of Education of the United Methodist Church, 1970.

English Country Dances of Today. Delaware, OH: Cooperative Recreation Service, 1948.

The English Folk Dance and Song Society. *Community Dance Manual, Books 1–7.* Princeton, NJ: Princeton Book Co., 1986.

Farwell, Jane. *Folk Dances for Fun.* Delaware, OH: Cooperative Recreation Service, n.d.

———. *The Folklore Village Saturday Night Book.* Dodgeville, WI: Folklore Village Farm, Inc., 1981.

Fillafer, Klaus, Rudi Hoi, and Mario Kanavc. *Tänze aus Kärnten.* Villach: Klagenfurt, 1997.

Flett, J. P., and T. M. Flett. *Traditional Dancing in Scotland.* Boston: Routledge and Kegan Paul, 1986.

Folklore Village Farm. *Folk Dances and Music.* Booklets Vol. 1, 1975; Vol. 2, 1976. Dodgeville, WI: Folklore Village Farm, Inc.

Gault, Ned and Marian. *Half a 100 and 1 More Easy Folk Dances.* 17632 Via Sereno, Monte Sereno, CA, 1983.

———. *100 and 1 Easy Folk Dances.* 17632 Via Sereno, Monte Sereno, CA, 1980.

Giurcheacu, Anca., and Sunni Bloland. *Romanian Traditional Dance.* Mill Valley, CA: Wild Flower Press, 1995.

Goldschmidt, Aenne. *Handbuch des deutschen Volkstanzes.* Wilhelmshaven, Germany: Heinrichshofen's Verlag, 1981.

Harris, Jane A. *File O'Fun.* Minneapolis: Burgess Publishing Co., 1970.

Hendrickson, Charles Cyril. *English Dances for the Dutch Court: Recvell de 24 Contredances Anglolse les Plus Usite, 1755 by G. Willsim.* Sandy Hook, CT: The Hendrickson Group, 1996.

Herman, Michael. *The Folk Dancer*, vol. 1. April 1941. Folk Dance House, P.O. Box 2305, North Babylon, NY 11703.

——. *Folk Dances for All.* New York: Barnes and Noble, 1947.

Hinman, Mary Wood. *Group Dances, Gymnastics and Folk Dancers.* Vol. IV. New York: A. S. Barnes and Co., 1930.

Holden, Rickey, and Mary Vouras. *Greek Folk Dance.* Newark, NJ: Folkraft Press, 1965.

Jackson, Rich, and George A. Fogg. *A Choice Collection of Country Dances: As Printed and Sold by John & William Neal in Christ Church Yard, Dublin, C. 1726.* Boston: Country Dance and Song Society, 1990.

Jankovic, Ljubica, and Danica Jankovic. *Dances of Yugoslavia.* New York: Crown Publishers, 1952.

Jensen, Mary Bee, and Clayne R. *Folk Dancing.* Provo, UT: Brigham Young University Press, 1973.

Joukowsky, Anatol M. *The Teaching of Ethnic Dance.* New York: J. Lowell Pratt and Co., 196

Katzarova–Kukudova, Raina, and Djener, Kiri *Bulgarian Folk Dances.* Sophia, Bulgaria: The Science and Art State Publishing House, 1958.

Keller, Kate Van Winkle, and Genevieve Shimer. *The Playford Ball, 103 Early English Country Dances.* North Hampton, MA: The Country Dance and Song Society, 1990.

Kennedy, Douglas, ed. Community Dances *Manual, Books 1–7.* London: English Folk Dance and Song Society, 1991.

——. *English Folk Dancing Today and Yesterday.* London: G. Bell and Sons, Ltd., 1964.

Khumer, Gertrude with Eliot Khumer. *The Golden Gate Book of Original Solo/Line Dances.* Vol.I. 1324 Bay View Place, Berkeley, CA.

Kraus, Richard G. *Folk Dancing: A Guide for Schools, Colleges, and Recreation Groups.* New York: Macmillan Pub. Co., 1962.

Lapson, Dvora. *Dances of the Jewish People.* New York: The Jewish Education Committee of New York, 1954.

LaSalle, Dorothy. *Rhythms and Dances for Elementary Schools,* New York: Ronald Press, 1951.

Lawson, Joan. *European Folk Dance: Its National and Musical Characteristics.* New York: Pitman Publishing Co., 1953.

Leeming, Joseph. *The Costume Book for Parties and Plays.* Philadelphia: J. B. Lippincott Co., 1938.

Lidster, Miriam D., and Dorothy H. Tamburini. *Folk Dance Progressions.* Belmont, CA: Wadsworth Publishing Co., 1965.

Lloyd, A. L. *Dances of Argentina.* London: Max Parrish and Co., n.d.

Lobley, Robert and Priscilla. *Your Book of English Country Dancing.* London: Faber and Faber, Ltd., 1980.

Longden, Sanna H., and Phyllis S. Weikart. *Cultures and Styling in Folk Dance.* Ypsilanti, MI: High Scope Press, 1998.

Marek, Jacek, and Bozena Marek. *Dance Poland.* Mansfield, MA: Jacek and Bozena Marek, 1997.

Martin, Phil. *Across the Fields. Traditional Norwegian-American Music from Wisconsin.* Dodgeville, WI: Folklore Village Farm, Inc., 1982.

Milligan, Jean C. *Won't You Join the Dance.* Available from: The Royal Scottish Country Dance Society, 12 Coates Crescent, Edinburgh, Scotland, EH3 7AF.

Mooney, Gertrude X. *Mexican Folk Dances for American Schools.* Coral Gables, FL: University of Miami Press, 1957.

Mynatt, Constance V., and Bernard D. Kaiman. *Folk Dancing for Students and Teachers.* Dubuque, IA: William C. Brown and Co., 1968.

The New Brunswick Collection of Scottish Country Dances. Fredericton, N.B., Canada: The Fredericton Scottish Country Dance Group, 1984.

O'Keefe, J. G. *A Handbook of Irish Dances.* Dublin: M. H. Gill and Sons, 1944.

Petrides, Ted P. *Greek Dances.* Athens, Greece: Lyeabettus Press, 1975.

Petrides, Theodore, and Elfleida Petrides. *Folk Dances of the Greeks.* New York: Exposition Press, 1961.

Pinon, Roger, and Henri Jamar. *Dances of Belgium.* London: Max Parrish and Co., 1953.

Playford, John. *The English Dancing Master: Or, Plaine and Easie Rules for the Dancing Country Dances, With the Tune to Each Dance.* Reprinted Princeton, NJ: Princeton Book Co., 1986.

Rohrbough, Lynn. *Treasures from Abroad.* Delaware, OH: Cooperative Recreation Service, 1938.

Rose, Marian. *Step Lively Dances for Schools and Families.* Vancouver, B.C., V5N 1H7: Community Dance Project, 1998.

Ross, F. Russel, and King, Virginia. *Multicultural Dance,* Box 18227, Cleveland Heights, OH: Russel & King, 1984.

Sedillo, Mela Brewster. *Mexican and New Mexican Folk Dances.* Albuquerque: University of New Mexico Press, 1948.

Shambaugh, Mary Effie. *Folk Festivals for Schools and Playgrounds.* New York: A. S. Barnes and Co., 1932.

Sharp, Cecil J., and Maud Karpeles. *The Country Dance Book.* London: Novello and Co., 1918. (Reissued, 1946.)

Sharp, Cecil J. and A. P. Oppé. *The Dance, An Historical Survey of Dancing in Europe.* London: Halton and Truscott Smith, Ltd.: New York: Murton, Balch and Company, 1924. (Republished EP Publishing Ltd., 1972.)

Spiesman, Mildred C. *Folk Dancing.* Philadelphia: W. B. Saunders Co., 1970.

Thurston, Hugh. "History of Scottish Dancing," *Viltis,* March 1964, p. 5.

Van Clef, Frank C. *24 Country Dances from the Playford Editions.* Princeton, NJ: Princeton Book Co., 1986.

Weikart, Phyllis S. *Teaching Movement and Dance.* Ypsilanti, MI: High/Scope Press, 1982.

———. *Teaching Intermediate Folk Dance.* Ypsilanti, MI: High/Scope Press, 1982.

Werner, Bob. *Scandinavian Folk Dances and Tunes. A compilation.* Dodgeville, WI: Folklore Village Farm, 1981.

Witzig, Louise. *Dances of Switzerland.* New York: Chanticleer Press, 1949.

TUNE BOOKS

Barnes, Peter, ed. *English Country Dance Tunes.* Massachusetts: Peter Barnes, 1986, 1996.

———. *A Little Couple-Dancemusik, 400 Waltzes, Polkas, Tangos, Hambos, Zwiesachers, and Other Traditional Dance Tunes.* Massachusetts: Peter Barnes, 1992.

Brody, David. *The Fiddler's Fakebook.* Oak Publications, 1983.

Cahn, David. *A Dozen Waltzes.* Seattle, WA: 1992.

Cole, M. M. *One Thousand Fiddle Tunes.* 1940, 1991.

Edelman, Larry. *Timepieces: Vintage Originals.* Baltimore, MD: Larry Edelman, 1989.

Geisler, Richard. *The Bulgarian Collection, The International Collection, The Yugoslav Collection.* The Village and Early Music Society, 15181 Ballantree Lane, Grass Valley, CA 95949.

Grossman, Dorothy. *An Index to Printed Sources of Folk Dance Tunes from the United States & British Isles.* Berea, KY: North American Imprints, 1995.

Kennedy, Peter, Ed. *The Fiddlers Tune Book: 200 Traditional Airs: Traditional Dance Music of Britain and Ireland.* 1994.

McQuillen, Bob. *Bob's Note Books: Jigs, Reels, and Other Tunes. Volumes 1–10.* Petersborough, NH: Bob McQuillen, 1982–1997.

Miller, Randy, and Jack Perron. *Irish Traditional Fiddle Music.* 1977.

———. *The New England Fiddler's Repertoire.* East Alstead, NH: Fiddlecase Books, 1983, 1986.

Songer, Susan, ed. *The Portland Collection, Contra Dance Music in the Pacific Northwest.* Portland, OR: Susan Songer, 1997.

Sweet, Ralph. *The Fifer's Delight.* Hazardville, CT: Ralph Sweet, 1964, 1981.

Williams, Vivian, ed. *Brand New Old Line Fiddle Tunes, Vol.1, 2, 3.* Seattle, WA: Voyager Recordings & Publication, 1992.

SQUARE DANCE

Beck, Donald H. *Out of Sight.* Stowe, MA: Donald H. Beck, 176 West Acton Road, 1983.

Burleson, Bill. *Square Dance Encyclopedia.* 2565 Fox Avenue, Minerva, OH 44657.

Casey, Betty. *The Complete Book of Square Dancing and Round Dancing.* Garden City, NY: Doubleday, 1976.

Clossin, Jimmy, and Carl Hertzog. *West Texas Square Dances.* El Paso, TX: Carl Hertzog Printing, 1949.

Dalsemer, Bob. *New England Quadrilles and How to Call Them.* Baltimore, MD: Bob Dalsemer, 1985.

———. *Smoke on the Water, Square Dance Classics.* Baltimore, MD: Traditional Caller Productions, 1989.

———. *West Virginia Square Dances.* New York: Country Dance and Song Society of America, 1982.

———. *When the Work's All Done: A Square Dance Party for Beginners and Old Hands.* Baltimore, MD: Traditional Caller Productions, 1990.

Damon, S. Foster. *The History of Square Dancing.* Barre, MA: Barre Gazette, 1957.

Durlacher, Ed. *Honor Your Partner.* New York: Devin–Adair Co., 1949.

Edelman, Larry. *Square Dance Caller's Workshop,* Fourth edition. Baltimore, MD: D & R Productions, 1991.

Everett, Bert. *Fifty Canadian Square Dances.* Toronto: Can–Ed Media, 1983.

Ford, Henry, and Mrs. Henry Ford. *Good Morning!* 3rd ed. 1941. 4th ed. 1943. Dearborn, MI: Dearborn Publishing Co.

Greene, Hank. *Square and Folk Dancing. A Complete Guide for Students, Teachers and Callers.* New York: Harper & Row, 1984.

Gunzenhauser, Margot. *Square Dancing at School.* Virum, Denmark: Square Dance Partners, 1991.

———. *The Square Dance and Contra Dance Handbook.* 1996.

Holden, Rickey. *The Square Dance Caller.* Newark, NJ: American Squares, 1951.

Howard, Carole. *Just One More Dance: A Collection of Old Western Square Dance Calls.* Chelsea, MI: Book Crafters, 1989.

The Illustrated Basic and Mainstream Movements of Square Dancing. Handbook Series. Official Publication of Sets in Order American Square Dance Society, 426 North Robertson Blvd., Los Angeles, CA 90048.

The Illustrated Plus Movements of Square Dancing. Handbook Series. Official Publication of Sets in Order American Square Dance Society, 426 North Robertson Blvd., Los Angeles, CA 90048.

Jensen, Clayne R., and Mary B. Jensen. *Square Dancing*. Provo, UT: Brigham Young University Press, 1973.

Kemper, Bob, and Janette Kemper. *Handbook for Square Dance Leaders*. Oak Ridge, TN: Bob and Janette Kemper.

Kraus, Richard G. *A Pocket Guide of Folk and Square Dances and Singing Games for Elementary School*. Englewood Cliffs, NJ: Prentice Hall Inc., 1966.

——. *Square Dances of Today and How to Call Them*. New York: Ronald Press, 1950.

Linnell, Rod and Louise Winston. *Square Dances from a Yankee Caller's Clipboard*. Nowell, MA: The New England Square Dance Caller, 1974.

Lyman, Frank Jr. *One Hundred and One Singing Calls*. Woodbury, NJ: American Squares, 1951.

Nevell, Richard. *A Time to Dance. American Country Dancing from Hornpipes to Hot Has??* New York: St. Martin's Press, 1977.

Owens, Lee, and Viola Ruth. *Advanced Square Dance Figures of the West and Southwest*. Palo Alto, CA: Pacific Books, 1950.

Page, Ralph. "A History of Square Dancing," *Square Dancing*. vol. XXVI, no. 1–5. 1974.

Pete, Piute. *Piute Pete's Down Home Square Dance Book*. New York: Grosset & Dunlap, 1977.

Ryan, Grace L. *Dances of Our Pioneers*. New York: Ronald Press, 1939.

Shaw, Dorothy. "The Story of Square Dancing: A Family Tree," *Sets in Order*, vol. XIII, no. 11, 1961, pp. 33–48.

Shaw, Lloyd, *Cowboy Dances*. Caldwell, ID: Caxton Printers, 1939.

Stultz, Sandra J. *Contemporary Square Dance*. Minneapolis: Burgess Publishing Co., 1974.

Trimmer, Gene. *Singing Thru Mainstream*. Marlborough, NH: Supreme Audio, Inc., 1995.

SOCIAL DANCE

Aldrich, Elizabeth. *From the Ballroom to Hell, Grace and Folly in Nineteenth-Century Dance*. Evanston, IL: Northwestern University Press, 1991.

Ancelet, Barry Jean. *Cajun Music: Its Origins and Development*. Lafayette, LA: University of Southwest Louisiana, 1989.

Bottomer, Paul. *Line Dancing*. New York: Anness Publishers, 1996.

Bottner, Paul. *Dance Crazy Series*. New York: Lorenz Books.

Boven, John. *South to Louisiana. The Music of the Cajun Bayous*. Gretna, LA: Pelican Publishing Co., 1992.

Boyd, Neville. *New Vogue Sequence Dancing*. North Star Publishers, 1989.

Buckman, Peter. *Let's Dance: Social, Ballroom and Folk Dancing*. New York and London: Paddington Press Ltd., 1978.

Casey, Betty. *Dance Across Texas*. Austin, TX: University of Texas Press, 1985.

Clark, Sharon Leigh. "What Do You Dance, America?" *Focus on Dance VI*. Jane Harris Ericson, ed. Washington, D.C.: American Association for Health, Physical Education and Recreation, 1972, pp. 51–55.

Collier, Simon, Artenis Cooper, Maria Susana Azzi, and Richard Martin. *Tango, The Dance, The Song, The Story*. London: Thames & Hudson Ltd., 1995.

Conrad, Glenn R. *The Cajuns: Essays on their History and Culture*. Lafayette, LA: University of Southwest Louisiana, 1983.

Dow, Allen, with Mike Michaelson. *The Official Guide to Ballroom Dancing*. Northbrook, IL: Domus, 1980.

——. *The Official Guide to Latin Dancing*. Northbrook, IL: Domus, 1980.

Duke, Jerry. *Social and Ballroom Dance Lab Manual*, San Francisco: Duke Publishing Co., 1988.

——. *Dance of the Cajuns*. San Francisco: Duke Publishing Co., 1987.

Elfman, Bradley. *Breakdancing*. New York: Avon Books, 1984.

Evanchuk, Robin. "Cajun Sight, Sound and Movement." *Ethnic and Recreational Dance: Focus on Dance VI*. Washington, DC: Dance Division of the American Association for Health, Physical Education and Recreation, 1972, pp. 43–46.

Fischer–Munstermann, Uta. *Jazz Dance and Jazz Gymnastics Including Disco Dancing*. New York: Sterling Publishing Co., Inc., 1978.

Franks, A. H. *Social Dance: A Short History*. London: Routledge and Kegan Paul, 1963.

Fresh, Mr., and the Supreme Rockers. *Breakdancing*. New York: Avon Books, 1984.

Fry, Macon, and Julie Posner. *Cajun Country Guide*. Gretna, LA: Pelican Publishing Co., 1992.

Goldman Albert. *Disco*. New York: Hawthorn Books, Inc., 1978.

Gould, Philip. *Cajun Music and Zydeco*. Baton Rouge, LA: Louisiana State University Press, 1992.

Gwynne, Michael. *Sequence Dancing*. London: A & C Black Publishers, 1985.

Hager, Steven. *Hip Hop: The Illustrated History of Break Dancing, Rap, Music, and Graffiti*. New York: St. Martin's Press, 1984.

Hampshire, Harry Smith, and Doreen Casey. *The Viennese Waltz*. Brooklyn, NY: Revisionist Press, 1993.

Heaton, Alma, and Israel Heaton. *Ballroom Dance Rhythms*. Dubuque, IA: William C. Brown Co., 1961.

Heaton, Alma. *Disco with Donny and Marie, Step by Step Guide to Disco Dancing.* CA and MT: Osmond Publishing Co., 1979.

———. *Techniques of Teaching Ballroom Dance.* Promo, UT: Brigham Young University Press. 1965.

———. *Techniques of Teaching Ballroom Rhythms.* Dubuque, IA: Kendall/Hunt Publishing Co., 1971.

———. *Fun Dance Rhythms.* Provo, UT: Brigham Young University Press, 1976.

Hostetler, L. A. *Walk Your Way to Better Dancing.* Rev. ed. New York: A. S. Barnes and Co., 1952.

Javna, John. *How to Jitterbug.* New York: St. Martin's Press, 1984.

Kilbride, Ann, and Angelo Algoso. *The Complete Book on Disco and Ballroom Dancing.* Los Alamitos, CA: Hwong Publishing Co., 1979.

Lane, Christy. *Complete Book of Line Dancing.* Champaign, IL, Human Kinetics, 1995.

Laird, Walter. *Technique of Latin Dancing: International Dance.* London: Book Service. New edition 1988. Reprint 1992.

———. *The Ballroom Dance Pack.* London: Dorling Kindersley. Publisher: Houghton Mifflin Co., 1994.

Livingston, Peter. *The Complete Book of Country Swing and Western Dance and a Bit About Cowboys.* Garden City, NY: Doubleday & Co., Inc., 1981.

Lustgarten, Karen. *The Complete Guide to Disco Dancing.* New York: Warner Books, Inc., 1978.

———. *The Complete Guide to Touch Dancing.* New York: Warner Books, Inc., 1979.

Marlow, Curtis, *Break Dancing.* Cresskill, NJ: Sharon Publications, Inc., 1984.

Monte, John. *The Fred Astaire Dance Book.* New York: Simon and Schuster, 1978.

Moore, Alex. *Ballroom Dancing: with 100 Diagrams and Photographs of the Quickstep, Waltz, Foxtrot, Tango.* London: A & C Clark Publisher, 1986.

National Association of Country Dancers. *Country and Western Dance Manual.* P. O. Box 9841, Colorado Springs, CO 80932.

Osborne, Hilton. *Line Dancing: Run to the Floor for Country Western.* Glendale, CA: Griffin Publisher, 1994.

Plater, Ormonde, Cynthia Speyrer, and Rand Speyrer. *Cajun Dancing.* Gretna, LA: Pelican Publishing Co., 1993.

Ray, Ollie Mae. *Encyclopedia of Line Dances.* Reston, VA: National Dance Association, American Alliance for Health, Physical Education, Recreation and Dance, 1992.

Rushing, Shirley, and Patrick McMillan. *Kicker Dancin' Texas Style.* Winston–Salem, NC: Hunter Textbooks, 1988.

Schild, Myrna Martin. *Social Dance.* Dubuque, IA: Wm. C. Brown, 1985.

Silvester, Victor. *Modern Ballroom Dancing: The Maestro's Manual.* London: Book Service, 1971.

Stephenson, Richard M., and Joseph Iaccarino. *The Complete Book of Ballroom Dancing.* New York: Doubleday, 1980.

Villacorta, Aurora S. *Step by Step to Ballroom Dancing.* Danville, IL: Interstate Printers and Publishers, 1974.

———. *Charleston, Anyone?* Danville, II: Interstate Printers & Publishers, Inc., 1978.

Wagner, Michael. "Swing Dance," *Viltis*, vol. 57, no. 5, September–October, 1997, p. 8.

White, Betty. *Teen Age Dance Book.* New York: David McKay Co., 1952.

———. *Teen Age Dance Etiquette.* New York: David McKay Co., 1956.

———. *Latin American Dance Book.* New York: David McKay Co., 1958.

———. *Ballroom Dancebook for Teachers.* New York: David McKay Co., 1962.

Wright, Judy Patterson. *Social Dance: Steps to Success.* Champaign, IL: Leisure Press, 1992.

Glossary

Above Contra Dance term. Refers to the next couple or the couples up the set from the actives.

Accent The stress placed on a beat that makes it stronger or louder than the others. The primary accent is on the first beat of the measure. Sometimes there is more than one accent per measure. Some dance steps have the accent on the off-beat, which makes the rhythm syncopated.

Active Couple Relating to Square Dance and Quadrilles, refers to lead couple. Relating to Contra Dance, refers to every other couple (1, 3, 5, and so forth) or every third couple (1, 4, 7, and so forth). Same as first couple, head couple, or top couple.

Alamo Style A Square Dance term. A variation of grand right and left. All eight dancers do an allemande left, hold on to the corner, but shift to a hands-up position and take partner by the right, making a complete circle with the men facing in and the ladies facing out. Dancers balance forward and back. They release the left hand halfway around so that the men now face out and the ladies face in. They join hands as before and repeat balance. Dancers release with the right hand and turn with the left hand halfway around. They join hands as before and repeat balance and right-hand turn. They repeat balance and left-hand turn and meet partner.

All Around Your Left-Hand Lady A Square Dance term. Corners move one time around each other in a loop pattern, the man starting behind the corner, continuing on around her and moving back to place. The woman starts in front of the man and continues on around him and back to place. As they move, both partners always remain facing the center of the square. This completes half of the loop. "See-saw your partner" is a similar action around partner that completes the other half of the loop.

All Eight A Square Dance term. Refers to all eight members in set.

Allemande Left A Square Dance term. Corners take a left-forearm grasp and turn each other once around and go back home. Left elbow is bent, and dancers pull away from each other to take advantage of the centrifugal force.

Allemande Right A Square Dance term. Man and woman designated to take a right-forearm grasp and turn each other once around. Right elbow is bent, and dancers pull away slightly as in allemande left.

Allemande Thar A Square Dance term. A star formation involving all four couples in the set. Dancers go allemande left, return to partner, give a right hand, pull by, and take the next with a left-forearm grasp. The man then turns this woman about a half-turn

counterclockwise until he can put his right hand into the box star position with all the other men. The men travel backward in the star; the women travel forward. To "shoot the star," the men release the box star position, turn the women on their left halfway around so that the women are facing clockwise and the men are facing counterclockwise. They release arm position, move forward to the next person, give a right hand, pull by, and take the next with a left-forearm grasp. The men turn as before into another box star, backing up. They shoot the star once more, pulling around to meet original partner.

All Jump Up and Never Come Down A Square Dance term. All jump into the air; usually followed by partner swing.

Along the Line A Square Dance term. This refers to the persons in the same line. If the call is "ladies chain along the line," each side of the line turns to face the other couple in the line and chains the women.

Anchor Step West Coast Swing term. Step right behind left (hook) (count 1), step left in place (count *and*), step right in place (count 2). Usually danced at the end of the slot.

Arch in the Middle A Square Dance term. The two persons in the center of a line take hands and make an arch for others to duck under. After the arch is made, the couple, if facing out, turns a California twirl to face the center of the set. Also called "make an arch."

Arm Around *See* Cast Off.

Around One or Two A Square Dance term used following split the ring, pass thru, or cross trail thru. Couples separate; one goes right, the other left around the outside of the set, just passing one person. They come into a line or into the middle of the set. Sometimes the call is "come around two," meaning the person going on the outside passes two persons before coming in.

Back Cross Position Man and woman stand side by side, the woman on the right. Arms are crossed behind them so that the woman's left arm is behind him and her left hand holds his left hand at his left side; his right arm is behind her and his right hand holds her right hand at her right side. *See* p. 60.

Back to Back *See* Face to Face.

Back Track A Square Dance term referring to a double turn back from a grand right and left. *See also* Single-File Turn Back; Turn Back.

Balance
1. *Contra.* The following is suggested.
   a. Step swing: step left (count 1) and swing right across in front of left (count 2). Repeat beginning right.

b. Refer to Folk Dance balance in 2/4 time.

2. *Folk Dance.* The balance may be done forward, backward, or sideward.

   a. *3/4 Time.* Step left (count 1); touch right to left, rising on balls of both feet (count 2); and lower heels in place (count 3). Repeat same movement, beginning right.

   b. *2/4 Time.*

      1) Step left (count 1); touch right to left, rising on balls of both feet (count *and*); lower heels (count 2); and hold (count *and*). Repeat, beginning right.

      2) Or step left (count 1) and touch right to left (count 2). Repeat same movement, beginning right. Omit the pronounced lift of the heel in this analysis. However, there should be a slight lift of the body as the movement is executed.

   c. *English Country Dance.* 3/4 Time. Balance forward. Step forward onto right, bring left close to right, step back on left (3 counts). Balance back. Step backward onto left, bring right close to left, step forward onto left. **Note:** Change of weight allows moving forward into a traveling figure (3 counts).

3. *Square Dance.* Partners face, inside hands joined; or man may hold woman's left hand in his right.

   a. Each takes two steps backward, dipping back on second step; then two steps forward to original position.

   b. Or man rocks back on left, taking weight on left, pointing right front (counts 1–2); then steps forward right to original position (counts 1–2). Woman's part reverse.

4. *Social Dance.* Same as the Folk Dance balance described above.

Balance in Line A Contra Dance term. Four in line, hands joined at shoulder height, elbows bent. Beginning right, balance to the right, then left. Look at the person with whom you are balancing.

Banjo Position *See* Right Parallel Position.

Basketweave Grasp A Square or Folk Dance term. Usually involves four or more people. Each puts the right hand into the center, and they all face left, one behind the other, and put the right hand on the wrist of the person in front of them.

Becket Formation Contra Dance formation, but couples stand side by side with partner. Each couple faces an opposite couple. Couples 1, 3, and 5 start as active on the women's line; couples 2, 4, and 6 start as inactive on the men's line. *See* p. 181.

Below Contra Dance term. Usually refers to the next couple or the couples down the set from the actives.

Bend the Line A Square Dance term. From any line of even numbers (four usually), the line breaks in the middle, the ends move forward, and the centers back up, so that one half of the line now faces the other half.

Bleking Step 2/4 time. A quick change of the feet, moving in place, in an uneven rhythm. Hop right (count *ah*); touch left heel forward (counts 1–2); leap onto left, bringing it back into place (count *ah*); touch right heel forward (counts 1–2); leap onto right in place (count *ah*); touch left heel forward (count 1); leap onto left in place (count *ah*); touch right heel forward (count 2); leap onto right in place (count *ah*); touch left heel forward (counts 1–2). The *ah* count comes on the pickup beat, and the heel touch on the accented beat of the music.

Bossa Nova A Social Dance from Brazil.

Bottom of Set In Contra and Longway sets, the end of the set is farthest from the caller and musicians.

Bow A Square and Folk Dance term. In Square Dance, it is the term that has replaced "honor." It is a slight turn to face partner while shifting the weight to the outside foot and pointing the inside foot toward partner. One may dip slightly as the weight shifts and one nods to partner.

Bow and Swing A Square Dance term. Bow, then step forward into swing position and swing once around. *See* Bow; Swing, item 3.

Box Star Position Also referred to as Pack Saddle Star and Basketweave Grasp. Each person places right (left) hand on wrist of the person in front to form a star.

Box the Flea A Square Dance term. Similar to box the gnat, except that both man and woman use the left hand instead of the right. The woman is turned clockwise under the man's right arm; the man walks around her counterclockwise. They end up facing each other, as they started, but they have exchanged places. Also called "swat the flea."

Box the Gnat A Square Dance term. A man and woman face each other, take right hands, and exchange places, the woman turning counterclockwise under the man's right arm while he walks around her clockwise. They end up facing each other, but they have exchanged places.

BPM Beats per minute. This is the measurement of tempo for dance music. Based upon the beats per minute, the instructor can quickly determine the best dance for a particular piece of music.

Break Drop clasped hands.

Break and Form a Line A Square Dance term. This occurs when two couples are in a circle. The lead man drops his left hand and pulls the others into a line square with the visited position. If first couple leads out to second couple, the man circles about two-thirds of the way to the left and breaks to form a line in the second position.

Break and Swing Drop clasped hands and partners swing with a waist swing.

Break and Trail Along that Line A Square Dance term. Drop hands, turn and face in opposite direction, move in single file to home position; the woman leads, the man follows.

Bridge Position *See* Yoke Position. *See* p. 29.

Broken Circle A single circle of dancers in which all hands are joined except two.

Brush A Clogging term. The Brush is a toe movement (*see* Toe Movement) occurring on the upbeat (count *and*). The leg performing the movement swings forward as the ball of the foot brushes the floor. No weight change occurs in the Brush. Brushes also may cross in front of the body or swing out to the side. Less frequently they are performed brushing backward. Both legs are straight on the Brush; on the following downbeat (accent), both knees bend slightly while performing the next movement.

Butterfly Position Couple faces, arms extended shoulder high and out to the sides, hands joined. In this position, couple may dance forward and backward or to the right or left, and in the line of direction and reverse line of direction.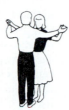

Buzz Step A turning step used in Contra, Folk, Square, and Social Dance. Done alone or with a partner, turning clockwise or counterclockwise in swing or shoulder-waist position. Buzz step may be used to travel sideways. The rhythm is uneven (long, short).
1. *Clockwise turn.* Step right (turn toe right), pivoting clockwise on ball of foot (long); push with ball of left foot placed slightly to side of right (short). Repeat as required. Reverse footwork for counterclockwise turn. **Note:** The weight remains on the right or pivot foot; the impetus for turn is given by left foot.

2. *Sideways.* Step left sideways (long); push with right foot as it moves to the left, displacing left foot (short). **Note:** The turning action of the pivot foot is omitted.

Buzz-Step Swing A Contra and Square Dance term. Use swing position for Contra and Square Dance. Folk Dance position as directed. Step right on long count into swing position; the left foot takes the short count in a pushing off motion to propel the turn. Couples generate centrifugal force by pulling away of upper torso. **Note:** Contra swings are usually eight measures; Square Dance swings usually two turns and open up to face center of set.

California Twirl A Square Dance term. Used by couples to change or reverse direction without changing relation of couple position. Woman's left in man's right, man walks around woman clockwise as woman executes a left-face turn, moving under raised right arm of man. If partners began movement side by side, facing center of set, they now are side by side, facing away from center of set. A repeat of the movement puts dancers in original position. Also referred to as "Frontier Whirl."

Canter Rhythm An uneven pattern in 3/4 time, resulting from a long beat (counts 1–2) followed by a short beat (count 3). A step is taken on count 1 and held over on count 2. Another step is taken on count 3. The three-step turn in canter rhythm is step left (count 1); pivot on left a half-turn counterclockwise (count 2); step right (count 3), pivoting almost a half-turn counterclockwise; step left (count 1), completing the turn; and hold (counts 2–3). Close right to left (count 3), but keep weight on left. It may be done clockwise by starting with the right foot.

Cast Refers to English Country Dance and Contra Dance. Partners turn away from each other and move outside the set to a new position; other dancers move up or down as indicated.

Cast Down A Contra Dance or English Country Dance term. Cast down means first or active couple face up, separate, and travel down the outside of the set one place.

Cast Off A Contra Dance term. Refers to one of the following ways to progress in the set:
1. *Walk Around.* Active couple separates, walks around the inactive and finishes below inactive, facing partner. Inactives do not turn.
2. *Arm Around.* Active couple separates and the inactive faces up the set; the active and nearest inactive put their nearest arm around each other's waist. May be same sex. The inactive person acts as a pivot or backs up, turning as the active moves forward, the two turning side by side. The active ends one position below, both facing partner.
3. *Unassisted, Two Dancers.* Like the arm around, the two dancers stand side by side, shoulders close together, but they do not touch. They turn as a unit, active ends one position below, with both facing partner.
4. *Hand Cast Off.* Coming up in a line of four, joined hands shoulder height, elbows down, active couple separates, active and inactive turn forward. The inactive acting as a pivot, the two turn; active ends one position below, with both facing their partners. Or active couple separates and joins hands with inactive, as in an allemande and the two turn.
5. *Two Couple.* Active couple leads up the set, followed by inactive. Active couple separates and travels in a small circle to one position below inactive. The inactive couple separates and turns almost in place, backing into the line above the active couple.
6. *Separately.* Sometimes one person casts off, as in a star figure, and the other person casts off in the next figure.

CCW Symbols referring to *counterclockwise*. *See* Counterclockwise.

Center The space in the middle of the square (set) or circle formed by dancers.

Centrifugal Force The force exerted outward from the center that is created by dancers rotating as in a buzz step swing or pivot turn.

Cha Cha Cha A Latin Dance from Cuba.

Chain For Contra and Square Dance, *see* Ladies Chain. For Folk Dance, *see* Grand Right and Left.

Challenge Position A Social Dance term. The man faces the woman at approximately arms distance. Hands are not joined. Also called Shine position.

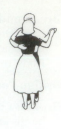

Charleston Step A step in 4/4 meter, accent on count *and*. Put weight on right bent knee, left foot in the air. Flip left foot up behind (count *and*); step forward left (count 1); bend left knee and flip right foot up behind (count *and*). Point right toe forward; straighten knees (count 2); bend left knee and flip right foot up behind (count *and*). Step back on right (count 3); bend right knee and flip left foot up behind (count *and*); point left toe behind and straighten knees (count 4).

Chassé A series of sliding steps; one foot displaces the leading one, moving forward, backward, or sideward. In Square Dance, called sashay.

Chug Step Move forward or backward on one or two feet or sideward on one foot. Moving backward on left foot, with weight on left foot and right foot slightly off the floor and knee flexed, the left foot pulls (drags) backward as the left knee straightens (count *and* 1). Body bends forward slightly with action.

Circle Four, six, eight, or more dancers join hands in a circle and move left or right as directions of the call or dance indicate. In a Contra or Square Dance call, if the direction is not indicated, circle left.

Circle to a Line—Line of Four Couples 1 and 3 lead to the right, join hands and circle three–quarters around, lead men (men 1 and 3) drop left hands with left–hand woman to form lines of four dancers. Couples 1 and 3 will be on the end of the line opposite their home position. Lines will be facing across the set from the side couples (couples 2 and 4) position. Also done with side couples 2 and 4, leading out to couples 1 and 3. Lines will be formed, facing from the head couple position.

Circle Wide Dancers join hands and circle left. In a Square Dance call, it may also mean that dancers enlarge circle as they circle left.

Circulate A Square Dance term. From two ocean–wave lines, dancers on the outside (or the inside) of the line circulate by moving forward to the next outside (or inside) position in a circle. Refer to diagram, p. 151.

Clockwise Refers to the movement of dancers around a circle in the same direction as the hands of a clock move or to a turning action of one dancer or couple as they progress around the floor. In directional terms, clockwise is to the left (e.g., "circle to the left").

Close Free foot is moved to supporting foot. Weight ends on free foot. Begin weight on left, move right (free foot) to left, and take weight on right.

Closed Position Partners stand facing each other, shoulders parallel and toes pointed directly forward. Man's right arm is around the woman and the hand is placed on the small of her back. Woman's left hand and arm rest on man's upper arm and shoulder. Man's left arm is raised sideward to the left, and he holds her right hand in his palm. For detailed description, refer to p. 373.

Coaster Step West Coast Swing term. Step back left (count 1), close right to left (count *and*), step forward left (count 2).

Contra Corners Turn (16 counts) Contra corners are diagonally across the set for each person. The *first contra corner* is diagonally right and the *second contra corner* is diagonally left. For the call "turn contra corners," active partners crossing set take right hands, turn halfway, take left hand of *first contra corner*, turn all the way around, take right hand of partner, turn three–quarters around in middle of set, take left hand of *second contra corner*, turn all the way around and return to center of set and await next call. The actives use their right and left hands alternately; the corners always use their left hands. Each turn is 4 counts.

Contra Dance Formation Parallel lines, men in one line or on one side and women in other line or on opposite side. Head or top of set to man's left, woman's right. Foot or bottom of set to man's right or woman's left when couples face partner. In Longway or Contra sets, dancers may face partners across lines; all dancers may face top or head of set; or couples 1, 3, and 5 may change sides or lines to put odd–numbered couples facing each other on opposite sides of set. *See* p. 181.

Contra Set *See* Longway Set.

Conversation Position As described for open position, but with the forward hand released and arm (man's left, lady's right) hanging at the side.

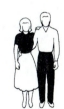

Corner The woman on the man's left. Also called left–hand lady. The woman's corner is the man on her right.

Corners An English Country Dance term. In duple minor formations, the *first corners* are the first man and second woman. *Second corners* are the first woman and second man.

Corner Swing Square Dance term. A waist swing or buzz–step swing with left–hand lady.

Corté Step back on foot indicated, taking full weight and bending the knee. The other leg remains extended at the knee and ankle, forming a straight line to the floor. The toe remains in contact with the floor. Also called a Dip.

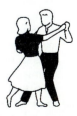

Counter Balance While holding on to one or both hands, partners lean away from each other with equal force.

Counterclockwise Refers to the movement of dancers around a circle in opposite direction from the movement of the hands on a clock or to a turning action of one dancer or couple as they progress around the floor. In directional terms, counterclockwise is to the right (e.g., "circle to the right").

Couple A man and a woman. Woman stands at man's right.

Couple Position Partners stand side by side, woman on man's right, inside hands joined, both facing in same direction. Also referred to as strolling, side-by-side, or open position, or inside hands joined.

Courtesy Turn A Contra Dance and Square Dance term. A couple is standing side by side, with the woman on the right of the man. They turn counterclockwise. The man takes the woman's left hand in his left. He puts his right arm around her waist and guides her forward as he moves backward. It is a spot turn in place.

Cross An English Country Dance term. Actives go directly across the set to the other side, passing right shoulders or as directed.

Cross Over A Contra Dance term. Two facing dancers exchange places, passing right shoulders.

Cross-Over Position Social Dance term for Cha Cha Cha. The couple is side by side, with inside hands joined. *See* Couple Position, p. 60.

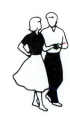

Cross Trail Thru A Square Dance term. Active couples meet, pass right shoulder to right shoulder, woman then crosses in front of partner to her left, man crosses behind woman to his right. Wait for caller's direction.

Cowboy Arch The man lifts up his left arm (forming an arch) and goes under as the woman goes behind him, trading places.

Cowboy Cross The man lifts up both hands keeping them together; he leads the woman to his right side going under his hands, ending with arms in a "crossed position."

Cuddle or Cowboy Cuddle The man leads the woman into a cuddle, or wrap position. *See* Wrap Position.

Curtsey The term used occasionally to refer to the action of honors in which the woman nods her head to partner, at the same time shifting her weight to the outside foot as she turns to face partner. Usually accompanied by a smile. *See also* Bow.

Cut-Step Step left (count 1); bring right quickly up to left and step right displacing left (count 2). Used in Mazurka.

Cut Time A rhythm that comes from 4/4 time. Refer to diagram on p. 44.

CW Symbols referring to clockwise. *See* Clockwise.

Dal Step A Swedish step in 3/4 time. Step left (count 1), swing right across in front of left (count 2), raise left heel from floor as weight rolls to ball of left foot, and complete swing of right across left (count 3). Repeat movement, beginning right.

Dance Walk A Social Dance term that describes the basic walking step. May move forward, backward, or sideward in Foxtrot, Waltz, or Tango.

Dig Step Place slight weight on the ball of one foot; usually followed by stepping on the foot.

Dip (Corté) Step back on foot indicated, taking full weight and bending the knee. The other leg remains extended at the knee and ankle, forming a straight line from the hip. The toe remains in contact with the floor.

Disco Dance A descriptive term that encompasses a wide variety of dance steps to many rhythms of recorded music. (*See* Disco Dance, p. 390).

Discotheque A French word referring to a place where records (disques) are stored. In common usage, it describes a place for contemporary dancing to records as opposed to live music.

Dish Rag Whirl A Square Dance term. Man and woman who are facing join both hands and turn under their joined hands, starting under man's left arm and woman's right. As they turn, their hands come up over their heads. They make one complete rotation and end up facing the side couples.

Dive Thru A Square Dance term. Active couple duck under an arch made by the couple they are facing. If the arching couple then faces the outside of the square, they turn a California twirl to reverse direction and end facing in.

Dixie Chain A Square Dance term. Two couples meet in single-file and move past each other as in a grand right and left. The first two to meet use right hands; the second two to meet use left hands. Remain in single-file; wait for caller's directions.

Docey Doe A Square Dance term. *See* Do-Si-Do, Shaw Style.

Do Paso A Square Dance term. Starting position is a circle of two or more couples. Partners face, take a left-forearm grasp, and turn each other counterclockwise until facing corner. They turn corner with right-forearm grasp until facing partner and take partner with the left hand. Man turns woman with a courtesy turn.

Do-Sa-Do A Square Dance term. The man and woman face, pass each other right shoulder to right shoulder, move around each other back to back, and return to original position. In Contra Dance, this is the correct action for the call "do–si–do."

Do–Si–Do

1. *Contra Dances.* The call "do–si–do" in Contra Dances is the same as defined by "do–sa–do."
2. *Shaw Style* (for two couples in a circle). A square Dance term. Form a circle of four and release hands; women pass left shoulders, turn left, and give left hand to partner. As the women move around behind partner, the men do **a** or **b**.
   a. Always facing partner and moving forward and backward to minimize the amount of space that the woman must travel, man releases partner's hand and gives right to opposite woman, who moves around behind him once.
   b. Partners pass back to back; man releases partner's hand, gives right to opposite woman, and turns once around until the partners again pass back to back. Then man takes partner's left hand and turns woman with a courtesy turn.
3. *Texas-Southwest Style* (for two or more couples in a circle). A Square Dance term. Partners face, join left hands, and turn once around to face corner; corners join right hands. Turn once around to face partner. Dancers describe a figure-eight pattern as they execute the figure. The Texas–Southwest style do-si-do is generally repeated until the caller calls "one more change and promenade." The last time the man turns his partner, the man puts his right arm around the woman's waist and turns her counterclockwise into place to promenade.

Double Pass Thru Starting position. Couple 1 stands with backs to couple 4; couple 3 stands with backs to couple 2. All couples move forward, passing right shoulders with two dancers (men pass two men; women pass two women), to end facing away from center of set. Couples 1 and 3 can get into starting position by circling couple 4 in center until backs are to designated couples. Danced also with couples 2 and 4 circling into positions with couples 1 and 3.

Double Pass Thru Formation Parallel lines. Outside couples face in or down the line. Inside couples face each other.

Double Progression A Contra Dance term. Each couple moves two positions within one dance sequence. *See* Progression.

Double-Toe A Clogging term. The Double–Toe is a toe movement (*see* Toe Movement) occurring on the upbeat (count *and*). The foot performing the movement makes two clicking sounds with the ball of that foot. A small brushing movement of the ball of the foot forward and a small brushing movement backward occur during the "and–ah" count. No weight change occurs in the Double-Toe. The knee of the supporting leg is straight; the knee of the leg performing the movement straightens on the small brushing movement forward and relaxes on the small brushing action backward. On the following downbeat (accent), both knees bend slightly while performing the next movement.

Double Turn Back from Grand Right and Left A Square Dance term. Dancers meet partner on grand right and left, take forearm grasp, turn halfway around to face reverse direction. Go grand right and left in reverse direction to meet partner for the second time, then turn halfway around to face original direction. Go grand right and left in original direction to meet partner for the third time. A promenade usually follows. Also called back track.

Down Contra Dance term. Refers to the foot of the set and away from the music.

Drag A Clogging term. The Drag is a toe movement (*see* Toe Movement) occurring on the upbeat (count *and*). A weight–bearing movement that may be performed on both feet simultaneously or on one foot. Similar to a chug step, the Drag is a movement that scoots *backward* a few inches as the weight is shifted to the balls of the feet. Heels skim the floor during the movement. Both knees are straight (not stiff) on the Drag; on the following downbeat (accent), both knees bend slightly while performing the next movement.

Draw Step In 2/4 time, step sideward on left (count 1) and draw right to left, transferring weight to right (count 2). To draw, the foot is dragged along the floor. In 3/4 time, step sideward on left (counts 1–2) and draw right to left (count 3).

Drop the Gate A Square Dance term. Called to form one circle of eight from two circles of four. Men of active couples release hands with corner woman in circle of four and join hands with original corner women to form a circle of eight.

Duple Minor A Contra set is divided into minor sets, two couples each.

Eight Chain Thru A Square Dance term. For starting position, first and third couples take the opposite person and face the side couples. Four couples are lined up across the floor. Two are on the outside facing in, while two are on the inside facing out. The action is like a grand right and left across the set and back, using a right and left thru when facing out. Refer to p. 149.

Eight Chain Thru Formation Parallel lines. Outside couples face down the line; inside couples face to outside. Example: Couple 1 faces couple 2 and couple 3 faces couple 4.

Elbow Swing Hook right elbows (or left) with person indicated and turn once around.

Ends Turn In A Square Dance term. Starting position is two lines of four, facing out. The two persons in the center of the line form an arch; the two persons on the ends of the line drop hands, walk forward, and go together under the arch, moving into the center of the square. The arching couple does a California twirl.

Escort Position Couple faces line of direction, woman to man's right. The woman slips her left arm through the man's right arm, which is bent at the elbow so that her left hand may rest on his right forearm. Free arm hangs to side.

Even Rhythm When the beats in the rhythm pattern are all the same value, the rhythm is said to be even.

Face Off Position A position used in the Lindy Hop. Partners are facing each other in closed position, bending slightly forward with the man's left foot forward and right foot back. Woman's footwork is opposite.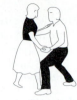

Face to Face, Back to Back A pattern of movement used by a couple moving in the line of direction or reverse line of direction. Partners face, inside hands joined. The basic steps most generally used to effect this movement are the Two–Step, Polka, or Waltz. For example, in the Two–Step, the man would begin left, the woman right. They would take the first Two–Step in the line of direction, turning toward each other. Inside joined hands are swung back and arms are extended. They would take the second Two–Step in the line of direction, turning away from each other. Inside joined hands are swung forward, and arms are extended. Repeat pattern.

Facing Position *See* Two Hands Joined Position.

Fan A term used to describe a manner of executing a leg motion, in which the free leg swings in a whip–like movement around a small pivoting base. Should be a small, subtle action initiated in the hip. *See* p. 423.

File A type of formation. Dancers stand one behind the other, all facing the same direction.

First Four Refers to the first and third couples in the set. Also called the head couples, first two couples, or heads.

First Position One of five basic positions of the feet used in classical ballet. The heels remain touching as the feet are rotated 180° to form one line.

First Two Couples Refers to the first and third couples in the set. Also called head couples, first four, or heads.

Flare An exaggerated lift of the foot from the floor accompanying a knee bend. It is often used in the Rock step of the Tango.

Flirtation Position Also called Swingout Position. Partners are facing; man's left hand and woman's right hand are joined. The arms are bent and are firm so as to indicate or receive a lead.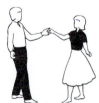

Foot Four In Longway sets, refers to the last two couples.

Foot of Set In Contra and Longway sets, the end of the set farthest from the caller and musicians.

Forearm Turn A Square Dance term. Partners grasp each other by the forearm just below the elbow with either right or left hand, as directions indicate. They press the palm of the hand against the person's forearm, pulling back slightly and keeping the elbow bent as the two people turn each other around. Avoid grasping with the fingers and thumb. This grasp is used in Square Dance for all arm turns, particularly for allemande left, back track, do paso, do–si–do, and allemande thar.

Form a Ring Join hands and circle left.

Forward and Back Move forward four steps and back four steps into place.

Four Gents Star A Square Dance term. All four gents go into the center, take a box star position with their right hand (or left hand), and turn the star as far as designated by the caller.

Four Sides A Square Dance term referring to all four couples in the set.

Four–Step Turn One complete turn is made in four steps. The turn may be made to the left (counter-clockwise) or to the right (clockwise). To right, step right to side (count 1); pivot clockwise on right and step left to face opposite direction (count 2); pivot clockwise on left and step right to side to face original direction (count 3); and step left across right in line of direction (count 4).

Foxtrot An American Social Dance.

Frontier Whirl *See* California Twirl.

Full Turn 'Round A Square Dance term meaning one full turn around from where the turn was started.

Gallop A basic form of locomotion in uneven rhythm, moving forward diagonally with a step close step close pattern (slow quick slow quick).

Gents Turn Back A Square Dance term. When couples are promenading in a circle, this call indicates that the man will drop promenade position, turn to his left, take four steps around to the next woman behind him, and take promenade position with her. It is a good means of changing partners quickly.

Get Outs Short calls that allow action in the square to be culminated with an allemande left to return couples to original positions. Typically used when the call sequence ends with the "key" couples out of sequence, i.e., not with partner or in position to move to home position.

Grand Right and Left A Square and Folk Dance term. Partners take right hands, move past partner, take next with the left hand, move past, take next with the right hand, move past, and so on until partners meet. In European Folk Dance, the term *chain* indicates the same movement.

Grand Square A Square Dance term. This is a no-patter, geometric figure that keeps all dancers in the set active at the same time. First and third couples have one action, while second and fourth couples have a different action. Refer to detailed instructions, p. 144.

Grapevine Step left to side (count 1), step right behind left (count 2), step left to side (count 3), and step right in front of left (count 4). Bend knees, let hips turn naturally, and keep weight on balls of feet.

Grapevine Schottische Beginning right, step right to side, step left behind right, step right to side, and hop right.

Gypsy (8 counts) Two dancers face each other and continuing to face each other with eye contact, move clockwise around each other once. "Left gypsy" travels counterclockwise.

Half Promenade Opposite couples take promenade position, pass each other to the right in the middle of the set (men pass left shoulders), and turn as a couple in the opposite position.

Half Right and Left A Contra Dance term. Same as right and left thru. Couples cross over with a courtesy turn but *do not* return.

Half Sashay *See* Sashay Halfway Around; Roll Away With a Half Sashay.

Half Square Thru A Square Dance term. *See* Square Thru.

Halfway Around Move in one direction, left or right, halfway around the circle (180°). In a circle of four couples, move left or right until on the opposite side of circle from original position.

Hammerlock Position Woman will be in the Hammerlock. Partners stand side by side with right hips together, facing opposite directions. Woman's left arm is behind her back at waist level. The woman's left hand is holding on to the man's right hand. The woman reaches in front of the man to hold his left hand with her right. This may be reversed to put the man in a hammerlock.

Hand Cast Off *See* Cast Off.

Head Couple Refers to first and third couples in a set of four couples. In Contra and Longway sets, head couple is the first couple (man's left shoulder is to top or head of the set).

Head Four Refers to first and third couples in a square.

Head of Set In Longway (Contra) sets, the end of the set closest to the caller and musicians.

Heads Refers to first and third couples in the set. Also called head four.

Heel A Clogging term. The Heel step is a weight-bearing heel movement (*see* Heel Movement) occurring on the downbeat (accent). Weight is shifted from the ball of the foot to the heel as it snaps to the floor.

Heel and Toe Polka Moving to the left, hop right (count *and*), place left heel close to right instep (count 1), hop right (count *and*), place left toe close to right instep (count 2), and take one Polka step to the left (counts *and* 1 *and* 2). Repeat beginning hop on left, moving to the right.

Heel and Toe Scottische Moving to the left, place left heel close to right instep (counts 1–2), place left toe close to right instep (counts 3–4), and take one Schottische step to the left (counts 1–4). Repeat, beginning right.

Heel Movement A Clogging term. The heel movements in clogging (step, slide, heel) take place on the downbeat (accent) of the music. Both legs are slightly bent. Heel movements are accented as the weight is transferred to the entire sole of the foot.

Hesitation A Social Dance step that cues "step hold, step hold."

Hey for Four An English dance figure, also used in Contra Dance. Four dancers in a line, center two facing, weave without touching hands, moving in a figure-eight pattern with an additional loop at end. For detailed analysis, refer to p. 185.

Hitch A Country Western Dance term. Swing right (left) knee almost waist height as one step hops on the other foot, slight chug back. Step hop is subtle.

Home Position Original position of each dancer or couple in the set.

Honey Partner.

Honors Man bows to woman, woman curtseys to man. "Honors right" means bow to partner; "honors left" means bow to corner. *See also* Bow.

Hop A basic form of locomotion in even rhythm. It is a transfer of weight by a springing action from one foot to the same foot. Refer to diagram on p. 48.

Hub Flies Out, Rim Flies In A Square Dance term called from star promenade position. The man, starting in the center, breaks the star and, with arm around partner, wheels counterclockwise around one full turn and a half more to put the woman into the center to form the star (rim flies in).

Hungarian Break Step (cross apart together). Hop left, touching right toe in front of left (count 1); hop left in place, touching right toe to right side (count 2); draw right foot to left, clicking heels together (count 3). Hold (count 4).

Hungarian Turn Partners face in opposite directions with right side to right side. Right hands on partner's right hip, left arm curved overhead. Turn using a push step, buzz step, or hop–step–step. Lean weight away from partner during turn. Reverse position for counterclockwise turn.

Improper A Contra Dance term. Refers to Contra Dances in which the active couples cross over (partners exchange places).

Inactive Couple In Contra Dance, refers to 2, 4, or 6 couples in duple minor dances; 2, 3, 5, 6, 8, or 9 in triple minor dances.

Indian Style A Square Dance term. *See* Promenade Single-File.

Inside Hands Joined Position Partners stand side by side, woman on man's right, inside hands joined, both facing same direction. Also referred to as side–by–side, open, or strolling position.

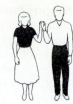

Inside Out, Outside In A Square Dance term. When two couples are facing, the couple designated by the call ducks under an arch made by the other couple. Immediately after they get under the arch, they stand up, make an arch, and back up, letting the other couple duck and move backward under that arch to starting position.

Jitterbug An American Social Dance done to jazz or swing music. *See* Lindy.

Jockey Position Partner stand side by side in open position. Man holds woman's right hand in his left hand at waist level. Knees are bent and couple is slightly bending over from the waist, mimicking the position of a jockey riding a horse.

Jody Position *See* Varsouvienne Position.

Jump A basic form of locomotion in which one or both feet leave the floor, knees bending; both return to the floor together, landing toe–heel with an easy knee action to catch body weight. Spring off the floor on the upbeat of the music and land on the beat.

Kolo Step Moving right: hop on left foot, leap onto right foot, step on left foot behind right, step on right in place, and hop on right foot. Moving left: hop on right foot, leap onto left foot, step on right foot behind left, step on left in place, and hop on left foot.

Ladies Chain

1. *Two Ladies Chain.* A Contra and Square Dance term. Women meet in center, clasp right hands, pass right shoulders, and give left hand to opposite man. Man puts his right arm around woman's waist and turns her with a courtesy turn. Women return to partner in the same manner.

2. *Four Ladies Chain.* A Square Dance term. All four women place right hands in the center, forming a star as they catch hands, and move to the left around circle to opposite man. He turns woman with a courtesy turn. Women return to partner in the same manner.

3. *Three-Quarters Chain.* A Square Dance term. Women chain three–quarters of the way around the ring instead of half of the way. Finish with a courtesy turn.

Ladies Line A Contra Dance term. When a Contra set is formed, the women are to the left of the caller. Even though they may cross over, this term refers to the original line.

Lady by Your Side A Square Dance term. Left–hand woman, corner, or woman on man's left.

Lady Go Gee. Gent to Haw A Square Dance term. Woman goes to right, man goes to left.

Latin Social Position Partners are in closed position with man's left elbow touching the woman's right elbow.

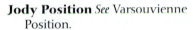

Lead Couple In Square Dancing, refers to the couple indicated to *move* (lead out) and progress through a figure. If two couples are requested to lead out, there are two lead couples. Also called active couple.

Leap A basic method of locomotion involving a transfer of weight from one foot to the other foot. Push off with a spring and land on the ball of the other foot, letting the heel come down; bend the knee to absorb the shock.

Left–Face Turn Dancer turns individually one full turn to the left, or counterclockwise.

Left–Hand Mini–Wave. Couples face in opposite direction. Left hands held above shoulders.

Left–Hand Two–Faced Line. Line of four dancers. Couples face in opposite direction. Center couples have left shoulders adjacent.

Left Parallel Position *See* Parallel Position.

Left Square Thru A Square Dance term. Same as square thru (full), except begin with left–hand grasp instead of right.

Lindy An American Social Dance done to jazz or swing music in 4/4 or cut time. There are three Lindy rhythms–single, double, and triple.

Lindy Hop An American Social Dance first done in the late 1920s in Harlem.

Line A type of formation. Dancers stand side by side, all facing in the same direction.

Line of Direction Refers to the direction of movement of dancers around the circle *counterclockwise*.

Little Windows Position Partners stand side by side with right hips together, facing opposite directions. Right arms are in front with a 90° bend at the elbow. The elbow is next to the partner's shoulder. Partners hold right hands on top and shake left hands in the window created by the right arm.

LOD Symbol for *line of direction*.

Long Lines, Join Hands Along the line, join hands with neighbor.

Longway Set Couples stand in a double line (file or parallel lines), men in one line and women in opposite line. Partners face in a double line or partners face head of set in a double–file. This is also known as Contra formation. *See* p. 63.

Magic Step A Social Dance term. A basic step of the American Foxtrot.

Major A Contra Dance term. The whole Contra set is referred to as the major set. The major set is divided into minor sets.

Make an Arch A Square Dance term. Any two dancers facing the same direction make an arch by raising their joined inside hands. The next call will be for someone to duck under, so arching couples need to separate slightly and make room for that, so that people do not bump each other. Also, if short people are making the arch, they may release hands in the arch in order to allow more room for the ducking couple to go under.

Mazurka Step left (slight stamp), bring right up to left with a cut step displacing left, and hop right while bending knee so that left foot approaches right ankle.

Measure One measure encloses a group of beats made by the regular occurrence of the heavy accent. It represents the underlying beat enclosed between two adjacent bars on a musical staff.

Men's Line A Contra Dance term. When a Contra set is formed, the men are to the right of the caller. Even through they may cross over, this term refers to the original side.

Meter Refers to time in music or group of beats to form the underling rhythms within a measure.

Minor or Minor Set A Contra set is divided into smaller sets that dance together. Two couples dancing together is called duple minor; three couples dancing is called triple minor.

Minuet Position Man extends right arm forward about waist high or to accommodate woman, bending elbow slightly and with palm down and fingers straight. Woman places her left hand, palm down, lightly upon his, keeping her forearm gracefully extended to side, palm down and fingers softly straight. Arms are horizontal; partners are side by side.

Motifs A short step pattern, for example, Two–Step. Several patterns (motifs) may be combined. Refer to Hungarian dances.

Neighbor A Contra Dance term. Same as the opposite person (different sex) or corner. It is not your partner.

Neutral Couple Relating to Contra Dance. A couple waiting out at either end of the set is called the "neutral couple."

Note Values A term used to refer to the relative value of the musical notes or beats that make up the rhythmic pattern.

Ocean Wave A Square Dance and Contradance term. A line of dancers–usually four, facing in alternate directions–join hands and balance (e.g., step or rock, forward and back). Count 1–2 for forward movement, counts 3–4 for backward movement.

Octopus Position With two hands joined, partners stand side by side with right hips together, facing opposite directions. The man's left hand is behind his head and his right hand is behind his partner's head.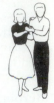

Open Position Partners stand side by side, woman on man's right, facing in the same direction. Man's right arm is around woman's waist. Woman's left hand rests on man's right shoulder. Man holds woman's right hand in his left. Arms extend easily forward.

Open the Gate A Square Dance call when four dancers are side by side in a line in the center of the ring. "Open the gate" will indicate that the two persons on the right of the line will step forward two steps and the two on the left will step back two steps, opening a space in the line. Usually the inactive couples will chain their women through the gate. The call "close the gate" will indicate that the active dancers will step back in line and wait for the next call.

Opposite The person standing in opposite position across the set.

Parallel Position Refers to right or left parallel position. Right parallel is a variation of closed position, in which both man and woman are turned one–eighth turn counterclockwise to a position facing diagonal. The woman is slightly in front of but to the right of the man. Also referred to as banjo position. In left parallel position, man and woman are turned clockwise to face diagonally on the other side. Woman is in front of and to the left of the man.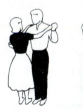

Parallel Two Faced Lines Parallel lines. Couples in each line face in opposite direction. Each line is in a right–hand two–faced line.

Partner Woman to immediate *right* of man and man to immediate *left* of woman. Also called taw and honey.

Pas de Basque
1. *3/4 Time.* Leap to side on left foot (count 1), step right in front of left (count 2), and step left in place (count 3).

2. *2/4 Time.* Leap to side on left (count 1), step right in front of left (count *and*), step left in place (count 2), and hold (count *and*).

Pas de Bourrée Step forward on left (count 1), step on right beside left or slightly forward of left (count 2), step on the left slightly forward (count 3). Step alternates. This step can be done in place.

Pass Thru A Square Dance term. Two couples face. They move toward each other, each passing his opposite by the right shoulder, and then wait for the next call.

Phrase A musical term that represents a short division of time comprising a complete thought or statement. In dance, it is a series of movements considered as a unit in a dance pattern. It is a group of measures, generally four or eight, but sometimes 16 to 32.

Pigeon–Wing Handhold Man and woman face each other and place their forearms, held vertically, close together. The palms are held together, open and upright, and elbows are almost touching.

Pirouette A turn clockwise or counter-clockwise. To go clockwise, step right foot across left and turn, pivoting on the balls of both feet halfway around until feet are uncrossed.

Pivot Turn clockwise or counterclockwise on balls of one or both feet.

Pivot Turn Closed or shoulder–waist position. Step left, pivoting clockwise (count 1), continuing in same direction step right (count 2); step left (count 3), and step right (count 4). Make one complete turn progressing in line of direction. May also be done counterclockwise. Refer to pp. 59 and 388.

Pivot Turn Dip Step left, turn clockwise (count 1); step back on right, continuing turn (count 2); step left, facing forward (count 3); dip back on right foot, still facing forward (count 4).

Polka Hop right, step left forward, close right to left, and step forward left. Repeat, beginning hop left.

Posture The position of the body. An easy, upright standing position is a tremendous advantage in helping one to move efficiently in dance.

Pressure Lead A lead in which extra pressure is exerted by the fingers, arm, or body in order to lead the woman into a particular position or step.

Pretzel A three–part move usually done in Cowboy Swing.

Progression A Contra Dance term. Refers to the movement of each couple to new positions during the dance. Active couples move down the set, inactive move up the set. A new minor set forms for each time through the dance. For most Contras, each couple progresses only one position.

Promenade Couples move counterclockwise around the set or large circle in promenade position. *See* Promenade Position. In Square Dance, the man may give his partner a finishing whirl, bow, and/or swing before resuming ready position facing the center of the set. *See also* Twirl.

Promenade But Don't Slow Down A Square Dance term. Couples continue promenading until caller gives the next call. They do not stop in home position.

Promenade Eight A Square Dance term. All four couples promenade once around the set and return to home position.

Promenade Inside Ring A Square Dance term. Promenade counterclockwise around the inside of the square.

Promenade Outside Ring A Square Dance term. Promenade counterclockwise around outside of square.

Promenade Position Partners stand side by side, facing line of direction. The woman stands to the right of the man. The man holds the woman's right hand in his right and her left in his left. The man's right arm is crossed above the woman's left arm. In some sections of the country, it is customary for the man to cross his right arm underneath the woman's left arm. The promenade position is also referred to as the skater's position.

Promenade Single–File A Square Dance term. Promenade one behind the other in single–file, woman in front, man behind. The line may move clockwise or counterclockwise or down the middle of the set. May also be referred to as Indian style.

Proper A Contra Dance term. Refers to Contra Dances in which the men and women remain on the original sides to start the dance.

Push Step Moving to the left, beginning left, step (chug) to the side (count 1); bring right toe close to left instep; and push right foot away from body (count *and*). Repeat pattern. The push step is similar to a buzz step, except that the action is taken to the side instead of in a turning or circling movement.

Q Symbol for Quick. Used for Rhythm Cue. For example, QQSS, Quick Quick Slow Slow.

Quadrille Formation *See* Square.

Quick A rhythm cue. For example, 4/4 time, 4 quarter beats to each measure; each beat is given the same amount of time, an accent on the first beats of the measure. When a step is taken on each beat (1–2–3–4), these are called *quick* beats. When steps are taken only on 1 and 3, they are twice as long and are called *slow* beats.

Red Hot A Square Dance term. Executed during a promenade by all four couples. Man releases woman's right and walks partner to center with left forearm grasp. Man moves forward to meet right–hand woman, with right forearm turns once around to meet partner, turns partner with left once and a half counterclockwise, faces corner, turns corner with the right once clockwise, moves back to partner with a left, and turns once around counterclockwise. Wait for caller's directions.

Reel A figure used in Longway dances. Head couple meets in middle of set and hooks right elbows, turns once and half around. Man faces women's line, woman faces men's line. Couple separates and head man hooks left elbows with second woman in line; head woman hooks left elbows with second man in line and turns once around. Head couple returns to middle of set. They hook right elbows, turn once, and return to respective lines to swing third dancer. Repeat the "reeling action" until head couple reaches the foot of the set.

Re-Sashay After having done a half sashay (*see* Half Sashay) dancers retrace steps to original position. Often the call "go all the way around" is given following a re-sashay. To "go all the way around" dancers, beginning in original positions, encircle each other once and go back to position. Men generally move behind partner first. Dancers usually face center of set while traveling on any variation of a sashay.

Reverse Line of Direction Refers to the direction of movement of dancers around the circle *clockwise*. Dancers move in the opposite direction from the line of direction.

Reverse Open Position From an open Social Dance position, facing line of direction, partners turn in toward each other to face reverse line of direction but do not change arm or hand positions.

Reverse Varsouvienne Position Couples are standing almost side by side, with the woman on the left side of the man. She is slightly behind him. The man reaches across in front of the woman to hold her left hand in his left. Her right arm is around his shoulders and her right hand grasps his right hand at shoulder level. For Social Dance, the right arm is sometimes extended behind partner at waist level and grasps his hand at the waist. Still a different concept of reverse Varsouvienne position is merely to turn half about from Varsouvienne position. Now woman is on man's left side but slightly in front of him, and his left arm is around her shoulders. Her right arm is across in front of him.

Rhythm Pattern The rhythm pattern in dance is the grouping of beats for the pattern of a dance step. The rhythm pattern must correspond to the underlying beat of the music.

Right and Left Eight *See* Grand Right and Left.

Right and Left Four *See* Right and Left Thru.

Right and Left Thru A Contra and Square Dance term. Two couples are facing each other. Both man and woman, using the right hand, pass by the opposite person on the right side and then immediately give the left hand to their own partner. The man, putting his right arm around his partner, turns her halfway around (courtesy turn) to face the same couple. The two couples have exchanged places.

Right-Face Turn Dancer turns individually one full turn to the right, or clockwise.

Right Hands Across Men or women join right hands in center and turn clockwise. Usually followed by the call "back with the left," which means break with the right, join left hands in the center, and turn counter-clockwise.

Right-Hand Lady A Square Dance term. The woman in the couple on the right, not partner.

Right-Hand Mini-Wave Couples face in opposite direction, right hand held above shoulders.

Right-Hand Two-Faced Line Line of four dancers. Couples face in opposite direction. Center dancers have right shoulders adjacent.

Right Parallel Position *See* Parallel Position.

Ringing Circle formed by two or more dancers joining hands, usually moving left, unless otherwise indicated.

Rip and Snort A Square Dance term. Four couples join hands in a circle. The designated couple, without releasing hands, leads down the center under an arch made by the opposite couple, pulling the whole circle with them. Once under the arch, the lead couple drop each other's hands. The woman pulls her line around to the right, and the man pulls his line around to the left until both man and woman are back to starting position. The arching couples turn under their own joined hands without letting go and face the center of the circle once more.

RLOD Symbol for *reverse line of direction*. *See* Reverse Line of Direction.

Rock A Clogging term. The Rock is a toe movement (see Toe Movement) occurring on the upbeat (count *and*). A weight-bearing movement in which the weight is taken on the ball of the foot. Both knees are straight (not stiff) on the Rock; on the following downbeat (accent) of the music, both knees bend slightly while performing the next movement.

Rock A dance term used when the dancer steps forward (or backward) a short step and then backward (or forward) a short step. With the body weight shifting forward and backward over the foot, this creates a rocking motion. The term is used in Social Dance and in American Round Dance and Folk Dance.

Rock-and-Roll When the second and fourth beats are accented in country western and folk blues music, it is referred to as rock-and-roll music. Contemporary fad dances are done to rock-and-roll music. Rock-and-roll is a rhythm; but the term *Rock Dance* is used.

Roll Away with a Half Sashay A Square Dance term. Partners are side by side, facing the same direction, woman on the man's right. The woman rolls across in front of the man to his left side. As she rolls, she makes one complete turn counterclockwise. The man guides the woman across with his right hand and simultaneously steps to his right so that they end up having exchanged places.

Roll Back A Square Dance term. From a star promenade position with the woman on the outside, the woman is released. She rolls out and around once to meet the man who is behind her. If the star is turning counterclockwise, she will roll back clockwise. If the star is turning clockwise, she will roll back counterclockwise.

Roll Promenade A Square Dance term. A man and woman meet with the left hand. The man rotates to face the same way as the woman with her on his right in promenade position. They wheel around until they face standard promenade direction.

Rumba A Latin–American Dance from Cuba in 4/4 time.

Run A basic form of locomotion in fast, even rhythm. It is similar to a walk, except that the weight is carried forward over the ball of the foot with a spring–like action.

Running Step A light, bouncy, dignified half–walk, half–run as in English dances. *See* Run.

Russian Polka The customary Polka hop is omitted. Step left (count 1), close right to left (count *and*), step left (count 2), and hold (count *and*), Repeat, beginning right.

S Symbol for slow. Used for Rhythm Cue. For example, SSQQ, slow slow quick quick.

Samba A Latin–American Dance from Brazil in 4/4 or cut time.

Sashay Dancers move once around each other. Man moves sideways to the right and behind the woman and the woman moves sideways to the left and in front of the man. Dancers face center of circle throughout the sashay.

Sashay Halfway Around *See* Roll Away with a Half Sashay.

Schottische Step left (count 1), step right (count 2), step left (count 3), and hop left (count 4). Repeat, beginning right.

Scissor Kick Kick the left leg (stiff–legged) forward (count 1) and exchange by kicking the right leg forward and left back to place (count *and*). Continue action.

Scoot A Country Western Dance term. *See* Chug Step.

Scuff A Country Western Dance term. A brush of the heel forward.

Second Corners An English Country dance term. Refer to Corners.

See Saw A Square Dance term. Man moves to his right around behind and then in front of partner and back to home position.

Semiopen Position A Social Dance position halfway between open and closed position.

Separate A Square Dance term meaning to turn one's back on the partner and do what the next call says. Couples frequently separate to go around the outside ring (man goes left, woman right) until they meet each other. Wait for next call.

Separate Go Around One Couple 1 moves into center, man goes left between couple 4 and around woman 4 and back to place; woman 1 goes right between couple 2 and around man 2 and back to place. Also done with two couples facing. Example: couple 1 leads out to couple 2, couple 1 moves between couple 2 man moving around woman and back to place as woman 1 moves around man 2 and back to place.

Set An English Country Dance term. Setting steps are done either in place, advancing toward or retiring from another dancer. A single set is to the right and the left. Dancer springs lightly on right, usually to side, steps onto left, then back onto right with a quick change of weight. Repeat to the left. (Slow, quick, quick, slow, quick, quick.)

Set Refers to a group formation for Square, Contra, and Longway formations. The term *set* is also used to describe a group of three people (i.e., "set of three").

Shine Position A Social Dance term. The man faces the woman at approximately arms distance. Hands are not joined. Also called the Challenge position.

Shoulder–Waist Position Partners stand facing each other, shoulders parallel and toes pointed directly forward. The man extends his arms in a "barrel shape" around the woman, both hands are placed below the woman's shoulder blades. Woman's raised arms rest gently on man's arms; her hands folding over his shoulder, point slightly toward each other. The woman supports the weight of her arms and give a firm pressure with her hands. Both lean slightly away from each other against the firm hand support of the other.

Shuffle An easy, light one–step, keeping feet lightly in contact with the floor as they move. Principal step used in Square and Contra dancing.

Sicilian Circle A double circle with *couples facing*, woman to man's right. Couples may be numbered 1, 2, 3, and so forth. All *even*–numbered couples face line of direction, while all *odd*–numbered couples face reverse line of direction. *See* p. 63.

Side Refers to second and fourth couples.

Side–by–Side Position *See* Inside Hands Joined Position.

Side Car Position *See* Left Parallel Position; Parallel Position.

Side Couples Refers to second and fourth couples in a set of four couples.

Side Four Refers to second and fourth couples.

Side Step Step to the left with the left foot (count 1). Close right to left, take weight on right (count 2).

Side Two Couples Refers to second and fourth couples in the set. Also called side four.

Single–File Promenade *See* Promenade Single–File.

Single–File Turn Back A Square Dance term. From a single–file promenade, traveling counterclockwise, either man or woman may be designated by the caller to step out of the circle, about–face to the right, and go the other way, making another circle on the outside, traveling clockwise.

Skater's Position Couple is standing side by side with the woman on the right side. The man reaches across behind the woman to hold her right hand in his right. Her left arm is in front of his waist, grasping his left hand. Also called Promenade Position.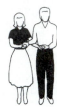

Skip A basic form of locomotion in uneven rhythm. The pattern is a step and a hop on the same foot in slow quick slow quick rhythm.

Slide A basic form of locomotion in uneven rhythm. The movement is sideward. It is a step close step close pattern (slow quick slow quick).

Slide A Clogging term. The Slide is a heel movement (*see* Heel Movement) occurring on the downbeat (accent). A weight-bearing movement that may be performed on both feet simultaneously or on one foot. Feet scoot *forward* a few inches as weight is shifted from balls of feet to heels. Heels skim along the floor. Both knees are slightly bent on the Slide; on the following upbeat (count *and*), both knees straighten while performing the next movement.

Slip the Clutch A Square Dance term. Starting from the allemande that star position, man will release partner on his left arm, move forward one place to the corner for an allemande left, and follow the call.

Slipping Step An English Country Dance term. Spring sideways to the right (or left) (count 1), bring trailing foot up taking weight (count *and*), spring again to right (or left).

Slow A rhythm cue. *See* Quick.

Social Swing Position A social dance position similiar to "semi–open". Man's right arm is around the woman and the right hand is placed in the center of the woman's back, just below the shoulder blades. The woman's left arm rests gently but definitely in contact with the man's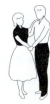

upper arm and the hand should lie along the back of the man's shoulder. Man's left, woman's right hands are joined with man's palm up and woman's palm down, arms lowered.

Split the Ring A Square Dance term. From square formation, the lead–off couple joins hands and goes between the couple they are facing, splitting them apart. After going through, they wait, facing out, for the next call.

Square The formation for Square Dancing. A square is composed of four couples, each standing on the imaginary sides of a square, facing the center. Each couple stands with their backs to one side of the room. Also called a set.

Square Sets A Square Dance term. At home: Man has his partner on the right and they are standing side by side, inside hands joined. Away from home: After a swing or promenade, man is on the left, woman is on the right, inside hands joined. The couple faces the center of the set.

Square Thru (full) A Square Dance term. The square thru is executed when two couples are facing. Couples move forward, take opposite's right hand, pull by; do quarter–turn to face partner, join left hands, pull by; do quarter–turn to face original opposite again, join right hands, pull by; make quarter–turn to face partner, join left hands, pull by; and wait for caller's directions.

Square Thru (half) A Square Dance term. The half square thru is executed when two couples are facing. Couples move forward, take opposite right hand, pull by; do quarter–turn to face partner, join left hands, pull by; do quarter–turn to face partner, join left hands, pull by; and wait for caller's directions. This is one half of a full square thru.

Square Thru (three–quarters) A Square Dance term. The three–quarters square thru is executed when two couples are facing. Couples move forward, take opposite's right hand, pull by; do quarter–turn to face partner, join left hands, pull by; do quarter–turn to face original opposite again, join right hands, pull by; and wait for caller's directions. This is three-quarters of a full square thru.

Stamp Place the ball of one foot firmly on the floor, accenting the placement. The weight is not usually transferred to the foot taking the stamp; however, in some instances, it does take the weight.

Star Promenade A Square Dance term. Either man or woman may be on the inside of the set, forming a star (box star position). The free arm is around partner, who travels in the same direction. If right hand forms the star, it will travel clockwise with left arm around partner. If left hand forms the star, it will travel counterclockwise with right hand around partner.

Star Thru A Square Dance term. When two couples are facing, each person works with the opposite. The man takes the woman's left hand in his right hand and turns her quarter–turn counterclockwise as he walks around her one–quarter of the way clockwise. They end up side by side. This woman is now his new partner and is on his right.

Step A Clogging term. The Step is a weight-bearing flat-footed heel movement (*see* Heel Movement) occurring on the downbeat (accent). Both knees are slightly bent on Step; on the following upbeat (count *and*) both knees straighten.

Step Close Step sideward left (count 1), and close right to left, take weight on right (count 2). The right foot does not draw along the floor, but moves freely into place beside left.

Step–Hop Step on the left foot (count 1) and hop on the same foot (count *and*). Even rhythm.

Step Swing Step left (count 1) and swing right across in front of left (count 2). Repeat movement, beginning right.

Strathopey Traveling Step A step used in Scottish reels and country dancing. 4/4 meter, the rhythm is slower than reel music. Beginning right, step forward closing left to right, step right forward, lifting right heel slightly as left foot swings through and reaches forward for next step. Alternate leads.

Stride Position A Social Dance term. Legs straight, feet apart.

Strut Walk forward, upper torso high and leading, left knee slightly bent, toe pointed, preparing to step. Step on *ball of foot first* and then lower heel gently.

Suzy Q Moving sideward, toes are together, heels apart, "pigeon toes." Weight on both feet, shift weight to left heel, right toe simultaneously, pivoting to "pigeon toe" position; shift weight to left toe, right heel, pivoting to toes out, "roach toe." Alternating toe heel, heel toe, move sideward.

Sweep Cue word for Varsouvienne and Country Western Line Dances as left heel swings across in front of right instep. Same as wing.

Sweetheart Modern Position Country Western dance position. Same as Varsouvienne.

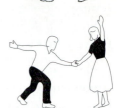

Swing
1. *Right- or Left-Hand Swing.* The woman and man clasp right (or left) hands and swing around clockwise. Forearm grasp may be used.
2. *Two-Hand Swing.* The woman and man face each other, join both hands, and one–step or shuffle once around clockwise. The elbows are held in close to the body.
3. *Waist Swing.* Couples take swing position (right parallel position) and turn clockwise with a shuffle, Two-Step, or buzz step. In Square Dance, make two turns. In Contra, turn for eight measures. Couples should lean back slightly for a swing.

Swing Out Position Also called Flirtation Position. Partners are facing; man's left hand and woman's right hand are joined. The arms are bent and are firm so as to indicate or receive a lead.

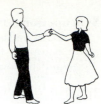

Swing Out Position – Lindy Style Partners are facing; man's left hand and woman's right hand are joined. Man's left foot is extended behind his right with bent knees. Woman's knees are bent and both feet swivel to her right or woman has the option of a right foot rock step.

Swing Position The man and woman step into right parallel position, the woman and man are almost right side to right side. The man's right arm is around the woman's waist, and his right hand is firm at her waist so that she may lead back against it. The woman places her left hand on his right shoulder. His left hand holds her right hand. The couple look at each other and lean back as they shuffle around in a clockwise direction.

Swing the Right–Hand Lady A Square Dance term. The women all stay in home position. The men pass in front of partner on the inside and move to the right to swing right–hand lady twice around and square the set in that position.

Swing Thru A Square Dance term. From an ocean-wave position, the two on each end of the line turn each other with right arm halfway around. Then the two in the center of the line turn each other with left arm halfway around. All balance forward and back and follow the next call.

Swing Your Opposite A Square Dance term. The women stay in home position. The men move straight across the inside of the set to the opposite woman, but the man must allow the man in the couple to his left to cross in front of him. He swings the opposite woman twice around and opens up to square the set from that new position. Another call to swing the opposite will take him back to his own original partner, but the caller may choose to get him back to his partner in another way.

Swivel Toes and heels move sideward, either weight on toes, pivoting heels, or weight on heels, pivoting toes. Also called Suzy Q. Or, pivoting on one toe and one heel simultaneously, then pivoting on the other toe and heel, alternating toe heel, heel toe, moving sideward; or, in place by shifting weight, feet are "pigeon-toed," then heels together, toes pointed out "roach toe."

Swivel Turn. In one spot, a complete turn on the ball of one foot, either direction. Free foot may be lifted, bending knee, or close to other heel.

Syncopation A temporary displacement of the natural accent in music. For instance, shifting the accent from the naturally strong first and third beat to the weak second and fourth beat.

Tango A Latin American dance from Argentina.

Tempo Rate of speed at which the music is played, or the speed of the dance.

Those Who Can A Square Dance term meaning that those who are in the right position should do what the next call says. Those who are not in the right position should just stand and wait.

Three–Quarter Chain *See* Ladies Chain.

Three–Step Turn One complete turn made in three steps. The turn may be made to the left (counter-clockwise) or to the right (clockwise). To turn right (clockwise), step right to side (count 1), pivot clock-wise on right, and step left to face opposite direction (count 2); pivot clockwise on left and step right to side to face original direction (count 1). Hold the last count of 2/4 or 4/4 music. For 3/4 time, *see* Canter Rhythm.

Throw in the Clutch A Square Dance term. Executed from an allemande thar or wrong way thar move-ment. On the call "throw in the clutch," dancers in the center retain hold on the star but release hand with outside dancers. The star changes direction and moves forward while the dancers on the outside (once released) continue in same direction (e.g., for-ward). Dancers then follow the next call.

Time Signature A symbol indicating duration of time. Example: In 2/4 time, the upper number indicates number of beats per measure, while the lower num-ber indicates the note value that receives one beat.

Tip A Square Dance term. One completed Square Dance call (sequence).

Toe A Clogging term. The Toe step in clogging is a weight-bearing toe movement (*see* Toe Movement) occurring on the upbeat (count *and*). Weight is placed on the ball of the foot, followed by a Heel step.

Toe Movement A Clogging term. The toe movements in clogging (rock, drag, toe, double–toe, brush) occur on the upbeat (count *and*) of the music. Both legs are straight (but not stiff).

Top of Set In Contra (Longways) sets, the end of the set closest to the caller and musicians.

Touch A Clogging term. The Touch is a variation of the Toe step. The Touch step involves no change of weight. The ball of the foot touches the floor on the upbeat (count *and*) and lifts on the downbeat (accent).

Trade By Formation Square Dance Term. Parallel lines. Outside couples face out and inside couples face each other.

Triple Allemande A Square Dance term. Men turn cor-ner women with a left allemande and send them to the center. Women form a right-hand star and move star clockwise, while men walk counterclockwise around star. Men again turn corners with left alle-mande one full turn, move to center, and form a right-hand star. Star moves clockwise, as women walk counterclockwise, around star. Men again, third time, turn corners (original always) with left allemande one full turn and move into a grand right and left or wait for caller's directions.

Triple Minor A Contra set is divided into minor sets, three couples each.

Triple Set A set of three couples.

Turn Dancers may move around individually clockwise or counterclockwise or with a partner. With a partner, dancers join right, left, or both hands as directed and move around clockwise (or counterclockwise).

Turn as a Couple A Contra Dance term. Hands may or may not be joined. Partners, side by side, turn as a unit counterclockwise, the woman moving forward, the man pivoting almost in place.

Turn Back A Square Dance term.

1. Sometimes used as "gents turn back and swing the girl behind you."

2. May be used as a single–file turn back.

3. *See* Back Track.

Turn Contra Corners *See* Contra Corners Turn.

Turn Single An English Country Dance term. One dancer turns clockwise (or counterclockwise) individ-ually, taking four walking steps.

Turn Thru A Square Dance term. Two dancers are fac-ing each other. They take a right forearm grasp and turn each other around clockwise 180°, so as to end up facing the direction they had their backs to when they started.

Twinkle Step A variation based on box rhythms for both Foxtrot and Waltz.

Twirl In Square Dance, the twirl may be used to get into and out of a prome-nade. To get into a promenade, part-ners face and join right hands. The man lifts his right hand, twirling the woman clockwise one time around under his right arm. As she comes around, he takes her left hand under-neath the right and they are ready to 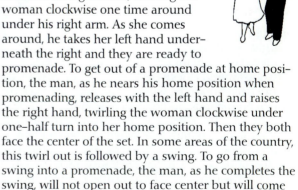 promenade. To get out of a promenade at home posi-tion, the man, as he nears his home position when promenading, releases with the left hand and raises the right hand, twirling the woman clockwise under one-half turn into her home position. Then they both face the center of the set. In some areas of the country, this twirl out is followed by a swing. To go from a swing into a promenade, the man, as he completes the swing, will not open out to face center but will come around to face the line of direction. He raises his left hand and twirls the woman clockwise under his left hand once around. As she comes around, he puts her right hand in his right and reaches underneath for her left hand. This needs practice so that the woman can be moving in the line of direction while twirling under because the total movement should be continuous.

Two–Hand Swing *See* Swing.

Two–Hand Turn *See* Swing, Two–Hand Swing.

Two Hands Joined Position Partners stand facing each other, shoulders parallel, and toes pointed directly forward. Two hands are joined, man's palms up, his thumbs on top of her hands. The elbows are bent and held close to the body.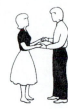

Two–Step Step left (count 1), close right to left (count 2), step left (count 3), and hold (count 4).

Tyrolian Waltz A series of Waltz steps taken in the line of direction. Beginning left, step diagonally forward left on first Waltz step, step diagonally forward to the right on the second Waltz step. Repeat pattern. Partners tend to face away and toward each other, with alternate steps, as they *glide* forward.

Unassisted, Two Dancers *See* Cast Off.

Uneven Rhythm When the beats in the rhythm pattern are not all the same value but are a combination of slow and quick beats, the rhythm is said to be uneven.

U Turn Back A single dancer, either man or woman or both, turn around in place 180°, ending facing in opposite direction.

Varsouvienne Position Couple faces in line of direction, woman in front and slightly to the right of man. Man holds woman's left hand in his left at shoulder level. Man's right arm extends back of woman's shoulders and holds woman's raised right hand in his right. In Social Dance, this is sometimes called jody position.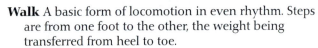

Walk A basic form of locomotion in even rhythm. Steps are from one foot to the other, the weight being transferred from heel to toe.

Walk Around *See* Cast Off.

Walking Waltz 3/4 time. Traveling forward, step on each beat.

Waltz Step forward left (count 1), step sideward right (count 2), close left to right, and take weight left (count 3).

Waltz Balance *See* Balance, 3/4 time.

Weave the Ring A Square Dance term. Same as grand right and left, except that dancers *do not* touch hands in passing each other.

Wheel and Deal A Square Dance term. From a line of four, facing out, the right–hand couple in line pivots counterclockwise halfway around the person nearest the center. The left–hand couple moves forward two steps and then pivots clockwise halfway around the person nearest the center and comes in behind the right–hand couple. Both end up facing the center, one behind the other.

Wheel Around A Square Dance term that is also used in Contra. From the promenade position, couples wheel around as a unit to face in opposite direction. Men back up, women move forward around men. Dancers retain the promenade position handhold.

Whirl Term used for waist swing in Square Dance. Also refers to several rather rapid individual right– or left–face turns.

Whirlaway With a Half Sashay *See* Roll Away With a Half Sashay.

Wrap Position The woman is at the right of the man. His right arm is around her waist and his hand holds her left hand. His left hand is holding her right hand in front.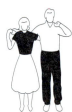

Yemenite Step In 4/4 meter. Begin left, with flexed knees, and step to left (count 1); step right behind left (count 2); step left in front of right (count 3); and hold (count 4).

Yoke Position Couple is standing side by side with the woman on the right side of the man. Man holds woman's left hand in his left hand, behind his shoulder. Man's right arm extends back of woman's shoulders and holds woman's raised right hand in his right hand.

Index of Mixer and Nonpartner Dances

MIXER

Den Toppede Høne   352
D'Hammerschmiedsg'selln   230
Doudlebska Polka   206
Familie Sekstur   353
Familjevalsen   354
Korobushka   345
La Bastringe   282
Levi Jackson Rag   124
Mexican Mixer   121
Mixers, Plain and Novelty   117
Mixers, Square Dance   134–135
Ninepin Reel   81
Oh Johnny   113
Oslo Waltz   271
Patty-Cake Polka   120
Paul Jones Your Lady   80
Red River Valley   123
Square Dance Mixers
   Big Circle Mixers   134
   Methods for Squaring Up   134
   Methods for Changing
    Partners   135
Tant' Hessie   227
Tennessee Wig Walk   121
Texas Schottische for Three   103
Totur   363

NONPARTNER

Alley Cat (Popcorn)   115
Amos Moses   114
Borborbor   223
Branle d'Ossau   289
California Hustle   447
Carnavilito   364
Charleston   393
Cherkessiya   305
Clogging   88
Cotton-Eyed Joe Line Dance   107
Cowboy Boogie   440
Cowboy Polka (Jessie Polka)   440
Eight Step Shuffle
   (Jessie Polka)   440
El Tango Sereno   449
Electric Slide   450
Four Corners   452
Freeze   451
Gahu   224
Harmonica   306
Hasápikos   246
Hineh Ma Tov   309
Hora   310
Hora De Mina   340
Itele   341
Las Chiapanecas   329

Lesnoto   247
Ma Na'avu   311
Mayim   312
Mon Père Avait un Petit Bois   294
Para Bailar   453
Pata Pata   226
Pljeskavac Kolo   250
Popcorn (Alley Cat)   115
Ranchera   365
Rondeau de Garein   296
Rumunjsko Kolo   251
Sarajevka Kolo   252
Saturday Night Fever
   Line Dance   454
Savila Se Bela Loza   253
Šetnja   255
Sira Din Cimpoi   342
Slappin' Leather   455
Syrtós   256
Tropanka   257
Twelfth Street Rag   116
Watermelon Crawl   456
Western Wind   458

Index of Folk Dances

Africa
    Borborbor 223
    Gahu 224
    Pata Pata 226
    Tant' Hessie 227
America (*see* United States)
Austria
    Spinnradl zu Dritt 241
Bolivia
    Carnavalito 364
Bosnia
    Sarajevka Kolo 252
Bulgaria
    Tropanka 257
Canada
    La Bastringe 282
    Saint John River 288
Czech and Slovakia
    Doudlebska Polka 286
    Tancuj 287
Denmark
    Bitte Mand I Knibe (Little Man in a Fix) 351
    Den Toppede Høne (The Crested Hen) 352
    Familie Sekstur 353
    To Ting 362
    Totur 363
England
    Butterfly Hornpipe–*Warwickshire* 265
    Dover Pier 266
    The First of April 267
    The Northdown Waltz 270
    Oslo Waltz *Scottish–English* 271
    The Ragg 272
    Three Meet 275
    Willow Tree 279
France
    Branle d'Ossau 289
    La Montagnarde 290
    La Tournijaire 292
    Mon Père Avait un Petit Bois 294
    Rondeau de Garein 296
Germany
    D'Hammerschmiedsg'selln 230
    Kanonwalzer 233
    Krüz König 234
    Man in the Hay 237
    Sonderburg Dopplequadrille 240
Greece
    Hasápikos 246
    Misirlou *Greek-American* 249
    Syrtós 256

Hungary
    Hungarian Motifs 299
    Csárdás Palócosan 300
    Kiskanásztánc 301
    Ugrós 302
Ireland
    The Bridge of Athlone 264
    Siamsa Beirte 274
Israel
    Cherkessiya 305
    Harmonica 306
    Hava Nagila 307
    Hineh Ma Tov 309
    Hora 310
    Ma Na'avu 311
    Mayim 312
    Vé David 313
Italy
    Il Codiglione 315
    Sicilian Tarantella 316
Lithuania
    Kalvelis 319
    Klumpakojis 320
Macedonia
    Lesnoto 247
Mexico
    El Jarabe Tapatío 323
    Jesucita en Chihuahua 325
    La Cucaracha 327
    La Raspa 328
    Las Chiapanecas 329
    Santa Rita 330
Norway
    Norwegian Polka (Scandinavian Polka) 357
    Seksmannsril 358
Poland
    Tramblanka–Polka Mazurka 335
    Walczyk "Ges Woda" 337
Romania
    Alunelu 339
    Hora De Mina 340
    Itele 341
    Sirba Din Cimpoi 342
Russia
    Alexandrovska 344
    Korobushka 345
    Troika 346
Scotland
    Bonny Prince Charlie Crossing the Frew 262
    Flowers of Edinburgh *Scottish Reel* 268

Gie Gordons 269
Oslo Waltz English–Scottish 271
Road to the Isles 273
The White Cockade *Scottish Reel* 277
Serbia
    Pljeskavac Kolo Serbian 250
    Rumunjsko Kolo *Serbian-American* 251
    Savila Se Bela Loza 253
    Šetnja 255
Sweden
    Familjevalsen 354
    Hambo 355
    Snurrbocken 359
    Swedish Varsouvienne 360
    Swedish Waltz 361
Switzerland
    Dr Gsatzlig 231

Uruguay
    Ranchera 365
United States
    Alabama Gal 96
    Amos Moses 114
    Big Circle Square Dance 84
    Blue Pacific Waltz 109
    Boston Two–Step 105
    Cajun Dances 413
    Clogging 88
    Contra Dances 187–215
    Cotton–Eyed Joe 107
    Cowboy Polka, Ten Step 440
    Garden Waltz 111
    Grand March 75
    Grand Square Quadrille 78
    Heel and Toe Polka 106
    Jiffy Mixer 119
    Levi Jackson Rag 124
    Mexican Mixer 121
    Mixers, Plain and Novelty 117
    Ninepin Reel 81
    Nobody's Business 97
    Oh Johnny 113
    Patty–Cake Polka 120
    Paul Jones Your Lady 80
    Ping–Pong Schottische 100
    Popcorn 115
    Portland Fancy 83
    Red River Valley 123
    Salty Dog Rag 104
    Schottische 98
    Square Dances 158–176
    Tennessee Wig Walk 121
    Texas Schottische 102
    Texas Schottische for Three 103
    Twelfth Street Rag 116
    Varsouvienne 112
    Virginia Reel 77

Subject Index

Aboriginal 18, 20
Accent 43
Acoustics 24
Africa 4
    Art and Dance 5
    Beo Dances 6
    Continent 4
    Environmental Influences 5
    European Influences 4
    Gnenon Dances 6
    Improvisation 5
    Instruments 5
    Slave Trade 4
    Spiritual World 5
    Traditional Dance 4
Afro–Americans 70
    Contributions 70
    Dances 70
Alpine Region (Switzerland, Austria, Germany) 228
American Folk Dance Society 219
American Dance Sampler
    Dress 73
    Music 72
    Origins 70
    Afro–American Influence 70
    Appalachian Clog Dance 72
    Cajun Dances 72, 413
    Contra Dances 72, 177
    Country Dancing, Revival 73
    Dress 73
    Etiquette 73
    European Courts 70
    Folk Traditions, Revival 73
    Melting Pot vs. Ethnic
        Identity 74
    Music 72
    Play Party Games 71
    Round and Novelty Dances 72
    Social Occasion 73
    Spanish–Mexican Influence 71
    Square Dances 71, 125
    Texas Square Dance, 127
    Teaching Suggestions 74
Allotey, Ardey 223, 224
American Square Dance Society, Sets in Order 130
Amerinds 20
Anderson, Kathy 213
Apache Fiddles 20
Appalachia, Dance 126

Appalachian Clog Dance 72. *See also* Clogging
Arabs 303
Armstrong, Don 191
Assemblé 48
Aztecs 20

Bali 15
Balkan Countries, Dance
    Characteristics 243
    Bulgaria 245
    Greece 243
    Yugoslavia, Former 244
Bannerman, Glen 84
Baris 16
Bartók, Béla 297
Basic Dance Steps 50
    Mazurka 52
    Polka 51
    Schottische 51
    Shuffle (Dance Walk
        or Glide) 50
    Two–Step or Triple Step 50
    Waltz 51
Basic Dance Steps, Teaching 55
    Analysis of Rhythm 55
    Method of Presentation 55
Basic Dance Turns
    Pivot 59
    Polka 53
    Schottische 52
    Two–Step 53
    Waltz 34
    Teaching 56
Bay Area Country Dance Society 180
Bayou Bedlam Contra Dance 180
Beat 43
Beliajus, Vytautas Finaden 319
Beo Dances 6
Berea 180
Berea College Mountain Folk Festival 124
Berutuk 16
Bharata 7
Bharata Natya 7
Bible 3
Binusan 17
Blue Bonnet Calls 101
Bogue, Erna–Lynne 210
Bon Festivals 13
Break Dance 368

Breunig, Fred 182, 204
Brigham Young Folk Dancers 218
British Isles, Dance
    Characteristics 258
    England 258
    Ireland 260
    Scotland 261
Buck Dancing 88
Bugaku 14
Bukhara 303
Bulletin Boards 38
Burchenal, Elizabeth 219

Cajun Dance 72, 413
California Folk Dance Federation 218
Callerlab 130
Calling Square Dances 131
Camcorder/VCR 26
Campbell, John C. Folk School 180
Camps 219
Card File 182
Carole 2
Cassette Sources 489, 491
CD 25
Cha Cha Cha 459
Chain 2
Chang, Soon 218
Charleston
    History 393
    Rhythm 394
    Style 394
    Teaching 394
Chestnut, New England. *See* New England Chestnut
China 9
Class Procedure 34
    Evaluation 37
    Strategies for Selecting
        Material 34
    Teaching Specific Dance 35
Climate 220
Cocke, Enid 128
Clogging 72, 88
    Basic Steps 91
    Costumes and Shoes 90
    History 88
    Music 90
    Style 90
    Teaching 95
Closed Circle 1

Closed Dance Position 60, 373
Combos
    Cha Cha Cha 466
    Foxtrot 390
    Merengue 472
    Rumba 479
    Samba 484
    Swing 407
    Tango 426
    Waltz 433
Communist Party 12
Community Centers 39
Community Resources 39
Compact Disc 25
Content Selection 30
Contradanza, La 178
Contra Dance 72, 178
    Basics 181
    Basic Step 183
    Basic, Figures 183
    Caller 182
    Card File 182
    Dance Structure 181
    Formation 181
    History 177
    Levels, Dance 185
    Music 182, 183
    Numbering Off 181
    Page, Ralph 179, 185
    Progression 181
    Record Sources 489, 491, 494
    Sources 182
    Teaching 184
    Timing 182
    Tunes 185, 501
Contra Set 63
Contredanse, French 69, 125
Contree–danse 69, 125, 133
Cook, Captain James 3
Corté 422, 508
Costumes, Dress 73
Cotillion 70, 125
Country Dance 73, 177
Counry Dance, English 295
Country Dance and Song Society 259
Country Dancing, Old Time 128
Country Western Dance 434
    Etiquette 434
    History 434
    Music 435
    Style 435
Court Dances 70
Cowboy Dances 128
Courtesy, Deportment. See Etiquette
Crampton, C. Ward 218
Crum, Dick 253, 255
Csárdás 297
Cue, Kinds 46, 370
Culminating Activities 38
Culture, Eastern and Western 234
Cusimano, Barbara E. 29
Cut Time 44

Cutting In 32
Czarnowski, Lucille 78, 178
Czech, Dance Characteristics 285
Czompo, Andor 297–302

Dalsemer, Bob 205
Dance Characteristics. See Specific
    Country
Dance–Drama 6, 228
Dance Formations 63
Dance Fundamentals 43
    Accent 43
    Analysis of a Basic Rhythm 46
    Beat 43
    Even Rhythm 45
    Line Values 45
    Measure 44
    Meter 44
    Note Values 44
    Phrase 45
    Rhythm Pattern 45
    Tempo 45
    Uneven Rhythm 46
Dance Lesson 29, 371
Dance Positions 60–62, 382
    Back Cross 60–505
    Banjo 62, 506, 516, 518
    Bridge 62, 507
    Butterfly 60, 507, 509
    Challenge 60, 508
    Closed 60, 373
    Conversation 60, 508
    Couple 61, 509
    Cuddle 60, 509
    Escort 60, 510
    Face Off 60, 511
    Facing 62, 511
    Flirtation 62, 511, 513
    Hammerlock 60, 512
    Inside Hands Joined 61, 513, 515,
    Jockey 61, 513
    Jody 513
    Latin Social 61, 513
    Left Parallel 61, 513, 516
    Little Window 61, 513
    Octopus 61, 514
    Open 61, 514
    Pigeon Wing 61, 515
    Promenade 61, 515
    Reverse Open 61, 516
    Reverse Varsouvienne 62, 516, 518
    Right Hand Star 61
    Right Parallel 62, 516
    Semiopen 62, 517
    Shine 60, 517
    Shoulder Waist 62, 517
    Side by Side 61, 518
    Side Car 61, 518
    Skaters (Promenade) 61, 51, 518
    Social Swing 62, 518
    Sweetheart (Modern) 62, 519
    Swing 62, 519

Swing Out 62, 519, 521
Swing Out–Lindy Style 62, 519
Two Hands Joined 62, 521
Varsouvienne (Traditional) 62, 521
Wrap 60, 521
Yoke 62, 521
Dance Steps, Basic 50–52
    Teaching 55
Dance Turns
    Pivot 59
    Polka 503
    Schottische 52
    Two–Step 53
    Waltz 34
        Box 58
        Running 58
        Teaching 55
Dance Unit 29
Dance Walk 50, 372
Danish Folk Dance Society 218
Daola Dance 12
David, Mihai 340–342
de Angeles, Señora Alura Flores 325
de Chavarria, Laura Zanzi 364–365
Death Dance 228
Denmark, Dance Characteristics 349
Diggle, Roger 206
Dillingham, Uncle Dave 107
Disabilities, students with 41
Disabled Person, Physically 390
Disco Dance 390
Double Time Swing 399
Dress, Costume 73
Drury, Nelda Guerrero 121, 126, 321,
    323, 325, 327, 329, 330
Dunsing, Gretel and Paul 240
Duple Minor Longways 181

East Coast Swing 405
Education, History 3
Edwards, Pru 283
English Country Dances 259
English Folk Dance and Song
    Society 279
Enrichment Activities 38
    Bulletin Boards 38
    Community Resources 39
    Culminating Activities 38
    Special Party 40
    Teacher Resources 39
Ericson, Jane Harris xviii, xx
Ethnic Lodges 41
Ethnic Museums 41
Etiquette 32
Evaluation 37
    Written Test 37

Facilities 24
Family Dances 39
Farandole 1
Farwell, Jane 219, 231
Feild, Fred 212

Fertility Rites 4
Fifth Veda 7
Finland, Dance Characteristics 350
Fix, Penn 181–185, 199
Floor 24
Fogg, George A. 259, 263, 266, 267, 270, 272
Folk Dance in America
    Camps 219
    Movement 218
    Performing Groups 219
    Trends 220. *See also* International
       Folk Dance
Folk Dance House 218
Folklore Village 219
Following, Techniques 374, 372
Foot 'n' Fiddle 129
Ford, Henry 129
Formations, Dance 63
Forms, Dance 2
    Chain 2
    Closed Circle 2
    Double Circle 2
    Processional 2
Foster, Brad xx
Foxtrot
    History 377
    Rhythm 377
    Style 378
France, Dance Characteristics 288
French–Canadian Influence, Contra
    Dance 178
French Contredanse 69, 125

Gadd, May 275
Gallemore, Sandra L. (Sandy) 88–95
Gallop 49
Gang of Four 12
Gaudreau, Herbie 188
Gavotte 70
Geography and Climate 220
German Dance 228
Glass, Henry "Buzz" 109, 449, 453
Glide 50
Golden, Kristina Waller 33
Gottier, Karin 241, 234
Grading. *See* Evaluation
Greece 243
Greene, Madelynne 294
Greggerson, Jr., Herb and Pauline
    101, 128
Guozhuang Dance 12

Han 9
Han Dynasty 12
Handicapped Students 33, 41
Hawaii 19
Hazelius, Arthur 218
Health 3
Helt, Jerry and Kathy 119
Henneger, Maurice 202
Herman, Michael and Mary Ann
    218, 250, 252, 286, 363

Hinds, Tom 202
Hinman, Mary Wood 219
Hip Hop 368
Hispanic 71, 321
History
    Afro–Americans 70
    Beginning 1
    Chain 2
    Colonial America 125
    Contra 177
    Cultural Significance 3
    Education 3
    Fertility Rites 4
    Forms, Dance 2
    Health 3
    International Folk Dance in
      America 218
      Camps 333
      Movement 218
      Performing Groups 219
      Programs 233
      Sources 218
      Trends 220
    Music 2
    New England Dance 3, 126, 178
    Play Party Games 71
    Religion 3
    Social Dance 367
      Cajun 413
      Cha Cha Cha 459
      Charleston 393
      Country Western 434
      Disco 390
      East Coast Swing 405
      Foxtrot 377
      Hip Hop 368
      Latin Dance 459–484
      Lindy Hop 410
      Mambo 467
      Merengue 469
      Reggae 368
      Rock and Roll 368
      Rumba 472
      Salsa 479
      Samba 480
      Swing 397
      Tango 418
      Vintage Dance 370
      Waltz 426
      West Coast Swing 407
    Southern Dance 126
    Square Dance 71
      American Square Dance
        Society, Sets in Order 130
      Antecedents 125
      Basic Plateau 136
      Black Dances 126
      Calls
        Singing Calls 169
        Keys to Good Calling 132
        Patter Calls 157
        Callerlab 13
        Early Leaders 128

Magazines 129, 130
New England 126
Post–World War II 126
South, The 126
Texas 127
Hoedown 71
Hofman, Huig 227, 230
Holidays, Festivals, Special
    Occassions 222
Hop 48
Hubert, Gene 195
Hula 19
Hula pa ipu 19
Hula pohu 19
Hungary, Dance
    Characteristics 298
Hurok, Sol 218

Inca 20
Ice Breakers
    See Mixers
Index of Dances. *See* inside front
    and back covers
Index of Mixer and Nonpartner
    Dances 523
India 6
Instruction 23. *See also* Teaching
    and Methods
    Assessing Group
      Variables 30
    Class Procedure 31
    Content Selection 30
    Curriculum 28
    Daily Lesson 29
    Dance Lesson 29
    Dance Unit 29
    Enrichment Activities 38
    Evaluation 37
      Practical Test 37
      Written Test 37
    First Class Meeting 31
    Goals 29
    Lesson Plan 30
    Objectives 29
    Presentation of Dances 34
    Projects 38
    Resources, Teacher 39
    Selecting Dances 34
    Social Aids 32
    Specific Dance, Teaching 35
    Students with Special
      Needs 33
    Total Dance Program 28.
      See also Teaching
      and Methods
Instruments, Percussion 221
Instruments, Wind 221
International Folk Dance 217
    Costumes 222
    Dance Characteristics
      Africa 223
      Alpine Region 228
        Switzerland 228

Balkan Countries 243
   Bulgaria 243
   Greece 243
   Yugoslavia, Former 243
  British Isles 258
   England 258
   Ireland 260
   Scotland 261
  Canada 281
  Czech and Slovakia 285
  France 288
  Hungary 297–298
  Israel 303
  Italy 314
  Lithuania 318
  Mexico 321
  Poland 333
  Romania 338
  Russia 343
  Scandinavia 348
   Denmark 349
   Finland 350
   Norway 349
   Sweden 350
  Eastern and Western
   Culture 220
  Geography and Climate 220
  Holiday, Festivals, Special
   Occasions 222
  Music 221
  Pacific Rim Countries 6–19
  Record Sources 489
  Religion 221
  Video Sources 491
Ireland, Dance Characteristics 260
Israel, Dance Characteristics 303
Italy, Dance Characteristics 314

Japan 13
Jensen, Mary Bee xx
Jews 303
Jitterbug (Swing) 397
Jump 48

Kabuki 14
Kalakaua 20
Kathak 7, 8
Kathakali 7, 8
Kaura 13
Keller, Kate Van Winkle 254
Kitch, Jim 211
Kopp, Carol 187
Korea 13
  Musical Instruments 13
  Traditional Dance 13
Kumu Lula 19

Lai Haraoba 9
Lalau 19
Lancers 125
Lapson, Dvora 306, 307, 312
Latin Dance Craze 368

Laufman, Dudley 180
Leading and Following 372, 374
Leading, Techniques 374
Leap 47
Legacy Weekend (Ralph Page) 180
Lesson Plan 30, 371
Library of Congress 487
Libre Arts 11
Lindsay, Mary McLaren 262
Lindy Hop 410
Line Dance 446
Line Values 45
Lion Dance 11
Lira Vase 1
Lithuania, Dance
  Characteristics 318
Locke, John 3
Locomotor Movements 47
  Exercises 50
  Longway Set 63, 181
  Duple Minor 510
  Triple Minor 520
Lovett, Benjamin B. 179
Lloyd Shaw Foundation, The
  128, 198

Magellan, Ferdinand 15
Mainstreaming 153
Manipuri 7, 8
Maori 17
Maoritanga 17
Marek, Jacek 333–337
Maria Clara 17
Mayan 20
Mayo, Monty 249
Maypole Dance 126
Mazurka 52
Measure 44
Mele Hula 19
Merengue 469
Mestiza 15, 17, 321
Meter 44
Mexico, Dance Characteristics 321
Microphones 25
Ming Dynasties 11
Minuet 70
Mixers and Icebreakers 117
Morris Dance 70, 258
Mountain Folk Festival 124
Music 2, 20, 26, 64, 72, 221
  CD and Tape Deck 26
  Countries/Region
   Bulgaria 245
   Czech and Slovakia 285
   England 260
   France 288
   Greece 243
   Hungary 298
   Ireland 261
   Mexico 321
   Romania 338
   Russia 343

Scandinavia 348
  United States 60
   Contra 182
   Square Dance, Calls 131
   Yugoslavia, Former 244
Instruments 2
Live Music 27
  Musicians 27
  Teaching with Music 28
Note Values 44
Primitive 2
Recordings 26
  Contra Dance 26
  Folk Dance 26
  Social Dance 26
  Square Dance 26
  Teaching with Recordings 27
Music in Relation to Dance 64
  Listening 64
  Recognizing 65
  Rhythm Training 65
Muslims 10, 19
Mynah Dance 11

New England 3, 126, 178
New England Chestnut 190, 194,
  198, 200, 203, 207
New England Folk Festival
  Association 179
New Hampshire Folk Dance
  Camp 179
New School of Social Research 218
New Zealand 17
Noh 14
Nordiskz Museet 218
Northern Junket 179
North Texas Traditional Dance
  Society 180
Norway, Dance Characteristics 349
Novak, Jeannette 286
Novelty Dances, Round Dances 72
Note Values 44

Obaon 13
Objectives 29
Odalan 17
O'Farrell, Una and Sian 274
Oglebay Folk Dance Camp 96, 219
Oli 19
Olson, Al 196
One-Night Stand 39
One-Step/Dance Walk 50, 372
Onnagata 15
Opera, Chinese 9
Orff-Schulwerk 65
Orientation to Dance Class 31
  First Class Meeting 31
  Setting the Stage 31
   Etiquette 32
   Fun with Cutting In 32
   Holding Hands 32
   Social Aids 32

Students With Special
    Needs 33
    Uneven Numbers 32
Osgood, Bob 78, 130

Pacific Rim 6
Page, Ralph 179, 180, 185, 198, 201,
    213
Ralph Page Library 180
Palestinian 303
Parkes, Tony 180, 209
Party, Theme 40
Parvati 9
Patter Call 157
Pavlova, Anna 9
Peacock Dance 9
Pearl, Dan 189
People's Government 12
Percussion Instruments 221
Periodicals 485
Peter, Paul, and Mary 180
Philippine 17
Phrase 45
Physical Disabilities 41
Pillay, Ponniah 9
Pillay, Vadiveda 9
Pittman, Anne 129
Pivot Turn, Step 59, 431
Pivot Turn, Teaching 59, 177
Playford, John 177
Playground and Recreation
    Association of America 219
Play Party Games 71, 127
Poi 17
Pokok 17
Polka 51
Polka Turn 53
Polynesia 17
Positions, Dance 60–62
Posture 66
Practical Test 37
Processional 2
Projects 38
Pyrrhic 3

Qing Dynasties 9
Quadrille 78, 125
Quadrille Sets 69

Ramsey, John 124
Ras Lila 9
Recordings 26
Record Players. See Turntable
Record Sources 489
    Calls 132
    Care 26
    Contra 27
    Folk 26
    Social Dance 27
    Sources 489
    Square Dance 26
    Teaching with Records 27

Regadon d'Honor 17
Reggae 368
Rejang 16
Religion 3
Resources, Community 39
Resources, Teacher 39
Retirement Homes 41
Revival of Folk Traditions 73
Rhythm and Meter 43
    Analysis of Basic Rhythm 46
    Beats 43
    Cue 46, 370
    Even Rhythm 45
    Line Values 45
    Measure 44
    Note Values 44
    Pattern, Rhythm 46
    Phrase 45
    Tempo 45
    Time Signature 44
    Uneven Rhythm 46
Rippon, Hugh 279
Rock and Roll 368
Round Dance Book 128
Round and Novelty Dances 72
Rotenberg, Tanya 197
Royal Scottish Country Dance
    Society 268, 277
Rudd, Helfrid 358
Rumba 472
Run 47
Running Set 126
Russia, Dance Characteristics 343

Salsa 479
Samba 480
Sanders, Olcutt 129
Sang Hyang Dedari 16
Sannella, Ted 179, 180, 192, 194,
    196, 213
Sanskrit 78
Scandinavia, Dance
    Characteristics 348
    Denmark 349
    Finland 350
    Norway 349
    Sweden 350
Schottische 51, 98
Schottische Turn 52
Schnur, Steve 193
Scotland, Dance Characteristics 261
Senior Dances 41
Sets in Order, American Square
    Dance Society 130
Sets in Order (Square Dancing
    Magazine) 129
Shang Dynasty 9
Sharp, Cecil J. 126, 258
Shaw, Lloyd and Dorothy 128
    Cheyenne Mountain School 128
Shaw, Lloyd Foundation 128
Shaw, Pat 124

Shinto 13
Shuffle 50
Sicilian Circle 63
Singh, Joy 8
Singing Quadrilles 126
Single Time Swing 397
Sissone 48
Shaw, Ed 196
Siva 6
Skip 50
Slide 49
Slovakia, Dance Characteristics 285
Smith, Marilyn M. (Walthen) 289,
    290, 292, 296
Smithsonian 287
Social Aids 32
Social Dance
    Break Dance 368
    Cha Cha Cha 459
        History 459
        Rhythm 459
        Style 459
    Charleston 393
        History 393
        Rhythm 394
        Style 394
        Teaching 394
    Combos
        Cha Cha Cha 466
        Foxtrot 390
        Merengue 472
        Rumba 479
        Samba 484
        Swing 407
        Tango 426
        Waltz 433
    Competition 368
    Country Western 368
        Etiquette 434
        History 434
        Style 435
    Dance Positions 373
    Dancesport 369
    Dance Walk/One Step 50, 372
    Disco Dance 390
        History 390
        Swing 391
    East Coast Swing 405
    Following, Techniques 372, 375
    Foxtrot 377
        History 377
        Rhythm 377
        Style 378
    Hip Hop 368
    History. See Specific Dances
    Hustle 392, 447
    Jitterbug. See Swing
    Leading, Techniques 374
    Lesson Plan 371
    Lesson Preparation 371
    Lindy Hop 410
    Line Dance 446

Merengue 469
    History 469
    Rhythm 469
    Style 469
Music 27
One Step/Dance Walk 50, 372
Phases 368
    Charleston Period 368
    Country Western 368
    Foxtrot Period 368
    Latin Dance Craze 368
    Rock and Roll 368
    Swing Era 368
    Vintage Dance 370
Positions, Dance 60–62
Record Sources 489, 491
Reggae 368
Rumba 472
    History 472
    Rhythm 473
    Style 473
    Teaching 474
Salsa 479
Samba 479
    History 480
    Rhythm 481
    Style 481
Style 371
    Dance Walk/One Step 50, 372
    Footwork 372
    International, Social Dance.
        See also Specific Dance
Swing 397
    History 397
    Rhythm 397
    Style 397
Tango 418
    History 418
    Rhythm 418
    Style 419
Teaching 370
    Cues 370
    Demonstration 370
    Formations 370
    Lesson Plan 371
    Teaching Progression 371
    Style 66, 371
    Walk Throughs 370
Touch Dancing 369
Video Sources 491
Vintage Dance 370
Waltz 426
    History 427
    Rhythm 427
    Style 427
West Coast Swing 407
Song Dynasties 9
Sound Systems 25
    Amplifier 25
    Camcorder/VCR 26
    Care of Turntable & Records 26

CD Player 25
Microphones 25
Speakers 25
Tapedeck 25
Spanish 17
Spanish–Mexicans 71
Speakers 25
Special Needs Students 33
Spivak, Joseph and Rajah 311
Spokane Folklore Society 180
Square Dance
    American Square Dance Society,
      Sets in Order 130
    Basic Movements 136
    Big Circle Method 134
    Caller 131
    Callerlab 130
    Calls
        Calling 131
        Calling Sequence 132
        Keys to Good Calling 132
        Patter 157, 164
            Breaks 164
            Breaks for Eights 165
            Breaks for Four 165
            Endings 164
            Openers 164
        Pre-Recorded Calls 132
        Pure Memory 131
        Sight Caller 131
        Singing Calls 169
    Early Leaders 128
    Fifty Basic Movements 136
    History 125
    Magazines 130
    Mainstream 130
    Maneuvering 139
    Methods for Changing Partners
      or Moving to a New
      Square 135
    Methods for Squaring Up 134
    Mixers, Square Dance 133
      Big Circle 134
    Planning Units and Lessons 133
    Progression and Analysis 136
      Additional Basics 51–59, 151
      Level 1A: Beginner Basics 137
      Level 1B: Orientation to
        Square 138
      Level 2: Beginner Basics 139
      Level 3: Beginner Basics 142
      Level 4: Intermediate
        Basics 146
      Level 5: Intermediate
        Basics 149
      Mainstream Movements
        60–78, 153
    Record Sources 489, 491
    Records with Calls 132
    Style 132
    Teaching Approaches 132

Teaching Progression
    and Analysis for Basic
    Movements 136
Texas Square Dance 126
Unit and Lesson Plans 133
Video Sources 489, 491
Visiting Couple Types 84–87
Western Cowboy Square
    Dance 166
Square Dancing Magazine 130
Streamline Waltz step 432
Step Dancing 82
Sturman, Rivka 313
Style 66, 371
    Posture 66
    Social Dance 371
    Teaching 66
Sui Dynasty 9
Sweden, Dance Characteristics 350
Swing
    Country Western 435
    Cowboy 435
    Disco 391
    Double Time 399
    History 397
    Lindy Hop 410
    Rhythm 397
    Triple Time 405
    Style 398
Swing (Jitterbug) 397
    East Coast Swing 405
    West Coast Swing 388, 399, 407
Switzerland, Dance
    Characteristics 228
Sword Dance 259
Ta Asobi 11
Taiping Music 9
Tang Dynasty 8
Tango 418
    History 418
    Rhythm 418
    Style 419
Tape Deck 25
Teaching and Methods. *See also*
    Instructor
    American Sampler, Dances 74
    Basic Dance Steps and
      Turns 56
        Analysis of Rhythm 50
        Box Waltz and Turn 58
        Method of Presentation 31
        Pivot Turn 59
        Polka and Turn 58
        Schottische and Turn 56
        Twirl 59
        Two-Step, Progressive and
          Turn 57
        Waltz and Turn 58
        Waltz, Running 58
    Contra Dance 184
    Live Music, with Teaching 28
    Presentation of Dances 31

Recordings, with Teaching 27
  Social Dance 370
  Specific Dances 35
  Square Dance 133
  Style 66, 371. *See also* Instruction
  Tape Deck 25
Tempo 45
Ternow 15
Testing. *See* Evaluation
Texas Square Dance 127
Theme Party 40
Thurston, Hugh 233
Ti Leaf 19
Tiananmen Square 12
Time Signature 44
Tinikling 17
Tolentino, Francisca Reyes 17
Touch Dancing 369
Tracie, Gordon E. 348–350, 354, 355,
    357, 359, 361
Trends (International) 220
Triple Step or Two–Step 50

Triple Time Swing 405
Turntable and Records, Care of 26
Trygg, Harry and Dia 122
Twirl 59
Two–Step or Triple Step 50
Two–Step Turn 53

Uneven Numbers 32
Unit Plan 29
University of New Hampshire 180

VCR/Camcorder 26
Verbunk 297
Video Sources 489
Viennese Waltz 432
Vintage Dance 370

Walk 47
Waller, Marlys Swenson 129
Waltz 51
  Box 52
  Canter 52

Running 52, 58
Rhythm 51
Social Dance 426
Streamline 432
Style 427
Turn 58
Wannadance 180
Wathen, Marilyn. *See* Smith, Marilyn
West Coast Swing 399, 407
Western Zhou 9
World Wide Web 487–488
Written Test 37

Yugoslavia, Former, Dance
    Characteristics 244

Zakon, Steve 223, 208
Zuobu Arts 9

Music to Accompany Dance A While:

Handbook for Folk, Square, Contra, and Social Dance, Eighth Edition

Jane A. Harris, Anne M. Pittman, Marlys S. Waller, Cathy L. Dark

Prepared by: Stew Schacklette, President, Kentucky Dance Foundation, Brandenburg, KY.*

1. Carnavalito
2. La Bastringue
3. Man in the Hay
4. Grand March
5. Nobody's Business
6. Tropanka
7. Ve'David
8. Alunelel
9. Doudlebska Polka
10. Hineh Ma Tov
11. Korobushka
12. Pljeskavac Kolo
13. Troika
14. Schottische
15. Crested Hen
16. D'Hammerschmiedsg'selln
17. Irish Washerwoman
18. Mayim
19. Polka
20. Savila Se Bella Loza
21. Siamsa Beirte
22. Sicilian Tarantella
23. Family Waltz

*Kentucky Dance Foundation, Folk Dancer Record Center, 6290 Olin Road, Brandenburg, KY 40108.

Dance A While CD: Notes on the Recordings

A Production of the Kentucky Dance Foundation 1999
Most dance tunes are produced by the late Michael Herman.

1. **Carnavalito.**   Bolivian.   p. 364
There are many Carnavalito dances, coming from the Andean highlands. This one is from Bolivia, from the town of Guadalquivir. **Carnavalito** is also known as **Guadalquivir.** The upbeat rhythm captivates the dancers as they flirt and snake down the streets.

    The native instruments of the Andean highlands that play throughout the tune are: *siku (sicu)*–a type of panpipe from the region of Lake Titicaca; *charango*–a 10-stringed guitar-like instrument tuned as 5 double strings (case commonly made of the shell of an armadillo or piece of hollowed out wood); *bambo*–a drum; *quena*–hollow tubes of bamboo, bone, or clay with a notch at the upper end; *tarka*–a whistle type mouthpiece made of wood (sound is shrill).

2. **La Bastringue.**   French-Canadian.   p. 282
La Bastringue music reflects the delightful and fun-loving people of Quebec who dearly love to sing and dance. French-Canadian fiddle tunes now mingle with Irish tunes. **La Bastringue** is played by Bob Hill and his Canadian Country Boys.

    The folk dance is choreographed to a French-Canadian party song.[1] An old man requests a young woman to dance with him but finally wants to stop dancing because his feet have corns!

3. **Man in the Hay.**   German.   p. 237
Man in the Hay from Northern Germany (Schaumpurg-Lippe) is a popular square dance (4 couples) at the Harvest festivals. The tune is an old German folk song, "A Farmer Had A Pretty Wife." The music has a strongly marked rhythm and dancers move briskly. When the music is accelerated, younger women's feet come off the ground in the swings (buzz step).

4. **Grand March.**   p. 75
The Grand March is 4/4 time!
    The spirit of a march permeates the dance hall as all promenade through the various figures. The drums, horns, tubas, trombones, clarinets, fifes, cymbals, sousaphones all sound wonderful and brave. An "Esprit de Corps" forms quickly.

5. **Nobody's Business.**   American.   p. 97
Nobody's Business is a fun-loving American Play Party Game. The accordion, banjo, piano, violin and bass harmonize together daring one to sit still. Singing the works adds playfulness/flirtation with the simple action.

    This peppy music may also be used for other mixers and circle two-steps.

6. **Tropanka.**   Bulgarian.   p. 257
Tropanka means "stamped," which describes the character of the dance. The 2/4 meter is most common in Bulgarian dance. It starts slow and gradually accelerates. The music sounds solemn as it moves through complex rhythms.

    The native instruments are: *gajda*–bagpipes; *kaval*–a long pipe; *duduk*–block pipe; *gădulka*–rebec–a Renaissance fiddle; sometimes *tambura*–a kind of mandolin; various sizes of drums and tympans. In the 19th–20th century, clarinets, violins, accordions, trumpets and drums became popular or the use of military bands in small villages.

7. **Ve'David.**   Israeli.   p. 313
The music is composed by M. Shelem (Weiner). The Israeli music for dance is a mixture of style and musical tradition coming from the Old Testament. The exposure to foreign folkways in centuries of exile blends. **Ve'David** is composed by Rivka Sturman and is similar to "Circassian Circle" and "Oh, Suzannah."

    The accordion, clarinet, drum, pipe, violin, bass, xylophone, block, all blend together. The melodic line is a definite 2/4 meter.

8. **Alunelul.**   Romanian.   p. 339
Alunelul came from Oltenia, Romania. The meter is duple (2/4), typical of some Romanian music, bright, energetic and syncopated. Gypsies have long been associated with Romanian folk music and affect the dynamics of the music. **Alunelul** accelerates as the music progresses.

    The violin dominates the piano, guitar, and bass. Two Romanian folk instruments, the *cimbalon*–a hammered dulcimer, and *nai*–a flute or panpipe, are frequently heard. Shrieks and whistles add to the spirit of the music.

---

[1] Party Song, La Bastringue, French and English words. Longden, Sanna H. And Phyllis S. Weikart. *Cultures and Styling in Folk Dance.* Ypsilanti, MI: High/Scope Press, 1998. P. 120.

9. **Doudlebska Polka.** Czech. p. 286
The Doudlebska music has three parts—polka, walking, and clapping. The festive mood changes from exuberant to a stroll, and moving back (clapping) to flirtatious to find a new partner. The Bohemian quality radiates.

Traditional bands are composed of a peppy accordion, clarinet, violin, double bass, horns and trumpets.

10. **Hineh Ma Tov.** Israeli. p. 309
Jacobsen composed the music for **Hineh Ma Tov** and Rivka Sturman choreographed the dance. The Yemenite influence is reflected in slow, flowing movements, then "quick prancing style" steps.

The violin, clarinet, mandolin, guitar, flute and piano present a thoughtful melody. And a vocal in Hebrew ties it together. Dancers are encouraged to sing.

11. **Korobushka.** Russian. p. 345
This delightful tune in 2/4 meter is a Russian folk song, **"Korobushka,"** meaning a "peddler's pack." It reflects its Slavic origin. The elegance of the ballroom seeps through the music and dance. The tempo starts slowly, stately and gradually accelerates.

The orchestra plays the balalaika, piano, accordion and tambourine. Refer to #13, **Troika,** for common Russian instruments.

12. **Pljeskavac Kolo.** Serbian. p. 250
Pljeskavac Kolo is danced to the melody of "Kjurdjevka"[2] played by the Banat Tamburizta Orchestra. It has all the original peasant flavor. The instruments are mandolin, balalaika, violin, and accordion. Clapping in the second part and occasional happy shouts add to the spirit of the dance.

13. **Troika.** Russian. p. 346
This exuberant Russian melody plays faster and faster. Dancers accelerate to keep pace with the music. The accordion, mandolin, balalaika and bass play with gusto.

Russian folk musicians play the *balalaika*–a three-stringed triangular lute; the *psaltery*–a zither; the *domra*–three-stringed mandolin; the shepherd horn and pipe; tambourine; and a variety of percussion instruments like wooden spoons.

14. **Schottische (Texas Schottische).** p. 101
The tune is Bummel Schottische, a Northern German folk song from Mecklenburg, Pomerania, and Schleswig-Holstein. "Bummel" means "strolling." The smooth flowing melody, 2/4 meter, is appropriate for the Texas Schottische, California Schottische, basic Schottische and Schottische mixers.

15. **Crested Hen (Den Toppede Høne).** Danish. p. 352
This spritely tune encourages the dancers to step lively and as the man goes through the arch, the woman playfully tries to snatch the man's red hat (the crested hen). The accordion, clarinet and guitar harmonize together, change keys, and challenge the dancers.

16. **D'Hammerschmeidsg'selln.** German. p. 230
This Bavarian tune and orchestra accompaniment radiates the "journeyman blacksmith" dance theme–especially the hand-clapping chorus. The playfulness and spontaneous antics are all part of the "clap" sequence. When the Journeymen completed their examinations, they would "whoop it up!"

The orchestra is comprised of many instruments–accordion, violin, trumpet, chimes, fife, clarinet, horns, drums and wooden blocks–together challenging the dancers.

17. **Irish Washerwoman (Virginia Reel).** p. 77
The Irish brought their folk music to America and one of the most-loved melodies, lilting dancing airs, is **Irish Washerwoman.** The tune is in "Jig" time, 6/8, and traditionally two parts, A and B, 8 bars each; each part is played twice (32 bars) to conform with the construction of the dance. Traditionally, musicians will play one tune, then shift to others for variety.

Irish Washerwoman is a favorite for the Virginia Reel, mixers, square, and contra dance because the steady decisive beat keeps the dancers together. As a general rule, any dance in jig or reel time may be danced to any regular jig or reel tune.

The Irish bagpipe is the most popular instrument and the violin was introduced later. In this recording, the accordion, violin, clarinet, bass or guitar keep the dancers wanting MORE!

18. **Mayim.** Israeli. p. 312
The music of **Mayim,** "water," is by Pugachov. This communal dance was created in 1938, celebrating the joy of discovering water in an arid country and their desire to establish a new cultural base–dance.

The musical accompaniment for Israeli dance reflects the "time" and "countries" from which the settlers came. The accordion, clarinet, drums, fifes, cymbals and violins blend together in this steady, pulsating melody

19. **Polka.**
This all purpose polka tune has a Scandinavian flair which may be used for the Scandinavian Polka (pivot), p. 357, or traditional turning polka (hop), p. 58. The accordion, violin, clarinet and bass combine for a rousing "romp."

---

[2] Kjurdjevka. Lidster, Miriam D. and Dorothy H. Tamburini. *Folk Dance Progressions.* Belmont, CA: Wadsworth Publishing Co., 1965. P. 76.

20. **Savila Se Bela Loza.**   Serbian.   p. 250
Today, Serbian musical instruments may vary from accordion, clarinet, balalaika, mandolin to native instruments–*svrala* or *frula*–shepherd's pipe; the *gaida*–bagpipe; the *gusle*–fiddle; and the *tupen*–drum.

Occasionally a dancer, caught up in the spirit of the dance, will shout. Singing the words of **"Savila Se Bela Loza"** is a common accompaniment and bonding of the dancers immediately emerges.

21. **Siamsa Beirte.**   Irish.   p. 274
The tune is "Bluebell Polka," a slow hornpipe tune. **Siamsa Beirte** may be danced to any evenly phrased Irish hornpipe tune.

22. **Sicilian Tarantella.**   Italian.   p. 316
The music of **Sicilian Tarantella** is gay, fast and exhilarating, in duple meter (6/8), 2 beats to the measure. The accordion and large tambourines dominate. The pipes, mandolin, piano, also accompany and dancers snap their fingers, clap their hands or shake and beat tambourines.

23. **Family Waltz (Familjevalsen).**   Swedish   p. 354
The **Family Waltz** dance is known throughout Scandinavia. It is an easy mixer and nice closing dance. There are many Scandinavian waltz tunes that are appropriate, but the tempo should not be too fast.

This music is especially suited to teach the waltz, p. 58, as well as the Swedish Waltz, p. 361.

La Bastringe 282
La Cucaracha 327
La Montagnarde 290
La Raspa 328
La Tournijaire 292
Las Chiapanecas 329
Lady of the Lake 200
Lady 'Round the Lady 86
Lesnoto 247
Levi Jackson Rag 124
Lindy Hop 410
Line Dance 446
Little Man in a Fix 351
Long Way Over, A 163

Magic Step 380
Mambo 467
Ma Na'avu 311
Man in the Hay 237
Mañana 170
Marianne 172
Mayim 312
Merengue 469
Mexican Mixer 121
Milagro Square 168
Misirlou 249
Mixers, Plain and Novelty 117
Mixers, Square Dance 133
Mon Père Avait un Petit Bois 294
Mountaineer Loop 86
Mucho Combo 162

New Star Thru 161
Ninepin Reel 81
Nobody's Business 97
Northdown Waltz, The 270
Norwegian Polka 357
Nova Scotian, The 201
Now Hear This 163

Ocean Wave–Circulate 164
Ocean Wave–Swing
   Thru Combo 1 164
Oh Johnny 113
Old–Fashioned Girl 172
One Step 379
Oslo Waltz 271
Other Mary Kay, The 202

Para Bailar 453
Pata Pata 226
Patty–Cake Polka 120
Paul Jones Your Lady 80
Petronella 203
Pierce's Hall Stroll 204
Ping–Pong Schottische 100
Pitt's Patter 2 162
Pitt's Patter 3 160

Pljeskavac Kolo 250
Popcorn 115
Pop Them Thru 86
Portland Fancy 83
Promenade the Outside Ring 159
Promenade the Ring 158

Queen's Highway 85

Ragg, The 272
Ranchera 365
Red River Valley 123
Road to the Isles 273
Roll Away Combo 1 160
Roll Away Combo 2 159
Roadblock Reel 205
Roll in the Hey 206
Rondeau de Garein 296
Rory O'More 207
Route, The 159
Rumba 472
Rumunjsko Kolo 251

Sail Away 161
Saint John River, The, 283
Sally Good'n 168
Salmonchanted Evening 208
Salsa 479
Salty Dog Rag 104
Samba 480
Santa Rita 330
Sarajevka Kolo 252
Saturday Night Fever Line Dance 454
Savila Se Bela Loza 253
Scandinavian Polka 357
Schottische 98
Seksmannsril 358
Šetnja 255
Shadrack's Delight 209
Shoo Fly Swing 85
Shoot the Owl 87
Siamsa Beirte 274
Sibra Din Cimpoi 342
Sicilian Tarantella 316
Sides Break to Line 162
Sides Divide 168
Silver Lake Waltz 210
Slappin' Leather 455
Small Potatoes 211
Smoke on the Water 175
Snurrbocken 359
Sonderburg Doppelquadrille 240
Spinnradl zu Dritt 241
Split the Ring Around Just
   One 158
Split the Ring Variation 1 159
Split the Ring, Variation 2 160
Square Dance Mixers 133

Star Thru–California Twirl 161
Star Thru and Square Thru
   Combo 161
Swedish Varsouvienne 360
Swedish Waltz 361
Sweetheart Schottische 445
Swing 397
Symmetrical Force 212
Syrtós 256

Take a Little Peek 87
Tancuj 287
Tango 418
Tant' Hessie 227
Tea Cup Chain 168
Ten–Step 440
Tennessee Wig Walk 122
Texas Schottische 101
Texas Schottische for Three 103
Texas Star 158
Texas Two–Step Swing 440
There's Your Corner 160
Three Meet 275
Tie Me Kangaroo Down 174
To Ting 362
Totur 363
Tourist, The 213
Tramblanka – Polka Mazurka 335
Traveling Cha Cha 444
Triple Time East Coast Swing 405
Troika 346
Tropanka 257
Turn Thru Combo 163
Twelfth Street Rag 116
Two–Step 442

Ugrós 302

Varsouvienne 112
Ve' David 313
Viennese Waltz 432
Virginia Reel 77

Walczyk "Ges Woda" 337
Waltz 42, 48, 426
Waltz, Streamline 432
Watermelon Crawl 456
Weave the Line 213
Westchester Box Step 385
West Coast Swing 407
Western Wind 458
White Cockade, The 277
Willow Tree 279
With Thanks to the Dean 214

Zydeco Two–Step 417